Stuttering and Behavior Therapy

Stuttering and Behavior Therapy

Current Status and Experimental Foundations

Roger John Ingham, PhD
Head, School of Communication Disorders
Cumberland College of Health Sciences
Sydney, Australia

College-Hill Press, San Diego, California

College-Hill Press
4284 41st Street
San Diego, California 92105

Library of Congress Cataloging in Publication Data

Ingham, Roger J.
Stuttering and behavior therapy.

Bibliography: p.
Includes index.
1. Stuttering—treatment. 2. Behavior therapy.
I Title. [DNLM: 1. Behavior therapy. 2. Stuttering—Therapy. WM 175-148s]
RC424.153 1983 616.85'5406 83-7593

ISBN 0-933014-72-4

Printed in the United States of America

Contents

10. Prolonged Speech, Its Variants, and Stuttering 273

Preface

Prefaces usually describe the purposes and influences that lead to the writing of a book. Presumably, this gives the reader some insight into the reasons why certain books are written. For what it is worth, I can only find one compelling reason for enduring the effort in writing this book; I was tired of writing up much of the material covered in this book for lectures to graduate and undergraduate speech pathology students. It seemed so much simpler to put the material together in one set form, rather than for it to continue as scattered notes and incidental comments that seem to have constituted my lectures on this book's topic.

There are, however, some ground rules that led to the structure of this book, and which have their origins in some quite transparent influences. The main ground rule was that the book should attempt to review and evaluate the contribution made by the principles and practices of behavior therapy to the treatment of stuttering. Another ground rule was that it should attempt to link the main treatment procedures to the now considerable and ever-growing body of research on stuttering. For it appeared to me that, at long last, there is increasing evidence that the huge amount of research on this disorder is beginning to have some substantial impact on the procedures and practices that clinicians use to help stutterers overcome this problem. One need only think of the enormous amount of research time that has been expended on the "adaptation effect," or the "consistency effect," to understand the frustration that many clinicians must have experienced in trying to relate their profession's research on stuttering to their therapy needs. In this respect, therefore, this book departs somewhat from its more obvious origins—two journal reviews on behavior therapy and stuttering that were written during the 1970s (Ingham & Andrews, 1973; Ingham & Lewis, 1978). These articles provided some of the format and material for this book. But, unlike these articles, this book has endeavored to review *both* the experimental and treatment literature that relates to current stuttering treatment.

In some ways the size of this book is not just testimony to my lack of editorial skill. It serves to reflect the quite enormous amount of stuttering therapy research, or related research, that has occurred over the past decade. In fact, my attempts to "control" and then organize this outpouring of literature were like trying to drink from a gushing firehose—somehow the output had to be brought to a brief halt, or slowed down, so that its content could be taken in. That "halt" took place in the middle of 1982. There are some later papers that dribbled into the text, but for those interested in dating this review it is fair to say that it is principally concerned with treatment research and related experimental studies published from the 1930s through to July 1982. In the future, I hope this task should be much more manageable now that some of the pertinent background material has been reviewed. And so I hope that this book will be the first of a series of editions designed to keep abreast of this literature.

I owe the impetus to write this book to the urgings of my late wife, Joan. She gave up much of, what turned out to be, precious little time during the last 2 years of her struggle with cancer to help me organize the early stages of this book. We spent far too much of our time together trying to finish something that I hope she would have been proud of. Fortunately she saw the end of the writing, but, tragically, not the result of our endeavors.

Numerous others contributed in various ways to the final product. I thank the many 2nd year students in the Bachelor of Applied Science (Speech Pathology) course at Cumberland College of Health Sciences who forced me to articulate many of the arguments contained in these chapters. In this respect, I also wish to express my gratitude to Ann Packman, Louise Ulliana, and Helen Southwood, my research assistants at Cumberland College, who also provided helpful "sounding boards" for some of the ideas contained in this book. The same gratitude is extended to David Prins, Mike McLean, and Howard Goldsmith at the University of Washington, Seattle, for their helpful comments on some of the issues in the later chapters. However, I am especially grateful to Jan Costello who is responsible for ensuring that I did not cut corners in covering the topic of this book. Our many discussions over the past year helped me to finish, what often seemed like, a never-ending task.

At least three other people need to be singled out for their indirect contributions to this book. In 1971 I had the good fortune to spend 9 months as a post doctoral fellow at the University of Minnesota. While there I was greatly influenced by three people; Pat Kuhl, Jerry Siegel, and Dick Martin. I will not saddle them with responsibility for any of the contents of this book. Nevertheless, so many of the ideas and issues that directed the shape of this book were the end products of our time together. They provided me with the most impressive academic experience of my life. Indeed, the foundation of this book is dedicated to Dick Martin, who I regard as the finest researcher I have known.

Last, but certainly not least, I want to give special thanks to Annette Uebergang, who labored constantly, and without complaint, on transforming my atrocious writing into a presentable typed product. Her efforts are largely responsible for ensuring that this book appears in reasonably close proximity to the time that this review ceased.

REFERENCES

Ingham, R.J., & Andrews, G. Behavior therapy and stuttering: A review. *Journal of Speech and Hearing Disorders*, 1973, *38*, 405-441.

Ingham, R.J., & Lewis, J.I. Behavior therapy and stuttering: And the story grows. *Human Communication*, 1978, *3*, 125-152.

1

The Arrival of a Behavioral Preparadigm in Stuttering Therapy

Introduction

Anybody who has anything to do with the treatment of problem behaviors would know that the past 2 decades have witnessed something of a revolution in this field. That revolution has been caused by the development of principles and practices in an area of clinical psychology generally known as behavior therapy. Like any revolution, its success is usually measured by the extent to which it overthrows an existing order and is accepted by the affected populace. In this respect, this therapy revolution cannot claim complete success, but its achievements have substantially altered many therapy practices. It has not been gleefully accepted by all practitioners, though by any measure of contribution to a field it can rightly claim an established status. It has certainly recruited a membership that would rival the subscribers to other therapy methods. Indeed, its development has been such that it now requires the dimensions of a book to track its contribution and appraise its current status in different therapy areas. Such is the reason for the following endeavor to review behavior therapy's contribution to stuttering.

One measure of a revolution's vitality is whether its effects spread beyond its frontline. By this measure, behavior therapy can certainly claim to have vitality. It is virtually impossible to gauge the size of its impact because its principles and practices have been taken up by clinicians in fields well beyond the domain of clinical psychology. For example, these practices are now fully employed in fields such as education, sport, welfare services, medicine (to name but a few), as well as speech pathology. But like any revolution, its arrival in most fields was eventful.

In many ways, the introduction of behavior therapy to speech pathology, and especially the area of stuttering, probably epitomizes the turbulent impact that this treatment orientation has had on many fields. In fact, there are probably few more vivid examples of the turbulence caused by a challenge to prevailing therapy systems than that which occurred in the area of stuttering. For behavior therapy was an approach to treatment that clashed with some long-held beliefs about this disorder. On the other hand, the use of many behavioral approaches in stuttering treatment vividly illustrates some other interesting problems that accompanied the introduction of much behavior therapy to various fields. For instance, it shows the types of problems produced when a new treatment system simply overlooks worthwhile knowledge derived from established systems. It also demonstrates how a system's principles can be subverted by its more zealous proponents—a typical problem in many revolutions. Other similar problems will emerge over the course of this attempt to chronicle behavior therapy's contribution to stuttering treatment.

The "Paradigm Era"

It is now almost commonplace to depict sudden developments in scientific fields as examples of Kuhn's (1962) argument about the role of paradigms in science. Yet, in many respects, this is a very credible framework to depict the changes that have occurred in stuttering treatment, and it provides a useful starting point for describing these events.

Over the past 2 decades, Thomas Kuhn's (1962) thesis on understanding the way in which scientists accumulate knowledge about their fields of practice has attracted massive interst. More often than not, Kuhn's interpreters have taken lavish liberties with his concepts in order to describe developments in their chosen field (Yates, 1975). In many instances their ill-disguised reasons have been to invest their fields with "respectability." On the other hand, Kuhn's concepts have certainly provided provocative reasons why certain research areas blossom while others seem to wilt in the shadow of disinterest.

Central to Kuhn's thesis is a concept which he described as the "paradigm." This much-used concept has now permeated behavioral science to such an extent that, as Peterson (1981) observed, virtually all of its areas claim to use "paradigms." Perhaps one reason for this enthusiasm is that Kuhn's concepts focused on the realities of science, rather than its ideals. In fact, probably unwittingly, it drew attention to some well-known but rarely mentioned aspects of science. The most important being that, more often than not, scientific activity is stimulated by clashing ideas and the building or preserving of reputations, rather than such lofty notions as the need to accumulate knowledge. Some interpreters of Kuhn's ideas have mistakenly regarded this process as an example of the "paradigm clash"—the centerpiece of Kuhn's thesis. And although this is a facile interpretation of the paradigm clash, it certainly resonates with the experiences of most researchers.

Kuhn argued that a paradigm[1] is formed by "accepted examples of actual scientific practice—examples which include law, theory, application, and ex-

[1] There continues to be much controversy surrounding the definitive features of a paradigm—much of the controversy being caused by Kuhn's (1962) varied use of the term. Masterman (1970) observed that the original text employed the term in 22 different ways; they varied between references to models, beliefs, and instrumentation.

perimentation together—[which] provide models from which spring particular coherent traditions of scientific research'' (Kuhn, 1962, p.10). Such examples are rare in science, but are found in Copernican astronomy, Newtonian dynamics, and corpuscular optics. Nevertheless, this view of the practice of some sciences nicely describes the way in which research activity is virtually dictated by a prevailing paradigm. Since the 18th century, at least, it has been generally accepted that knowledge is gained by research based on theoretical models. Kuhn's important contribution was to highlight the events that occur when the methods and practices of a current paradigm begin to fail—especially the events that surround the appearance of an alternative paradigm.

Kuhn postulated that the great advances in science tend to occur when a prevailing paradigm is found wanting. This usually occurs when that paradigm's capacity to generate predictable and valid concepts is challenged by alternative theories and practices, alternatives that may also form a coherent framework for "normal science." In such circumstances there occurs a dramatic upsurge in research aimed at resolving this conflict.

The idea that knowledge advances in a climate of conflict is very appealing. Such climates certainly typify some of the most exciting periods of research activity. This makes it easy to understand why the notion of paradigmatic conflict has been equated with the argumentative climate that pervades so much scientific practice. The competitive struggle to design crucial experiments that will support or reject hypotheses, and the formulation and testing of competing theories, is the very essence of science and, even more significantly, the basis of reputations. Perhaps the most graphic recent example of these activities was the resolution of the DNA molecule's structure by Watson and Crick. Watson's (1968) engrossing account of how the structure was resolved vividly describes the realities of much scientific activity.

Most research activity is related to the more usual meaning of a paradigm, that is, it follows a pattern or a model. This means that there are binding rules on theory testing: hypotheses are formulated in order to test the stability of a theory, and only the methods and measurement procedures acceptable to a scientific community can be used to test a theory. In the Kuhnian paradigm, the bulk of scientific activity can be likened to puzzle-solving; the researcher always feels confident that a solution will be found because of the paradigm's strength. Ironically, its strength is best demonstrated when solutions are not found. If the paradigm is robust, then such a failure is regarded as a reflection on the scientist's skills, rather than a reflection on the paradigm: it is the scientist who is inadequate, not the paradigm.

The resemblance that all this has to clinical research is striking. It too may be depicted as a conglomeration of activities by clinical researchers who often seek to demonstrate their competence by providing unique solutions to clinical puzzles. And the puzzles are normally based on paradigmatically defined assumptions about the disorder. Thus an acceptable solution must be seen to be logically derived from the methodological rules generated by peers. In other words, the clinical researcher faces a set of rules that the clinical community has decreed (either implicitly or explicitly) must be followed if a solution is to be regarded seriously.

At present, neither the field of speech pathology nor behavior therapy operates within a paradigm. For, as yet, no completely accepted laws or theories of human behavior exist. In consequence, Kuhn claims that such fields are better described as passing through a "preparadigm" phase, or a phase in which there exist competing models and theories. But even in this developmental phase there are many practices or rules that are the only ones acceptable for testing models and theories in such fields. So, in what follows, an endeavor will be made to examine the practices that form this new preparadigm in the area of stuttering treatment. It will be seen that this preparadigm has challenged the practices of a previous preparadigm, thereby introducing many of the characteristics that Kuhn anticipated would typify such circumstances.

The "Behavioral Preparadigm"

There are numerous excellent accounts of the origins of behavior therapy. Perhaps the most extensive and most interesting of these is Kazdin's (1978a) recent attempt to record its history. For this reason, the following sections will draw freely from Kazdin's contribution to the topic.

In general, behavior therapy's origins may be traced to at least three identifiable sources that partially merged to form the essential principles of this form of therapy. The first source was an approach to treatment which sought to develop therapeutic practices using the principles of learning theories, particularly the principles of classical conditioning. The second source was the experimental analysis of problem behavior using atheoretical concepts derived from operant-conditioning methodology. The third source was the development of a social-learning theory of human behavior, and, to some extent, the analysis and modification of cognition via self-management procedures. In behavior therapy's developmental years, the first two sources were identified with certain treatment techniques found to be useful for changing many problem behaviors. But within these different developing areas there also emerged a great number of treatment methods that have less and less in common with their foundations.

Over recent years, the definitive features of behavior therapy have become increasingly detached from particular "schools" of treatment and their attendant theoretical foundations. For example, it is now inappropriate to describe behavior therapy as based upon the laws of modern learning theory (Eysenck, 1964), or that it be especially concerned with the genesis of abnormal behavior (Yates, 1970). Despite this, it is still true that certain types of treatment techniques tend to characterize behavior therapy. For example, systematic desensitization (Wolpe, 1958), reinforcement procedures (Krasner & Ullmann, 1965), and modeling (Bandura, 1969), are almost exclusively identified as behavior therapy techniques. But what unites these and other procedures are the distinctive methodological approaches that accompany their use in therapy practice. It is now generally agreed that common to their methodologies is the application of the principles of scientific method to treatment. For example, Thoresen and Coates (1978) recently reviewed the wide range of practices described as behavior therapies and concluded that they are only united to the extent that "they attempt to apply the methods and procedures of experimental science to clinical practice [and that what is referred to as] good therapy is the practice of good science" (Thoresen & Coates, 1978, p. 7). In other words, concepts and procedures are stated explicitly, able to be tested empirically, and subject to continuous revision. Research and treatment are therefore virtually one and the same thing.

Before discussing the ramifications of this methodology on therapy practice, it is worth pondering the circumstances that surrounded the emergence of behavior therapy—circumstances that have particular relevance to developments in stuttering therapy. Yates (1970) has given one of the most-quoted accounts of these circumstances. He argues that something resembling a crisis prevailed in the field of clinical psychology during the period preceding the development of behavior therapy. That crisis had three features. The first was growing disaffection with a "medical model" explanation of problem behaviors. This model was embodied in the notion that problem behaviors were the manifestations, or symptoms, of an underlying problem condition. The term "medical model" implied that these behaviors were merely byproducts of a more fundamental diseased state. This interpretation of problem behavior is also found within the underlying parameters (for example, "traits") postulated by many personality theories (see Hall & Lindzey, 1957), and which influenced almost all clinical psychology from the 1920s to the 1950s. The most prominent of these theories was, of course, psychoanalytic theory with its emphasis on unconscious conflict between psychic structures. This conflict was the underlying disease condition which revealed itself in various disabilities. Personality theories also contributed a "trait" and "attitude" approach to diagnosis which, in turn, also dictated much clinical practice.

The second aspect of this crisis was the ineffectiveness of treatments for neuroses or problem behaviors. This was exemplified by Eysenck's (1952) well-known survey on the efficacy of psychotherapy. The essential finding of this survey was that over a 2-year period, approximately the same number of patients recovered from their neuroses after treatment (mainly with psychoanalytically oriented procedures) as did those who were untreated, or only received custodial care. There have been many criticisms of this study (Bergin, 1971). But these criticisms did not blunt the impact of Eysenck's findings. The belief grew that the available therapy procedures could not achieve a better result than that which occurs without such therapy.

Yates (1970) suggests that the final aspect to this crisis was a role problem. Clinical psychologists were increasingly dissatisfied with their clinical role, which involved little more than a passive diagnostic contribution towards patient welfare. The assessment procedures provided a hypothetical description of the source of the patient's problem but they had little (if any) relevance to any treatment that followed the diagnoses.

This combination of role dissatisfaction and inadequate treatment provided a climate that was tailor-made for the arrival of a radically different approach to treatment. It was particularly suited to the appearance of treatments based on practices for which psychologists are more appropriately trained—the systematic investigation of behavior. What emerged was an approach to therapy fostered by psychologists which, according to Kazdin (1978b), contained the following shared characteristics:

1. Focus on current rather than historical determinants of behavior,
2. Emphasis on overt behavior change as the main criteria by which treatment is to be evaluated,
3. Specification of treatment in objective terms so as to make replication possible,
4. Reliance upon basic research in psychology as a source of hypotheses about treatment and specific therapeutic techniques, and
5. Specificity in defining, treating and measuring target problems in therapy. (1978b, p.35).

It should be added that these approaches accompanied a growing commitment to a social-learning theory of behavior. This theory postulated that much problem behavior is under environmental control and, therefore, is modifiable by the manipulation of environmental conditions. These appear to be the general ingredients that blended to form what will be termed "the behavioral preparadigm."

The "Preparadigm Clash" in Stuttering Therapy

It is indisputable that behavior therapy has had a profound effect on treatments for stuttering. The extent and nature of that effect should become evident as these treatments are reviewed. The treatments will be shown to have many limitations, but, thus far, this has failed to dampen a growing and influential comitment to this "preparadigm" by many practitioners. For, in keeping with Kuhn's prediction, there is a firm belief that the solution to providing viable and effective treatments for stuttering will be solved if the principles of scientific methodology are carefully applied within an environmental management framework. But, before the implications of this approach for stuttering therapy are discussed it is worth considering the circumstances that surrounded behavior therapy's introduction to stuttering treatment.

A reasonable case can be made to support the argument that the crises Yates (1970) associated with behavior therapy's arrival in psychology were also evident within speech pathology. This case also rests on three principal grounds. The first is the overriding influence of a medical model approach within theories of stuttering that influenced most stuttering treatments in the 1930-1960 period. The second was the limited effectiveness of the existing treatment procedures; there was scant evidence that durable fluency ever resulted from these treatments.

Finally, there was the evident fear that clinicians had in dealing with this disorder, especially when it occurred in children. The parallel between these circumstances and those that occurred in clinical psychology is striking. But it is not entirely coincidental. For most theories and therapies in clinical psychology have ultimately found their way into stuttering therapy (as well as other areas of speech pathology).

The commanding influence that a select band of clinician/theorists have had on stuttering theories and therapies is really quite remarkable, if not unique. This may be due to the relatively brief history of speech pathology as a distinctive profession, particularly in America. But it is almost certainly due to, perhaps, five impressive individuals who developed theories and therapies that have enormously influenced all work on stuttering: Lee Travis, Bryng Bryngelson, Wendell Johnson, Charles Van Riper, and Joseph Sheehan. Johnson (1955) has provided an intriguing account of the history of the development of therapy and research that emerged under most of these figures, a development that was virtually identified with the University of Iowa during the 1930 to 1960 period.

Travis had a founding influence on many stuttering theories and therapies. He was the first academic head of an American department that trained speech pathologists. Among his first students were Bryngelson and Johnson—and one of their students was Van Riper (he was actually supervised by Bryngelson). In conjunction with Samuel Orton, Travis was responsible for the Orton-Travis theory of stuttering. The essence of this theory was that stuttering was a byproduct of the speaker's failure to achieve cerebral dominance. This decidedly medically based theory quite naturally led to a disease-based approach to treatment. The favored treatment involved exercises in handedness or sidedness training, and also psychoanalysis. Travis was, perhaps, the most prominent and influential exponent of psychoanalytic treatment for stuttering. And his influence continues in various forms, even among clinicians who ultimately developed a more symptomatic approach to stuttering therapy.

Bryngelson was also much influenced by the Orton-Travis theory and a "mental hygiene" model for therapy. The therapy procedures promoted by Bryngelson required both attitude change and social adjustment to enable the stutterer to cope with the assumed emotional consequences that arise from stuttering. One significant therapy procedure that Bryngelson introduced was "voluntary stuttering"; a procedure borrowed from the Negative Practice technique introduced by Knight Dunlap in the 1930s. Dunlap's procedures will be discussed later.

Johnson's contributions to the theory and therapy of stuttering have had an inestimable impact on treatment and research approaches to this disorder. His theory of stuttering departed from those advocated by Travis and Bryngelson. It was based on the belief that there was little organic basis to stuttering and that the disorder had a "diagnosogenic" origin. That is, stuttering was largely a consequence of listener reaction and labeling—it was also the result of trying to avoid stuttering. The therapy that Johnson advocated was aimed at reducing emotional reactions to the disorder by encouraging the patient to freely stutter—even using voluntary stuttering—and altering the stutterer's perceptual and evaluative response to his speech. It was assumed that as the speaker became less concerned about his speech, he would lose the fear-induced reactions to his problem—in turn, this would remove the problem itself. Johnson's approach to the disorder was extremely influential with respect to the role of parents of stutterers; he encouraged the notion that the disorder would most likely disappear if it was not the object of attention. Conversely, the problem would be exacerbated if it became the object of attention. It was advice that has had an incalculable effect on the management of the disorder in children.

Van Riper's principal contribution to stuttering treatment was the development of procedures designed to modify the speaker's actions leading up to, during, and following the moment of stuttering. Among the techniques he devised to control these actions were the well known "preparatory sets," "cancellations," and "pullouts." The skillful use of these techniques was designed to help the speaker achieve "fluent stuttering." By these means, also, the stutterer could overcome fears and abnormal attitudes about his problem.

Sheehan's principal contribution was the proposition that stuttering should be viewed as an example of approach-avoidance conflict. In other words, the speaker wishes to speak, but also wishes to avoid stuttering. Sheehan theorized that the factors associated with avoiding speaking, however, may also involve unconscious conflicts, or repressed needs, as much as learned fears with a more conscious origin. Accordingly, his treatment procedures were (and are) based upon a combination of "fluent stuttering" and psychotherapy. These procedures are mainly designed to alleviate conscious and unconscious fears about stuttering.

The general purpose of the therapies advocated by all five clinicians was to remove the fear and avoidance of stuttering, and also alter the amount of difficulty that the stutterer experiences with all aspects of speaking. It also required the subject to carefully analyze the types of activities associated with speech and avoid using "crutches" to temporarily remove stuttering.

It is probably more than significant that three of the main proponents of this approach to stuttering therapy were (or are) themselves stutterers (Johnson, Van Riper, and Sheehan). Each has written at length about experiences with older techniques of stuttering treatment, and the distrust that this produced towards similar techniques. All grew up in an era which saw the proliferation of "stuttering schools." These were commercial enterprises, run by allegedly exploitive individuals who advertised almost instant "cures" for stuttering. Their treatments are described in a number of places (see Clark, 1964; Van Riper, 1973), and appear to have relied upon variations on rhythmic stimulation or changed vocal inflections. The effect was tantalizingly successful in the short term, but exasperatingly transient (a not uncommon feature of many recent therapies). The consequence of this form of "symtomatic" or "distraction" treatment appears to have left an indelible impression on many clinicians of this era. It also contributed greatly to the search for more theoretically sound and clinically sensitive approaches to the problem. These approaches were based upon almost total mistrust of any method that produces fluency by manipulating the subject's speech pattern, or by employing unusual stimulation. The extensive influence of these major figures on many clinicians inevitably produced a "ruling system" in stuttering therapy and research. It is a system which contains all the hallmarks of a Kuhnian preparadigm, in that it developed and sustained assumptions about stuttering that have influenced generations of clinicians and researchers.

The most developed form of this "ruling system" can be found in many publications from the Speech Foundation of America. This is an organization that was developed and is supported by Malcolm Fraser. The Foundation mainly promotes the practices and theories of the previously mentioned clinicians, but particularly the theory and therapy approaches advanced by Van Riper. The features of the preparadigm, which this Foundation generally supports and promotes, are enunciated in the group's objectives for stuttering therapy:

1. To restore or increase the stutterer's ability to speak normally in any situation.
2. To enable the stutterer to achieve knowledge of the process of speaking and of things he is doing to interfere with speaking.
3. To enable the stutterer to achieve a reversal of these evaluations which motivate the reactions which are included in his stuttering.
4. To enable the stutterer to achieve necessary changes in the attitudes, beliefs, and feelings that affect the interpersonal relationships involved in speaking. (Speech Foundation of America, 1960, p.13).

It will be seen that these criteria assume the stutterer will probably retain at least part of his problem, even if these treatment goals are attained. Presumably, this reduced stuttering would cease to be a problem since it should not restrict the speaker's ability to live a fulfilling existence. These criteria typified an approach to therapy that was not principally concerned with the restoration of normal fluency. It thereby provided fertile ground for therapy approaches that did just the opposite: gave the total primacy to the achievement of stutter-free fluency.

Stuttering therapy's limitations during the prebehavioral period were evident by the paucity of data that accompanied most therapy reports (these will be reviewed shortly). The consequences of this state of affairs on clinical services for stutterers was graphically described by Van Riper (1970) in the following way:

> Unfortunately for the stutterer, no unified program of experimental therapy exists. Communication between training centers, so far as therapy is concerned is practically nil. Indeed, the state of stuttering therapy in this country generally is inadequate, largely in the hands of untrained graduate students, superficial and confused in goals and methods. Therapy time is woefully inadequate. Follow-up is almost non-existent. Criteria for evaluating therapeutic progress are unsystematic. Protocols are missing. A few isolated workers are experimenting with therapy, but their accomplishments are seldom written up or available. Most of the research on stuttering has been descriptive and, for therapy, rather sterile. With more than a milion and a half victims of the disorder in this country (U.S.A.) alone, some integrated attack on the problem is sorely needed. (Van Riper, 1970, pp.53-54)

It is not surprising, therefore, that this situation eventually reduced the confidence many clinicians had in their dealings with this disorder. For example, at about the same time as Van Riper expressed his concerns, Wingate (1971) gave the following portrayal of the attitudes of many clinicians towards the treatment of stuttering in children:

> It is legitimate to contend that a substantial majority of public school speech clinicians have a fear of stuttering. In fact . . . one could even develop impressive substantiation for the claim that most speech clinicians are in their own way, more afraid of stuttering than many of the stutterers they are called upon to treat. (Wingate, 1971, p.3)

It does not require much of an inferential leap to view this situation as a byproduct of the prebehavioral "ruling system." The system promoted nonintervention with children and a reaction against anything that attracts attention to the problem. For the most part, therefore, it can be described as characterized by an indirect and even passive approach to treatment. In this respect it stands in stark contrast to the behavioral approach.

Further Considerations of the Behavioral Preparadigm

With the arrival of behavior therapy approaches to stuttering treatment there occurred something of a return to the approaches of an earlier era. On first appearances, long-discarded treatments were simply revived and employed in a different context. But it was the context, as such, that distinguished this new approach to treatment. In general terms, this context promoted the use of experimental method and, thereby, continuous evaluation within treatment. In doing so, it defined yet another "ruling system" for stuttering therapy: clinicians who used this system were obliged to utilize treatment techniques or procedures with operationalized concepts, in order to achieve equally specifiable objectives. The general manner in which this "system" was promoted was to present examples of the technique's role in achieving a treatment's objective. Unfortunately, this has also served to misrepresent a number of aspects of behavior therapy—the most important of these being that demonstrations of a particular technique's effectiveness in modifying stuttering were often incorrectly characterized as examples of therapy.

The emphasis on a technique-oriented, rather than a problem-oriented, approach to therapy typified many of the early behavioral treatments. To some extent this was fostered by the distinction between process and outcome evaluation of therapy. This was an important distinction, for it served to establish the functional value of many "therapeutic" activities, but in some respects it also separated these activities from their ultimate purpose—sustained behavior change. During its infancy, behavior therapy was characterized, even caricatured, by its emphasis on process analysis, rather than outcome analysis. And, as will be seen, this trend was very evident in early applications of these procedures to stuttering therapy.

Another distinguishing feature of behavior therapy was (and is) the systematic analysis of the variability of a problem behavior (Hersen & Barlow, 1976). It has been presumed that the careful analysis of factors that might contribute to this variability should yield viable techniques for controlling or modifying this variability. In other words, if a procedure results in only short term maintenance of reduced variability (such as improved fluency) then the problem-oriented approach demands the investigation of additional procedures to achieve sustained control over variability. This data-based investigative process, with its emphasis on systematic management of variability, virtually identifies this form of therapy. Thus, a treatment's failure to procure sustained benefits is not regarded as a weakness of behavior therapy, but, rather, the use of ineffective technology for controlling variability. In this respect, therefore, behavior therapy bears all the earmarks of a preparadigm.

Of course, therapies are ultimately judged by the durability of their effects—and nothing that is said with respect to a problem-oriented approach is meant to deny this. The concern is that any consideration of the technique's efficacy should take into account whether it has been fully investigated with a problem-oriented therapy.

The data-based decision-making process, which characterizes behavior therapy, is frequently used to distinguish it from a medical-model approach to treatment. A feature of most medical treatments is that a therapeutic agent is administered for a fixed period (this is almost equivalent to a "dosage" of treatment), and its effects are presumed to be evident at a later time. Hence, the "ongoing performance" of the subject need not prescribe the treatment's duration or "dosage." By contrast, in behaviorally based treatments the subject's problem behavior is monitored throughout treatment and the behavior's response pattern determines variation in the treatment. Specified behavior-change criteria are used to indicate whether the treatment should be continued, withdrawn, or simply judged to be ineffectual. In some ways, the distinguishing features of behavior therapy have resulted in a move away from group study approaches to therapy evaluation, and a move towards single-subject methods of assessment. The identification of a treatment's efficacy may be estimated from group data, but the clinical utility of the procedure is far more evident by carefully assessing its effect on individuals over the course of their therapy. Of course, this move is synonymous with the focus on specificities, rather than generalities, in the formulation of treatment.

The obligations attached to the use of experimental methodology in treatment are quite demanding. The most pressing of these is that a treatment should be shown to be related unambiguously to changes in specified and valid measures of a problem behavior. The methodology must be entirely replicable, including the operations involved in obtaining these relevant measures. In effect, its datum must be observable (by some means), and demonstrably reliable.

All of these therapy operations must also be amalgamated with clinically valid treatment objectives. In the case of stuttering treatments, it is clear that there are at least two objectives. The first, and presumably ideal objective, is that the treatment must achieve normal-sounding stutter-free speech that is durable across a suitable array of speaking situations and over an adequate period of time. The number of situations and the length of time are rarely defined, although it is almost self-evident that these situations should represent the speaker's normal daily environment. The temporal criteria tend to range between 6 months and 2 years after the cessation of formal treatment conditions. The second objective is somewhat less demanding: the resulting improved speech may not be normal sounding and/or may not involve a total absence of stuttering. Actually, the measurement operations used to evaluate a treatment may well determine whether its objectives are the former or the latter. In short, either objective is clinically valid (though not necessarily equally desirable), but only measurement methodology will finally determine which has been attained.

Summary

This chapter has given a general overview of the context that surrounded the introduction of behavior therapy to stuttering treatment. This context contained a number of ingredients that could be expected to produce much conflict with treatment approaches that were favored during the 1930s through the late 1950s, and beyond. The resemblance between Kuhn's analysis of developments in science and the developments that occurred in stuttering therapy in recent years was noted. This development is probably best described as a "preparadigm clash." In the following chapters, various forms of this clash will be observed as the strengths and weaknesses of recent developments in stuttering therapy are critically reviewed.

The structure of subsequent chapters will be as follows: The next chapter will review the features of stuttering that must be recognized in any endeavor to employ behavior therapy with this disorder. This will begin with an overview of the procedures that are used to measure stuttering and its necessarily related behaviors. Then follows a brief review of factors that may easily confound a treatment effect within a therapy context: these are conditions that are well known modifiers of stuttering, and which need to be controlled within an experimental treatment design. One of the important factors which could be confounded with treatment is spontaneous remission. The evidence that has been gathered to demonstrate spontaneous recovery from stuttering will be reviewed in some detail. In the course of this review particular attention will be directed towards those aspects of the recovery process that may be relevant to treatment. Thereafter, the principal treatments will be reviewed along with their experimental foundations. Finally, the reader is invited to consider issues in treatment evaluation and the development of a general therapy evaluation format.

References

Bandura, A. *Principles of behavior modification.* New York: Holt, Rinehart & Winston, 1969.

Bergin, A.E. The evaluation of therapeutic outcomes. In A.E. Bergin & S.L. Garfield (Eds.), *Handbook of psychotherapy and behavior change: An empirical analysis.* New York: John Wiley, 1971.

Clark, R.M. Our enterprising predecessors, and Charles Sydney Bluemel. *Asha,* 1964, *6,* 107-114.

Eysenck, H.J. The effects of psychotherapy: An evaluation. *Journal of Consulting Psychology,* 1952, *16,* 319-324.

Eysenck, H.J. The nature of behavior therapy. In H.J. Eysenck (Ed.), *Experiments in behavior therapy.* London: Pergamon, 1964.

Hall, C.S. & Lindzey, G. *Theories of personality.* New York: John Wiley, 1957.

Hersen, M., & Barlow, D.H. *Single-case experimental designs.* New York: Pergamon, 1976.

Johnson, W., & R. R. Leutenegger (Eds.). *Stuttering in children and adults.* Minneapolis: University of Minnesota Press, 1955.

Kazdin, A.E. *History of behavior modification. Experimental foundations of contemporary research.* Baltimore: University Park Press, 1978 (a).

Kazdin, A.E. Behavior therapy: evolution and expansion. *The Counseling Psychologist,* 1978 (b), *7,* 34-37.

Krasner, L., & Ullmann, L.P. *Research in behavior modification.* New York: Holt, Rinehart & Winston, 1965.

Kuhn, T.S. *The structure of scientific revolutions.* Chicago: University of Chicago Press, 1962.

Masterman, M. The nature of paradigm. In I. Lakatos & A. Musgrave (Eds.), *Criticism and the growth of knowledge.* Cambridge: Cambridge University Press, 1970.

Peterson, G.L. Historical self-understanding in the social sciences: The use of Thomas Kuhn in psychology. *Journal of the Theory of Social Behaviour,* 1981, *11,* 1-30.

Speech Foundation of America. *On stuttering and its treatment.* Memphis: Speech Foundation of America, Publication No. 1, 1960.

Thoresen, C.E., & Coates, T.J. What does it mean to be a behavior therapist? *The Counseling Psychologist,* 1978, *7,* 3-21.

Van Riper, C. Historical approaches. In J.G. Sheehan (Ed.), *Stuttering: Research and therapy.* New York: Harper & Row, 1970.

Van Riper, C. *The treatment of stuttering.* Englewood Cliffs, NJ: Prentice-Hall, 1973.

Watson, J.D. *Double helix: Being a personal account of the discovery of the structure of DNA.* New York: Mentor, 1968.

Wingate, M.E. The fear of stuttering. *Asha,* 1971, *13,* 3-5.

Wolpe, J. *Psychotherapy by reciprocal inhibition.* Stanford: Stanford University Press, 1958.

Yates, A.J. *Behavior therapy.* New York: John Wiley, 1970.

Yates, A.J. *Theory and practice in behavior therapy.* New York: John Wiley, 1975.

2

Identification, Measurement, And Modification of Stuttering

Identification of Stuttering

The Search for a Definition

One of the recurring issues about stuttering has been the failure to settle on an agreed definition of the disorder. It is not a major issue since clinicians seem confident that they can recognize stuttering; they certainly have no difficulty in assigning subjects to stuttering and nonstuttering groups. The problem is that they are unable to agree on the types of behaviors lumped under the label "stuttering," and whether the label refers only to speech behavior. In essence there is as yet no agreement on what necessarily distinguishes "stuttering" from normally nonfluent speech. To a large extent, this issue has been amplified by some of the more influential stuttering theories. Wendell Johnson (1955; 1959) probably complicated the issue by postulating that stuttering is primarily a problem caused by listener judgments rather than a special form of speech behavior. He argued that stutterers and nonstutterers actually exhibit similar speech features, disfluencies, but persons labeled as stutterers simply exhibit more of them. Also, with the revived interest in the organic foundations of stuttering (including genetically based factors), there have been other influential theories that have suggested that more than speech is involved in stuttering. In a very real sense, these different concepts of stuttering have supported the view that the disorder is symptomatic, or indicative of something the speaker "has"—as determined by either listener judgment or by behavior.

A symptomatic definition of stuttering is understandably appealing in a clinical context. People seek assistance for a speech problem they are unable to solve themselves. The nature of this problem may even compel a decision that it cannot be removed. It may not be surprising, then, that it appears to be a disability which involves "more than" poorly controlled fluency. But does it? Certainly stuttering is usually considered an involuntary behavior. It appears to occur constantly, yet may vary in "severity" according to circumstance. It may also be associated with other disabilities which prevent the speaker living a relatively happy life. But there are also numerous disabilities not usually regarded as symptoms. They are simply recognized as problems that need to be removed if the patient is to live a fulfilling existence. For example, an odd-shaped nose or a broken leg are disabilities which may be symptomatic of little more than the events that produced them. They are not usually regarded as symptoms of some less-evident condition. They may recur because of subsequent experiences or accidents, but their successful treatment is normally regarded as all that was necessary to remove the problem. On the other hand, there are numerous problems that require treatment and *are* symptoms of less evident and, possibly, more serious conditions. Although these might be risky comparisons, since they refer to problem conditions rather than behaviors, they have relevance to the problem of defining stuttering. They will also be seen to be particularly important issues when we come to the problem of evaluating treatments for this problem.

Numerous attempts have been made to find an acceptable definition of stuttering. None has been entirely successful. This is because the definition either fails to embrace what some theorists judge to be essential parts of the disability, or it has included what others regard as nonessential. One depiction of this argument is to view these definitions as falling at different points along a symptomatic-nonsymptomatic continuum. For example, at the symptomatic end are definitions that regard the stutterer's speech as virtually incidental to the problem. Thus, Sheehan (1970) claims that "stuttering is a disorder of the social presentation of the self. Basically, stuttering is not a speech disorder but a conflict revolving around self and role, an identity problem" (p.4). Similarly, Murphy and Fitzsimons (1960) argued:

> Stuttering can be defined as "what a person is." It tells us that self defensive processes are in action, that anxieties or fears of diffused or specific character are operating, that the person is attempting not only to protect himself but to prove and improve himself also. (p. 172)

In other words, for some theorists stuttering is a symptom of a disabled or abnormal personality.

But "symptomatic definitions" do not identify the types of behaviors that unambiguously identify a stutterer, or a person exhibiting stuttering-type behaviors. It is surely undeniable that stuttering refers in the first instance to speech. But the type of speech that specifically describes stuttering is still a source of controversy. Indeed the type of speech that is described as stuttering may not be the same as that which causes a person to be described as a stutterer. This was illustrated in studies by Voelker (1942) and Villarreal (1945). They found that many speakers accept that they may have "been stuttering" at some time in their lives, but they would not agree that either they or others referred to them as "stutterers." In essence there are stutterings that are identified as such, but which may not be a problem.

If we wish to define stuttering by reference to specific behaviors, then we must move to the nonsymptomatic end of the definition continuum. Just what are these behaviors? Possibly the most frequently cited definition is that provided by Wingate (1964) which includes

> (a) Disruption in the fluency of verbal expression, which is (b) characterized by involuntary, audible or silent, repetitions or prolongations in the utterance of short speech elements, namely: sound, syllables, and words of one

> syllable. These disruptions (c) usually occur frequently or are marked in character and (d) are not readily controllable (p. 488).

The virtue of this definition is that it has been durable—probably because it refers to aspects of the disorder that many clinicians and researchers use when describing stuttering. The definition's main problem is that it contains too many qualifiers and too many imprecise terms (Woolf, 1967). In spite of this, it continues to be the most-referenced definition of stuttering, and for this reason alone it probably comes close to being an acceptable definition.

Frequency and Form Considerations

The search for an agreed-upon definition of stuttering has also been complicated by the "frequency versus form" issue. Some behaviors only become problems because they occur frequently. We can easily tolerate one or two sneezes per day, but if they occur 100 to 200 times per day, then they become intolerable problems. We may search for their cause, perhaps judging them to be a symptom of some allergy, but the form of the behavior may remain unchanged. Thus, a high frequency of some disfluency (even when it is produced by normal speakers) may, as Sander (1963) and Hegde and Hartman (1979a; 1979b) have found, cause listeners to judge a speaker to be a stutterer. Although it is equally apparent that the form of a behavior may also be a problem—regardless of its frequency. Stuttering provides a perfect example of this issue. This writer has described (Ingham, 1981) a subject who had three stutterings in about 5,000 syllables. But the duration of these stutterings — one lasted 3¼ minutes and the others were 1 and 2 minutes long—was sufficient to judge it a problem. (Incidentally, two trained clinicians and the subject had no difficulty in describing them as stutterings.) But if these behaviors were defined as disfluencies or repetitions, then their frequency would not have been unusual among persons described as nonstutterers.

Thus, the problem of defining stuttering is partly complicated by certain behaviors that are only problematic if they occur frequently. A worthwhile definition should identify features that listeners agree distinguish stuttering from all other features of speech. And therein lies probably the most functional solution indeed the essence of any definition. They are those behaviors that listeners agree are stutterings and not some other type of behavior. Bloodstein (1981) has summarized this with what he regards as the "best definition" at present—that it is:

> whatever is perceived as stuttering by a reliable observer who has relatively good agreement with others. If we want to be guided by a more "objective" definition we must not ask questions about "stuttering" but about repetition, prolongations, broken words, speech rate, and the like, and must be content with answers that are not about stuttering, but about repetitions, prolongations, and so forth (p.9).

In other words, in the final analysis observer agreement is the essence of a satisfactory definition. That should not deter the search for those features that judges agree are stutterings. These features could be useful, if only to improve observer reliability. For even expert observers have difficulty in agreeing on instances of stuttering during ongoing speech (Tuthill, 1946). And in the context of treatment or research, that is exactly what a clinician must do if stutterings, rather than all disfluencies, are to be measured. On the other hand Martin and Haroldson (1981) reported that stutterings were judged less reliably by listeners who were provided with a definition (Wingate's) than by listeners who were simply asked to count stutterings.

Stuttering Behaviors

A considerable amount of research has been conducted in order to find the distinguishing features of stuttering. Van Riper (1971) has made much of the temporal aspects of the disorder. He contends that the

> essential feature that distinguishes a stutterer from a person with an articulatory disability is the former individual's apparent inability to perform the motor sequencing of a given sound or syllable or word at the proper moments in time. . . . When this sequencing of a word utterance is noticeably disrupted in a certain way and evaluated as undesirable, the person is said to possess the disorder of stuttering (p. 19).

But is this timing problem common only to stuttering? Prins and Lohr (1972) provided some support for this viewpoint. They identified 10 factors from an analysis of correlation between measures made on 23 stutterers. The measures derived largely from a frame-by-frame analysis of 10 moments of stuttering obtained from each of 19 stutterers (four were not measured on other variables). A principal components solution found the first factor included moments of stuttering, slow rate of speech, frequency of lip oscillations, revisions, word repetitions, and incomplete phrases. This was interpreted as a severity factor. All other factors included either disfluencies or facial movements. The first factor certainly involved a combination of rate and disfluency variables, however. Prosek, Walden, Montgomery, and Schwartz (1979) used multidimensional scaling techniques to identify the dimensions used by clinicians to judge severity. The dimensions were then correlated with measures of disfluency obtained from 13 stutterers. They found that two dimensions accounted for approximately 50% of the variance: reading rate and the number of pauses within a sentence. Both of the abovementioned studies obtained findings resembling those obtained in an earlier study by Young (1961). Using multiple regression analysis, Young found that the number of "repetitions" ("number of words involving part-word repetitions, prolongations, broken utterances, and apparent unusual stress or tension") and reading rate could predict severity. Thus, the reference to temporal features in the stutterer's speech appears to align with the findings from intercorrelation studies. But there is also recurring reference to certain classes of disfluent behavior.

Part of the problem about defining stuttering in terms of disfluency categories has been that the disfluencies that fit into these categories also describe the speech of nonstutterers. But when these disfluency categories are refined so that there is interest in only certain types of disfluency, then it becomes evident that stutterers exhibit a disproportionate number of these behaviors. This does not mean that these disfluencies should be regarded as the necessary characteristics of stuttering. Rather, they are the features that occur sufficiently often for them to be regarded as typifying stuttering.

Young's (1961) reference to part-word repetitions, prolongations and broken utterances accords with other descriptions of stuttering. It also relates to findings from research aimed at distinguishing between the disfluencies of stutterers and nonstutterers. Johnson (1959) compared 246 stutterers and 246 nonstutterers (2-14 years), and found that the stutterers had significantly more syllable repetitions and prolongations. Subsequently, Johnson (1961) provided supportive data in a study of 100 college-age stutterers and their nonstuttering counterparts. These data clearly showed significantly more part-word repetitions, prolongations, and broken words among the stutterers. Essentially similar findings were reported by Voelker (1944) and Egland (1955).

Summary

Repetition of part-words, particularly the first sound (see Sander, 1963), prolongations, and broken words are the disfluency types that typify most stutterings. This is not to say that each of these disfluencies will be described as a stuttering. These disfluency categories probably provide the clearest description of the behaviors that typify the speech of most persons who stutter, although they have less measurement validity than stuttering judgments made by groups of listeners, or even a sole listener.

Measuring Stuttering

A measure estimates an object's or event's magnitude by reference to some standard. Thus, a valid measure of stuttering should reflect the magnitude of its distinguishing features. For this reason, there is general agreement that a suitable measure of stuttering must be multidimensional. These dimensions should include the frequency of occurrence and some estimate of the extent to which it impedes or disrupts communication. There should also be some means of measuring the so-called accessory features of stuttering. In short, a useful and valid measure will describe how often stuttering occurs and how severe it is.

The methods of measuring stuttering have shown some interesting changes over the years. They clearly reflect the changes in the "ruling systems" that direct both clinical and research practices. So, before the currently used measures are described their antecedents will be briefly reviewed.

Earlier this century, a number of influential clinicians began to assess stuttering by using frequency counts of "moments of stuttering." This index appears to have been introduced by either Johnson and/or Knott in the 1930s (see Johnson, 1955). Initially, the "moment" was partitioned by Johnson (1933) into "pre-spasm," "spasm," and "post-spasm" phases, in order to identify the reactions and responses to the central spasm phase. But, in later reports, a "moment of stuttering" referred to each identifiable "stuttering" that could be counted in a speech sample. Presumably, this measure referred only to the spasm phase. In the 1950s, a number of rating scales were developed in order to measure stuttering severity. These scales usually required the clinician to rate speech samples on a 5- or 7-point scale. Some scales related a scale number to descriptions such as "no stuttering" through to "very severe stuttering," while others were description-free. Both types of scales were used to identify behaviors that correlated with severity judgments. These behaviors included disfluency categories, durations of stutterings, and speech rate. Some other scales permitted subjects to self-rate their form of speech, reactions to speaking situations, and their attitudes.

In recent years, more prominence has been given to the use of frequency counts of either stutterings or disfluencies during different speaking conditions. These have been accompanied by measures of speech rate and, occasionally, the duration of intervals of stuttering. The moment of stuttering, or disfluency, has also been fragmented into disfluency categories such as part-word repetitions, prolongations, interjections, etc. The modality of speech and the setting in which it is measured have also been used to assess variability in the subject's speech behavior.

The influence of certain treatment procedures have also produced a range of measurement strategies. Some have been designed to assess speech "normalcy." These include rating scales for assessing features such as prosody, rate, and fluency as well as perceptual judgment methods. Other rating scales have been designed to assess changes in nonbehavioral or cognitive factors associated with stuttering. These scales assess stuttering severity, communication attitudes, and self-identified criteria of successful treatment.

In general, the measurement of stuttering has become increasingly multidimensional. The measures currently used seek to reflect the frequency, severity, and variability of stuttering. They also appear to be reliable and clinically valid. But measurement methodology continues to change. The development of measurement procedures is allied to developments in sound and visual recording technology. It is now possible for clinicians to record speech over lengthy periods in conditions that closely approximate the subjects' "real world." Other developments have permitted more refined measures of many seemingly pertinent variables such as laryngeal behavior, skin conductance, muscle tension, and phonatory activity. Computer technology is also beginning to play a significant role in measurement methodology. The advantages of very rapid analysis of the voice signal are becoming increasingly obvious. The clinical application of more sophisticated measurement technology is inevitable; perhaps eventually making it possible to automatically measure "stutterings." Such a development would totally revolutionize stuttering treatment. But for the present, and probably for some time, stuttering measurement will continue to depend on the ears and eyes of reliable observers.

The measures currently used to assess stuttering will now be reviewed. This review will consider frequency measures, severity measures, speech rate measurement, mediums of measurement, measures of normalcy, and reactive measures of stuttering.

Frequency Counts

Frequency counts are the most common method of assessing stuttering. They are also the oldest and to some extent the most contentious. The point of contention is in the choice of what should be counted. Some argue that it should be stutterings, while others incline towards measuring all disfluencies. Ironically, Johnson popularized measuring the "moments of stuttering," and, in spite of its critics, this measure has survived to become the most frequently used index of the disorder. In practice, the moment of stuttering usually refers to the audible and visible features that observers agree form a stuttering incident.

It is evident that observers are able to count total moments of stuttering with a high level of interjudge and intrajudge agreement. Tuthill (1946) and Young (1975), for instance, have shown that observers are able to listen to recordings of stutterers reading orally, and mark stutterings on a transcript with high levels of agreement—at least in terms of total stuttering counts. But this level of agreement does not always extend to the actual words judged as "stutterings." This finding has been obtained regardless of whether the judges use audio or audiovisual recordings to make their assessments (Coyle & Mallard, 1979). Nevertheless, this does not mean that judges are unable to agree on instances of stuttering. MacDonald and Martin (1973) found that observers could agree that certain instances in recorded samples of spontaneous speech were "stutterings" and these instances differed from those marked as "disfluencies"—although Curlee (1981) failed to obtain an equally decisive result using a slight variation on MacDonald and Martin's procedure. Nevertheless, Hulit (1978) found that when judges observed a video recording of a stutterer's spontaneous speech, they, too, agreed that certain words were stutterings, even if they "received no training prior to seeing the tape, and they were not given a definition of stuttering" (Hulit, 1978, p. 361). Indeed, Martin and Haroldson (1981) reported that when listeners *were* given a definition, their reliability suffered. Hence, the task of counting stuttered words, or moments of stuttering, *may* be conducted with a high degree of reliability. The variability in this skill is probably due to observer skill and the differences among subjects.

In many recent studies, stuttering counts are converted to either a percentage of words stuttered or percentage of syllables stuttered, thereby relating stuttering frequency to speech output. The advantage of counting either words or syllables has not been determined. Numerous clinical studies have been reported, however, in which either syllables or words stuttered were counted with high levels of reliability (for examples, see Ingham, Martin & Kuhl, 1974; Ingham & Packman, 1977). Percentage of syllables stuttered has been used more often in recent years largely because it takes account of more aspects of the subject's utterances. It also allows for the possible occurrence of stuttering on more than one syllable in a word. In some clinical procedures, such as rhythmic speech, this has practical value, since each syllable is given equal emphasis. In this circumstance, it is obviously much easier to count syllables than words.

Some other clinical researchers, such as Ryan (1974), have used stuttered-words-per-minute as a frequency measure. This is a much easier method of recording stuttering because it does not involve concurrent word or syllable counts. It is also evident from Ryan's reports (Ryan, 1971; 1974) that such counts can be made with impressive reliability. But its disadvantage is that it is insensitive to the possibility that reduced or increased stuttering may simply reflect reductions or increases in the number of words spoken. For this reason, more recently, Ryan (1981) has chosen to accompany stuttered-words-per-minute scores with words-spoken-per-minute data. Of course, this means that the clinician would need to count both stutterings and words concurrently, in order to derive both measures, thereby increasing the complexity of Ryan's measurement method.

Frequency counts of disfluencies, rather than stutterings, is often preferred, because it allegedly provides a more accurate description of both the form and the frequency of stuttering. It may also be useful in analyzing changes in stuttering. Webster (1968), for example, analyzed the types of disfluencies that occur within moments of stuttering and found that some (but not all) tend to interact. During a treatment condition, certain behaviors the subject described as involuntary stutterings were found to increase, while those described as voluntary showed decrease. This is consistent with Brutten and Shoemaker's (1971) Two-Factor Theory of stuttering, where Factor I is composed of word repetitions and prolongations, and Factor II includes the so-called avoidance responses, such as arm swinging, head turning, word changing, and interjecting. It should also be mentioned that in some of the early response-contingent studies, various types of behaviors were used as measures of stuttering (for example, 'nose-wrinkling,'' ''uh-uh-uh,'' in Martin and Siegel's 1966 study).

A number of researchers have also measured the frequency of certain types of disfluencies, in order to provide a more detailed analysis of stuttering. Johnson (1961) used eight disfluency categories to compare their frequency of occurrence in the speech of stutterers and nonstutterers. Williams, Darley, and Spriestersbach (1978) suggest that the following categories provide the most comprehensive analysis of disfluent speech: interjections of sounds, syllables, words, or phrases; part-word repetitions; word repetitions; phrase repetitions; revisions; incomplete phrases; broken words; prolonged sounds; dysrhythmic phonation in words; and tension pause. Hood (1974) has suggested that a molar analysis should be made on the moment of stuttering, using four descriptive categories; ''audible-vocalized, audible-nonvocalized, inaudible-nonvocalized and avoidance escape'' (p. 27). Similarly, Sakata and Adams (1972) identified the frequency of subclasses of disfluencies in the speech of two stutterers. Of most interest was their finding that one subject had speech which was devoid of syllable repetition or prolongations, the very disfluencies that are so often alleged to characterize stuttering. Arguably, the main purpose of measuring disfluency categories appears to have been to explore particular theoretical issues about stuttering, rather than to assist with its treatment.

Many studies have suggested that sound and syllable repetitions or prolongations are probably the definitive disfluency behaviors that describe stuttering. Boehmler (1958) and Williams and Kent (1958) found that sound and syllable repetitions and prolongations are more likely to be judged as stutterings, while revisions and interjections are more likely to be judged as normal disfluencies. However data from Hegde and Hartman (1979a; 1979b) tend to contradict these findings. They assessed some effects of varying the numbers of interjections ("a grammatically obtrusive schwa") and word repetitions on listener judgments of stuttering. Their results show that the frequency of these disfluencies could influence listeners to judge the speech (of a normal speaker) as that of a stutterer.

One unusual method of measuring disfluencies was reported in a study by Rickard and Mundy (1965). They counted the number of repetitions of a sound or syllable to derive a measure of "repetition errors." No other types of stutterings or disfluencies were used to measure the subject's disorder.

There appears to be no virtue in identifying one class of disfluency if the object is to obtain a measure of stuttering. In fact, if the purpose is to provide an account of disfluencies in stutterers' speech, then it may be necessary to use all available categories. It should be noted, however, that this measurement method may only shift the definition problem to another locality; identifying the defnitive characteristics of a disfluency requires the same listener judgment process that is required to identify stuttering. It is also equally likely that other nonstuttering behaviors may be classified within these categories (Wingate, 1976) when used with stuttering or any other speech problems. In other words, the advantages of the procedure may be disadvantaged by its plunge toward reductionism.

Severity

The measurement of severity of stuttering is usually based upon a listener-judged global assessment of the overall form of the speaker's stuttering. In recent years, however, the concept of severity has also been extended to describe different frequencies of stuttering, speech rate, and the duration of moments of stuttering. These measures are reviewed in this section.

Numerous rating scales have been used to estimate stuttering severity. They involve either 5-, 7-, or 9-point scaling systems. On some scales, a description of the type of behavior to be related to each scale point is included (see, for example, Johnson, 1961; Johnson, Darley, & Spriestersback, 1963; and Lewis & Sherman, 1951). Cullinan, Prather, and Williams (1963) compared the ratings of severity that were obtained by different groups of undergraduate students using seven different forms of these rating scales. They used each type of scale to rate

20-second speech samples from stutterers. The results indicated that intrajudge reliability was about the same for either of the 5-, 7- or 9-point scales, those that did not have point definitions (direct magnitude scales), or a 7-point scale with and without point definition. But Cullinan et al. also observed that "there is not sufficient reliability to suggest the use of a single rating from a single judge as an individual predictor" (1963, p. 193). In effect, these scales were essentially similar, though none was really satisfactory for use by an individual clinician with a subject. It should be noted that this conclusion was derived from undergraduate raters and may not apply to experienced clinicians.

The findings by Cullinan and his colleagues suggested that scales using nondefined or defined points provided about the same ratings. Thus, the rather popular Scale for Rating the Severity of Stuttering (Johnson, Darley, & Spriestersbach, 1963) may make unnecessary demands on clinicians. This 7-point scale requires the subject's speech to be rated under four features: frequency of stuttering (in percentage of spoken words); tension-struggle; average duration of moments of stuttering; and frequency of postponement and avoidance. The difficulty with this scale is that it lumps together different behaviors that may not occur in concert. For example, it is possible to conceive of a stutterer who displays a high frequency of stutterings of short duration with no evidence of severe tension or struggle. Another problem is that these ratings are derived from different tasks (talking about the subject's job, describing a TAT card, and oral reading) which may be associated with quite different patterns of severity.

Johnson (1961) also developed a measure of severity known as the Iowa Speech Disfluency Test. This test required counts of eight different types of disfluency, plus rate of utterance, during an oral reading (300-word passage) and a spontaneous speech task (describing a job). From this assessment, a decile score for severity ratings correlated 0.68 with speech rate and 0.85 with total disfluencies. Sander (1961) found a high correlation between rate of utterance and total disfluencies on this test, which also suggests that these two measures are probably integral to judgments of severity.

The evident relationship between speech rate, disfluency counts, and judgments of stuttering severity has found its way into a number of different measures. For example, Minifie and Cooker (1964) recommended their Disfluency Index; it divides the total number of syllables uttered (including those repeated in disfluencies) by the words spoken per minute. This was found to correlate 0.86 with severity ratings (on a direct magnitude scale) of stuttering. Another measure is the Alpha Score derived by Neilson and Andrews (see Guitar, 1976), which provides a weighted combination of percentage of stuttered syllables and syllables-spoken-per-minute scores. Prosek, Walden, Montgomery, and Schwartz (1979) also found oral reading rate to be an important parameter in clinician ratings of severity.

Other clinician-rated severity scales have been developed to distinguish between frequency and form when assessing stuttering severity. Van Riper (1971) has suggested that this may be achieved if the Scale for Rating the Severity of Stuttering (Johnson, et al., 1963) is scored so that subjects obtain a severity score on each of the scale's four dimensions. Riley (1972) has developed a similar scale, in that it independently measures frequency of stuttering, average duration of blocks, and physical concomitants during spontaneous speech and oral reading. Not surprisingly Riley found this Stuttering Severity Instrument correlated 0.89 with Johnson and colleagues' scale.

Severity scores have also been derived from self-ratings made by stutterers. Naylor (1953) had stutterers rate their severity of stuttering on a nine-point scale and found that these ratings were significantly correlated with severity ratings made by graduate students. But since only 50% of variance was accounted for by this correlation it also indicated that subjects and clinicians may respond to related, but different, dimensions when assessing severity. This difference may also be important in considering scores from other scales that use subject judgments to measure severity. For example, Lanyon (1967) developed a Stuttering Severity (SS) Scale which asks the subject to answer "true" or "false" to items that describe different forms of stuttering. And Woolf (1967) reported the construction of a multidimensional self-report scale which measures avoidance, expectancy, and struggle. It is possible that both of these scales identify dimensions of stuttering severity that are either unrecognised or not measured within a clinician-scored test.

The practice of measuring the severity of stuttering in treatment and clinical research has declined in recent years. To a large extent, it has been replaced by frequency-count measures. Perhaps the principal reason for their decline has been that scales are quite cumbersome to administer and provide relatively imprecise scores. They are also of limited value during the course of treatment. By contrast, frequency counts of stuttering are easy to administer, relatively precise, and may make a direct contribution to treatment. Nevertheless, some aspects of severity, such as duration of moments of stuttering, have been measured in treatment-related studies on stuttering. Cherry and Sayers (1956) employed duration of moments of stuttering as a measure of stuttering within their masking and shadowing experiments. Martin and Haroldson (1979) also used this measure during experiments on a variety of procedures known to modify stuttering. They established that this was a reliable and independent measure of stuttering behavior.

The purpose in measuring severity of stuttering is to describe the form of stuttering rather than its frequency. Consequently, the clinical value of a severity score is that it may help identify variability in the more disfiguring and disruptive features of stuttering. For this reason alone, clinicians should be familiar with reliable and practical methods for measuring this dimension.

Speech Rate

The review of severity measurement shows that speech rate measures usefully indicate the extent to which stuttering disrupts the ongoing flow of speech. Many studies, for instance, have shown that speaking rate and oral reading rate are negatively correlated with stuttering frequency. Bloodstein (1944) found a correlation of -0.88 between reading rate and stuttering frequency. The highest reported correlation between speaking rate and stuttering frequency is -0.81

(Sander, 1961). These may not be particularly surprising findings, but they carry the implication (Andrews & Ingham, 1972) that if stuttering frequency is reduced, then, on average, this should be associated with an increased rate of utterance. If this does not occur, then stuttering may not be the only factor that has retarded a stutterer's speech rate.

Speech-rate data are also considered essential in measuring the effects of a stuttering treatment. This is to control for the possibility that improved performance may simply be a byproduct of reduced speech rate. For example, there is now ample evidence (Adams, Lewis, & Besozzi, 1973; Ingham, Martin, & Kuhl, 1974; Johnson & Rosen, 1937) that when stutterers are induced to reduce their customary rate of speaking, this may also reduce their percentage of words or syllables stuttered.

The most common measures of speech rate are words-per-minute, syllables per minute, or the time taken to utter a prescribed number of words or syllables. The advantage of syllable-counts over word-counts is that the former probably provides a more constant measure, or one that is unaffected by variations in the syllable size of words spoken. This is supported in part by Umeda and Quinn's (1980) finding that in reading material, at least, syllables tend to carry approximately the same number of phonemes regardless of the density of the material (i.e., length of sentences, number of polysyllables, size of content/function ratio). For this reason, Umeda and Quinn suggest that syllables-per-unit-of-time may provide a more universal measure of speech rate.

The difficulties in obtaining reliable measures of speech rate are often considerable—particularly in conversational speech. Ingham and Packman (1977), for example, reported that reliable syllable-per-minute measures could be made in nonconversational speech, but were difficult to obtain in conversational speech. The reasons are quite obvious: much conversational speech is composed of single-syllable or word utterances that do not permit meaningful measures of speech rate. The same problem may also occur when measuring speech rate in uninterrupted speech; pause intervals may be either complete cessations of speaking or part of the speaking process. Consequently, the lack of general agreement on what represents an "acceptable" pause in speech-rate data is a continuing source of measurement error.

Perkins (1975) has introduced a measure which partly overcomes the pause problem. He advocates the measurement of articulation rate. This is found by counting stutter-free syllables uttered and ignoring or eliminating pause intervals. This may provide a more accurate assessment of syllable rate, especially in the context of treatments that manipulate this variable (for example, the "prolonged speech" treatments). This has been partly demonstrated by Perkins, Bell, Johnson, and Stocks's (1979) finding that an identical measure, "phone rate," could be obtained with adequate reliability during oral reading.

Speech-rate data are often regarded as important in determining whether a stutterer has achieved normal-sounding speech after treatment. While there exists considerable overlap between the speech rate of populations of stutterers and nonstutterers (Johnson, 1961), there are also relatively significant differences between their rates. Darley (1940) reported that the oral-reading rate of a population of normal (American) speakers (n=200) was 167 words-per-minute, with a range of 129 to 222 words-per-minute. Bloodstein (1944) had a group of stutterers (n=30) read material similar to that used by Darley, but found they produced a mean of 123 words-per-minute with a range of 42 to 191 words-per-minute. This has led to the view that post-treated stutterers should speak at close to the mean speech rate of nonstutterers in order to achieve at least one aspect of normalcy. In Australia, it has been reported by Bernard (1965) that normal speakers (around age 17 years) have a mean-utterance-rate during spontaneous speech of approximately 222 utterances (or identified syllables)-per-minute with an "average diversion from the mean" of 32 utterances-per-minute. Some practical use has been made of these data in the context of treatment programs. For instance, Ingham and Andrews (1973) used the lower end of this range, 190 syllables-per-minute, as their target speech rate in a treatment program. Similar target rates have been used in other stuttering treatment programs (see, for example, Boberg, 1980; Perkins, 1973). But, of course, the restoration of statistically normal speech rate does not necessarily ensure that a subject has acquired normal-sounding speech (Ingham, 1981).

Mediums of Measurement

The medium in which a stutterer's speech is measured may have much influence on evaluation. The most important factors in this measurement parameter include the type and amount of speech, plus the method of assessment. An important additional factor is the speaking situation. This will be considered in more detail in the following section.

One method of categorizing speech behavior is to consider it in terms of three common types of speaking: oral reading, monologue, and conversational speech. Each has been found to be associated with quite different frequencies of stuttering among individual stutterers (Ryan, 1974). For this reason, many clinicians and researchers now favor part of Ryan's (1971; 1974) assessment procedure. This requires the subject to read orally, provide a monologue, and converse with another person for 5 minutes under each condition. The assessment is conducted in a common setting, such as the clinic. Occasionally, the content of the reading material and the topics for the monologue and conversation are also prescribed. Johnson (1961), for example, suggested the Job Task, describing TAT pictures, and the Rainbow Passage (Fairbanks, 1960) were suitable for this purpose. Other passages, such as those provided by Fairbanks (1960), are also useful oral reading tasks.

The choice of an appropriate method for assessing the speech of a young child stutterer presents a number of special problems. Ryan (1974) has outlined a series of speaking tasks that are designed to obtain suitable speech samples from children. These include echoic reading, picture naming, speaking with a puppet, monologue, sampling difficult words, talking while drawing, telephoning, and observing in a natural setting. Other methods have been described by Hood (1978), and, for the most part, these involve sampling speech across a variety of situations—also highly desirable in any pretreatment assessment. Williams

(1978) has outlined a procedure which involves altering the social complexity of the clinic situation; in essence, the child is introduced to, and speaks with, a range of familiar and unfamiliar people.

The amount of speech that should be sampled is also a matter for debate. Young and Prather (1962) found that a 20-second sample of connected speech (not including initial segments) was highly correlated with much larger samples when assessing stuttering severity. But this finding emerged from group data, and may not be relevant to individual data. For this reason, most assessments are made on the basis of 200- to 400-word samples, or 5-minute units (Van Riper, 1971). Perhaps the most useful sampling procedure is to have the subject talk long enough to produce at least 10 moments of stuttering (Van Riper, 1971). This has the advantage of providing an estimate of the number of words or syllables required in different modalities. This, then, provides a firmer basis for assessing the effects of a treatment procedure. Far larger samples are often required in the context of certain treatment procedures. For example, in treatments that use operant-conditioning methodology, the subject's speech is sampled in either time intervals or speech units until a stable frequency of stuttering and speech rate are identified. In some studies, this has involved samples of many thousands of syllables or words.

Another measurement medium issue is whether audio-visual or audio-alone conditions should be used to measure stuttering. The research findings on this issue are not particularly helpful. Tuthill (1946) found that different groups of judges produced similar frequency counts of "stutterings" during audio and audio-visual conditions. Williams, Wark, and Minifie (1963) also obtained an essentially similar result for judgments of stuttering frequency and stuttering severity. By contrast, Luper (1956) found that frequency counts of stuttering from visible samples were somewhat higher than were frequency counts from audible samples. Martin (1965) also reported differences between audio-visual and audio-only ratings of stuttering severity. It has been suggested by Van Riper (1971) and others that the differences between the findings from these studies may simply reflect differences in the overt features of stuttering in the speech samples used in these studies. Perhaps the most obvious conclusion from these findings is that audio assessment should be satisfactory for most rating purposes. From time to time, however, audio assessments should be supplemented by measures derived from audio-visual conditions.

Measures of Normalcy

In recent years, a number of treatments for stuttering have been developed that involve altering the subject's customary manner of speaking. These procedures appear to achieve reductions in stuttering at the cost of normal sounding speech—mainly via reduced speech rate and altered phonatory behavior. Older procedures, such as rhythmic speech, may also procure reduced stuttering at the expense of normalcy. As a result, measures have been designed to determine whether a subject's post-treatment speech has achieved a "normal-sounding" quality.

Jones and Azrin (1969) described speech-quality assessment of rhythmic speech. They had their observers judge one-minute samples of the subject's speech as either "natural" or "unnatural": the total percentage of "natural" judgments was then used to make a comparative assessment of speech quality. Perkins (1973) also used one-minute samples for listeners to rate fluency, speech rate, and prosody on a 4-point scale. The difficulty with both of these procedures is that they do not indicate when "normalcy" has been achieved. Ingham and Packman (1978) attempted to solve this problem by using a perceptual judgment method in which listeners attempted to identify stutter-free samples of the subject's speech from among similar size speech samples of "normal" speakers. An almost identical procedure was described by Runyan and Adams (1978). Both procedures were based on a method used by Wendahl and Cole (1961) and Young (1964) to determine differences between fluent speech samples from stutterers and nonstutterers. The procedure assumes that if listeners are unable to distinguish the stutterer's speech from that produced by normal speakers, then the subject has achieved normal-sounding speech. A variation on this procedure involves a forced-choice technique: paired samples are presented and the listener is asked to decide which is the treated-stutterer sample (Ingham and Packman, 1978). But the flaw in this type of procedure is that it assumes that the nonstutterer's speech is normally fluent. This is not necessarily true, and so failure to distinguish the stutterer's sample does not mean that it is thereby equivalent to normal-sounding speech. For this reason, Martin (1981) has proposed a method in which observers rate speech samples for "naturalness" on a 5-point scale. The origin of the sample is not mentioned, since the object is to measure the relationship between the ratings.

An alternative, though related, approach to evaluating the normalcy of nonstuttered speech has been proposed by Hegde (1978). He has suggested that treatments should be designed to achieve only fluent intervals (free of all disfluencies). If this were to occur, then the problems of rating scales and speech-rate criteria of fluency are bypassed. This is difficult to accept if the object of treatment is to produce normal fluency: totally fluent speech is not necessarily normal-sounding speech. In fact, a normal speaker's fluency may be better described as "normally fluent speech," since, as Johnson (1961) found, it may contain an acceptable sprinkling of disfluencies.

Many treatment programs specify goals or criteria of "success" that one might assume are equivalent to normally fluent speech. But there is a vast gap between some of these "success" criteria and normally fluent speech. For instance, many clinicians specify goals that include an absence of stuttering and a speech rate resembling that found among normal speakers. But these features are sufficient to describe a wide variety of unusual forms of speaking. For this reason, there is an urgent need to find procedures that will assist clinicians in operationalizing or programming for normally fluent speech. At present, normal-sounding speech appears to be a "hoped for" consequence rather than a programmed feature within most treatments.

Reactive Measures

For many clinicians, the targets of normal speech include an absence of avoidance behavior, reduced negative reactions to speech situations, and acceptable communication attitudes. This orientation produces measurement procedures that claim to estimate whether the subject continues to react in ways typified by stuttering populations, reaction patterns that should not be evident if a treatment is successful.

A variety of questionnaires have been developed to measure stutterers' reactions to their problems. These attitudes and patterns of behavior have been a source of theoretical interest and investigaton since the 1930s. For some researchers and clinicians, these aspects of stuttering are regarded as crucial to treatment, and even responsible for retarding treatment gains. Others argue that it would be surprising if stuttering did not manifestly alter attitudes and interpersonal behavior. In other words, if these reactions are a problem, then they should diminish if stuttering is reduced or removed (Boberg, 1981). It is probable that the differences between stutterers will provide support for both viewpoints.

Perhaps the most commonly used assessment of a stutterer's reaction to speech situations is the Stutterer's Speech Situation Rating Sheet (see Johnson, Darley, & Spriestersbach, 1963), devised by Johnson in 1943. This self-rating scale asks the subject to provide four modes of response to 40 speaking situations. Each response is measured on a 5-point scale. The modes of response are (1) the tendency to avoid each situation, (2) reactions as to enjoyment of speaking in the situaton, (3) severity of stuttering in the situation, and (4) the frequency of involvement in the situation. Shumak (1955) reported the results of administering the scale to 95 stutterers (17-46 years). She found that the Avoidance and Reaction scores were highly correlated (0.84), while the Severity of Stuttering was moderately but signficantly correlated with Avoidance (0.52) and Reaction (0.57) scores. The frequency of contact with a situation was somewhat less related to Avoidance and Reaction scores but did not correlate with severity. The findings suggest that stutterers' affective responses to situations are partly, though not completely, related to their judgments on the severity of their stuttering in those situations.

The Perceptions of Stuttering Inventory devised by Woolf (1967) also measures some affective aspects of stuttering by self-assessing its struggle, avoidance, and expectancy effects. Woolf argues that these features actually define stuttering. Hence, the extent to which these features occur in a subject's speech is the extent to which the Inventory probably measures stuttering severity. No data are provided, however, that would permit estimation of either the validity or reliability of this scale.

The attitudes that stutterers possess towards speaking situations is currently regarded as an important dimension of stuttering—particularly with respect to treatment. Interest in this parameter began in the 1940s with the then considerable concern for "mental hygiene." Ammons and Johnson (1944) at that time devised the Iowa Scale of Attitude Towards Stuttering, which asks stutterers to indicate their level of agreement with statements about stuttering. The scale is not widely used and has been largely replaced by a scale devised by Erickson (1969), which claims to measure "communication attitudes." Erickson's S Scale asks the subject to respond ("true" or "false") to 39 statements about different features of stuttering. The scale was standardized on groups of stutterers and nonstutterers, in order to permit the indentification of items that distinguished a significant majority of stutterers from nonstutterers. The stutterers' scores on this scale were reported to be not substantially correlated with severity of stuttering. A modification of the S Scale was made by Andrews and Cutler (1974), so that items were included only if they were responsive to changes in stuttering during treatment. The use of this 24-item S24 Scale has been reported in a number of studies. It has also been claimed by Guitar and Bass (1978) to be a good predictor of long-term outcome from treatment. However, the extent to which scores on the S24 Scale are actually independent of speech behavior, especially since it was designed to be responsive to changes in stuttering, is a source of some controversy (Guitar, 1979; 1981; Ingham, 1979; 1981).

The extent to which nonspeech behavior can be regarded as an essential source of measurement for stuttering is a debatable issue. For instance, some clinicians regard avoidance and communication attitudes as important to assessment, but not entirely necessary to treatment. This is reflected, in an interesting manner, through a study reported by Silverman (1980). Twenty-six authorities on stuttering (representing a wide spectrum of theoretical positions) were asked to rate 288 statements about stuttering on a seven-point scale, in order to determine whether each statement was related to improvement in treatment ("1 representing *least* improvement and 7 representing *most* improvement; 4 represents the midpoint between 1 and 7"). The statements covered (1) modification of speaking behavior; (2) reduced avoidance of words or of speaking situations; (3) modification of attitudes and feelings related to speaking; (4) modification of attitudes and behaviors in the personal-social sphere; (5) unclassified. No item in categories (2), (3), and (4) achieved a mean score greater than 4.25, while nine items in category (1) and two items in category (5) were given scores higher than 4.25. All the higher items in categories (1) and (5) referred to reduced stuttering or improved ability to speak in situations.[1] In effect, these authorities generally agreed that nonspeech aspects of stuttering are less than essential dimensions for measuring and determining improvement.

There are a number of other reactive measures that are used in specific areas of stuttering research and treatment. These include measures of trait and state anxiety, physiological measures, and personality scales of different types. They will be described in connection with specific treatment procedures. In general, the previously mentioned self-rating measures have been used in a variety of treatment contexts and provide data that are largely of supplementary value.

[1]It is noteworthy that the item reading, "My speech is now normally fluent in all situations and has been for the past three years" could only attract a mean of 6.38 (it was the highest-rated item). It is surprising that this item was not judged to represent most improvement and suggests that some authorities regard this seemingly demanding criterion as an insufficient measure of improvement.

Perhaps the principal use of their information is in the identification of problem areas that may need investigation and therapy during the course of treatment. However, there is no evidence which indicates that they supplant speech performance data.

Some General Comments on Measurement

By now, it should be clear that there has emerged a variety of measurement procedures for both treatment and research which suits the various features of this problem and the complexities involved in measuring and evaluating changes in stuttering. It will be seen that measurement technology is intimately, if not inextricably, connected with treatment methodology. Many measurement procedures were developed in order to assess particular aspects of treatment and have waned in their use as the treatment's popularity has declined. Others show more prominence because of their relationship with treatments currently in use.

At present, there is an increasing amount of emphasis on treatment-outcome evaluation and maintenance procedures. As a result, measurement strategies are beginning to emerge that provide their own peculiar indices. Included among these are covert assessment and self-evaluation of speech performance. The indices they require will be discussed in connection with treatments that use these strategies.

Perhaps the most notable recent development in stuttering therapy has been the integration of treatment research and therapy programming. A variety of research designs, particularly those suitable for single-subject research (Hersen & Barlow, 1976) have found their way into general treatment methodology. These designs have the advantage of providing a data-base for decision-making during treatment. The point at which a decision is made about a therapy's effectiveness (or ineffectiveness) is increasingly based on a formalized schedule of data collection and trend analysis. The quasi-experimental time-series designs (Campbell & Stanley, 1963) have been particularly suited to this purpose, but they also involve special measurement considerations.

Among the most useful single-subject experimental designs for therapy are those that involve multistimulus baseline analysis (Hersen & Barlow, 1976). They require that measures be made of stuttering during a pretreatment period and across a variety of stimulus conditions or situations. A treatment for stuttering is introduced to one of these situations, while the behavior is concurrently measured in other situations. This procedure is repeated across further situations, and treatment effects are assessed according to specified criteria. Such a design calls for a system of regular recordings of prescribed amounts of speech behavior across a range of speaking situations. Typically, this includes counts of syllables, stutterings, and speech rate. But these measures are occasionally supplemented by assessments of speech quality, reactions to speaking situations, and, perhaps, attitudes.

The subject's speech data can now be collected quite easily from a variety of conditions because of the vast developments in recording technology. But parents and significant others can also provide a valuable avenue for obtaining formal and informal data. Regularly obtained information from different sources within the subject's environment, as well as the subject's own assessments, are providing the means for therapy decision-making as well as treatment evaluation.

The conversion of recorded data into clinically useful scores has also been assisted by the development of manually operated event counters. Some light-weight electronic button-press units are now commercially available, and, provided clinicians are adequately trained, they may be used with adequate reliability to obtain measures such as percentage of syllables stuttered and syllables spoken per minute. One such unit, the "Kabtronic Disfluency Counter," has been used in numerous studies by this writer.

Ultimately, the choice of a measurement system will be governed by the therapy format which is chosen to treat a stutterer. In any event, a clinician is generally advised to systematize a pattern of repeated speech recordings across time and over situations. This should be supplemented by such other measures as the clinician and subject deem suitable to identify the efficacy (or otherwise) of treatment. It is to be hoped that the reasons for this rather cursory account of measurement methods will become apparent when the stuttering treatments are reviewed. Suffice to say, at this point, that the increasing complexity of these methodologies is a response to the dubious credibility of stuttering treatment as much as the vagaries of the disorder. The rationale and features of a therapy measurement and evaluation procedure suitable for most stuttering treatments will be outlined in Chapter 12.

Common Conditions that Modify Stuttering

Introduction

Thus far, we have considered the commonly used methods for measuring stuttering behavior. In the course of this consideration, it was noted that there exist some sources of error posing potential threats to the reliability and validity of many measurement and (necessarily) treatment procedures. Many of these are related to conditions known to modify stuttering. Consequently, unless these conditions are adequately controlled within an experimental or treatment setting, they may compromise the internal and external validity of stuttering treatment effects. This section will generally review the better-known conditions that are reported to modify stuttering. They will also be considered in the review of each treatment that employs some of these conditions for therapy purposes.

The most commonly described feature of stuttering is its variability. Numerous texts on stuttering have given descriptions of the remarkable variations that may occur in both its severity and frequency. It seems clear that there are occasions and situations that many stutterers find cause a high frequency and/or severity of stuttering, and others where their problem might be completely absent. These changes are also reported to occur in all age groups, but they are more commonly associated with stuttering in adulthood. The problem facing the clinician (and subject) is to identify predictability in this variability.

There are a number of factors involved in assessing sources of variability in stuttering. Among the more prominent is the source of the data. If stuttering is potentially present in all of a subject's speech behavior, then it is easy to understand why its impact on communication could be inconsistent. For instance, a disruption to communication on certain important occasions might be far more impactful on a speaker than it would be at other less important times. Understandably, this may cause stutterers to judge their problem as more severe in those important and more easily remembered situations. In other words, observers may judge the subject's stuttering to change minimally, whereas stutterers, themselves, could have a different perception of their speech. Another consideration is the size of the task involved in identifying sources of variability. How are the distinguishing features of conditions defined so that changes in stuttering may be related to observable or measureable conditions? For instance, it is possible that variability may in itself be variable: a consistent association between stuttering and certain circumstances during one period of time may not remain that way (Ingham, 1981). To some extent, both of these considerations can be allowed for in an adequate therapy design. But these issues require assumptions about measurement and assessment that may be intrinsic sources of error.

There are numerous ways of partitioning speech in order to discern factors that produce variability in stuttering. For most practical purposes a broad division can be made between environmental factors and factors that relate to alterations in the subject's speaking behavior. These factors may overlap but the principal variables are usually related to one of these categories. However, in reviewing the sources of variability in these categories, our interest will be mainly restricted to those that are commonly reported to reduce, rather than increase, stuttering. The reason for this limitation is to identify ameliorative conditions that might confound treatment or therapeutic benefits.

Environmental Factors

Audience Size and Type

The literature on stuttering is peppered with examples of unusual environmental conditions that seemingly reduce stuttering in certain individuals. Although these examples are rarely accompanied by careful documentation, their frequency should be a matter of interest. It is probably prudent, therefore, to have subjects identify and record their speaking circumstances so that they may be "controlled" within a treatment evaluation. However, many of these circumstances share much in common and are almost predictably associated with reduced stuttering.

The audience size and type is one environmental category that has been the subject of much research. The findings of studies by Porter (1939), Shulman (1955), and Siegel and Haugen (1964) have shown that an increase in the number of listeners (mainly during oral reading) may increase the severity and frequency of stuttering. When subjects are not forewarned of the audience size, however, this effect is less likely (Young, 1965). On the other hand, many studies (for example, Langova & Svab, 1973; Porter, 1939; Quinn, 1971) have shown that when stutterers are recorded speaking alone, their problem is substantially reduced or absent.

Some studies have also supported the often-reported statement that stuttering may be reduced if the subject speaks with people he judges to be "easy" listeners or not "authority-laden." Porter (1939) found somewhat less stuttering occurred when subjects read orally before "easy," rather than "hard" listeners (although there was even less stuttering when they read to "neutral" listeners). Berwick (1955) reported that when subjects read orally to a photograph of a person rated an "easy listener," they had comparatively less stuttering than when the photograph was that of a "hard listener." A related effect was reported by Sheehan, Hadley, and Gould (1967), who had subjects read orally before those who were casually attired and introduced as a peer. This resulted in less stuttering than with someone dressed more formally and introduced by the title "Doctor."

Chorus Reading or Shadowing

One of the most remarkable features of stuttering is the apparent immediacy with which it is reduced if the subject reads aloud with an accompanist. Johnson and Rosen (1937) and Barber (1939), among others, have shown the extent of this effect. A similar effect occurs when stutterers repeat, or shadow, words spoken by a lead speaker (Cherry & Sayers, 1956). The amount of similarity between the subject's and accompanist's reading material (in the case of chorus reading) may also influence this effect. However the necessary temporal interval between the leader and shadower has not been defined. It should be noted that one common explanation for the benefits caused by these procedures is that they alter the subject's customary manner of speaking (Wingate, 1969).

Rhythmic Stimulation

Another fluency-inducing condition, whch may also involve an altered speech pattern, is rhythmic stimulation. When stutterers are instructed to speak to the accompaniment of rhythmic stimulus there is ample evidence that their stuttering may be reduced (Bloodstein, 1981). Greenberg (1970) reported that when school children who stuttered were recorded speaking in the presence of a rhythmic signal, there was a significant reduction in stuttering. This also occurred when they were not instructed to attend to the signal. More systematic applications of this procedure will be reported in Chapter 5, but most of these applications involve instructions to alter the speech pattern.

Masking

It is evident from many studies that when stutterers speak in the presence of either bilaterally or unilaterally presented noise (either filtered or unfiltered), there is likely to be a reduction in stuttering (Barr & Carmel, 1969; Cherry &

Sayers, 1956). The masking effect is evident at very low noise levels (Maraist & Hutton, 1957), and may even occur when only the silent intervals between the voice signal are masked (Sutton & Chase, 1961; Webster & Dorman, 1970). This raises the possibility that if the subject is recorded speaking in relatively noisy conditions, be it during treatment or assessment, then stuttering may be "artificially" reduced.

Adaptation Effect

When stutterers orally read the same material on successive occasions they may markedly reduce their stuttering. The effect is remarkably specific and is one of the most researched aspects of stuttering (see Bloodstein, 19[illegible]. For most subjects, stuttering is decreased by about 50% after five successive readings. This level of reduction is most evident if the subject is not judged severe, if the time between readings is minimized, and if the reading situation remains constant. Virtually all departures from these conditions have been shown to temper the adaptation effect.

A related effect has been reported to occur within spontaneous speech tasks. Bloom and Silverman (1979), for instance, reported that some stutterers' disfluencies were reduced by roughly 50% after five successive telephone calls to the same person. In some cases this improvement trend was reported over successive days, but others showed no evidence of this effect, either within or across days.

The evidence of the adaptation effect indicates that for some stutterers repeated readings of the same material, or speaking on regular occasions under identical conditions, may substantially (though not completely) reduce stuttering.

Punishment

There is considerable evidence that stuttering may be reduced under conditions containing aversive stimulation. A number of studies (see Chapter 9) have shown that when an electric shock or loud noise is delivered contingent on stuttering, then there may be a substantial, if not complete, reduction in stuttering—at least in some subjects. Even under conditions in which aversive stimulation is delivered noncontingently, stuttering may also be reduced or absent (Toomey & Sidman, 1970). Although, in the last-mentioned condition, it is likely that this effect is accompanied by an altered speech pattern.

Measurement Reactivity

When stutterers have been assessed covertly and overtly in relatively similar conditions, there is some evidence of clinically significant differences in their stuttering. This effect is often observed during the later stages of therapy programs when stutterers have achieved ostensibly stutter-free speech. For instance, Ingham (1975; 1980) found that when "fluent" subjects were unaware they were being recorded, their speech was far from stutter-free. This suggests that some reductions in stuttering may occur simply because the subject is aware of assessment.

Altered-Speaking-Behavior Factors

It may be trite to suggest that stutterers have much reduced stuttering behavior if they change their usual way of speaking. It seems quite logical that if stuttering is removed, the subject will not have a customary manner of speaking. But there are some characteristic ways of speaking that are known to eliminate stuttering—at least for short intervals—and these are usually quite unlike the stutterer's nonstuttered intervals of speech. The extent of this effect is such that almost any novel manner of speaking may reduce stuttering. However, the nature of this effect is usually known through anecdotal reports rather than systematic investigation.

Altered Inflection

This phenomenon is also generally reported within case studies, rather than controlled studies. The effect is most apparent if the subject introduces an accent, or changes his or her speech pattern. Bloodstein (1949) reported that more than 85% of stutterers stated that the following conditions reduced their stuttering: "swearing," "imitating a regional dialect," "imitating another person's manner of speaking," "imitating a foreign dialect," "when putting on a jocular manner," "speaking through closed teeth," "speaking in a sing-song manner," and "speaking on a lower pitch." Some of these effects have been investigated in a research context. For example, Johnson and Rosen (1937) instructed subjects to alter their manner of inflection by using a "sing-song" method of oral reading. They found that 15 of their 18 subjects reduced their stuttering to zero in this condition. By contrast, no more than four subjects were stutter-free during any "ordinary" oral reading condition.

Singing and Whispering

Both of these alternatives to speaking are rather extreme departures from normal speech behavior, but they show ameliorative effects. Bloodstein's (1949) report found that 100% of surveyed subjects reported that singing achieved substantial reductions in stuttering. Indeed, the effect is so common that more interest has been shown in finding subjects who do stutter when they sing (Wingate, 1969). Some recent experiments by Healey, Mallard, and Adams (1976) and Colcord and Adams (1979) have shown that quite a number of stutterers produce low but evident stuttering while singing.

There is some relatively substantial evidence that when stutterers whisper, or fail to use voicing, they also reduce their stuttering, although these speech behaviors generally produce less reduced stuttering than that found during singing. For instance, Johnson and Rosen (1937) found that only four of their 18 subjects were stutter-free in this condition. Nevertheless, their subjects produced only 72 stutterings across all 500-word passages during whispered reading, but at least 316 when they read normally. Adams (1955) reported that whispering was more effective in reducing stuttering in severe rather than mild stutterers.

These changes in customary methods of speaking involve infrequently used methods of speaking. It is possible, however, to conceive of a manner of speaking which involves singing or whispering, but which is not too dissimilar from normal-sounding speech. In effect, some of these patterns could be blended with normal speech and be sufficient to modify stuttering.

Rhythmic Speech

There is overwhelming evidence that stuttering is reduced when speakers introduce a rhythmic emphasis to their speech (Bloodstein, 1981; Van Riper, 1971). The effect is most obvious when subjects are asked to speak so that each syllable accompanies a rhythmic stimulus. Syllabized or unaccompanied rhythmic speech may also achieve the same effect (Brady, 1969). The magnitude of this effect has been shown in many studies on metronomic stimulation, but it is equally evident when subjects are instructed to use an identical unassisted speech pattern (Andrews & Harris, 1964). In most of these studies it has been shown that quite severe stutterers may cease stuttering whenever they use this speech pattern.

DAF/Prolonged Speech

This is another speech pattern which emerged from external stimulation conditions, but which may also be adopted without assistance. The stutterer's speech during delayed-auditory-feedback conditions has been found to be stutter-free, but characterized by emphasized phonation and reduced articulatory stress (Goldiamond, 1965). It may also involve reduced speech rate, although this appears to be unnecessary. Prolonged speech is one of the currently favored methods in stuttering treatment, again, because it generally removes stuttering whenever it is used (Ingham & Lewis, 1978). This rather "slurry" type of speech may be adopted with little formal assistance, and could conceivably yield stutter-free speech under the demand conditions of treatment.

Slow Speaking

Almost every stutterer reports being advised to "slow down." And despite the understandable resistance of most stutterers to such "folk remedies," the beneficial effects of reduced speech rate on stuttering are at times striking. Studies by Johnson and Rosen (1937) and Ingham, Martin, and Kuhl (1974) have shown that when stutterers are instructed to reduce their oral reading or spontaneous speech rate, there can be considerable reductions in stuttering, although Ingham et al. (1974) found this was not common to all stutterers. It should also be noted that some stutterers claim that reduced speech rate was the main reason for their recovery without professional assistance. This issue will be discussed in Chapter 4.

Spontaneous Recovery

It is claimed in many texts (for example, Beech & Fransella, 1968; Van Riper, 1971) that by early adulthood around 80% of stutterers will recover from stuttering without assistance. It is also reported that some children experience relatively brief periods of stuttering. These claims carry the additional implication that these subjects ultimately achieve normal fluency. However, at present, there are no data available to help predict which stutterer might recover without assistance. Thus, it is occasionally claimed that any long-term treatment, especially one that includes a lengthy follow-up period, may achieve improved fluency because it has "chimed in" with spontaneous recovery.

Spontaneous remission (or spontaneous recovery) from stuttering will be considered in some detail in Chapter 4. At this point it should be noted that when such recovery occurs, it may be due to a variety of conditions that are known to change stuttering.

Word Avoidance

One of the more bizarre features of stuttering, and also the least researched, is the stutterer's ability to substitute words or use circumlocution in order to avoid stuttering. Both Van Riper (1971) and Bloodstein (1975) have described stutterers who are, ostensibly, completely fluent whenever they manipulate their language behavior. The success of this tactic is alleged to be short-lived, although in the absence of any systematic investigation of this phenomenon, that is open to question. Some analogue research has been conducted on word avoidance during oral reading. Johnson and Sinn (1937) provided one of the earliest studies. During oral readings, their adult subjects omitted words on which they expected to stutter and thereby achieved a 98% reduction in stuttering. Silverman and Williams (1972) conducted a similar study with children and adolescents, and found that they were only able to predict correctly about 50% of words subsequently stuttered or spoken fluently. Taken together, these studies suggest that avoidance may achieve a substantial, though not complete, reduction in stuttering. The problem is that these analogue studies may have only partial relevance to spontaneous speech.

The task of assessing word avoidance is immense. In many ways the concept of word avoidance refers to a motive rather than a behavior: it can only be inferred from absence of stuttering. Nevertheless the clinical descriptions of word avoidance are such that it should be obvious when the subject is doing something unusual in order to reduce stuttering. This is a fascinating aspect of stuttering which is long overdue for careful investigation. It is undoubtedly necessary to develop some method for controlling its effects on therapy.

Conclusion

This has been a brief overview of the environmental and speech change variables that may substantially or completely reduce stuttering. Some of these variables may also be closely related (Wingate, 1976), a possibility that has led to the suggestion there may be more similarities than differences between stutterers. Wingate (1969; 1970), for instance, has argued that the apparent universality of the altered-speaking effect is one of few common features in a disorder remarkable for its complexity and variability.

In view of the many variables that may reduce or eliminate stuttering, it is incumbent on clinicians to find methods of therapy evaluation that ensure these conditions are *not* responsible for any resulting benefits. A number of workers are currently investigating the parameters of fluency (for example, Adams, 1982). Perhaps this research will eventually yield methods for deciding whether or not a subject is displaying artificial or true fluency. In the meantime, the most useful approach to this problem is through carefully collected assessments of the subject's speech. Williams (1978) has suggested that the following situations should be included in any clinical assessment: different numbers of listeners, different types of listeners, different types of speaking situations, conditionally changed situations, and specific subject-identified problem situations. But, in order to control for factors that might "demand" subjects alter their usual way of speaking, then, perhaps, covert or unprepared assessments (either with stooges or helpful associates) might help determine whether the subject's assessed speech is typical speech behavior. The methods suitable for assessing "typical speech" are contentious mainly because they involve ethical problems. As yet, an acceptable solution to these problems has not been found, although some attempted solutions will be discussed in connection with some recent treatment procedures.

References

Adams, L.H. A comparison of certain sound wave characteristics of stutterers and nonstutterers. In W. Johnson & R.R. Leutenegger (Eds.), *Stuttering in children and adults.* Minneapolis: University of Minnesota Press, 1955.

Adams, M.R. Fluency, nonfluency, and stuttering in children. *Journal of Fluency Disorders,* 1982, *7,* 171-185.

Adams, M.R., Lewis, J.I., & Besozzi, T.E. The effect of reduced reading rate on stuttering frequency. *Journal of Speech and Hearing Research,* 1973, *16,* 671-675.

Ammons, R., & Johnson, W. Studies in the psychology of stuttering: XVIII. The construction and application of a test of attitude toward stuttering. *Journal of Speech Disorders,* 1944, *9,* 39-49.

Andrews, G., & Cutler, J. Stuttering therapy: The relation between changes in symptom level and attitudes. *Journal of Speech and Hearing Disorders* 1974, *39,* 312-319.

Andrews, G., & Harris, M. *The syndrome of stuttering.* Clinics in Developmental Medicine No. 17. London: Heinemann, 1964.

Andrews, G., & Ingham, R.J. An approach to the evaluation of stuttering therapy. *Journal of Speech and Hearing Research*, 1972, *15*, 296-302.

Barber, V. Studies in the psychology of stuttering, XV. Chorus reading as a distraction in stuttering. *Journal of Speech Disorders*, 1939, *4*, 371-383.

Barr, D.F. & Carmel, N.R. Stuttering inhibition with high frequency narrow band masking noise. *The Journal of Auditory Research*, 1969, *9*, 40-44.

Beech, H.R., & Fransella, F. *Research and experiment in stuttering.* Oxford: Pergamon, 1968.

Bernard, J.R.L. Rates of utterance in Australian dialectic groups. Occasional Paper No. 7, The University of Sydney, Australian Language Research Centre, August, 1965.

Berwick, N.H. Stuttering in response to photographs of selected listeners. In W. Johnson & R.R. Leutenegger (Eds.), *Stuttering in children and adults.* Minneapolis: University of Minnesota Press, 1955.

Bloodstein, O. Studies in the psychology of stuttering: XIX. The relationship between oral reading rate and severity of stuttering. *Journal of Speech Disorders*, 1944, *9*, 161-173.

Bloodstein, O. Conditions under which stuttering is reduced or absent: A review of literature. *Journal of Speech and Hearing Disorders*, 1949, *14*, 295-302.

Bloodstein, O. *A handbook on stuttering* (2nd ed.). Chicago: National Easter Seal Society, 1975.

Bloodstein, O. *A handbook on stuttering* (3rd ed.). Chicago: National Easter Seal Society, 1981.

Bloom, C., & Silverman, F. Stability of performances of individual stutterers on oral reading adaptation tasks. *Journal of Fluency Disorders*, 1979, *4*, 39-44.

Boberg, E. Intensive adult therapy program. *Seminars in Speech, Language and Hearing*, 1980, *1*, 365-373.

Boberg, E. *Maintenance of fluency.* New York: Elsevier, 1981.

Boehmler, R.M. Listener responses to non-fluencies. *Journal of Speech and Hearing Research*, 1958, *1*, 132-141.

Brady, J.P. Studies on the metronome effect on stuttering. *Behaviour Research and Therapy*, 1969, *7*, 197-205.

Brutten, G.J., & Shoemaker, D.J. A two-factor learning theory of stuttering. In L. Travis (Ed.), *Handbook of speech pathology and audiology.* New York: Appleton-Century-Crofts, 1971.

Campbell, D.T., & Stanley, J.C. *Experimental and quasi-experimental designs for research.* Chicago: Rand McNally, 1963.

Cherry, C., & Sayers, B. McA. Experiments upon the total inhibition of stammering by external control, and some clinical results. *Journal of Psychosomatic Research*, 1956, *1*, 233-246.

Colcord, R.D., & Adams, M.R. Voicing duration and vocal SPL changes associated with stuttering reduction during singing. *Journal of Speech and Hearing Research*, 1979, *22*, 468-479.

Coyle, M.M., & Mallard, A.R. Word-by-word analysis of observer agreement utilizing audio and audiovisual techniques. *Journal of Fluency Disorders*, 1979, *4*, 23-28.

Cullinan, W.L., Prather, E.M., & Williams, D.E. Comparisons of procedures for scaling severity of stuttering. *Journal of Speech and Hearing Research*, 1963, *6*, 187-194.

Curlee, R.F. Observer agreement on disfluency and stuttering. *Journal of Speech and Hearing Research*, 1981, *24*, 595-600.

Darley, F.L. A normative study of oral reading rate. Unpublished masters thesis, University of Iowa, 1940.

Egland, G.O. Repetitions and prolongations in the speech of stuttering and non-stuttering children. In W. Johnson & R.R. Leutenegger (Eds.), *Stuttering in children and adults.* Minneapolis: University of Minnesota Press, 1955.

Erickson, R.L. Assessing communication attitudes among stutterers. *Journal of Speech and Hearing Research,* 1969, *12,* 711-724.

Fairbanks, G. *Voice and articulation drillbook.* New York: Harper & Row, 1960.

Goldiamond, I. Stuttering and fluency as manipulatable operant response classes. In L. Krasner & L.P. Ullmann (Eds.), *Research in behavior modification.* New York: Holt, Rinehart, & Winston, 1965.

Greenberg, J.B. The effect of a metronome on the speech of young stutterers. *Behavior Therapy,* 1970, *1,* 240-244.

Guitar, B. Pretreatment factors associated with the outcome of stuttering therapy. *Journal of Speech and Hearing Research,* 1976, *19,* 590-600.

Guitar, B. A response to Ingham's critique. *Journal of Speech and Hearing Disorders,* 1979, *44,* 400-403.

Guitar, B. A correction to "A response to Ingham's critique." *Journal of Speech and Hearing Disorders,* 1981, *46,* 440.

Guitar, B., & Bass, C. Stuttering therapy: The relationship between attitude change and long-term outcome. *Journal of Speech and Hearing Disorders,* 1978, *43,* 392-400.

Healey, E.C., Mallard, A.R., & Adams, M.R. Factors contributing to the reduction of stuttering during singing. *Journal of Speech and Hearing Research,* 1976, *19,* 475-480.

Hegde, M.N. Fluency and fluency disorders: Their definition, measurement and modification. *Journal of Fluency Disorders,* 1978, *3,* 51-71.

Hegde, M.N., & Hartman, D.E. Factors affecting judgments of fluency: I. Interjections. *Journal of Fluency Disorders,* 1979, *4,* 1-11. (a)

Hegde, M.N., & Hartman, D.E. Factors affecting judgments of fluency: II. Word repetitions. *Journal of Fluency Disorders,* 1979, *4,* 13-22. (b)

Hersen, M., & Barlow, D.H. *Single-case experimental designs.* New York: Pergamon, 1976.

Hood, S.B. Clinical assessment of the moment of stuttering. *Journal of Fluency Disorders,* 1974, *1,* 22-34.

Hood, S.B. The assessment of fluency disorders. In S. Singh & J. Lynch (Eds.), *Diagnostic procedures in hearing, speech, and language.* Baltimore: University Park Press, 1978.

Hulit, L.M. Inter-judge agreement for identifying stuttered words. *Perceptual and Motor Skills,* 1978, *47,* 360-362.

Ingham, R.J. A comparison of covert and overt assessment procedures in stuttering therapy outcome evaluation. *Journal of Speech and Hearing Research,* 1975, *18,* 346-354.

Ingham, R.J. Comment on 'Stuttering therapy: The relation between attitude change and long-term outcome.' *Journal of Speech and Hearing Disorders,* 1979, *44,* 397-400.

Ingham, R.J. Modification of maintenance and generalizaton in stuttering treatment. *Journal of Speech and Hearing Research,* 1980, *23,* 732-745.

Ingham, R.J. Evaluation and maintenance in stuttering treatment: A search for ecstasy with nothing but agony. In E. Boberg (Ed.), *Maintenance of fluency.* New York: Elsevier, 1981.

Ingham, R.J., & Andrews, G. Details of a token economy stuttering therapy programme for adults. *Australian Journal of Human Communication Disorders,* 1973, *1,* 13-20.

Ingham, R.J. & Lewis, J.I. Behavior therapy and stuttering: And the story grows. *Human Communication,* 1978, *3,* 125-152.

Ingham, R.J., Martin, R.R., & Kuhl, P. Modification and control of rate of speaking by stutterers. *Journal of Speech and Hearing Research,* 1974, *17,* 489-496.

Ingham, R.J., & Packman, A. Treatment and generalization effects in an experimental treatment for a stutterer using contingency management and speech rate control. *Journal of Speech and Hearing Disorders*, 1977, *42*, 394-407.

Ingham, R.J., & Packman,A. Perceptual assessment of normalcy of speech following stuttering therapy. *Journal of Speech and Hearing Research*, 1978, *21*, 63-73.

Johnson, W. An interpretation of stuttering. *Quarterly Journal of Speech*, 1933, *19*, 70-77.

Johnson, W. The time, the place, and the problem. In W. Johnson & R.R. Leutenegger (Eds.), *Stuttering in children and adults*. Minneapolis: University of Minnesota Press, 1955.

Johnson, W. *The onset of stuttering*. Minneapolis: University of Minnesota Press, 1959.

Johnson, W. Measurements of oral reading and speaking rate and disfluency of adult male and female stutterers and non-stutterers. *Journal of Speech and Hearing Disorders*, Monograph Supplement No. 7, 1961, 1-20.

Johnson, W., Darley, F.L., & Spriestersbach, D.C. *Diagnostic methods in speech pathology*. New York: Harper & Row, 1963.

Johnson, W., & Rosen, L. Studies in the psychology of stuttering: VII. Effect of certain changes in speech pattern upon frequency of stuttering. *Journal of Speech Disorders*, 1937, *2*, 105-109.

Johnson, W., & Sinn, A. Studies in the psychology of stuttering: V. Frequency of stuttering with expectation of stuttering controlled. *Journal of Speech Disorders*, 1937, *2*, 98-100.

Jones, R.J., & Azrin, N.H. Behavioral engineering: Stuttering as a function of stimulus duration during speech synchronization. *Journal of Applied Behavior Analysis*, 1969, *2*, 223-229.

Langova, J., & Svab, L. Reduction of stuttering under experimental social isolation: The role of adaptation effect. *Folia Phoniatrica*, 1973, *25*, 17-22.

Lanyon, R.I. The measurement of stuttering severity. *Journal of Speech and Hearing Research*, 1967, *10*, 836-843.

Lewis, D., & Sherman, D. Measuring the severity of stuttering. *Journal of Speech and Hearing Disorders*, 1951, *16*, 320-326.

Luper, H.L. Consistency of stuttering in relation to the goal gradient hypothesis. *Journal of Speech and Hearing Disorders*, 1956, *21*, 336-342.

MacDonald, J.D., & Martin, R.R. Stuttering and disfluency as two reliable and unambiguous response classes. *Journal of Speech and Hearing Research*, 1973, *16*, 691-699.

Maraist, J.A., & Hutton, C. Effect of auditory masking upon the speech of stutterers. *Journal of Speech and Hearing Disorders*, 1957, *22*, 385-389.

Martin, R.R. Direct magnitude-estimation judgments of stuttering severity using audible and audible-visible speech samples. *Speech Monographs*, 1965, *32*, 169-177.

Martin, R.R. Appercus. In E. Boberg (Ed.), *Maintenance of fluency*. New York: Elsevier, 1981.

Martin, R., & Haroldson, S.K. Effects of five experimental treatments on stuttering. *Journal of Speech and Hearing Research*, 1979, *22*, 132-146.

Martin, R.R., & Haroldson, S.K. Stuttering identification: Standard definition and moment of stuttering. *Journal of Speech and Hearing Research*, 1981, *46*, 59-63.

Martin, R.R., & Siegel, G.M. The effects of response contingent shock on stuttering. *Journal of Speech and Hearing Research*, 1966, *9*, 340-352..

Minifie, F.D., & Cooker, H.S. A disfluency index. *Journal of Speech and Hearing Disorders*, 1964, *29*, 189-192.

Murphy, A.T., & Fitzsimons, R.M. *Stuttering and personality dynamics*. New York: Ronald Press, 1960.

Naylor, R.V. A comparative study of methods of estimating the severity of stuttering.

Journal of Speech and Hearing Disorders, 1953, *18,* 30-37.

Perkins, W.H. Replacement of stuttering with normal speech: I. Rationale. *Journal of Speech and Hearing Disorders,* 1973, *38,* 283-294.

Perkins, W.H. Articulatory rate in the evaluation of stuttering treatments. *Journal of Speech and Hearing Disorders,* 1975, *40,* 277-278.

Perkins, W.H., Bell, J., Johnson, L., & Stocks, J. Phone rate and the effective planning time hypothesis of stuttering. *Journal of Speech and Hearing Research,* 1979, *22,* 747-755.

Porter, H.V.K. Studies in the psychology of stuttering: XIV. Stuttering phenomena in relation to size and personnel of audience. *Journal of Speech Disorders,* 1939, *4,* 323-333.

Prins, D., & Lohr, F. Behavioral dimensions of stuttered speech. *Journal of Speech and Hearing Research,* 1972, *15,* 61-71.

Prosek, R.A., Walden, B.E., Montgomery, A.A., & Schwartz, D.M. Some correlates of stuttering severity judgments. *Journal of Fluency Disorders,* 1979, *4,* 215-222.

Quinn, P.T. Stuttering: Some observations on speaking when alone. *Journal of the Australian College of Speech Therapists,* 1971, *21,* 92-94.

Rickard, H.C., & Mundy, M.B. Direct manipulation of stuttering behavior: An experimental clinical approach. In L.P. Ullmann & L. Krasner (Eds.), *Case studies in behavior modification.* New York: Holt, Rinehart & Winston, 1965.

Riley, G.D. A stuttering severity instrument for children and adults. *Journal of Speech and Hearing Disorders,* 1972, *37,* 314-322.

Runyan, C.M., & Adams, M.R. Perceptual study of the speech of "successfully therapeutized" stutterers. *Journal of Fluency Disorders,* 1978, *3,* 25-39.

Ryan, B.P. Operant procedures applied to stuttering therapy for children. *Journal of Speech and Hearing Disorders,* 1971, *36,* 264-280.

Ryan, B.P. *Programmed therapy for stuttering in children and adults.* Springfield, IL: Charles C. Thomas, 1974.

Ryan, B.P. Maintenance programs in progress - II. In E. Boberg (Ed.), *Maintenance of fluency.* New York: Elsevier, 1981.

Sakata, R., & Adams, M.R. Comparisons among various forms of individual stutterers' disfluency. *Journal of Communication Disorders,* 1972, *5,* 232-239.

Sander, E.K. Reliability of the Iowa Speech Disfluency Test. *Journal of Speech and Hearing Disorders,* Monograph Supplement No. 7, 1961, 21-30.

Sander, E.K. Frequency of syllable repetitions and "stutterer" judgments. *Journal of Speech and Hearing Disorders,* 1963, *28,*, 19-30.

Sheehan, J.G. *Stuttering: Research and therapy.* New York: Harper & Row, 1970.

Sheehan, J.G., Hadley, R.G., & Gould, E. Impact of authority on stuttering. *Journal of Abnormal Psychology,* 1967, *72,* 290-293.

Shulman, E. Factors in influencing the variability of stuttering. In W. Johnson & R.R. Leutenegger (Eds.), *Stuttering in children and adults.* Minneapolis: University of Minnesota Press, 1955.

Shumak, I.C. A speech rating sheet for stutterers. In W. Johnson & R.R. Leutenegger (Eds.), *Stuttering in children and adults.* Minneapolis: University of Minnesota Press, 1955.

Siegel, G.M., & Haugen, D. Audience size and variations in stuttering behavior. *Journal of Speech and Hearing Research,* 1964, *7,* 381-388.

Silverman, F.H. Dimensions of improvement in stuttering. *Journal of Speech and Hearing Research,* 1980, *23,* 137-151.

Silverman, F.H., & Williams, D.E. Prediction of stuttering by school-age stutterers. *Journal of Speech and Hearing Research,* 1972, *15,* 189-193.

Sutton, S., & Chase, R.A. White noise and stuttering. *Journal of Speech and Hearing Research*, 1961, *4*, 72.

Toomey, G.L., & Sidman, M. An experimental analogue of the anxiety-stuttering relationship. *Journal of Speech and Hearing Research*, 1970, *13*, 122-129.

Tuthill, C.E. A quantitative study of extensional meaning with special reference to stuttering. *Speech Monographs*, 1946, *13*, 81-92.

Umeda, N., & Quinn, A.M.S. Some notes on reading: Talkers, material and reading rate. *Journal of Speech and Hearing Research* 1980, *23*, 56-72.

Van Riper, C. *The nature of stuttering*. Englewood Cliffs, NJ: Prentice-Hall, 1971.

Villarreal, J. The semantic aspects of stuttering in nonstutterers: Additional data. *Quarterly Journal of Speech*, 1945, *31*, 477-479.

Voelker, C. On the semantic aspects of stuttering in nonstutterers. *Quarterly Journal of Speech*, 1942, *28*, 78-80.

Voelker, C.H. A preliminary investigation for normative study of fluency: A clinical index to the severity of stuttering. *American Journal of Orthopsychiatry*, 1944, *14*, 285-294.

Webster, L.M. A cinematic analysis of the effects of contingent stimulation on stuttering and associated behaviors. PhD dissertation, Southern Illinois University, 1968.

Webster, R.L.,& Dorman, M.F. Decreases in stuttering frequency as a function of continuous and contingent forms of auditory masking. *Journal of Speech and Hearing Research*, 1970, *13*, 82-86.

Wendahl, R.W., & Cole, J. Identification of stuttering during relatively fluent speech. *Journal of Speech and Hearing Research*, 1961, *4*, 281-286.

Williams, D.E. The problem of stuttering. In F.L. Darley & D.C. Spriestersbach (Eds.), *Diagnostic methods in speech pathology*. New York: Harper & Row, 1978.

Williams, D.E., Darley, F.L., & Spriestersbach, D.C. Appraisal of rate and fluency. In F.L. Darley & D.C. Spriestersbach (Eds.), *Diagnostic methods in speech pathology*. New York: Harper & Row, 1978.

Williams, D.E. & Kent, L.R. Listener evaluations of speech interruptions. *Journal of Speech and Hearing Research*, 1958, *1*, 124-131.

Williams, D.E., Wark, M., & Minifie, F.D. Ratings of stutterings by audio, visual and audiovisual cues. *Journal of Speech and Hearing Research*, 1963, *6*, 91-100.

Wingate, M.E. A standard definition of stuttering. *Journal of Speech and Hearing Disorders*, 1964, *29*, 484-489.

Wingate, M.E. Sound and pattern in "artificial" fluency. *Journal of Speech and Hearing Research*, 1969, *12*, 677-686.

Wingate, M.E. Effect on stuttering of changes in audition. *Journal of Speech and Hearing Research*, 1970, *13*, 861-873.

Wingate, M.E. *Stuttering: Theory and treatment*. New York: Irvington, 1976.

Woolf, G. The assessment of stuttering as struggle, avoidance, and expectancy. *British Journal of Disorders of Communication*, 1967, *2*, 151-171.

Young, M.A. Predicting ratings of severity of stuttering. *Journal of Speech and Hearing Disorders*, Monograph Supplement No. 7, 1961, 31-54.

Young, M.A. Identification of stutterers from recorded samples of their "fluent speech." *Journal of Speech and Hearing Research*, 1964, *7*, 302-303.

Young, M.A. Audience size, perceived situational difficulty and stuttering frequency. *Journal of Speech and Hearing Research*, 1965, *8*, 401-407.

Young, M.A. Observer agreement for marking moments of stuttering. *Journal of Speech and Hearing Research*, 1975, *18*, 530-540.

Young, M.A., & Prather, E.M. Measuring severity of stuttering using short segments of speech. *Journal of Speech and Hearing Research*, 1962, *5*, 256-262.

3

The Nonbehavioral Preparadigm's Contribution to Stuttering Treatment

Introduction

The state of stuttering therapy under the nonbehavioral preparadigm has been mentioned generally in the first chapter. It is evident from a number of reviews of therapy throughout the period from 1930 to 1960 that treatment efficacy was a continuing source of concern to the profession. It was also a period in which therapy was largely dictated by some influential theoretical models of human behavior and this theory-influence promoted an overriding concern to avoid "artificial treatments," that is, well-known methods that provide only brief benefits. They were regarded as methods which fostered the avoidance of stuttering and did not deal with the essence of the problem.

Stuttering therapy during the 1930-60 period, particularly in the United States, was dominated by the Iowa School, a dominance that reverberated throughout the speech pathology profession in English-speaking countries. This therapy was largely characterized by procedures designed to reduce anxiety about stuttering, improve nonavoidance behavior, analyze symptomatic implications, and reduce stuttering by gradually simplifying its abnormal aspects. Its therapists, as Bloodstein (1981) has noted, were not especially concerned to seek the achievement of normal speech:

> The total elimination of stuttering was generally viewed as a long-term goal. Some of the foremost Iowa therapists even believed that it was unrealistic for adult stutterers to aim for perfectly normal speech. In a certain percentage of cases, for various reasons, even a moderate reduction in stuttering failed to occur. Certain gifted clinicians unquestionably did much better. But some with modest gifts and limited training did worse. With the old methods the problem had been that fluency often did not last. Now the problem was the slowness with which fluency appeared in the first place (p. x.).

The rest of this chapter will review the treatment procedures that are generally described as forming the "traditional approach" to stuttering treatment.

The "traditional approach" is a rather gratuitous description of these therapies to which Sheehan (1978), with some justification, has raised objections. His principal objection is that it implies that the procedures are ineffective. That implication is not intended here; nevertheless, it does beg the very question raised in Bloodstein's comment. What is the evidence that indicates the contribution these procedures have made to stuttering therapy? Or conversely, what is the evidence to suggest that the nonbehavioral preparadigm was unable to yield predictable solutions to the treatment puzzle?

There are many ways of recounting and examining the nonbehavioral treatment literature. None is likely to give an easily digested account which does justice to the diversity of these therapy practices. In fact, much stuttering literature only alludes to this diversity (this is also true of current therapy practices). From a very broad perspective, it now appears that most of these therapies have either "indirect" or "direct" orientations. The indirect approach is characterized by procedures that are not primarily directed at changing stuttering, but usually at theoretically related features in the subject's personality or behavior. It is usually postulated that if these features are altered, this will lead, sooner or later, either to reduced stuttering or to an improved ability to cope with this disability. The direct approach to treatment is, by implication, principally aimed at stuttering, but it may also be supplemented by "indirect" methods.

The Indirect Treatments

The most obvious example of an indirect approach in stuttering treatment is psychoanalysis. Freud's analysis of psychopathology led to a belief that much human behavior is under the control of unconscious motives which seek to resolve unconscious conflicts. Such conflicts were thought to be expressed in abnormal patterns of behavior, particularly in the recurring and seemingly self-destructive problem behaviors termed neuroses. It is interesting to recall that much of the evidence which Freud used to support his theory of human behavior was based upon unusual speech behavior. Certain verbal errors, or "Freudian slips," were judged to reflect relatively unconscious wishes. Psychoanalysis was the treatment that was devised to resolve these unconscious conflicts. The purpose in this treatment was to lead the subject ultimately to "give up" these destructive behaviors; behaviors which were regarded as the subject's defense against even more destructive feelings and behaviors. In other words if the symptom (or problem behavior) was removed before the underlying conflict had been dealt with successfully, then the symptom would either recur or be substituted by yet another problem.

The Freudian concept of problem behavior is an excellent example of a Kuhnian preparadigm. Undoubtedly, it led to a virtual revolution in psychology. The effect of this revolution was far-reaching—and remains so. It changed the focus of treatment for almost all nonorganic disorders, and firmly established an approach to therapy based on the analysis of feelings and thoughts associated with past and present events. In essence, the object of treatment moved from the symptom and centered on a theorized diseased psychological state within the patient. With respect to stuttering, it led to the contention that this disorder was the result of a neurotic personality which required far more than speech therapy.

Stuttering has been described in a variety of ways by psychoanalytic theorists (Barbara, 1962; Fenichel, 1945; Glauber, 1958). It has also been the object of a variety of psychoanalytically oriented therapies. Freud (see Glauber, 1958) actually reported on treatment of at least one stutterer (female) by a combination of psychoanalysis and hypnosis, although it appears that the subject's speech problem was not her reason for seeking treatment.

Other psychoanalysts have reported carefully delineated accounts of their therapy, but with little evidence of its effect on stuttering behavior. Coriot (1927; 1943) wrote at length on psychoanalytic treatment of stutterers and also included some innovative indirect but "active therapy." This included the requirement that the subject should cease indulging in orally gratifying activities, such as smoking and gum chewing. Unhappily, no information was reported on the consequences of this treatment. This is also true for the psychoanalytic treatment approaches outlined by Travis (1940), Glauber (1958) and Barbara (1962). Harle (1946), however, described a psychodynamic approach in the treatment of a three-year-old female stutterer who, it is claimed, stuttered only occasionally when assessed eight months after treatment.

The relatively small amount of data available on the long-term effects of psychoanalysis on stuttering have not been encouraging. Brill (1923) reported treating 69 stutterers (15-51 years) for periods of a few months to over a year. He used an extraordinarily long follow-up period (11 years) and reported that only five of these subjects remained improved at the end of that time. Somewhat better results were implied in a report by the Berlin Psychoanalytic Institute. Knight (1941; see Bergin 1971) provided a summarized account of the results of treatment for 13 stutterers within the Institute from 1920 to 1930. Four subjects were reported to have been "cured" or "much improved." But the main difficulty with these data is that there is no indication about the criteria used for determining a successful outcome. In fact, it is entirely possible that the "bench mark" may not have been reduced stuttering, but some form of agreement that the source of the stutterer's neurosis had been removed.

A number of indirect therapies, based either totally or closely on psychodynamic principles, were also used in the treatment of stuttering. These include group psychotherapy (Brody & Harrison, 1954), psychodrama (Honig, 1947), and Adlerian therapy (Nystul & Muszynska, 1976). But in each report of these therapies, there is virtually no evidence that treatment was responsible for improved fluency.

The principles of psychoanalytic treatment were largely based upon the person becoming aware of, and resolving, unconscious motives which controlled much of his problem behavior. This principle has been central to some other "indirect treatments." Among those which have been used in stuttering treatment are Gestalt therapy (Kaplan & Kaplan, 1978) and confrontation therapy (Gendelman,

1977). Gendleman's report, for example, describes a therapy strategy designed to assist the persons's awareness of the distinction between rational and irrational (conditioned) fears. The stutterer must then confront the situations associated with those fears. In this respect, it shares with psychoanalysis a concern to have the subject recognise and cope with fears and destructive feelings alleged to control the problem behavior. Gendelman reported that 90 stutterers were treated with this therapy system, and 29 were followed up 2 to 36 months later; 22 were then claimed to be either normally fluent or had improved—but no speech behavior data were collected in support of this claim.

During the late 1940s, another mild revvolution occurred in the area of psychotherapy. This was occasioned by the widespread acceptance of Carl Roger's (1942; 1951) nondirective counseling technique and its later development into client-centered therapy. This procedure regarded the relationship between therapist and patient as "person-oriented" rather than "patient-oriented." A relationship was formed which permitted the person the opportunity to achieve "psychological growth" and, as a result, the ability to find solutions to problem behaviors. This form of counseling has probably influenced the therapy process almost as much, or more, than has conventional psychoanalysis. The specific use of this therapy for stuttering treatment, however, has been limited—at least as judged by the published reports. Rogers (1942) and Hejna (1963) reported a nondirective type of counseling treatment with some stutterers, but failed to provide clear evidence of its effect on speech behavior. The only available reports in the speech-disorders literature describe approaches that have combined nondirective counseling with other procedures. Clark (1948) outlined a procedure in which subjects received individual and group counseling, and this was supplemented by their written autobiography; but not even a case report was used to justify the procedure. Schultz (1947) described combined group and individual nondirective counseling with 20 adult stutterers, but also provided no information on the effect that this procedure had on either their speech behavior or other behaviors. Both of these clinicians described their procedures as forming part of the "mental hygiene" approach to the treatment of stuttering.

The "mental hygiene" approach to stuttering treatment appeared in the early 1930s with the work of Travis (1931) and the Blantons (1936). It appears to have been a description for all counseling or therapy procedures which were designed to assist the subject to adjust to the social or personal difficulties associated with stuttering. It also became an integral feature of Bryngelson's (1931; 1938) therapy which combined mental hygiene counseling with symptomatic therapy procedures. Some descriptions of the use of mental hygiene therapy were provided by Brown (1933) and Cypreansen (1948). Brown reported some success in the treatment of three adolescent stutterers, although no data were collected to support this claim. Cypreansen (1948) described group-counseling treatment for 14 stutterers (18-22 years), which involved 15, 1½-hour sessions. The only data in the effects of this treatment did not refer to speech behavior; they were scores on the California Personality Inventory for three of the 14 subjects. These scores indicated that the three subjects had achieved improved "adjustment."

This overview of indirect approaches within stuttering treatment suggests that there is little evidence supporting the effectiveness of these procedures in reducing stuttering. There is certainly plenty of information, mainly in the form of case descriptions, to indicate that some benefits must have been reflected in the stutterers' speech. But these are far from satisfactory indicators of the contribution of treatment. One relatively general indication of the efficacy of psychotherapy is provided by Webster's (1977) brief account of the outcome of group or individual psychotherapy with 648 stutterers. These subjects were treated at the New York Speech and Hearing Institute between 1969 and 1972. Their treatment did not include speech therapy, and it can only be assumed that it involved the more conventional approaches to psychotherapy. The reported findings are quite telling: 92% of the patients "showed either no improvement or only slight improvement in their fluency characteristics after psychotherapy as independently judged by certified speech pathologists" (Webster, 1977, p.254). Even allowing that the method of assessment is not described in a satisfactory manner, it does suggest that this form of treatment is relatively ineffectual—at least as far as stuttering is concerned.

The Direct Treatments

The direct approach to the treatment of stuttering has involved a wide variety of methods. Historical accounts of stuttering treatment (Clark, 1964; Rieber & Wollock, 1977; Van Riper, 1973) provide many graphic descriptions of the techniques that have been used to alter or treat stuttering. These accounts also provide some interesting examples of early applications of many procedures that have been used widely at different times throughout this century, and particularly within the context of behavior therapy.

The "Remedialists"

Some striking examples of the early use of many recently employed treatment procedures may be found in the reports of many stuttering treatment methods used in America during the 1930s and 1940s. For example, Bender and Kleinfeld (1938) described a treatment which was built around speech rate control. The stutterer was instructed to read orally certain sounds, followed by syllables, words, and finally sentences at a rate that allowed the subject to "speak smoothly." Also, Stoddard (1939) described a range of therapy activities based upon relaxation, voice training ("particularly the attack upon the consonants"), mental hygiene, oral reading, and spontaneous speech. Gifford (1940) recommended a somewhat similar range of "remedial procedures" which have been graphically outlined in Hahn's (1941) report on a remedial treatment program.

Hahn's treatment study involved 22 adult stutterers who were treated for 3 months on "two evenings a week." The program included "bodily relaxation, physical control, emotional control, disruption of old habits of speaking and substitution of a new speech pattern, positive suggestion, and change of attitudes" (1941, pp.30-31). In view of some of the more recent treatment procedures within the behavioral framework, it is most interesting to relate Hahn's description of the "new speech pattern" to prolonged speech (see Chapter 10). The treatment proceeded through a series of structured speech situations, so that subjects could learn to use this new pattern under all conditions. Furthermore, the subject was required to evaluate speech performance at different times during the day and provide a score for self-rated performance. The results of this treatment are presented in terms of numbers of stutterings on a 550-word passage which was orally read before and after treatment across a variety of reading conditions (reading alone, with an unseen listener, before the listener, and before a group). The data show that there was a mean reduction in stuttering of about 90% across all situations; four subjects did not appear to change, and three were recorded as stutter-free after treatment.

Hahn's (1941) study is one of the most data-filled treatment reports to emerge during this period. It is quite interesting that the seemingly promising findings of this study did not ensure the survival of this form of therapy—at least according to the literature on stuttering treatment. It is also quite amazing that the recent treatment literature has virtually ignored a report which appears to contain almost all the elements of some currently advocated behavioral procedures.

The remedialist trend apparently influenced some therapy practices that continued during the 1940s and 1950s, but the extent of this influence diminished with the arrival of the Iowa School's approach to stuttering. With the emerging influence of behavior therapy in stuttering therapy, however, it will be seen that many of its practices are reappearing in different guises.

Dunlap's Negative Practice

As mentioned above, the antecedents of many behavior therapy approaches to stuttering appeared well before the 1950s and 1960s. Actually, most of the earlier techniques for modifying stuttering are still used in various ways in many current behavioral treatments. One of the interesting exceptions is negative practice. Paradoxically, it was one of the first techniques for modifying problem behaviors that was derived from traditional learning theory concepts. Yet, strangely enough, it almost disappeared from use just as this conceptual approach to therapy was developing the early features of behavior therapy.

Knight Dunlap appears to have been first to recognize the untenability of earlier theories which had postulated that a response repeated under similar stimulus conditions increases the probability of recurrence of that response. Dunlap (1928) introduced two alternative hypotheses which were intrinsic to the theory of negative practice. The first hypothesized that past appearances of the response may have no effect on the probability of the same stimulus producing the same response ("beta hypothesis"). The second contended that the past appearance of the response may decrease the frequency of future responses ("gamma hypothesis").

Stuttering was one of the first disorders that Dunlap (1928) used to test the negative practice hypotheses. To do so, he stressed that the subject must learn to practice repeating the exact features of involuntary responses, such as stuttering. Even in later descriptions of negative practice, Dunlap (1942) stressed this, "The essential point is to bring under voluntary control the behavior pattern which has been involuntary. It is a very difficult task to teach a stammerer voluntarily to reproduce his involuntary pattern, but unless this is done, the method of negative practice is not applied" (p.270). But the most significant feature of the method was the procedure followed in therapy:

> At first, nothing should be done in the daily practice except the practice of stammering. After three or four weeks, a part of the time may be occupied in trying to speak correctly. The *modus operandi* of this is to have the patient practice stammering a phrase until he stammers it well, and then immediately speak it correctly. If he succeeds on first trial, he may repeat it once or twice. If he fails, he should be stopped at the first appearance of stammering, and stammering practice should be immediately renewed. Avoid, above all, during the practice period, having the patient trying to speak incorrectly and failing (Dunlap, 1932, pp.205-206).

If the subject succeeded with oral reading practice, he was then instructed to follow the same procedure with conversation.

A confusing feature of Dunlap's procedure is that it is not clear whether the subject was required to "stutter" on all words, or only those that typified his stuttering. This was not clarified in later writings (for example, Dunlap, 1942), and contributed to the many differences between the negative practice procedures used in later studies. Although, it is clear that the subject was required to stutter voluntarily on more than the expected stuttered word after attempting to speak correctly. Yet another difficulty was Dunlap's failure to specify the amount of phrase repetition or stuttering practice that should follow a failed fluent production; actually, he did consider this a research issue.

Dunlap (1928; 1930) incidentally noted that negative practice had improved some stutterers, but Fishman (1937) provided the first results of negative practice use with stutterers. He employed a method which closely resembled Dunlap's procedure with five adolescent and adult stutterers. The speech of three of these subjects was described as characterized by repetitions and the other two experienced "severe speech blockage." Subjects were assessed before treatment on the number of words orally read or spoken in a 10-minute period. The words stuttered were recorded and inserted into 10 sentences. The subject was then required to "stutter" the inserted words. This procedure was continued with new sentences being added from time to time. Treatment was conducted for varying periods and produced decreased percentages of stuttering on a second test passage for the three "repetition" stutterers, and increased percentages for the "speech blockers."

Case (1960) drew on Fishman's (1937) findings to design a therapy program for 30 stutterers (8-39 years), of whom five were described as "speech blockers." Thus, one aim of this study was to compare the effects of negative practice on the speech blockers and 25 nonspeech blockers. It was also proposed to assess the effect of "positive adjustment techniques" separately or in conjunction with negative practice. Case additionally reported accompanying Dunlap's (1932) procedure with a faradic punishment shock whenever there was a mistake in the voluntary stutter attempt.[1]

Treatment was not clearly described, but varied in duration and type from patient to patient. Most subjects received 1½ hours therapy per week for up to 13 months. The five "speech blockers" apparently deteriorated under negative practice, and so their treatment was changed to a form of directive counseling; they were instructed to participate in increasingly demanding social situations. In some cases, subjects were forbidden to speak in order to induce an attraction to talking. Some other subjects also received social adjustment counseling. The results were assessed on the basis of reports by the patient or patient's parents and friends. Case claimed that 10 of the patients were "cured" and 15 showed "improvement."

Fahmy (1950) reported using negative practice in treating eight young stutterers (8-14 years). This study included assessment on a reading test before treatment and every 2 weeks for 6 weeks of therapy. If subjects improved, they were retained for another 8 weeks of treatment, and were finally assessed after another 9 weeks. Fahmy used a slightly modified version of Dunlap's procedure:

> Each subject was made to repeat the error several times either during a period of reading aloud from a text, or whilst being encouraged to talk about a topic which interested him. By hearing the command "again," the subject was to repeat his "stammer" and then to the command "right" he may be able to say it correctly. If he made the same error, further practice on the words was given before going on. At least three repetitions of the error were required before the command "right" was given (p.25).

The results showed that four of the subjects worsened during the first six weeks of treatment. These were described as having a stutter characterized by blockages. The other four "repetition" stutterers reduced their percentages of stutterings after the first 6 weeks, and this was generally maintained at the final follow-up assessment.

The most interesting feature of Fahmy's study is that the procedure is actually much more than a slight modification of negative practice. Since the patient was halted after each stuttering and instructed to repeat the involuntary stammer until he could continue, he was thereby subjected to a response-contingent

[1]Case (1960) justified this by claiming:

> It is essential that the emotional content of the situation surrounding the condition of stuttering by the patient be reproduced as accurately as possible during the negative practice situation. This is just as important as accurate reproduction of the specific manner of stuttering by the individual patient. In fact the more accurate the emotional situation induced, the less difficult it is for the patient to accurately reproduce his stuttering (p.209).

Quite apart from the dubious assumption that shock will induce the emotional environment accompanying a stutter, this purpose also departs from the aims of negative practice as enunciated by Dunlap (1942):

> What is repeated in negative practice of a motor habit is not the total response involved in the habit, but a new response in which only the behavior pattern of the habitual response is repeated, with affective and ideational components quite different from those involved in the habit (p.270).

procedure. Thus it is more likely that this treatment was an example of response-contingent punishment rather than negative practice. It may also mean, of course, that the procedure reinforced rather than punished "speech blockage."

A part of the reason for differences in the "negative practice" methodology in stuttering may reside in a review of this technique by Lehner (1954). Stuttering was one of a number of disorders which Lehner concluded had benefited from the use of negative practice. But in reviewing factors he considered important in applying this technique, Lehner also appeared to favor Fahmy's (1950) procedure:

> In practice sessions with the therapist the patient must be cautioned and aided (verbally, with the aid of mirrors, by various demonstrations, etc.) to reproduce in the practiced response a response as nearly like the involuntary responses as possible. This may take the form of repeating responses which occur spontaneously in the sessions or of reproducing characteristic responses upon command of the therapist. The former method seems preferable whenever possible (Lehner, 1954, p.77).

Numerous variations of Dunlap's negative practice appeared in the 1940s and 1950s; particularly prominent were the voluntary stuttering techniques used by the Iowa School's clinicians. Meissner (1946), for example, investigated one form of voluntary stuttering, the "bounce." The subjects were instructed to use this technique in the following fashion: "What is wanted is an easy obvious repetition of the first sound of the word until the word is said without tension. The rate can be as fast or as slow as you can handle without getting tense and going into 'blocking.' Maintain as good control as you can" (p.15). Sheehan (1951) also used a variation of voluntary stuttering in a study that will be described in more detail in Chapter 9. His subjects were instructed to orally read while "repeating every stuttered word until you have said it once normally" (p.56).[2]

At least three different types of voluntary stuttering appear to have emerged during the 1940s. These were imitation of stuttering instances, the "bounce" (voluntary syllable repetition), and the "slide" (voluntary prolongations). Oxtoby (1955) had 24 stutterers orally read passages under either control conditions, when they were instructed to avoid stuttering, or using easy stuttering, or using "bounce" whenever stuttering was expected. The data are difficult to evaluate, but they were claimed to show significant reductions in stuttering during the "bounce" condition. Sheehan and Voas (1957) conducted a rather similar investigation on 24 stutterers who were divided into three equal groups. Essentially, one group had to "imitate" their stutterings in line with Dunlap's technique, another was required to use "bounce," and the third was instructed to use the "slide." On a final control reading (following four "treatment" readings), the results show that the "imitate" group produced significantly more stuttering than either of the other groups. But the performance of the last two groups was

[2] Yates (1970) has claimed that "massed practice does not appear to have been used with stutterers in any genuine sense" (p.123). This claim is challenged by Sheehan's study which seems to fulfill most of the requirements of massed practice rather than negative practice.

not significantly different from that achieved by repeated control readings. In short, Dunlap's procedure was not found to produce beneficial effects, at least in this experimental setting.

In retrospect, it now seems that the failure to adequately specify or identify the treatment characteristics of negative practice has contributed much to its demise. This is unfortunate because it may have had quite beneficial effects on persons who were not described as "speech blockers." Nevertheless, the history of this technique has much relevance to many later developments in stuttering therapy, where lack of specificity has contributed to many problematic aspects of the behavioral approach to therapy.

The Iowa School Influence

The remarkable influence of the Iowa School on stuttering treatment, which began during the 1940s, appears to have almost swept aside the use of all other therapy approaches. This school introduced and formalized almost all the treatment methods that formed the foundations of the nonbehavioral pre-paradigm. Indeed, a strong case can be made for the argument that the methods advocated by Bryngelson, Johnson, Van Riper, and Sheehan provided not only the techniques for much stuttering therapy during the past 3 or 4 decades, but, also, an orientation towards therapy evaluation. For during a period in which the therapy for many disorders was the focus of considerable research (see Bergin, 1971, for a review of psychotherapy evaluation), stuttering treatment was subjected to remarkably little evaluation. In retrospect, it appears that much of this therapy was directed towards assisting or coping with the disorder rather than its treatment. At the same time, many procedures were employed with the express purpose of modifying stuttering behavior, though their efficacy was assessed in very limited ways.

Bryngelson's (1943; 1950) approach to therapy owed much to both the Orton-Travis therapy of cerebral dominance and to mental hygiene. The most significant features of this therapy were "sidedness training" and voluntary stuttering. The principle behind sidedness training was to strengthen cerebral dominance in order to reduce the effects on stuttering caused (allegedly) by unresolved dominance of the cerebral speech centers.[3] Voluntary stuttering was used with a dual purpose; it was designed to bring the problem behavior under voluntary control and also reduce the stutterer's concern about displaying his problem. Carlson (1940), Read (1940), and Spates (1940) have provided some excellent descriptions of the use of Bryngelson's approach in the treatment of school-age

[3] Sidedness training often involved remarkably demanding controls over the subject's bodily functions. While this writer was working at the University of Minnesota in 1971, he had the benefit of many fruitful conversations with the late Dr. Bryngelson, who was then a retired professor at the University. He provided some graphic descriptions of sidedness training. For example, subjects were required to wear slings on one arm, usually an eye patch, and often hop for many hours on one unstrapped leg. A photograph of a stuttering-therapy group from this period was more reminiscent of a battlefield hospital than a speech therapy facility.

stutterers. Their reports claim some lessening in the problem, but this was not based upon anything resembling an appropriate evaluation.

Johnson (1948) also used voluntary stuttering, but in a somewhat different fashion. His therapy approach was built around procedures aimed at reducing anxieties about stuttering and the speaker's semantic misinterpretations of his problem. Various methods were used to improve the subject's awareness of his capacity to speak normally and also control feelings that might inhibit stuttering. For example, the subject was encouraged to stutter openly in order to remove any attempts to avoid nonfluency. He was also encouraged to use effortless repetitions such as the "bounce," or stress-free prolongation of sounds, to produce "easy stuttering." These techniques were also combined with nondirective counseling. In the case of children, much of the therapy was directed towards their parents, the purpose being to reduce the ways in which parents might promote the child's concern about the speech problem.

To the best of this writer's knowledge, Johnson never provided a systematic account of the effectiveness of these therapy procedures. That appears to have been left to some other clinicians. Jameson (1955) reported some findings from a parent-counseling program structured along the lines suggested by Johnson. She found that among 23 children (under 16 years), whose parents accepted the counseling advice, 70% were assessed as "normal or near normal" at their follow-up evaluation a year later. Some of the children did receive therapy but it is difficult to identify the contribution that this made to their outcome. Rotter (1942) reported on a treatment program (actually supervised by Travis and Johnson) which apparently included substantial amounts of Johnsonian therapy. Five adult stutterers (18-25 yrs.) were treated over a 3-month period in a program which is described with limited detail. It did involve counseling on attitudes towards speaking situations, oral reading in order to demonstrate that fluency was possible, and a 2-hour-per-week group therapy session. No data are provided, but at the end of the study it is claimed that:

> Two of the cases did not stutter at all and had not stuttered after a period of one and a half years. Both after the conclusion of the therapy and after a period of one and a half years cases 1 and 5 are described by themselves and by the head clinician as no longer regarding themselves as stutterers nor feeling the need for any work on their speech, although they occasionally still have slight interruptions (Rotter, 1942, p.287).

Williams (1955) also reported a treatment program conducted under the supervision of Johnson. This program involved four stutterers (17-29 years) who received 3 hours a week of "counseling and direct modification of the stuttering behavior pattern" for either 6 weeks (two subjects) or 8 weeks (two subjects). In addition, the subjects attended group meetings with other speakers. This amounted to informational lectures, speech practice, and group discussion about common problems. The individual treatments were not detailed, but they involved treatment for attitudes and evaluations regarding stuttering. The results were reported in terms of scores obtained from self-ratings for attitudes, speech situation reactions, and stuttering severity. In addition, subjects orally read a 250-

word passage (five consecutive times) every 2 weeks. Comparisons between the beginning and end of therapy show positive reductions on each of the self-rating scales and also in the number of stuttered words on each of the 250-word passages: one subject was reported stutter-free on this task at the end of treatment.

Subsequently, Williams (1957) went on to develop his own approach to a stuttering therapy. His procedure involved concentrating on and modifying the "things he [the stutterer] does which interfere with normal speech production." Each individual is trained to be more objective about stuttering and to modify feelings and behaviors which prevent normal fluency. It is difficult to identify precisely what procedures were used, either by the clinician or the stutterer, but they appear related to Johnson's approach. Kent (1961) applied this procedure in a treatment context and claimed that the subject's awareness of normal fluency was enhanced by the use of chorus reading, shouting, and talking in noise conditions. No data were provided, however, to illustrate the method's efficacy.

Rubin and Culatta (1971) presented some results from a treatment program which they based on Johnson, Williams, and Kent's approach to therapy. They reported on 15 stutterers (13-40 years) who were treated individually and in groups over periods ranging from about 2 weeks to 1½ years. Six subjects were followed up for periods of 4 to 19 months, and five were reported to have "normal fluency now." No information is provided on where or how these data were collected, however.

Van Riper's description of his treatment procedures and endeavors have literally filled volumes. Perhaps the most complete and easily disgested account of the more developed version of his treatment approach is outlined in a chapter appositely titled "Symptomatic Therapy for Stuttering" (Van Riper, 1971). This outlines the way in which his therapy procedures emerged from those developed by Bryngelson, Johnson and, to a lesser extent, Sheehan. Apart from a reliance upon various forms of psychotherapy, the principal feature of Van Riper's therapy has been the modification of stuttering by "cancellations" (pausing after a stuttering, and then repeating the stuttered pattern with "less struggle and avoidance"), "pull-outs" (preventing the block from continuing its course by various articulatory strategies), and "preparatory sets" (patterns of responses which permit the speaker to retain control over tremors that precede a moment of stuttering). The overall aim of this therapy has been to achieve "a type of fluent stuttering which could be used as a replacement for the abnormal symptoms presented by the stutterer" (1970, p.50).

The development of Van Riper's treatment procedures can be seen in a remarkable account of therapy programs which he conducted over a period of 20 years (Van Riper, 1958). Many of the procedures described by Bryngelson and Johnson found their way into this program, as did the techniques mentioned above. Approximately 10 stutterers, mainly adults, were treated in groups over a substantial portion of each year from 1936 to 1956. A 5-year follow-up period was used for most of the subjects and assessment was based upon the following criteria:

> First of all, the stutterer must be speaking better than this author in all situations . . . We might perhaps define this as 0.5 on the Iowa Scale of Severity. Secondly, the stutterer must not be avoiding words or speaking situations. Thirdly, his stuttering must not be interfering with his social or vocational adjustment. Fourthly, his situation and word fears must be pretty close to zero. Finally, his stuttering must present no concern to himself or others (Van Riper, 1958, p.390).

Based on these peculiar criteria, one can estimate that approximately 50% of all subjects were judged successful. It is difficult to draw any firm conclusions from this study, however. It is not at all clear, for example, just what factors within this package of therapies were associated with the success of any group of subjects, let alone individual subjects. There is also a notable lack of data on the methods used to assess stuttering either before, during, or after treatment. But it does provide an unusually rich account of the numerous types of approaches that have been tried to treat stutterers.

The literature on stuttering is brimming with accounts of allegedly successful uses of Van Riper's treatment procedures (for example, Speech Foundation of America, 1968; 1974). But they are rarely accompanied by even rudimentary treatment evaluations. One useful attempt in this direction is a report by Irwin (1972) on individual treatments using "easy stammering." The therapy used Van Riper's procedures over at least 10 therapy sessions. Eighty-seven adult stutterers received treatment, though data are only available for 26 subjects. These subjects completed a rating scale (identical to the Iowa Scale for Stuttering Severity) at the end of an unstated period following treatment. Seventy-five percent of the subjects rated the frequency, duration, and serverity of their "stammering," and their attitude towards "stammerers," as "good" to "complete improvement." No other data were reported, and it is noteworthy that the sample represented only 30% of those treated. Nevertheless, these subjects reported their obvious satisfaction with their treatment.

Various other "direct therapies" have also been described in the literature. One of the most interesting was a procedure devised by Froeschels (1941), which involved practicing a chewing action. The method was first reported in a therapy context by Despert (1942), who described the treatment of two children (5 and 10 years) by a combination of psychotherapy and "chewing speaking" practice. No data were provided in this report, nor in the only other report on this therapy, by Kastein (1947). The method received wide publicity but was never evaluated. Later Froeschels (1950) suggested that the altered articulation used in the chewing action could be varied to resemble the manner of speaking used by a ventriloquist. Quite obviously, both of these techniques relied upon radically altered ways of speaking yet no indication was given as to whether or not the speaker was supposed to retain this rather bizarre speech.

The Gregory and Prins Evaluations of Traditional Treatments

At least two programs of therapy research have endeavored to assess the efficacy of some nonbehavioral treatments. The first was carried out by Gregory (1972), and the second involved a series of studies under the direction of David Prins (1970; 1976; Prins & Miller, 1973; Prins & Nichols, 1974). These research programs involved the most controlled endeavors yet reported to evaluate the traditional therapy approaches.

Gregory (1972) employed a therapy evaluation design which required the subject to be assessed on four occasions: nine months before treatment, immediately before treatment, immediately after treatment (which lasted nine months), and nine months following cessation of treatment. The treatment procedure involved 1 hour of individual therapy and 1 hour of group therapy each week. The methods used were derived from those used by "Bryngelson (1950), Johnson (1956), Sheehan (1958) and Van Riper (1963)," as well as relaxation procedures described by Gregory (1968). Two groups of eight stutterers were treated, and they formed a "less severe" and a "more severe" group. Assessments were made of each subject's oral reading and spontaneous speech in front of individuals or groups of listeners. These assessments were supplemented by self-ratings using the Stutterers' Self Rating of Reactions to Speech Situations form and the Iowa Scale of Attitudes Toward Stuttering. Ratings of severity of stuttering were obtained using a method devised by Young (1969). The latter ratings revealed a significant reduction in stuttering severity as a result of treatment in the "more severe" group, but *not* in the "less severe" group. In other words, the treatment was quite ineffective for one group of subjects. There was also some evidence of relapse in stuttering severity in the "more severe" group. The self-rating data showed some significant improvements were associated with treatment. These were judgments of avoidance, reaction to speaking situations, and frequency of stuttering. This was also true for the attitude-change measures. Gregory (1972) also indicated the clinical limitations of these findings: "The ratings of stuttering severity at the post-therapy and follow-up testing sessions ... revealed that the group were still showing means which are characteristic of mild to moderate stuttering" (p.331). Another significant finding from this study, which Gregory reported earlier (1969), was that measures made of state anxiety (palmar sweat print indices) on each of the assessment occasions showed no significant change.

A final comment by Gregory (1972) indicates that he was less than satisfied with these procedures and encouraged movement towards a quite different treatment approach:

> The findings for Group II [the less severe group] imply more strongly that the therapy program needs to be modified to make it maximally effective. In the author's more recent work with stutterers he has extended his work in the therapeutic area of building up a new psychomotor speech pattern using delayed auditory feedback and other approaches to blending and motor

> speech planning. It is concluded that the results from both groups indicate that along with work on attitudes and the modification of instrumental avoidance behavior, greater emphasis in therapy needs to be placed on instating a smoother, more flexible speech pattern and generalizing this modified behavior to various situations. The less severe group would possibly have shown a significant change if this approach had been emphasized more (p.331-332).

The treatment programs reported in the Prins studies describe the evaluation of an increasingly systematic and behaviorally oriented approach to therapy. At the same time they provide a rather general, though sometimes obscure, account of the effects of applying Van Riper's treatment procedures in a group setting. The principal reason for this obscurity is that, like Gregory's study, much of the data are derived from self-rating scales and, therefore, they have a questionable relationship to speech data.

In 1970, Prins reported the description and evaluation of treatment for 94 male stutterers (8-12 years) who were enrolled for 8 weeks in the well-known "Shady Trails" Michigan Speech and Hearing Camp Program. During this time, subjects lived in a 16-person cabin which forms a "self-contained therapeutic group with a clinical staff assigned to it for the entire session" (Prins, 1970, p.124). The treatment involved both group and individual sessions and included a wide range of procedures. It seems fair to conclude that they represented many of the procedures described by Van Riper, Sheehan, and Williams. The total treatment time involved 120 hours. The evaluation procedure was designed to estimate improvement and regression following completion of treatment. This evaluation was based largely on a questionnaire which provided scores in each of the five problem areas specified by Van Riper's (1963) formula for stuttering severity; (1) speech penalties, frustrations, anxiety, guilt, hostility and communicative stress, (2) situation fears, (3) word fears, (4) morale and, (5) fluency. The answers to these questions were then scored for ratings "during camp," "since the end of camp," and "now." A huge array of data were reported but the ratings of fluency are of most interest. The main finding was that the extremes of improvement and regression ratings occurred on the fluency scale. Only 42% of the fluency responses showed little or no regression, and 20% indicated "much or complete regression" during the after-treatment period. By contrast, 77% of respondents indicated "much or complete" improvement in fluency "during camp." This does not do complete justice to the findings of this study, but, since no speech data were provided, it is difficult to do more than conclude that most subjects appeared to improve their fluency during treatment, but most also showed substantial regression over the 6-to-42 month follow-up interval.

One indication of the amount of relapse that followed the Prins (1970) program is contained in a report by Prins and Miller (1973). They reported findings from a group of 16 subjects (10-18 years) who were assessed before treatment, following the 8-week residential program, and then 10 months later. On Johnson's (1961) Job Task, these subjects recorded means of 30%, 9%, and 21% stuttered words on each of these respective assessment occasions. It was also reported that the social skills subscale of the California Test of Personality (Thorpe, Clark, & Tiegs, 1953) was significantly correlated (0.65) with posttherapy regression.

The Prins and Nichols (1974) study compared the performance of nine subjects (11-15 years) treated in a nonresidential therapy program with a selection of subjects (N=23) treated in the previously described residential conditions (Prins, 1970). The nonresidential program involved 36 hours of direct therapy, using procedures described by Sheehan, Van Riper, and Williams. In addition, there were 9 hours of group therapy sessions and social situation practice, which were designed to aid carry-over. The treatment time in this nonresidential setting was considerably less than the 120 hours in the residential setting. The subjects in both groups were matched for a follow-up interval, however, after which they completed the questionnaire used in the Prins (1970) study. The nonresidential group also provided video-tape speech samples made at the beginning and end of treatment. These were assessed by the Riley Stuttering Severity Instrument. The results indicated that subjects rated their fluency as less-improved by the nonresidential program, although the graphed data suggest that they showed more reports of "little or no" regression in fluency. The video data reveal that the nonresidential group showed a similar trend of reduction in the Riley scores for frequency, duration, and physical concomitants of stuttering. At the end of this report, Prins and Nichols anticipated making a number of modifications in this treatment; the most important being that criteria for speech behavior change were to be established within treatment, and the program would include transfer procedures based on performance criteria. In effect, they foreshadowed the replacement of a nonbehavioral treatment with a behavioral treatment.

The previously mentioned proposals were effected in the most recent treatment report by Prins (1976). This program represents a radical departure from the traditional approach to stuttering therapy and should be regarded as an example of behavior therapy. The aim of this treatment, as stated by Prins, best describes this change:

> A traditional, symptomatic stuttering therapy program for school-age children was modified to (1) focus more upon self-therapy activities while reducing group work emphasis; (2) specify more precisely the target responses used to replace stuttering; (3) establish clearly the criteria for client programs; and (4) provide well defined activities for the transfer of speech change" (p.452).

Procedures are described which fit these criteria and the program was conducted with eight children (10-15 years) over a 6-week period. No information is provided on the number of treatment sessions, but the program timetable appears to resemble the one described by Prins and Nichols (1974). Indeed, treatment outcome is assessed by comparison with the findings from that study. These indicate a higher level of improvement on the fluency ratings and an overall Riley SSI mean score which was superior to that achieved by subjects in the Prins and Nichols study. However, the data do not indicate whether any subjects achieved sustained fluency or whether their improved performance extended beyond the treatment setting. Nevertheless, there is some justification for concluding that this alternative treatment program resulted in markedly improved performances.

There are some interesting sidelight issues mentioned in the Prins (1976) report. Prins suggests that the findings of his study indicate that the present writer's earlier comment (Ingham & Andrews, 1973, p.436) that behavior therapy has not "made a major contribution towards providing clinicians with effective and reliable therapeutic procedure" is challenged by the results of the 1976 study. To some extent this seems justified. But in the absence of evidence that treatment procured stutter-free speech—which was durable beyond treatment conditions—it is difficult to decide whether this claim is warranted.

Another remark in Prins's (1976) discussion is also of interest here. It is inferred that the overall evidence from the studies directed by Prins indicates that "the development of more effective programs of therapy is seen primarily as an evolutionary and cumulative process rather than as a revolutionary new discovery" (p.462). Of course, that is very much a question of judgment, but it seems that the Prins study introduced a radical change in his approach to therapy. It is an approach which is disavowed by most traditional clinicians (see, for example, Sheehan, 1978), and which places his later treatment firmly within the behavioral preparadigm. For instance, the decisions about therapy progress were altered from client-clinician agreements, or predetermined periods of treatment, to those made on the basis of behavioral or observable criteria. Such an approach owes its origins to a radically different concept of treatment. In fact, there is something of a problem for those who claim to be able to place Van Riper's therapy program within a behavioral context: in almost every account of this symptomatic treatment procedure, Van Riper insists that it must be supplemented by psychotherapy which is directed towards a cognitive reappraisal of the subject's self-concept (see, for example, Van Riper, 1973). In fact, Van Riper has constantly advocated a distinct mistrust of behavior as an indicator of the acquisition of improved fluency. This makes it difficult to accept that clinicians will ever be able to truly represent Van Riper's therapy system within a behavioral preparadigm.

Conclusions

This overview of the "indirect" and "direct therapies" that have formed part of the nonbehavioral preparadigm provides some indication of the limitations of those treatment procedures. For the most part, their findings are weakened by the absence of one important feature that the behavioral orientation has endeavored to bring to treatment—the use of systematic evaluation. In the absence of relevant and appropriately gathered speech data, all of these therapy endeavors have provided remarkably little substance for their claims. The varibility of stuttering, which most traditional clinicians regard as integral to the problem, is given cursory consideration. This is made evident by the failure of their treatment reports to provide public and representative data. There is sufficient evidence to suggest that substantial numbers of stutterers must have benefited by many of the traditional approaches to treatment. But it seems fair to conclude that the gains, particularly for adults, have been in the form of improved speech, rather than the acquistion of normal fluency.

References

Barbara, D. *The psychotherapy of stuttering*. Springfield, IL: Charles C. Thomas, 1962.

Bender, J.F., & Kleinfeld, V.M. *Principles and practices of speech correction*. New York: Pitman, 1938.

Bergin, A.E. The evaluation of therapeutic outcomes. In A.E. Bergin & S.L. Garfield (Eds.), *Handbook of psychotherapy and behavior change: An empirical analysis*. New York: Wiley, 1971.

Blanton, S., & Blanton, M.G. *For stutterers*. New York: Appleton, 1936.

Bloodstein, O. *A handbook on stuttering*. (3rd ed.) Chicago: National Easter Seal Society, 1981.

Brill, A.A. Speech disturbances in nervous and mental diseases. *Quarterly Journal of Speech Education*, 1923, *9*, 129-135.

Brody, M.W., & Harrison, S.I. Group psychotherapy with male stutterers. *International Journal of Group Psychotherapy*. 1954, *4*, 154-162.

Brown, F.W. Personality integration as the essential factor in the permanent cure of stuttering. *Mental Hygiene*, 1933, *17*, 266-277.

Bryngelson, B. Treatment of stuttering. *Journal of Expression*, 1931, *5*, 19-26.

Bryngelson, B. Treatment of stuttering in children. *Speech*, 1938, *3*, 7-10.

Bryngelson, B. Stuttering and personality development. *The Nervous Child*, 1943, *2*, 162-166.

Bryngelson, B. *Know yourself: A workbook for those who stutter*. Minneapolis: Burgess, 1950.

Carlson, S.M. Varied case histories. *Journal of Speech Disorders*, 1940, *5*, 368-370.

Case, H.W. Therapeutic methods in stuttering and speech blocking. In H.J. Eysenck (Ed.), *Behaviour therapy and the neuroses*. Oxford: Pergamon, 1960.

Clark, R.M. Supplementary techniques to use with secondary stutterers. *Journal of Speech and Hearing Disorders*, 1948, *13*, 131-134.

Clark, R.M. Our enterprising predecessors and Charles Sydney Bluemel. *Asha*, 1964, *6*, 107-114.

Coriot, I.H. *Stammering: A psychoanalytic interpretation*. New York: Nervous and Mental Disease Monographs, 1927.

Coriot, I.H. The psychoanalytic concept of stammering. *The Nervous Child*, 1943, *2*, 167-171.

Cypreansen, L. Group therapy for adult stutterers. *Journal of Speech and Hearing Disorders*, 1948, *13*, 313-319.

Despert, J.L. A therapeutic approach to the problem of stuttering in children. *The Nervous Child*, 1942, *2*, 143-147.

Dunlap, K. A revision of the fundamental law of habit formation. *Science*, 1928, *37*, 360-362.

Dunlap, K. Repetition in the breaking of habits. *Scientific Monthly*, 1930, *30*, 66-70.

Dunlap, K. *Habits: Their making and unmaking*. New York: Liveright, 1932.

Dunlap, K. The technique of negative practice. *American Journal of Psychology*, 1942, *55*, 270-273.

Fahmy, M. The theory of habit control and negative practice as a curative method in the treatment of stammering. *Speech*, 1950, *14*, 24-30.

Fenichel, O. *The psychoanalytic theory of neurosis.* New York: W.W. Norton, 1945.

Fishman, H.C. A study of the efficacy of negative practice as a corrective for stammering. *Journal of Speech Disorders,* 1937, *2,* 67-72.

Froeschels, E. Differences in the symptomatology of stuttering in the United States and Europe. *Journal of Speech Disorders,* 1941, *6,* 45-46.

Froeschels, E. A technique for stutterers—"Ventriloquism." *Journal of Speech and Hearing Disorders,* 1950, *15,* 336-337.

Gendleman, E.G. Confrontation in the treatment of stuttering. *Journal of Speech and Hearing Disorders,* 1977, *42,* 85-89.

Gifford, M.F. *How to overcome stammering.* New York: Prentice-Hall, 1940.

Glauber, I.P. The psychoanalysis of stuttering. In J. Eisenson (Ed.), *Stuttering: A symposium.* New York: Harper & Row, 1958.

Gregory, H.H. *Learning theory and stuttering therapy.* Evanston, IL: Northwestern University Press, 1968.

Gregory, H.H. An assessment of the results of stuttering therapy. Final Report. Research and Demonstration Project 1725-S USDH, 1969.

Gregory, H.H. An assessment of the results of stuttering therapy. *Journal of Communication Disorders,* 1972, *5,* 320-334.

Hahn, E.F. A study of the effect of remedial treatment on the frequency of stuttering in oral reading. *Journal of Speech Disorders,* 1941, *6,* 29-38.

Harle, M. A dynamic interpretation and treatment of acute stuttering in a young child. *American Journal of Orthopsychiatry,* 1946, *16,* 156-162.

Hejna, R.F. *Interviews with a stutterer.* Danville, IL: Interstate, 1963.

Honig, P. The stutterer acts it out. *Journal of Speech Disorders,* 1947, *12,* 105-109.

Ingham, R.J., & Andrews, G. Behavior therapy and stuttering: A review. *Journal of Speech and Hearing Disorders,* 1973, *38,* 405-441.

Irwin, A. The treatment and results of 'easy-stammering.' *British Journal of Disorders of Communication,* 1972, *7,* 151-156.

Jameson, A.M. Stammering in children—some factors in the prognosis. *Speech,* 1955, *19,* 60-67.

Johnson, W. Stuttering. In W. Johnson & S.F. Brown, J.F. Curtis, C.W. Edney, & J. Keaster (Eds.), *Speech handicapped school children.* New York: Harper & Row, 1948.

Johnson, W. Stuttering. In W. Johnson, S.J. Brown, J.F. Curtis, C.W. Edney, & J. Keaster (Eds.), *Speech handicapped school children.* New York: Harper & Row, 1956.

Johnson, W. Measurements of oral reading and speaking rate and disfluency of adult male and female stutterers and non-stutterers. *Journal of Speech and Hearing Disorders,* Monograph Supplement No. 7, 1961, 1-20.

Kaplan, N.R., & Kaplan, M.L. The gestalt approach to stuttering. *Journal of Communication Disorders,* 1978, *11,* 1-9.

Kastein, S. The chewing method of treating stuttering. *Journal of Speech Disorders,* 1947, *12,* 195-198.

Kent, L.R. A retraining program for the adult who stutters. *Journal of Speech and Hearing Disorders,* 1961, *2,* 141-144.

Lehner, G.F.J. Negative practice as a psychotherapeutic technique. *Journal of General Psychology,* 1954, *51,* 69-82.

Meissner, J.H. The relationship between voluntary non-fluency and stuttering. *Journal of Speech Disorders,* 1946, *11,* 13-33.

Nystul, M.S. & Muszynska, E. Adlerian treatment of a classical case of stuttering. *Journal of Individual Psychology,* 1976, *32,* 194-102.

Oxtoby, E.T. Frequency of stuttering in relation to induced modifications following expectancy of stuttering.In W. Johnson & R.R. Leutenegger (Eds.), *Stuttering in children and adults*. Minneapolis: University of Minnesota Press, 1955.

Prins, D. Improvement and regression in stutterers following short-term intensive therapy. *Journal of Speech and Hearing Disorders*, 1970, *35*, 123-135.

Prins, D. Stutterers' perceptions of therapy improvement and of posttherapy regression: Effects of certain program modifications. *Journal of Speech and Hearing Disorders*, 1976, *41*, 452-463.

Prins, D., & Miller, M. Personality, improvement, and regression in stuttering therapy. *Journal of Speech and Hearing Disorders*, 1973, *16*, 685-690.

Prins, D., & Nichols, A. Client impressions of the effectiveness of stuttering therapy. A comparison of two programs. *British Journal of Disorders of Communication*, 1974, *9*, 134-139.

Read, L.F. Varied case histories. *Journal of Speech Disorders*, 1940, *5*, 365-367.

Rieber, R.W. & Wollock, J. The historical roots of the theory and therapy of stuttering. *Journal of Communication Disorders*, 1977, *10*, 3-24.

Rogers, C.R. *Counseling and psychotherapy*. Boston: Houghton Mifflin, 1942.

Rogers, C.R. *Client-centered therapy*. Boston: Houghton Mifflin, 1951.

Rotter, J.B. A working hypothesis as to the nature and treatment of stuttering. *Journal of Speech Disorders*, 1942, *7*, 263-288.

Rubin, H., & Culatta, R. A point of view about fluency. *Asha*, 1971, *13*, 380-384.

Schultz, D.A. A study of non-directive counseling as applied to adult stutterers. *Journal of Speech Disorders*, 1947, *12*, 421-427.

Sheehan, J.G. The modification of stuttering through non-reinforcement. *Journal of Abnormal Psychology* 1951, *46*, 51-63.

Sheehan, J.G. Conflict theory of stuttering. In J. Eisenson (Ed.), *Stuttering: A symposium*. New York: Harper & Row, 1958.

Sheehan, J.G. Current issues on stuttering and recovery. In H.H. Gregory (Ed.), *Controversies about stuttering therapy*. Baltimore: University Park Press, 1978.

Sheehan, J.G. & Voas, R.B. Stuttering as conflict: A comparison of therapy techniques involving approach and avoidance. *Journal of Speech and Hearing Disorders*, 1957, *22*, 714-723.

Spates, E.S. Varied case histories. *Journal of Speech Disorders*, 1940, *5*, 370-374.

Speech Foundation of America. *Stuttering: Successes and failures in therapy*. Memphis: Speech Foundation of America, Publication No.6, 1968.

Speech Foundation of America. *Therapy for stutterers*. Memphis: Speech Foundation of America, Publication No.10, 1974.

Stoddard, C.B. A public school approach to treatment of stuttering. *Journal of Speech Disorders*, 1939, *4*, 219-222.

Thorpe, L.P., Clark, W.W., & Tiegs, E.W. *California Test of Personality (Manual)*. Monterey: California Test Bureau, 1953.

Travis, L.E. *Speech pathology*. New York: Appleton-Century, 1931.

Travis, L.E. The need for stuttering. *Journal of Speech Disorders*, 1940, *5*, 193-202.

Van Riper, C. Experiments in stuttering therapy. In J. Eisenson (Ed.), *Stuttering: A symposium*. New York: Harper & Row, 1958.

Van Riper, C. *Speech correction: Principles and methods*. Englewood Cliffs, NJ: Prentice-Hall, 1963.

Van Riper, C. Historical approaches. In J.G. Sheehan (Ed.), *Stuttering: Research and therapy*. New York: Harper & Row, 1970.

Van Riper, C. Symptomatic therapy for stuttering. In L.E. Travis (Ed.), *Handbook of speech pathology and audiology*. Englewood Cliffs, NJ: Prentice-Hall, 1971.

Van Riper, C. *The treatment of stuttering*. Englewood Cliffs, NJ: Prentice-Hall, 1973.

Webster, L.M. A clinical note on psychotherapy for stuttering. *Journal of Fluency Disorders*, 1977, *2*, 253-255.

Williams, D.E. Intensive clinical case studies of stuttering therapy. In W. Johnson & R.R. Leutenegger (Eds.), *Stuttering in children and adults*. Minneapolis: University of Minnesota Press, 1955.

Williams, D.E. A point of view about stuttering. *Journal of Speech and Hearing Disorders*, 1957, *22*, 390-397.

Young, M.A. Observer agreement: Cumulative effects of repeated ratings of the same samples and of knowledge of group results. *Journal of Speech and Hearing Disorders*, 1969, *12*, 144-155.

4

Spontaneous Remission Of Stuttering[1]

Introduction

Perhaps the most interesting example of the preparadigm clash in stuttering research is the recent reassessment of the role of "spontaneous remission." It may not be the most vivid example of a clash between stuttering research ruling systems, but it does reveal the powerful influence that one system has had on this research and the interpretations of its findings. In essence the clash has been between a theoretically acceptable explanation for changes in stuttering behavior and the challenge to that acceptance by an opposed concept of stuttering.

The very term "spontaneous remission" incorporates certain assumptions: it generally refers to the disappearance of a problem without the assistance of formal treatment. When it is used in the context of a disability, it also has a medically oriented connotation. It usually describes the lessening in some condition or the "abatement of the symptoms of a disease" without any apparent cause. In some respects it is almost an antideterministic label: it carries the connotation of a mystical intervention. Perhaps clinical researchers have not intended the term to have this connotation, but the manner of its use, particularly over the past few decades, suggests otherwise. In fact, this connotation alone has influenced the interpretation of much stuttering research. In the course of this chapter, it will be shown that it has tended to cause many investigators to bypass a variety of factors that could justify as "treatments," even though they are not administered formally or professionally.

Spontaneous remission in the stuttering literature is usually a shorthand description for the permanent cessation of this problem without the intervention of formally managed speech therapy (Andrews & Harris, 1964, p.33). Recently, however, many of the research findings used to justify its occurrence have been reappraised (Ingham, 1976; Wingate, 1976; Young, 1975). This has led to the view that perhaps a conceptual error has been committed if the findings of most of these studies are examined from an alternative perspective. These examinations have been concerned to identify the incidence of putative therapy procedures, particularly self- or patient-administered procedures, that occur informally in many of these studies. If these procedures appear with any prominence, then this

[1] An earlier version of this chapter by the author appears in Prins and Ingham's (1983) book.

would, at the very least, compromise a "spontaneous remission" explanation of recovery. It will be argued that most of these studies now appear to support diametrically opposed explanations of changes in stuttering. One explanatory model regards the evidence as an account of the "natural history" of the disorder; it provides the expected trend of stuttering within a population—at least over the first part of the life span. The other explanatory model seeks a more casual explanation for the duration and cessation of stuttering; it regards "unassisted" recovery from stuttering as worthy of investigation for procedures which may usefully treat stuttering.

Our knowledge about the rate of spontaneous recovery[2] from stuttering is derived from either longitudinal or cross-sectional studies. The longitudinal studies involve regular assessments over time of a population of stutterers, in order to identify changes in their disorder. The cross-sectional method surveys, at one time, a population of stutterers, and/or those who claim to have recovered from stuttering, in order to identify factors associated with recovery or non-recovery. As a result of both types of studies, the belief has grown that approximately 80% of stutterers will spontaneously lose their problem by early adulthood. The significance of this belief is immense. It has largely supported the view that most children who stutter will "grow out" of the problem, and if they are treated, their natural recovery could be impeded. Of course, it has also implied that any evaluation of a stuttering treatment with children, especially long-term outcome assessment, is likely to be confounded by this high recovery rate.

General Methodological Issues in Recovery Studies

There are now quite a few studies concerned with measuring the rate of spontaneous recovery among stutterers. They have produced a variety of recovery rates. One explanation for this variety is that it reflects the age of the population in these studies. For instance Bloodstein (1981) reviewed some of these studies and concluded that stuttering will "disappear of its own accord" for between 36% and 79% of stutterers, depending on the age group on which the study was conducted—the wider the age range, the higher the percentage. But this rather cursory explanation certainly invites some questioning. Indeed, the questioning becomes compelling when stutterers and their families are surveyed to find reasons for recovery, and when the methodology in these studies is examined.

Rather obvious methodological weaknesses abound in almost all the recovery studies. For example, the reliable identification of stutterers within the cross-sectional and longtitudinal studies would appear to be a straightforward task, yet

[2] For the duration of this chapter, the term "spontaneous recovery" will be used in preference to "spontaneous remission," because the former term is used in most research studies.

only one study (Panelli, McFarlane, & Shipley, 1978) reports that its subjects were tape-recorded, or that a subject's "diagnoses" were made by independent assessors. The cross-sectional studies have mainly relied on the subject's responses to a questionnaire, with only infrequent attempts at cross-validation. These questionnaires have sought relatively general information on the role of speech therapy in recovery and have rarely provided information on the content or duration of that therapy. This leaves ample room to speculate about what type of therapy might have contributed to the presence or absence of recovery. These are some of the more prominent methodological problems that should be noted as we survey the available research on recovery.

Review of Recovery Studies

Recovery In Below 9-Year-Olds

One of the limitations about the cross-sectional and longitudinal studies of recovery from stuttering is that they have been mainly directed at the below-adult-age group of stutterers. Arguably, this fact alone may have increased the probability that recovery is regarded as a characteristic of younger, rather than older, subjects. Nevertheless, when some studies have ascertained the number of former or active stutterers in a population, then the age factor becomes evident. For instance, Johnson reported on a series of surveys (Johnson, 1955; Johnson & Associates, 1959) which identified children under eight years of age who were "allegedly stuttering." In the first study (Study I), 46 children, with a median age of 4 years, 2 months at the beginning of the study, were intermittently observed over approximately 2.5 years. At the end of that time, 72% were considered to have recovered (that is, they were rated as either "nearly normal," "indefinite," or "normal"). In the subsequent studies (II and III), 118 of 150 "allegedly stuttering" children (ages 2.5 to 7 years) were assessed 2.5 years after initial interview. Yet, only 36% of these children were found to have "no problem" according to parents' judgments. Why such a huge disparity?

One plausible answer appears in Studies II and III. It was reported that 50 children were assessed separately by the interviewers, and they judged 46 to have "normal speech," yet only 17 of these children were given the same assessment by their mothers! So whose data should be used to assess whether subjects have "recovered"? If the parents' judgments are given priority (as they are in some studies), then perhaps Johnson's data on the 7.5-year-olds should be regarded as showing about a 36% rate of recovery. This also turns out to be a more plausible figure if an 80% recovery rate is expected by adulthood. This low recovery rate among children also seems to be corroborated in a cross-sectional study by Bryne (1931). In an evaluation of 315 stutterers who (in the main) had attended a speech therapy clinic in their first three school grades, she found that 32% had recovered when they were assessed up to 12 years later. However, the role of therapy (such as it was) in this study raises some problems: it could be interpreted as retarding the recovery rate; it could also imply that, despite therapy, the recovery rate in children will be not much greater than 32%.

The age factor is also partly evident in studies that have consulted stutterers' parents for evidence regarding recovery. Glasner and Rosenthal (1957) surveyed the parents of children "approaching the first grade level," and found 153 parents who said their child had "stuttered at some time." They reported that 54% of their children had stopped stuttering, and the others were either still stuttering or only stuttered occasionally. Dickson (1971) surveyed the parents of an older age group of children (approximately 9 years) and found 364 who said their child had either ceased or continued stuttering. It was reported that 53.8% were recovered. Intriguingly, Dickson's survey also revealed that approximately 38% of these children had recovered by 6 years of age—remarkably similar to the 36% identified by parents in Johnson's Studies II and III.

In short, the findings of both cross-sectional and longitudinal studies on younger children tend to suggest that approximately 40% to 50% of children described as stutterers will recover by 6 to 9 years of age.

Recovery in Below-12-Year-Olds

Any endeavor to estimate the rate of recovery among children over the age of 9 must allow for the number of children who might begin stuttering at this time. This factor would tend to depress the recovery rate when compared with that found in younger children. After a fairly detailed survey of the available evidence on the development of stuttering, however, Young (1975) concluded that there are "essentially no new cases of any significant number after the age of nine" (p.51). Consequently, an analysis which anticipates identifying an age factor in the spontaneous recovery process should produce some evidence of this effect across the age groups "below-9 years," "below-12 years," and "below-adulthood." Such a step-wise analysis should show a systematic increase in recovery rates and end with close to the alleged 80% recovery rate in adulthood.

The below-12-year group may contain a higher reported recovery rate than that reported in the below-9 group. But the evidence is certainly not decisive. Milisen and Johnson (1936) reported on a questionnaire-survey of 132 subjects, plus their parents, relatives, neighbors, and school teachers. They provided data on 56 stutterers, aged 3 to 22 years, and 32 former stutterers (ages not specified). They also reported, however, that these subjects were drawn from 201 stutterers and former stutterers, and that 42% of these were in the latter group. (They were reported to have an age range of 5 to 20 years!) Inconsistencies in Milisen and Johnson's data make this a difficult study to review. Nevertheless, their findings suggest that the recovery rate in the below-9-years group was not increased by adding the higher age group. This is confirmed in a later study by Milisen (1936), which surveyed 741 children (aged 6 to 18 years) who were either stutterers or former stutterers. She found that 32% were former stutterers, and that 99% of this group reported recovering by 14 years of age.

By contrast, Andrews and Harris (1964) obtained data from a longitudinal study which claimed to have involved at least annual assessment of 43 stutterers from birth to 16 years. They reported that 34 subjects, or 79% of their group, had recovered by their 12th year. However, as this writer has noted (Ingham, 1976), not all of the recovered stutterers were followed beyond their seventh year, and a portion may not have been judged as "stutterers." In other words, there is ample reason to suspect that this high recovery rate may be exaggerated.

The only other study that provides a clue to the recovery rate in the below-12-year group is the previously mentioned study by Dickson (1971). His findings (though based on parent assessment) suggested a rate of around 54% among children aged 9 years. This is probably the most reliable figure in the light of other studies, and the increased rate of recovery which is reported to occur from adolescence onwards. This figure also resembles the recovery rate that Wingate (1976) derived from a review of relevant studies on this age group.

Recovery in Below-Adult-Age Subjects

Quite surprisingly, the recovery rate in this age group is also not substantially higher than the below-12-years group. The cut-off point for studies on this population is difficult to establish because most describe their subjects as "senior high school" students, or "freshmen." So their true age can only be an estimate. This problem is evident in a study by Cooper (1972) which involved a survey of 5054 "junior and senior high school" students in order to identify "active" and recovered stutterers.

Cooper's study was a replication of a series of survey-type studies on an older age group by Sheehan and Martyn (1966; 1970) and Martyn and Sheehan (1968). Cooper's very substantial survey identified 119 active stutterers and 68 who claimed to have recovered from stuttering. This means that only 36% of their group had recovered, although this was composed of a 44% recovery rate in the senior high school group, and a 30% rate in the junior high school group. Nevertheless, these figures are in stark contrast to the 79% recovery rate among 16-year-olds suggested by data from Andrews and Harris (1964). At the very least, it implies that there must have been very significant differences between the populations used in these studies.

If Cooper's finding is reliable, then it follows that the rate of recovery from childhood to adolescence does not change very much at all. Some apparent support for this is provided in a study by Fritzell (1976) on 91 children who stuttered when assessed at ages 7 to 9 yuears. These children were followed for 10 years, and during that time all received some form of therapy—although Fritzell claimed that it was not particularly influential therapy. Nevertheless, by the time these children reached the end of the study, only 46.7% did not stutter. Once again, this may suggest that their allegedly ineffective therapy actually impeded the recovery rate; a possibility that could not be established definitely because of the absence of a control group.

Contrasting findings were reported by Panelli, McFarlane, and Shipley (1978) who assessed 15 children and adolescents (7-14 years) who had been evaluated as stutterers when they were younger (2-5 years). They claimed that 80% of these children had "recovered spontaneously from stuttering" by their final assessment. At that time they were recorded within the clinic (via spontaneous speech, counting, reciting, and oral reading) and were judged by themselves or a clinicians as either a "stutterer" or a "nonstutterer." The difficulties with these findings are that the assessment failed to include parent judgments as to whether they were definitely nonstutterers (the importance of this assessment was illustrated by Johnson's data on children) or information on what activities during the intervening years might have contributed to their "recovery." The significance of failing to include "beyond clinic" data is also illustrated by incidental information that two subjects "expressed their feeling that they were still stutterers" (1978, p. 45).

Recovery in Adult Subjects

In view of the foregoing, we should expect quite a dramatic increase in the recovery rate among adults. And there is some evidence that fulfills this expectation. One example occurs in Wingate's (1976) account of a study by Patricia Johnson on 23 former stutterers. She found that more than 50% of her subjects (17-31 years) reported their age of recovery as 15 years or older. In a similar study on 50 recovered stutterers (17-54 years), Wingate (1964) reported that 54% of his subjects recovered after they were 17 years of age. Also, Shearer and Williams (1965) reported that 31% of their 58 "ex-stutterers" (17-21 years) recoverd at 15 to 17 years of age. However, any reliance on these "recovery rates" must recognize that most of these subjects had received treatment. Nevertheless, the findings do suggest that the recovery, by whatever means, will be increasingly frequent when late adolescent and adult age groups are considered.

The most complete survey on an older age group was conducted by Sheehan and Martyn. It was reported in three principal studies (Martyn & Sheehan, 1968; Sheehan & Martyn, 1966) which involved 116 recovered stutterers and 31 active stutterers. They were identified from a survey of 5138 California university students. The findings were based on an oral reading, and the "recovered stutterer's" response to questions which determined whether he or she knew the "inside of stuttering." This required the subjects to describe their stuttering and its accompanying features; they also answered a questionnaire on the history of their problem. The findings suggested (see Sheehan, 1979) that 52% of subjects recovered from 15 years of age onward. In fact, about 26% reported they had recovered after 19 years of age.

Sheehan and Martyn's reports are perhaps the most significant and provocative, with respect to spontaneous recovery. For instance, their findings suggested that most recovered stutterers regarded themselves as having been "mild" stutterers, and their recovery was not associated with attendance in public school therapy. Sheehan and Martyn reached a number of other conclusions from their findings that will be considered shortly. But the finding regarding therapy is of most interest, especially when related to an almost identical study by Cooper, Parris, and Wells (1974).

Cooper, Parris, and Wells assessed the incidence of speech problems, and self-reported recovery from these problems, among 7090 University of Alabama students. It is possible that these students were, on average, 4 or 5 years younger than Sheehan and Martyn's subjects (see Sheehan, 1979, p. 198). Nevertheless, the stutterers and ex-stutterers were given virtually the same assessment procedure as that used by Sheehan and Martyn. Cooper et al. reported that 81% of the combined active and ex-stutterers had recovered (compared with 79% in Sheehan and Martyn's studies), but when the subjects who received therapy are excluded from this group, then the percentage drops to 52%. Unfortunately, it is not clear in the study by Cooper and his associates whether the subjects actually attributed their recovery to therapy—especially since this was not reported to be the case in Sheehan and Martyn's study.

Probably a similar-aged population was used in a cross-sectional study by Porfert and Rosenfield (1978). They questioned 2107 students at the University of Massachusetts on "whether they were or had been stutterers," and found that 61.7% of the 115 positive respondents claimed to have recovered. Unhappily, no information was collected on the respondent's therapy history, or their view as to why they had recovered.

Perhaps for the sake of completeness it should be added that recovery may occur among much older subjects. Shames and Beams (1956) sent questionnaires to clergymen in an endeavor to estimate how many stuttrers were among their parishioners. They found a substantially smaller percentage of stutterers among the older-age (above 50 years) groups of this second-hand reported population. The relatively small numbers of stutterers that this method identified, however, (64 or 0.57% of the population) highlights the need for a more extensive survey of this age group.

Longitudinal Studies on Recovery

The most obvious problem with most of the previously reported studies is that they rely on recall data—be it by subjects, parents, or relatives. This should not be an issue in longitudinal studies. But, unhappily, it emerges that two of the principal longitudinal studies contain some problems that make it difficult to place any confidence in their findings, especially with respect to spontaneous recovery.

Andrews and Harris (1964) claim to have followed 43 stutterers from the onset of their problem until they reached the age of 16 years. The fact is, however, that not all subjects were followed throughout this period. In reviewing this study, the present writer (Ingham, 1976) noted that 16 of their subjects were described as "transient nonfluents" (not "stutterers"), and all were not followed beyond the 7th year. Moreover, the 18 stutterers, who were described as "spontaneous remitters," were not followed after the 12th year. More importantly, on inquiry it was found that at least eight of the "spontaneous remitters" were independently reported (Morley, 1972) to have received "at least one form of therapy endeavour." The failure to include this information raises serious questions about Andrews and Harris's claim that "in none of these children could it be claimed that the remission was induced by treatment" (1964, p. 33). This is especially significant, since no information was given on the temporal relationship between these "treatments" and remission, nor was it reported (see below) that some of these treatments actually did reduce stuttering in these children.

The second longitudinal study was reported by Fritzell (1976). Ninety-one stutterers (identified at 7 to 9 years of age) were followed for 10 years in this study, and almost 47% were reported recovered. However, these findings are hopelessly confounded by the fact that all subjects were enrolled in therapy programs throughout this period. Fritzell regarded their therapy as relatively ineffectual, but the absence of a control group means that the number who recovered may simply reflect the rate of therapy success.

The previously mentioned study by Panelli, McFarlane, and Shipley (1978) on 15 adults and adolescents (7-14 years) also qualifies as a longitudinal study, since these subjects had been assessed as stutterers between 2 and 5 years of age by a practicing speech pathologist. The problem with this study is that it is not clear that the parents, or, indeed, the subjects, concurred with the final clinician judgments.

Conclusions

What can be deduced from the foregoing? Perhaps very little more than a range of interesting issues which qualify whatever findings that emerge. But on the basis of this relatively brief review, it becomes clear that the putative unassisted recovery rate from childhood to adolescence is likely to range between approximately 30% and 50%. It is almost certain that it is not as high as the generally accepted figure of 80%. After adolescence it may rise considerably but the reasons for this rise need to be examined. These reasons may also be very important to recovery in childhood, and raise further questions about the nonspecific nature of the term "spontaneous recovery."

Treatment Variables in Recovery Studies

As mentioned earlier, the role of therapy in recovery studies, whether self- or clinician-managed, appears to have received only cursory consideration. Obviously, the very notion of "spontaneous remission" becomes confusing if recovery is associated with treatment, regardless of who directs it. It may be possible to control for the effects of therapy, if its point of introduction and, perhaps, its content are known. But this is difficult (if not impossible) to know in retrospect, particularly if the therapy is self-managed, intermittantly administered, and vaguely reported. And by unfortunate coincidence, it is just this set of circumstances that intrudes, either directly or indirectly, into most recovery studies. At the same time, this type of evidence is also of dubious worth if it is reported imprecisely. Therefore, while it is interesting to probe these studies for therapy or therapy-related activities, it can do little more than draw attention to factors that might be relevant to "spontaneous recovery" findings.

Wingate's (1976) review of the literature on recovery from stuttering has contributed a very different perspective on its findings. His review found ample reason to question the much-accepted notion that if a child's stuttering is either highlighted or "treated," then it will be exacerbated. In particular, Wingate claimed there was little evidence that "unfavorable critical evaluation" of stuttering by parents of stutterers will worsen their problem. Indeed, the weight of evidence actually suggests that methods used by parents and stutterers to prevent stuttering have been quite successful and could have contributed much to the recovery role in childhood. A brief overview and appraisal of the evidence which contributes to this reanalysis of the recovery studies will now be considered.

It flies in the face of almost everything we know about human behavior to accept that parents of a child displaying stuttering problems would not endeavor to "do something." Yet that is precisely the implication to be drawn from those studies which have ignored (usually by default) the contribution of parent behavior to the high rate of recovery from stuttering among their children. It is also inconceivable that a good portion of older-aged—even younger-aged stutterers would not seek techniques (readily described in the literature on the disorder) or not use advice offered by others to alleviate their disorder. Yet, once again, that is the implication in studies that have not offered at least a caution about the role of this variable in recovery—particularly among adults.

Parent Intervention

The relevance of parent intervention in recovery from stuttering must be considered in relation to certain procedures that are known to reduce stuttering within a clinic or research setting. These studies will not be described in detail at this stage; however, it is sufficient to point out that when some stuttering children have been briefly (but consistently) stopped from speaking or asked to "slow down" immediately after stuttering (Martin, Kuhl, & Haroldson, 1972; Reed & Godden, 1977), their stuttering has been reduced or removed both within and beyond the clinic setting. Other procedures also draw attention to, or alter, the subject's manner of speaking, and have been reported to reduce stuttering in children (Egolf, Shames, Johnson, & Kasprisin-Burelli, 1972; Greenberg, 1970). Suffice to say, at this point, that if these procedures are used by parents or children, then it is difficult to discount their ameliorative possibilities—even allowing that they might have been used in an uncontrolled, or even inconsistent, fashion. For, although these procedures may not be effective when employed inconsistently, there is, as yet, no evidence that their efficacy is impeded by haphazard usage. Of course, there is also no evidence that these procedures are necessarily effective for all children. All that we have to look to is some evidence that they may be effective with some children who stutter. This should be borne in mind as we review, once again, some of the recovery studies. On this occasion, however, attention will be directed towards parent behavior.

In Johnson and Associate's (1959) study on 150 stuttering children, it was reported that around 36% of the subjects' parents confidently described 118 of them as having "no problem" 2.5 years after an initial diagnosis, and that 52% showed some improvement. Yet, during this 2.5-year period it was reported that:

> two-thirds of the fathers and three-fourths of the mothers indicated that something had been said to the child about what was referred to as his stuttering, and of these about three-fourths reported that something had been said either immediately or soon—that is, within one month. ... These persons had made a great variety of comments to the child ... the most common of which were suggestions that he slow down, take it easy, and stop and start over. Such comments or suggestions were said to have been made as often as from 5 times a day to 25 times a month in roughly one-third of the cases in the experimental group (p.149).

In effect, these children lived in an environment which fairly bristled with intervention methods that could have contributed towards their recovery. Yet, under these "undesirable" conditions only 11.8% of the children were unchanged or worsened, according to their parents. However, when parents were asked to give reasons for their child's recovery, most attributed the change to the child's growth, maturity, and confidence, or because they either allowed their child to talk more, offered less criticism, or ignored their stuttering. About 30% of parents could not provide a reason for the improvement.

A related finding occurs in a study by Glasner and Rosenthal (1957), which found a 54.6% recovery rate among 5- to 6-year-olds (as reported by their parents). In this group, about 58% received "active correction." Their parents "told him to speak more slowly and to take his time; made him repeat; made him stop and start over; said the word for him; reminded him not to stutter; told him to speak more softly; got angry; corrected him; emphasized the sound of proper speech, etc." (1957, p.291). About 40% of parents reacted minimally, that is, by virtually ignoring their child's disorder. These data must also be related to the finding that the parents mainly responded actively when more than one type of disfluency pattern (that is, repetitions, hesitations, prolongations, or combinations) was evident in their child's speech. It is noteworthy that out of approximately 30% of subjects who were reported to be "still stuttering," about 80% also received "active correction" from their parents. Consequently, these "active" procedures cannot be easily related to an increased rate of recovery.

Dickson (1971) also compared the method of "active correction" used by parents with children (around 9 years of age) who failed to recover and those who had recovered. It was reported that "admonishments" were used by 65% of parents in the recovery group and 84% of the nonrecovered group. "Slow down" and "take a breath" were used equally often by both groups of parents, but, in the nonrecovered group, the parents used "start over" and "think before you speak" more frequently. This led the author to the rather questionable conclusion that the use of "start over" and "think before you speak" may impede recovery because they interrupt rather than modify the child's speech pattern. Nevertheless, Dickson's findings show that about 71% of the nonrecovered stutterers were also described as "improved." In addition, 33% of the recovered stutterers' parents had obtained "professional advice" (it was not clear whether this included treatment), but 42% of the nonrecovered stutterers' parents sought the same type of assistance—although this is not at all surprising, because of the duration of the problem in the latter group.

Therapy Intervention

Some studies have endeavored to identify therapy-related activities within the background of recovered and nonrecovered adult stutterers. Sheehan and Martyn's (1966; 1970) studies, for instance, questioned subjects on the reasons for their recovery, including the extent to which they could attribute their present condition to speech therapy. When their findings were collated (see Wingate, 1976), approximately 61% of the recovered group attributed their improved speech to "self therapy," "slowing down and relaxing," or "speaking more, and improved self-concept." Martyn and Sheehan (1968) also provided data which compared the nonrecovered and recovered stutterers on this variable.[2] They found that 62% of recovered stutterers said this was due to "self-therapy or taking some action," but this was true for only 30% of the nonrecovered group. The authors observed that "those who found self-therapy to be helpful seemed to approach their problem directly, by talking more, slowing down, or taking speech courses. Those who did not seemed to be running away from their problem" (Martyn & Sheehan, 1968, p.305).

The Cooper et al. studies (Cooper, 1972; Cooper, Parris, & Wells, 1974) do not provide the reasons that subjects gave as explanations for their recovery. Lankford and Cooper (1974) did collect this information, however, from the parents of the recovered stutterers in the Cooper (1972) study. They reported that 79% of the parents admonished their child most frequently with " 'start over' closely followed ... by 'slow down.' Other suggestions frequently offered were reported to include: 'think before you speak,' 'take your time,' 'wait a minute,' and 'stop and start over' " (Lankford & Cooper, 1974, p.178).

Sheehan and Martyn reported that speech therapy was negatively correlated with recovery. Most of their subjects who failed to recover were reported to have received speech therapy, but those who did recover failed to indicate this as a reason for their recovery. This is perhaps the most surprising finding to have emerged from the "recovery studies," and for this reason alone it merits close examination.

The complete series of studies by Sheehan and Martyn comprise their 1966 and 1970 reports and a 1968 report by Martyn and Sheehan. Across the three studies,

[2]These data are from disproportionate samples of the recovered and nonrecovered stutterers. Forty-eight recovered stutterers were compared with 37 active stutterers, even though the ratio of recovered to active stutterers was reported to be four to one.

there were 116 recovered stutterers and 31 active stutterers. Surprisingly, the aspect of these studies which is concerned with this issue involves fewer than the total number of recovered stutterers, and either more or less than the total number of active stutterers. For example, the Martyn and Sheehan (1968) report involved 37 active stutterers, and the 1970 Sheehan and Martyn report used only 21 active stutterers. (It is claimed that their numbers were reduced as a control for severity.) But if the therapy was counterproductive, then it would be interesting to learn about the type and content of their treatment. Presumably the authors did not wish to imply that all types of therapy (including their own) are ineffectual. The only indication provided is that:

> Speech therapy as reported by the respondents, included many instances of quite brief contact, and many instances of obviously incompetent and irrelevant speech therapy, as judged by either current or the then contemporary standards. Hence caution should be exercised in condemning ... speech therapy for young stutterers from these data. For example, there were very few instances of the kind of speech therapy for stuttering outlined in the Speech Foundation of America's recent publication, *The Treatment for the Young Stutterer in the Schools* (Sheehan & Martyn, 1966, p.128).

In the light of this information, it is difficult to decide whether the active or recovered stutterer's speech therapy should be considered seriously in relation to recovery: On the one hand, it suggested that therapy was brief and irrelevant, while on the other, absolutely no information is provided on subjects who received what the authors judged to be suitable therapy. For this reason, prudence would suggest that the negative "therapy factor" in these studies has been considerably overemphasized.

The effect of therapy on the recovery rates reported in studies by Cooper and colleagues is also virtually impossible to assess. Cooper (1972) reported a nonsignificant relationship between recovery from stuttering and therapeutic intervention, when severity was held constant. But Cooper's relatively abbreviated report did not include information on the duration or content of treatment; presumably, this means that "therapy" may have been little more than a brief supportive-type contact with a clinician. Indeed, there is good reason to believe (Wingate, 1971) that much stuttering therapy during the 1960s was really supportive counseling designed to assist the subject to cope with, rather than overcome, the disorder. But this may not have been true in all of Cooper's data. Cooper, Parris, and Wells (1974) provided a very brief report on a partial replication of the Cooper (1972) study, using students enrolling at the university. They found 12 active stutterers, plus 54 who reported that they had recovered from stuttering. Twenty of the 54 recovered stutterers reported that they had received therapy. The difficulty in deducing the efficacy of this therapy is that similar information was not provided for the active suttterers. Ironically, the only way in which the therapy's contribution can be gauged is to note that the overall recovery rate in this study (81%) is high when related to other recovery studies. Yet, this high rate is remarkably similar to that reported ty Sheehan and Martyn, which, in turn, suggests the intriguing possibility that therapy may have contributed substantially to the high rate of recovery reported in Sheehan and Martyn's study.

From the preceding review, it becomes clear that when studies involving both recovered and active stutterers are considered, the contribution of "parent intervention" on recovery rates is not at all obvious. It may be that their contribution is more evident in the milder, rather than severe, stuttering children (Glasner & Rosenthal, 1957), but it is evident that their advice is offered freely and frequently to most of the children in these studies. At the same time, among older age stutterers, there is some evidence that when subjects employed some of these suggestions, they judged that they contributed significantly towards recovery. This possibility is strengthened by the findings in studies on recovered stutterers only. But before they are considered, it is important to highlight some methodological issues that emerged in the previously mentioned studies.

Some Methodological Considerations

The main weakness in the cross-sectional studies on recovery is that they hinge on the subject's ability to recall events that occurred possibly 1 or 2 decades previously. If cross-validating data or information are not provided as a control, the only method of checking the validity of their findings is via related studies. Thus, when cross-validation provides nonsupportive or contradictory data, the findings of studies which have not used this control are brought into question. Such an issue arises in connection with the Cooper et al. studies. It will be recalled that Cooper (1972) reported finding 68 self-diagnosed recovered stutterers. Subsequently, Lankford and Cooper (1974) wrote to the parents of all the recovered stutterers in Cooper's study and found that two-thirds of the subjects' parents "did not feel that their child had ever stuttered." The implication is fairly obvious: the true recovery rate might be much less than what has been suggested by this type of study. Of course, it is also equally possible that parents have a poor ability to accurately recall their child's speech quality. It is rather surprising, however, that such a high proportion of parents would fail to recall such a distinctive feature in their child's development.

The reasons for differences between the parents' and the subjects' responses in Cooper's study may be related to what they refer to as "stuttering." In reviewing some of these studies, Young (1975) drew attention to the findings in studies by Villarreal (1945), Voelker (1942) and Sander (1963; 1965; 1968) which indicate that "there is much more complexity than realized in assigning individuals to the categories of nonstutterer, recovered stutterer or active stutterer" (Young, 1975, p.57). For instance, 29% of nonstuttering subjects in the Villarreal and Voelker studies were "said to have been stuttering," but only about 10% had "called themselves a stutterer." In effect, subjects recalled behaviors that others might describe as "stuttering," even though these behaviors may not have bothered them sufficiently to warrant describing themselves as a "stutterer." Similarly, Sander found that mothers would classify some recordings of a child's speech behavior as "stuttering," yet, up to a third of these women would not regard the child as a "stutterer." This difference in the basis of classification might explain the disparities among the findings of Cooper's studies. It may also explain the relatively higher recovery rates in Andrews and Harris's (1964) longitudinal study: it will be recalled that about half their recovered "stutterers" had a bout of nonfluency which lasted for less than 6 months. A bout of this type and duration may not have been recalled by parents or subjects as stuttering, nor indicate to either that they were stutterers.

Another problematic measurement issue is that in many studies the so-called "recovered stutterers" were reported to be still stuttering at certain times. Recall, for instance, in the Johnson and Associates (1959) studies that 46 out of 50 children were assessed by interviewers as having "normal speech," but only 17 of the mothers agreed with that assessment. Similarly, Wingate (1964) and Shearer and Williams (1965) conducted studies on "recovered" stutterers, but noted that around 50% of their subjects still had evident, though infrequent, stutterings. This suggests the possibility that many of the "recovered stutterers" in these and other studies were still active stutterers, but were either not detected at interview, or were judged to be normal speakers. In any event, this is a much overlooked factor which might contribute much to the variation among the findings of recovery studies.

Therapy Effects in Studies on Recovered Stutterers Only

Thus far, it has been argued that a relatively conservative interpretation of the evidence on the effects of parent intervention in the recovery process is that it is at best ambiguous. But in the case of studies using adult stutterers and recovered stutterers, there is considerable evidence that "self-therapy" procedures, such as slowing down, relaxing, and talking practice, might be quite useful. This is also evident in those studies that assessed only recovered stutterers. These studies are of more than usual interest because the researcher's theoretical posture with respect to self-therapy or parent intervention is often evident and antagonistic.

One can confidently argue that during the period when many recovery studies were conducted, the prevailing belief was that the child's family environment could sustain and/or aggravate stuttering. Furthermore, parental anxiety about the child's speech, or any effort to correct the problem—especially by admonishment—could cause chronic stuttering. On the other hand, if the problem was ignored and the child's speech skills were not placed "under pressure," then stuttering was likely to disappear. Indeed, one could argue that, during this time, the inducement of this pattern of family behavior was actually the preferred treatment for stuttering. It follows, therefore, that if recovery does occur under these preferred conditions, it may be more appropriate to describe it as a result of a treatment, rather than "spontaneous recovery." This issue is well illustrated by Morley's (1972) consideration of the findings of the 1000 Family Study (also described by Andrews and Harris, 1964):

> The part that correction of the stammer plays in its persistence is important but difficult to ascertain without constant association with the family and even with our frequent contacts it was not possible to assess entirely the part played by parental correction in the persistence of the stammer. In the children seen by us the mother was advised to ignore the hestitation in its early stages and to accept it as a phase through which many children pass during their progress towards stable speech. Again it is impossible to be certain how far this advice was actually carried out, and if so, what effect it had on the eventual achievement of fluent speech (Morley, 1972, p.68).

Quite obviously, Morley inclined to the view that this counseling could be regarded as a treatment agent. But from an alternative viewpoint, there is ample evidence in the 1000 Family Study that "correction" could have contributed much to recovery. For, as this writer observed (Ingham, 1976), the case descriptions of some of the recovered subjects were especially revealing. They show subjects received "directives to 'speak slowly,' speech therapy, and [there was] even evidence from a mother that her child's stuttering 'stopped when corrected' " (p.281). This type of family behavior was reported for more than half the 14 subjects for whom case descriptions were provided. It is possible, therefore, that these correctives could have also contributed much to the recovery process. This issue is resolved more easily if comparisons can be made between children who have been exposed to different types of environments.

A comparative study by Jameson (1955) provides perhaps the only known support for the claim that parental correction may impede recovery. She surveyed 69 children ("still under the age of 16 years") who had not attended a clinic for advice or treatment for at least a year. Evidence was provided that 70% of the children whose parents did not offer correction were "normal or near normal" at assessment, but only 62% of children whose parents used correction fell into this category. In the case of parents who used "persistent correction, and in a few cases actual punishment," only 10% were judged in the same category. But unfortunately these data are confounded by potential therapy effects. Eighty-two percent of the children under 5 years of age were assessed as "normal or near normal" after treatment, and only 37% over 5 years of age reached this level. Since no other information is provided, it is possible that the noncorrective parents were mainly parents of those under 5 years of age. But if one accepts that the treated children were randomly distributed, then there is some support for the argument that correction impedes recovery. The point is even more significant when related to Jameson's claim that their treatment was virtually nondirective.

Unfortunately, it is impossible to learn whether the parents' corrective advice for stuttering had been employed beneficially or otherwise by their children. There may be some indication of the effect that it had by gleaning opinions from older-age stutterers on what they judged to be beneficial. Horowitz (1962) asked 14 nonrecovered stutterers and one recovered stutterer what they would advise to assist other stutterers. "[T]he subjects offered up such well-worn homilies as 'Don't think about it'; 'take your time'; 'stop and start over'; 'slow down'; 'take a deep breath'; 'relax'; 'buy a tape-recorder'; and 'think that you have a right to speak as well as anybody else' '' (p.31). Similar comments have surfaced in other studies on recovered stutterers—and also at apparent odds with the researchers' theoretical positions.

Shearer and Williams (1965) questioned 58 self-described recovered stutterers (ages 17 to 21 years) who claimed their improved speech was obtained without "professional assistance." There was "some remaining tendency to stutter" in all subjects, particularly those who said they recovered after 13 years of age. It was reported that the "factor which most of the subjects (69%) felt had helped or would help in the recovery from stuttering was speaking more slowly (p.289). Interestingly, reduced speaking rate was usually mentioned in connection with some other activity. Typical responses were: 'I tried not to speak until I was ready to slow down', 'I began to realise the problem at that age and tried to talk slower', 'I slowed down and tried to pronounce things more deliberately', and 'speak more slowly and think about what you are going to say' '' (p.289). The relationship between these reasons and some procedures currently used in stuttering treatment is, as was mentioned, quite striking. Among the other factors that subjects reported to be of assistance were: "Thinking before speaking (43%); achieving greater self-confidence (26%); becoming more aware of the problem (22%); speaking more deliberately (20%) and relaxing (19%)" (1965, p.289). Against this background, it is fascinating to find that the authors concluded that their data supported treatments which use "development of adequacy and self-confidence, relaxation, and particularly with older children—greater understanding of the problem" (1965, p.290). Almost unbelievably, the gains possible from speech rate control procedures were literally ignored, seemingly to the benefit of more theoretically acceptable methods.

In a somewhat older group of recovered stutterers, Wingate (1964) reported generally similar findings to those obtained by Shearer and Williams. Nevertheless, these studies differed in important ways. The most important was that 28 of the 50 subjects (17-54 years) in Wingate's study had received professional assistance: 22 reported that it was "beneficial," although only seven (25%) said that it was "the important factor in recovery." But, since almost half the recovered stutterers indicated that therapy was an aid, it is difficult to disentangle the contribution of treatment to the recovery rate. Wingate concluded that there were "major" and "secondary" factors that subjects said aided their recovery. The main factor appeared to be a "change in attitude." This was followed by speech practice in either varying situations or by use of control methods, changing the environment, and relaxation. (Incidentally, more subjects nominated speech practice rather than therapy as being most helpful to recovery.) Wingate (1976) observed that: "For most of these subjects recovery was not a passive process, and there are many clear assertions of commitment and application. The obvious implication is that personal motivation was one important factor common to efforts of many of these subjects" (pp.102-103). Speech control procedures, such as speaking slowly, were certainly mentioned by some subjects, but they were not prominent reasons, although they may have been involved in the therapy procedures that were reported to aid many subjects.

In contrast to Wingate's finding is a report by Quarrington (1977) on 27 recovered stutterers who had not received professional assistance. The report revealed a high incidence of subjects who used a modified manner of speaking to aid their recovery. Twenty of these subjects attributed their recovery to either a changed attitude or a "new approach to the mechanics of speaking." But all 20 said they had made some specific change in their method of speaking. These changes were "speaking slowly," "talking more clearly," or "speaking in a deeper and firmer voice."

Conclusions on Recovery-Only Studies

When the studies on recovered stutterers are compared, it becomes clear that speech control procedures figure largely among the reasons that subjects have identified as responsible for their improved speech. This factor is not always identified as the sole factor and may be closely related to a change in the subject's attitude towards his or her difficulty. This is particularly evident among adult subjects, which suggests that the high rate of "spontaneous recovery" in adult subjects is a byproduct of a self-managed (often self-designed) treatment based on a modified method of speaking. Another frequently mentioned factor in these studies is that the recovery process was usually very gradual: some of the most interesting anecdotal accounts of recovery refer to a constant and systematically managed program. In this respect, they share a great deal in common with many currently advocated therapy programs.

General Conclusion

The general conclusion that emerges from the so-called spontaneous recovery literature is almost inescapable—for many stutterers a program of specific speech modification, constantly managed and associated with substantial practice, probably aids recovery and is largely responsible for "spontaneous remission." The self-assisting aids that adult subjects claim to use with success are also frequently advocated by the parents of many children who stutter. These aids may well be largely responsible for recovery in adulthood, although this is less likely to be the principal reason for recovery in childhood. Presumably, the motives that older-age stutterers have for improving their speech are not found as commonly among children. That should not be surprising. But whatever the crucial factor is in childhood recovery, it is obvious that a direct attack on the problem is not necessarily deleterious.

The implications of these findings are quite important for treatment. To begin with, it is apparent that treatment in childhood is not likely to exacerbate the problem, and may even be desirable. Parents should be told that drawing attention to their child's problem will not result in irreparable (or even repairable) damage. In fact, it is probably wiser for parents to be told how to manage their direct "interventions" in a much more systematic and effective fashion. The evidence that "slowing down," careful articulation, and speech practice are likely to be beneficial is an important element in the management of stuttering in all age groups. It could be embodied in advice that is given to parents, and recognized as a useful ingredient within treatment programs. It will be seen in the following chapters that many of the apparently successful treatment procedures have employed very much related methods. It is surely time to reject the notion that recovery may be a passive, spontaneous process. There is quite sufficient evidence that it is anything but spontaneous.

References

Andrews, G.J. & Harris, M. *The syndrome of stuttering.* London: Heinemann, 1964.

Bloodstein, 0. *A handbook on stuttering.* (3rd ed.), Chicago: National Easter Seal Society, 1981.

Bryne, M. A follow-up study of one thousand cases of stutterers from the Minneapolis Public Schools. *Proceeding of the American Society for the Study of Disordered Speech,* 1931.

Cooper, E.B. Recovery from stuttering in a junior and senior high school population. *Journal of Speech and Hearing Research,* 1972, *15,* 632-638.

Cooper, E.B., Parris, R., & Wells, M. Prevalence of and recovery from speech disorders in a group of freshmen at the University of Alabama. *Asha,* 1974, *16,* 359-360.

Dickson, S. Incipient stuttering and spontaneous remission of stuttered speech. *Journal of Communication Disorders,* 1971, *4,* 99-110.

Egolf, D.B., Shames, G.H., Johnson, P.R., & Kasprisin-Burelli, A. The use of parent-child interaction patterns in therapy for young stutterers. *Journal of Speech and Hearing Disorders,* 1972, *37,* 222-232.

Fritzell, B. The prognosis of stuttering in school children. A 10-year longitudinal study. *In XVIth International Congress on Logopedics and Phoniatrics, Interlaken 1974.* Basel: Karger, 128-131, 1976.

Glasner, P.J., & Rosenthal, D. Parental diagnosis of stuttering in young children. *Journal of Speech and Hearing Disorders,* 1957, *22,* 288-295.

Greenberg, J.B. The effect of a metronome on the speech of young stutterers. *Behavior Therapy,* 1970, *1,* 240-244.

Horowitz, E. A follow-up study of former stutterers. *Speech Pathology and Therapy.* 1962, *5,* 25-33.

Ingham, R.J. "Onset, prevalence, and recovery from stuttering": A reassessment of findings from the Andrews and Harris study. *Journal of Speech and Hearing Disorders,* 1976, *41,* 280-281.

Ingham, R.J. Spontaneous remission of stuttering: When will the emperor realize he has no clothes on? In D. Prins & R.J. Ingham (Eds.), *Treatment of stuttering in early childhood: Methods and issues.* San Diego: College-Hill Press, 1983.

Jameson, A.N. Stammering in children—some factors in the prognosis. *Speech.* 1955, *19,* 60-67.

Johnson, W. A study of the onset and development of stuttering. In W. Johnson (Ed.), *Stuttering in children and adults.* Minneapolis: Univeristy of Minnesota Press, 1955.

Johnson, W., & Associates. *The onset of stuttering.*Minneapolis: University of Minnesota Press, 1959.

Lankford, S.B., & Cooper, E.B. Recovery from stuttering as viewed by parents of self-diagnosed recovered stutterers. *Journal of Communication Disorders,* 1974, *7,* 171-180.

Martin, R.R., Kuhl, P., & Haroldson, S.K. An experimental treatment with two preschool stuttering children. *Journal of Speech and Hearing Research,* 1972, *15,* 743-752.

Martyn, M., & Sheehan, J.G. Onset of stuttering and recovery. *Behaviour Research and Therapy,* 1968, *6,* 295-307.

Milisen, R. A comparative study of stutterers, former stutterers, changed handedness normal speakers and articulation cases. *Proceedings of the American Speech and Hearing Association,* 1936, *6,* 168-177.

Milisen, R., & Johnson, W. A comparative study of stutterers, former stutterers and normal speakers whose handedness has been changed. *Archives of Speech,* 1936, *1,* 61-86.

Morley, M.E. *The development and disorders of speech in childhood.* Edinburgh: Churchill Livingstone, 1972.

Panelli, C.A., McFarlane, S.C., & Shipley, K.G. Implications of evaluating and intervening with incipient stutterers. *Journal of Fluency Disorders,* 1978, *3,* 41-50.

Porfert, A.R., & Rosenfield, D.B. Prevalence of stuttering. *Journal of Neurology, Neurosurgery and Psychiatry,* 1978, *41,* 954-956.

Prins, D., & Ingham, R.J. (Eds.), *Treatment of stuttering in early childhood: Methods and issues.* San Diego: College-Hill Press, 1983.

Quarrington, B. How do the various theories of stuttering facilitate our therapeutic approach? *Journal of Communication Disorders,* 1977, *10,* 77-83.

Reed, C.G., & Godden, A.L. An experimental treatment using verbal punishment with two preschool stutterers. *Journal of Fluency Disorders,* 1977, *2,* 225-233.

Sander, E.K. Frequency of syllable repetitions and "stutterer" judgments. *Journal of Speech and Hearing Disorders,* 1963, *28,* 19-30.

Sander, E.K. Comments on investigating listener reaction to speech disfluency. *Journal of Speech and Hearing Disorders,* 1965, *30,* 159-165.

Sander, E.K. Interrelations among the responses of mothers to a child's disfluencies. *Speech Monographs,* 1968, *35,* 187-195.

Shames, G.H., & Beams, H.L. Incidence of stuttering in older age groups. *Journal of Speech and Hearing Disorders,* 1956, *21,* 313-316.

Shearer, W.M., & Williams, J.D. Self-recovery from stuttering. *Journal of Speech and Hearing Disorders,* 1965, *30,* 288-290.

Sheehan, J.G. Current issues on stuttering and recovery. In H.H. Gregory (Ed.), *Controversies about stuttering therapy.* Baltimore: University Park Press, 1979.

Sheehan, J.G. & Martyn, M. Spontaneous recovery from stuttering. *Journal of Speech and Hearing Research,* 1966, *9,* 121-135.

Sheehan, J.G. & Martyn, M. Stuttering and its disappearance. *Journal of Speech and Hearing Research,* 1970, *13,* 279-289.

Villarreal, J. The semantic aspects of stuttering in nonstutterers: Additional data. *Quarterly Journal of Speech,* 1945, *31,* 477-479.

Voelker, C.H. On the semantic aspects of stuttering in nonstutterers. *Quarterly Journal of Speech,* 1942, *28,* 78-80.

Wingate, M.E. Recovery from stuttering. *Journal of Speech and Hearing Disorders,* 1964, *29,* 312-321.

Wingate, M.E. The fear of stuttering. *Asha,* 1971, *13,* 3-5.

Wingate, M.E. *Stuttering: Theory and treatment.* New York: Irvington, 1976.

Young, M.A. Onset, prevalence, and recovery from stuttering. *Journal of Speech and Hearing Disorders,* 1975, *40,* 49-58.

5

Rhythmic-Stimulation Procedures

Introduction

The literature on the history of stuttering treatment makes for enlightening and sobering reading. It should be almost mandatory reading for any clinician who believes that the current procedures represent significant and original advances in stuttering treatment. This should have become evident during the course of the brief review of procedures that formed the nonbehavioral preparadigm. But it becomes starkly obvious by reading accounts of earlier treatments in sources such as Klingbeil (1939), Clark (1964), and, especially, Van Riper (1973). Among the procedures that are currently employed in the behavioral preparadigm, none has had a longer and less illustrious career than those using rhythmic stimulation or syllabized speech. It has been known for centuries that almost all stutterers completely lose their problem (at least temporarily) whenever they are induced to speak in time to a rhythmic stimulus (usually 90 beats-per-minute or less). The same effect occurs when they are asked to alter their customary speech pattern so that each word or syllable is emphasized to form a distinctive rhythmic speech pattern. One form of speech pattern that uses this procedure is quite descriptively known as "syllable-timed speech."

The use of rhythmic stimulation in treatment has been traced back to the third century B.C., when Satyrus the Greek actor was said to have treated Demosthenes by, among other things, declaiming while walking uphill (Klingbeil, 1939). Van Riper (1973) suggsts that this meas that he was required to speak to the accompaniment of a regular stimulus—his footsteps. There are more definitive descriptions of the use of rhythm within stuttering treatments, reportedly in use during the late eighteenth and early nineteenth centuries. Klingbeil (1939) reviewed many of the therapy reports from that era and suggests that two Frenchmen, Serre d'Atais and Dupuytren were independently using rhythmic stimulation to treat stuttering. This appears to have been affected via a foot-tapping technique. At about the same time in England, John Thelwall, who was himself a stutterer, devised a treatment based on speaking in time to a self-imposed rhythm. Another Frenchman, Colombat de L'Isère, is usually credited with the development of the first mechanical rhythmic stimulation device for the treatment of stuttering. This predecessor to the metronome was known as the "muthonome." It even received the Monthyon prize from the French Academy.

Thereafter, similar devices appear to have been used in different ways by various clinicians, including those who managed the much-maligned commercial "Stuttering Schools" (Clark, 1964). Subsequently, rhythm appears to have had waves of interest for clinicians. The latest began in the 1960s with interest in its therapeutic possibilities for a behavior therapy. Some experimental investigations were also designed to determine whether the rhythm effect is related to other conditions known to modify stuttering. Currently, this latest wave has broken and a trough of disinterest is returning. Van Riper's observations on the recurring interest in rhythmic stimulation treatment is quite pertinent:

> Any method which for at least a century and a half has failed so consistently to produce any real cure for stuttering and still manages to be used so widely must have something pretty vital in it. We think that vitality resides in the fact that it works. Yes, temporarily and unfortunately it works! (Van Riper, 1973, p. 63)

So, what is the evidence that it works, and what are the explanations for its ameliorative, though transient, effects?

Review of Experimental Studies

There is overwhelming evidence in the literature that stuttering is reduced when stutterers speak in rhythmic stimulation conditions. Stutterers are also well aware of this effect. Bloodstein's (1950) survey of stutterers found that more than 90% of his respondents said that speaking in time to arm swinging, walking, a rhythmic twist of the wrist, or rhythmic foot tapping produced "hardly any stuttering. . .[or] no stuttering at all."

The extent to which rhythmic stimulation reduces stuttering is also evident in Johnson and Rosen's (1937) evaluation of different speech patterns during oral reading conditions. They had 18 stutterers orally read different 500-word passages under such conditions as fast and slow reading rate, whispering, vocal level changes, singing, changes in inflection, chorus reading, accompanying a metronome, and accompanying an arm swing. During oral reading conditions, the stutterers produced a median percentage of words stuttered which ranged from 7.6% to 3.5% (across three readings). When the subjects spoke to the accompaniment of a metronome beat, their stuttering was reduced to 0.06%. During the arm-swing condition, they were asked to speak one syllable at a time, and reduced their stuttering to 0.01%. They were also asked to speak so that they alternated a high and low pitch pattern on consecutive syllables. This rather rhythmical, syllable-timed pattern achieved a reduction to 0.09%. During the metronome condition, the subjects actually spoke at a 59.1% slower rate than during their control readings, although there was only a 45.3% reduction during the slow-reading conditions. Slow reading produced 1.3% words stuttered.

The Johnson and Rosen (1937) study is rather remarkable in many respects. It is something of a landmark report on the effects of speech pattern alterations on stuttering behavior. It also provides data that relates to most of the parameters that have been examined with respect to rhythmic speech; these include altered speech rate, accompanied and unaccompanied stimulus conditions, and accompanying words or syllables to a rhythmic stimulus. The experimenters also suggested that the effect is due to distraction.

In later studies which used oral reading under rhythmic stimulation conditions, similar reductions in stuttering have been reported. Barber (1940) assessed the effect of a variety of rhythmic stimulation conditions (walking, foot tapping, arm swinging, wrist movement, sing-song rhythm, accenting every word, and accenting every third word). She also compared the effect of a metronome set at 92 beats-per-minute (bpm) and at 184 bpm on oral reading of 500-word passages. It was reported that both bpm rates achieved about a 98% reduction in stuttering. Fransella and Beech (1965) used only a 50-word passage, and Brady (1969) employed three-minute readings with bpm rates in approximately the same range. Not surprisingly, both of these studies reported more modest reductions in stuttering (54.9% and 49% respectively).

During spontaneous speech conditions, the effect of rhythmic stimulation is also reported to be substantial. Azrin, Jones, and Flye (1968) found an average 85% reduction in stuttering across four subjects using a 90 bpm vibrotactile stimulus, while Martin and Haroldson (1979) found a mean 75% reduction in stuttering across 20 adult subjects, during 90 bpm audio stimulus conditions.

By now, it should be evident that the rhythm effect appears to be independent of the stimulus medium. Experimentally contrived comparisons have confirmed that this is so. Barber (1940) compared an audio, visual, and tactile system of delivering rhythmic stimulation during oral reading and found no significant differences[1] between the mean percentage of words stuttered among 19 subjects. Unhappily, Barber did not control the bpm rate in any of these conditions. However, Brady (1969) did so, and found that a 90 bpm stimulus, which was delivered either auditorily, visually or tactilely, produced on average no difference in the rhythm effect on oral reading (although two subjects failed to respond to the tactile conditions).

A comparison between internally (or self-generated) rhythmic conditions and externally delivered rhythmic stimulation on speech was partially investigated by Johnson and Rosen (1937) and Barber (1940). In both studies, their subjects used arm swinging or a sing-song speech pattern as the self-generated condition. These conditions produced reductions in stuttering that were comparable to those obtained using a metronome.

The duration of stimulus conditions does not appear to be a significant factor in the rhythm effect. In some studies, the comparisons between metronome and nonmetronome conditions have yielded effects when as few as 50 words (Fransella & Beech, 1965) or three minutes of oral reading (Brady, 1969) have been required. At the other extreme, Silverman and Umberger (1974) had subjects speak for between four and eight hours, and 75% of that time was spent

[1]It is important to note that a large number of comparisons were made using *t* tests. This could have inflated the probability that some significant differences would be found.

wearing an earpiece metronome. This study found no evidence that the rhythm effect (on disfluency categories) "carried over" to nonmetronome conditions in any substantial way. The clinical implications of such a finding are fairly obvious.

Some other aspects associated with the modality of stimulus conditions have been assessed. These include the effects of an audience and instructions. Barber (1940) found that five of her subjects produced roughly the same metronome effect when reading orally before a class of students as when they read alone. In another group setting, Greenberg (1970) demonstrated not only the effect of rhythmic stimulation, but, also, that the effect may not depend upon instructions. A group of 20 stutterers (9-11 years) were asked to describe a display of toys. Half of the subjects were instructed to pace their speech for five minutes to a 98 bpm metronome, and the other half were given no instructions other than to continue their description while an auditory metronome was active. They were recorded for five minutes in this condition and three minutes in nonmetronome conditions (these preceded and followed the metronome conditions). The results are shown in Table 5.1 along with results of a replication of this experiment which Greenberg conducted with 20 nonstuttering children.

TABLE 5.1
Summary of results in Greenberg's (1970)* experiment on the effect of instructing and not instructing stutterers or nonstutterers to speak to the accompaniment of a metronome (98 bpm).

Subjects	*Conditions*	*% DYSFLUENCIES*		
		No Metronome (3 min.)	*Metronome (5 min.)*	*No Metronome (3 min.)*
Stuttering Group	No Instructions (n=10	6.33	3.32	7.45
	Instructions (n=10)	8.08	3.80	7.39
Nonstuttering Group	No Instructions (n=10)	0.30	0.17	0.10
	Instructions (n=10)	0.70	0.29	0.36

* Adapted from Greenberg (1970, p. 242).

The two stuttering groups did not show a difference in "metronome effect" on their dysfluent (sic) speech. The overall effect amounted to a reduction of more than 50% in percent dysfluencies. However both of the nonstuttering groups showed no evidence of a metronome treatment effect. Greenberg also reported that the reductions in dysfluencies during metronome conditions were not associated with reductions in speech rate.

Explanations for the "Rhythm Effect"

The explanations that have been offered for the rhythm effect have included "distraction," simplified motor planning, altered speech rate, predictability of response, and altered vocalization. The research evidence which has been mustered in support of these explanations will be considered below. First, it is worth taking into account what is sought by an "explanation of the rhythm effect."

The usual notion of an explanatory model is that it provides a common factor(s) which interrelates a number of different findings. In effect, what appears to be a unique phenomenon may simply be a predictable response to a more common factor. The difficulty in applying this type of model to the rhythm effect is that it assumes that the effect is a unitary one, and that the sought-after common factor is also unitary: neither is necessarily true. Indeed, this will become quite evident with respect to the explanatory models which have been offered on behalf of the rhythm effect. On the other hand, the virtue of a viable explanatory model, particularly with respect to this type of phenomenon, is that it offers the prospect of predicting the most useful application of the model. This would obviously have a great deal of clinical value.

The "Distraction" Hypothesis

The "distraction hypothesis" has been used by many researchers (for example, Barber, 1940; Johnson & Rosen, 1937) to explain the rhythm effect. it is not at all clear where this hypothesis emerged from (maybe Fletcher, 1928), or what it actually involves. Van Riper (1973), for example, points out that it refers to any effect that is produced when the speaker's attention to his speech is diverted by a novel way of speaking. Presumably, the novel speech pattern, or its unusual sound, diverts the subject's attention from his customary manner of speaking. The difficulty with this explanation is that it is vulnerable to circularity: in the absence of independent measures of the focus of attention, the only evidence we have of "distracted attention" are the novel speech pattern and changed stuttering. Another problem with this explanation is that there are striking differences in the amounts of reduction in stuttering which occur with different speech patterns. At least one of these patterns, fast speaking (Johnson & Rosen, 1937), may not even reduce stuttering. The retort offered to save the distraction hypothesis (Bloodstein, 1975) is that any differences in reductions in stuttering among the various novel conditions may simply reflect different levels of distraction. In other words, some conditions such as rhythm and singing, may be more powerful distractors than are others—such as masking. Masking reduces stuttering, but it rarely produces reductions as great as those achieved by rhythm (Martin & Haroldson, 1979). This saving retort also reeks of circularity: it presumes the very conditions it is supposed to prove. It presumes that these conditions are more or less distracting. Incidentally, it is also difficult to accept that masking (sometimes at 140 dB SPL) would not completely remove the subject's attention from his speech.

Some attempts have been made to test the distraction hypothesis by having the stutterer perform a task while speaking, and then comparing the subject's performance with that found during rhythmic stimulation. Fransella (1967) had stutterers (n=18) write down numbers, which were fed through a headset at 1- to 4-second intervals during oral reading of a 50-word passage. The subjects' "speech errors" in this condition were compared with those found during readings with either no auditory stimulation, or while speaking to the accompaniment of a metronome (bpm rate not specified). The results indicated that the subsidiary task and the nonmetronome conditions were not significantly different, while the metronome condition produced a 61% reduction in speech errors. Brady (1969) essentially replicated Fransella's (1967) study using 10 subjects, a 90 bpm metronome condition, and an identical subsidiary task: he obtained an identical finding. The criticism that Bloodstein (1975) has ably directed at these tests of the distraction hypothesis is that distraction may have occurred in the opposite direction—it is entirely possible that the subjects' speaking behavior may have distracted the writing task, rather than vice versa.

Another test of the distraction hypothesis has been through comparisons between the effects of arhythmic and rhythmic stimulation conditions. It is presumed that both conditions should be equally diverting, and any differences in their effects on stuttering would be due to differences in the stimulus pattern. Three studies have reported this type of comparison: Fransella & Beech (1965), Azrin, Jones, & Flye (1968) and Brady (1969).

Fransella and Beech (1965) assessed the effect of a rhythmic stimulus (set at individually calibrated silent-reading rates), a comparable arhythmic stimulus rate, and a nonstimulus condition on the oral reading of 18 adult stutterers. Each of these conditions was also compared under "usual" oral reading speed and a "slow" oral reading speed (not specified). Azrin, Jones, and Flye (1968) had four adult stutterers read orally under rhythmic and arhythmic tactile stimulus conditions. These conditions were also compared with no-stimulus conditions. The results of both of these studies are shown in Table 5.2, along with those reported by Brady (1969). In Brady's study, 12 adult stutterers spoke spontaneously under a 120 bpm auditory metronome rhythmic condition, an arhythmic condition, and a nonmetronome condition. The important difference between Brady's study and the other studies is that Brady's subjects were "instructed to pace one syllable of speech to each tick." But in the Fransella and Beech study, and the Azrin et al. study, subjects were told to accompany either words *or* syllables to the stimulus. This appears to be an obvious explanation for Brady's finding that the arhythmic and the rhythmic conditions did not produce significant differences in the number of dysfluencies. (But it should not be overlooked that the subjects in Brady's study used spontaneous speech, while subjects in the other studies used oral reading).

The above mentioned findings suggest that the distraction hypothesis is under considerable pressure. It can resist this pressure in the argument that the syllabized pattern, which must have been evident in Brady's arhythmic condition, is just as "distracting" as the rhythmic condition. But it seems far more expedient at this point to bypass the distraction hypothesis and look at these findings as providing evidence of another dimension in the rhythm effect.

TABLE 5.2
A comparison between the findings reported by Fransella & Beech (1965), Azrin, Jones, & Flye (1968), and Brady (1969) on the effects of arhythmic and rhythmic stimulation on stuttering.

STUDY	*MEASURE*	*SPEECH MODE*	*MEAN SCORES IN EACH TREATMENT CONDITION*		
			No Stimulus	*Rhythmic Stimulus*	*Arhythmic Stimulus*
Fransella & Beech (1965) (n=18)	"Errors"	Oral Reading "usual rate" "slow rate"	23.06 20.11	10.83 9.06	19.06 17.83
Azin, Jones,& Flye (1968) (n=4)	"Percent Stutterings"	Oral Reading	28.42	2.67	30.05
Brady (1969) (n=12)	"Dysfluencies"	Spontaneous Speech	12.58	1.58	2.58

Some Multidimensional Aspects in a Rhythm Effect Hypothesis

The effect on stuttering of syllabizing, or using syllable-timed speech, obviously does not depend upon an external stimulus, such as a metronome. It is quite possible that this is yet another speech pattern which may occur within the rhythm effect. Indeed, it might be one of many patterns. This becomes apparent when some of the rhythm effect experiments are examined closely.

It appears that the amount of "patterning" in the subject's speech during some rhythmic stimulation conditions may vary greatly, but the effect still occurs. Jones and Azrin (1969) had four stutterers read orally for five minutes under nine different stimulus duration conditions. They used vibrotactile stimulus (250 Hz) of different duration on the bony portion of each subject's wrist. In the first condition, the subject experienced a rhythmic stimulus that had 0.1 seconds duraton and was then followed by a one-second pause interval. The other eight conditions all used a one-second pause interval between the stimulus events, but the stimulus duration was either 0.5, 1.0, 2.0, 3.0, 5.0, 10, 20, or 300 seconds. One-minute speech samples were rated as "natural" or "unnatural" by a group of 12 judges. The findings showed that the percentage-of-naturalness ratings reached a peak with stimulus duration levels that ranged from one to five seconds. The subjects' stuttering was at zero or close to zero during most of these condition (1.0 to 5.0 seconds stimulus duration).

Jones and Azrin (1969) provide some graphic indications of the markedly different speech patterns that subjects adopted under each of these duration conditions in their experiment. One subject's printout shows that at a duration of 0.1 seconds, one word accompanied each pulse, while at 2.0 seconds duration, between two and 10 words accompanied a stimulus pulse.

The only data available on self-regulated change in a rhythmic pattern is provided in Barber's (1940) study. In one condition, subjects were asked to read with an accent on every third word (a waltz time!). This condition produced more than a 50% reduction in stuttering, but this was much less than that achieved during other rhythmic stimulation conditions.

In general, therefore, when we "look across" the rhythm effect, it is possible to discern effects associated with syllabizing, melodic stressing of words, and, perhaps (as demonstrated by Jones and Azrin), intermittant pausing between clusters of words. There can be little doubt, however, that all these patterns involve an alteration in the speaker's customary manner of speaking.

The Speech-Rate Hypothesis

Another factor that has been thought to explain rhythm effect is reduced speech rate. But there is now ample evidence that the effect is independent of speech rate —either slow or fast. Fransella and Beech (1965), as previously mentioned, compared the effect of a "slow" and "usual" rate of oral reading under comparable "slow" and "usual" rhythmic stimulation rates. It was found that substantial reductions in stuttering were associated with the "slow" condition, but they were independent of reduced speech rate (see Table 5.2). Brady (1969) also conducted an experiment in which the bpm rate was calibrated to each subject's usual reading rate. Under these conditions (the subject's speech rate was virtually unchanged by the rhythmic conditions), there was a reduction of more than 50% "dysfluencies" during the rhythmic stimulus conditions. Azrin, Jones, and Flye (1968) also reported that one of their four subjects actually increased his oral reading rate during rhythmic stimulus conditions. Hanna and Morris (1977) compared the effects of metronome rates set at 25% above each subject's (n=6) basal articulation rate (Perkins, 1975), at their base rate, and at 50% below their base rate during oral-reading conditions. They found that the slow, normal, and fast metronome conditions produced nonsignificant differences in mean number of stutterings, and all were at least 65% below the stuttering rates found in nonstimulus conditions.

The Predictability Hypothesis

Yet another explanatory model was offered by Beech and Fransella (1968). They argued that the regular stimulus signal increases the "predictability" with which the stutterer must utter a sound. Fransella (1971) tested this proposition by comparing the frequency of speech errors both when the subject knew he would have to produce a word and when he did not know it would be required. The "predictability condition" was associated with a marginally lower level of stuttering, but not sufficient to regard it as likely to explain the substantial reductions that occur during rhythmic stimulation.

The Modified-Vocalization Hypothesis

The most popular explanation for the rhythm effect is the modified vocalization hypothesis offered by Wingate (1969). The essence of this hypothesis is that rhythm, and many other fluency-inducing conditions, share in common the characteristic of inducing the stutterer to alter his customary manner of speaking and emphasize vocalization. With respect to rhythmic stimulation, Wingate claims that the speaker

> (a) is induced to express a pattern of stresses which he (b) executes in at least a partially intentional manner, (c) guided by focusing on syllable nuclei and (d) implemented through emphasis on phonation. In short, the process is organized around the production of a melody which is actualized through emphasis on vocalization (p. 680).

The mention of emphasized phonation in this description has been responsible, in part, for a stream of research evaluating the extent to which abnormal phonation is associated with stuttering. More particularly this research has been concerned to determine whether modified phonatory behavior is related to the rhythm effect and other fluency-inducing conditions.[2]

There is little doubt that rhythmic stimulation does induce an alteration in the customary manner of speaking. The distinguishing feature of rhythmic speech is that it is an unusual manner of speaking, although it is not altogether clear that it need be unnatural sounding (see Jones and Azrin, 1969). Some attempts have been made, however, to identify the parameters of speech behavior that are significantly associated with any changes that occur during rhythmic stimulation. Brayton and Conture (1978) assessed the effects of noise and rhythmic stimulation on vocal fundamental frequency, vowel duration, and vocal level. They had nine stutterers (15-22 years) read different 1,000-word passages under a control condition, during rhythmic stimulation conditions (a 60 bpm auditory stimulus), and noise stimulation (95dB SPL continuous white noise). Only the rhythmic stimulation and control condition data will be dealt with at this time. Comparisons were made between the subjects' production of 16 monosyllabic CVC target words that occurred in each passage (i.e., in each condition). The results showed that rhythmic stimulation condition was associated with a significantly greater reduction in frequency of stuttering than was the noise condition. It was

[2] Wingate (1979) has recently pointed out that many of these endeavors have assumed a direct association between phonation and vocalization and this has led to a misguided interpretation of his original hypothesis. In operational terms, it would appear that Wingate argues that "altered vocalization" involves more than a modification in the manner of producing a glottal sound.

also found that vowel duration increased by more than 90% in the rhythmic stimulation condition (the increase was nonsignificant in the noise condition).

In another study on the effect of rhythmic stimulation on speech parameters, Hutchinson and Navarre (1977) measured five aerodynamic dimensions in the speech of five adult stutterers and five adult nonstutterers during oral reading in control and metronome pacing conditions (60 bpm auditory stimulus). The five dimensions were (1) peak intraoral air pressure, (2) intraoral air pressure onset duration, (3) intraoral air pressure offset duration, (4) total intraoral air pressure duration, and (5) peak air flow rate. From comparisons between consonants (12 consonants, each in three syllable-initial stressed positions), it was found that stutterers and normals tended to demonstrate lower peak pressures and greater pressure durations during the metronome conditions. But there was also a tendency for the air flow rates of the normal subjects to increase, and to decrease for stutterers. The results are consistent with the notion that the duration of the phonated element in the subject's speech is increased during the metronome conditions, although no explanation is offered for the different pattern of airflow rates in both groups. There are, however, some problems with both the Brayton and Conture, and the Hutchinson and Navarre studies which make it difficult to know whether changes they found are relevant to metronome pacing.

The Hutchinson and Navarre (1977) study is characterized by a complete absence of analyses of the differences between the measures obtained under the metronome pacing and control conditions. The graphic presentation of the data[3] reveals ample overlap between the range of scores except in the case of the air pressure onset duration. But more importantly, both the Hutchinson and Navarre study and the Brayton and Conture study failed to control for the substantial changes that may have occurred between the control reading and the metronome condition, because of reduced speech rate. Both studies used a 60 bpm treatment rate. This rate is equivalent to the word-per-minute rate which Adams, Lewis, and Besozzi (1973) imposed on stutterers in assessing the effect of reduced rate on stuttering. They found that this rate produced a 50% reduction in the median amount of stuttering during oral reading. In other words, at this very slow rate of reading reduced stuttering would be expected, and any changes in speech parameters may be due to a reduced reading rate rather than rhythmic stimulation.

Andrews, Howie, Dozsa, and Guitar (1982) used a 90 bpm stimulus to train three adult male stutterers to use "syllable-timed rhythmic speech," and reported that this produced a mean 91% decrease in stuttering. They produced some confusing data relative to the notion that the procedure would emphasize phonation. The subjects' speech was analysed for phonation duration and pause proportions via an apparatus developed by Goldman-Eisler (1968). The combined data revealed that, relative to base rate, their phonation duration was markedly reduced, but the proportion of pausing remained unchanged. On closer examination, however, one of the subjects actually increased mean phonation duration and used about the

[3]These data are difficult to interpret since three of the figures in this chapter are incorrectly labeled.

same pause proportions. Of course, these data do not yield information on vocal intensity, which may well be involved in Wingate's notion that the procedure emphasizes phonation.

It is worth mentioning at this point that research in this area almost cries out for the use of carefully managed single-subject experimentation. There is a need to look at the effect, on all parameters, of systematic alterations to the rate of rhythmic stimulation, and, perhaps, the duration of the stimulus. This seems to be the only way in which it will be possible to disentangle the multitude of variables which appear to be associated with the "rhythm effect."

Some Other Explanatory Hypotheses

At least two other hypothesis have also been offered to explain the rhythm effect. Van Riper (1971) has hypothesized that it works "because it facilitates the timing of motoric patterns which are prone to asynchrony." In other words, the external timing device seems to integrate the motoric patterning necessary to perform any skill. A typical example would be the way a golf swing or music helps to keep a sequence of motor movements smoothly organized. This explanation is also related to one offered by Azrin, Jones, and Flye (1968), who claim that because stuttering is essentially a disorder of rhythm, then a procedure which restores this rhythm should thereby improve fluency. They argue that both verbal and nonverbal behavior has a tendency to respond to rhythmic stimulation. Therefore, when such stimulation occurs in the presence of stuttering, the normal rhythmic character of the speech is achieved. The experimental assessment of both hypotheses awaits a researcher who is sufficiently inventive to operationalize these concepts.

Speech Quality and Rhythmic Speech

One final issue that merits comment is the abnormal sound quality of rhythmic speech. The clinical implications of this characteristic are obvious, and will be considered in relation to therapy applications of this method. But some experimental studies have provided useful information on this matter. The previously-mentioned Jones and Azrin (1969) study revealed that certain types of rhythmic stimulation conditions may be associated with either more or less natural-sounding speech (at least in the case of four stutterers). Evidently, when the duration of the rhythmic stimulus interval is less than one second (in conditions where the pause between each stimulus is one second), then the subject's speech may be stutter-free, but definitely "not natural." At duration intervals of between one and five seconds, these ratings showed a rise to around 60% to 80% "natural" judgments.

Silverman and Trotter (1973) made a rather questionable comparison between the levels of "adverse reaction" to rhythmic speech and stuttered speech. The subjects (four adult stutterers) used a self-chosen bpm rate and the observers

(N=8) rated video samples of their speech (with and without the metronome assistance) on the Iowa Scale of Stuttering and the Semantic Differential Scale. However, even though their fluency improved in the rhythm condition, at least one subject was rated to have more adverse qualities in his speech during this condition. A rather identical result was reported by Mallard and Meyer (1979) in a similar videotape study with three stutterers. They had 23 naive judges rate their preference for samples drawn from conditions in which the stutterers were either not accompanied by rhythmic stimulation, or the stimulus beat was set at either 70 or 100 bpm. Once again, the judges found that in one subject the unaccompanied sample (presumably with more stuttering) was the preferred sample. But, in general, they indicated a preference for the samples drawn from 100 bpm conditions.

Both of the above-mentioned studies suggest that listeners regarded the stuttered speech of some stutterers as more acceptable than the speech pattern which removed their problem. It is quite likely that stutterers have similar reactions to this speech, and, in turn, this may influence its acceptability in clinical conditions.

Conclusions on Experimental Studies

The overall conclusion from this review is that rhythmic stimulation or speech patterns which emphasize a rhythmic pattern may be responsible for either partial or complete elimination of stuttering among adults and children. The effect appears to be unrelated to alterations in speech rate, but may depend on a number of different patterns that have been found to accompany these conditions. These include syllabizing, pausing, and clustering of phrases between regular pauses. The explanations for its effect remain unclear. It undoubtedly depends on an altered manner of speaking, but the extent of alteration which is critical to its effect is still obscure. To some extent, the speech pattern which occurs under this condition may be distinguished by degrees of "naturalness." It appears to vary from an acceptable to an unacceptable alternative to stuttering, at least as far as listeners are concerned. But this probably depends upon the form of rhythmic stimulation used. There is an obvious need to isolate the parameters of the voice signal that are associated with improved fluency under the different forms of rhythmic stimulation.

Therapy Procedures

As mentioned earlier, it would appear to any dispassionate observer of stuttering therapy practice (at least in the English-speaking world) that treatment procedures have a habit of appearing, disappearing, and reappearing in new forms. A good case can be made to support Van Riper's (1973) argument that many therapists, or, more specifically, publication-oriented clinicians, have a tendency to revive procedures which history would tell them have been found ineffectual. Such a case can be made for rhythmic speech and Van Riper (1971; 1973) has forcefully provided the argument line. His most recent argument against rhythmic stimulation was a response to the re-emergence of this procedure during the 1960s within the context of behavior therapy. It is perhaps not too early to say that he will also witness its declining use within behavior therapy. This review will attempt to trace the relatively recent rise and demise of rhythm stimulation procedures in stuttering treatment.

Many recent reviews of behavior therapy and stuttering (for example, Ingham & Andrews, 1973b; Hutchinson, 1976) have traced the emergence of rhythmic stimulation treatments in the behavioral preparadigm to a report by Van Dantzig (1940). This report of a finger-tapping technique is almost a caricature of behavior therapy, and was probably an apt comment on the many ways in which rhythmic speech was being used by clinicians during the 1930s and 1940s. In fact, there was serious interest in rhythmic procedures during this period. This is quite apparent in the previously mentioned studies by Johnson and Rosen (1937) and Barber (1940). Indeed, far from rejecting rhythmic stimulation techniques, many of the Iowa-trained clinicians actually promoted its use as a means of demonstrating to stutterers that they could achieve fluency. For example, in 1948, Johnson recommended that in treating school-age children the clinician should "try experimenting with rhythmic speech. . .to demonstrate to the speaker that his speech mechanism is in good working order — not that he should immediately expect to talk that way" (Johnson, 1948, p. 308). It is not surprising, therefore, that the method was retained by many clinicians and stutterers as a means of sustaining at least some semblance of fluency—no matter how abnormal sounding —in spite of Johnson's advice to the contrary. This advice was based on the first-hand knowledge of many of these premier clinicians that this speech was not only disfiguring, but also achieved only transient fluency. The significant point is that it never really left the clinical armamentarium of even the staunchest opponents to its use in therapy.

By tracing the origins of many recent influential rhythmic stimulation studies in stuttering therapy, it would seem that it was the practices of some English and Scottish clinicians that substantially encouraged the revival of rhythm. Brandon and Harris (1967), for example, have indicated that the methods of many "less orthodox practitioners" in that country included syllable timed speech. The effects they achieved appear to have profoundly influenced a group of researchers who were working at that time in Newcastle-upon-Tyne. This appears to be one of the two localities where rhythmic stimulaton sprang to life as a procedure used by more "orthodox" practitioners, such as Andrews, Harris, and Brandon. The other locality was London, where, at about the same time, Meyer and Mair began experimenting with a hearing-aid style electronic metronome.

Thus emerged two principal streams of clinical research on rhythmic stimulation that eventually found their way into behavior therapy approaches to stuttering. The first stream was concerned with procedures which relied on essentially unaided rhythmic speech as a method of modifying stuttering. The second stream employed either continuous or intermittent use of an electronic metronome.

Unaided Rhythmic Treatments

The report by Andrews and Harris (1964) on the use of syllable-timed (ST) speech in the group treatment of stuttering in children and adults revived interest in this type of therapy. Both the treatment format and method of evaluation have been described in other places by Andrews and some associates (Andrews, Holgate, Hopper & Ingham, 1967; Brandon & Harris, 1967; Holgate & Andrews, 1966). It also provided a description of a structure and method of stuttering therapy that appears in many behavior therapy contexts. In this structure, the group is treated in conditions where a substantial amount of their speech behavior is controlled for a short, but intensive period (perhaps 10 to 20 days). This period is followed either by weekly, bi-weekly, or monthly sessions for up to a year. This is not a new format, but it is the foundation for many stuttering treatments.

The Andrews and Harris program should not be considered seriously as an example of behavior therapy, since it was built around a rather classical medical model of treatment. Essentially this treatment had a predetermined duration, even though the subject's treatment was monitored via speech behavior measures. Neither these measures, nor any other behavior measures, however, were specified as treatment criteria. At the same time, the Andrews and Harris program has much relevance for behavior therapy, as it contains a treatment format which has been used in many behaviorally oriented treatments.

The Andrews and Harris (1964) study was based on 35 subjects who were allocated to four groups, according to their age. There were two adult groups (A1 and A2), an adolescent group (B), and a children's group (C). Each group received treatment for 10 hours each day over 10 days, within a 2-week period. During this time, they were taught ST speech by example, and then practiced it with oral reading and conversational practice at a very slow speech rate. Thereafter, their rate was incresed by clinician guidance to between 100 and 150 syllables per minutes. Certain exercises were arranged so that the subjects could gain experience in previously "difficult" speech situations. In one of the groups (A2), and in subsequent programs, subjects received a daily 1-hour session of group psychotherapy. At the end of the 10-day intensive treatment period, subjects met for 10 one-hour weekly sessions of practice or discussion. In later programs, subjects received three hours of speech therapy and group psychotherapy per week for 40 weeks.

The speech performance data collected for the Andrews and Harris study were 200-word samples made before and at the end of the 10-day treatment, and then at three-month intervals for between 6 and 12 months. The percentages of words stuttered and words spoken per minute were calculated on each of those occasions, although without the benefit of reliability data. The results indicated that the children's group (n=5) was the most successful group. They had pretreatment means of 20.4% words stuttered and 86 words per minute. Nine months after the end of the intensive phase, the corresponding scores were 0.8%

words stuttered at 108 words per minute. This result was also close to that group's performance over the three postintensive-phase assessment occasions. The adult and adolescent groups did not fare as well. The graphed data (Andrews & Harris, 1964, p. 154) suggest that the adolescent group showed a 55% reduction in mean percentage of words stuttered, with a change from 63 to 83 words per minute by the end of the 9-month postintensive phase. The data also suggest that group A2 performed better than group A1 at the 6-month assessment point (the last point of assessment for group A2). But a two-factor analysis of variance with repeated measures (Winer, 1971) conducted on these data (Ingham, 1972) reveals that this was not significant. Both of these groups reduced their mean percentage of words stuttered by 76% (A1) and 84% (A2), and achieved a mean word-per-minute rate of 89.8 (A1) and 100 (A2). From data provided in Holgate and Andrews (1966), it is possible to determine that group A2 completed their 12-month assessment with eight subjects speaking less than 5% words stuttered, but group A1 had only three subjects at this level.

The performance of group A2 led to the inclusion of group psychotherapy in the Andrews and Harris format. This was used by Holgate and Andrews (1966) throughout a 42-week program. They only reported data at the end of this treatment period, however. A comparison between data from this adult group (n=10) and that provided for group A2 indicates approximately the same level of performance. To some extent, this may also suggest that the follow-up program of group psychotherapy and speech practice was ineffectual—a finding which has some significance with respect to later research on this program.

Andrews, Holgate, Hopper, and Ingham (1967) replicated part of the Andrews and Harris (1964) study in a treatment of 10-year-old stutterers (n=10). All began treatment with over 6% words stuttered and received the intensive treatment phase, plus 90 minutes of speech practice, once a week for 13 weeks. At 12 months after treatment, seven of the 10 subjects had less than 6% words stuttered. Like the Holgate and Andrews study, however, these data were neither assessed for reliability of scoring, nor accompanied by details on how they were collected.

Brandon and Harris (1967) reported a treatment based on procedures almost identical to those reported by Andrews and Harris. The main difference was that after the intensive phase, their subjects (n=28) attended twice-weekly for 3 months, "then weekly and latterly every 3 months." Unfortunately, the duration of the treatment is not specified, nor is the method used to collect the subjects' speech data at each assessment point. It was indicated that the subjects were followed for at least 18 months, but it is not possible to deduce what part of this time was free of treatment. Unhappily, the researchers chose to report their data in terms of a peculiar measure of "success"—60% reduction in the percentage of stuttering recorded before treatment. By this liberal criterion, 64% of their subjects were "successful" at follow-up. But, again, these data were not favored with an independent assessment. Brandon and Harris also indicated that certain personality factors were likely to be associated with success. This is of questionable value in view of the dubious criteria used to judge treatment outcome.

In 1968, this writer (Ingham, 1972) established a behavioral format on the Andrews and Harris treatment program by introducing a token economy schedule. This was based on the observation that much of the activity that transpired during the 2-week intensive phase of this treatment could be scheduled to reinforce the maintenance of ST speech. Moreover, the program lent itself to systematic programming of each of the principal treatment stages under a performance-contingent schedule. The subjects received tokens for completing a prescribed number of syllables at less than a variable level of stuttering. When a criterion of fluency was achieved, subjects were then reinforced for speaking these syllables at above a prescribed syllable-per-minute speech rate. This rate was then systematically increased as the subject succeeded in speaking fluently at a criterion rate during a prescribed number of rating sessions (rating sessions were 45-minute intervals of group conversation in which each speaker had to speak a specified number of syllables). When a criterion of fluency—0% syllables stuttered (SS%) at 180 to 220 syllables per minute (SPM)—was achieved, the subject entered a sequence of speaking tasks within the hospital setting and nearby shopping areas. These speaking tasks were recorded, and the subject earned tokens for completing a prepared number of syllables within the criterion of fluency range. The tokens could be cashed for all food and drinks the subject received while in hospital. It should also be mentioned that tokens were redeemed for departures from the target behavior.

The token economy schedule used in the Andrews and Harris treatment format has been outlined in a number of places (Andrews & Ingham, 1972; Ingham, 1975; Ingham & Andrews, 1973a; Ingham, Andrews, & Winkler, 1972). It was based upon similar systems developed by Ayllon and Azrin (1965), in particular, for modifying problem behavior in hospitalized psychotic patients. These systems are now widely used and are based upon operant conditioning methodology. For this reason, many of the within-treatment findings that emerged with the application of a token economy to stuttering treatment will be considered in Chapter 9.

The token economy procedure was first employed in a series of group treatment studies reported initially by Ingham and Andrews, (1968), and then, in more detail, by Ingham, Andrews, and Winkler (1972). These reports described comparisons between groups of subjects that received different combinations of four treatment procedures. These were the token economy, syllable-timed speech, group-psychotherapy, and a variation on negative practice termed "increased stuttering." This last-mentioned technique was introduced as a method of reinforcing the use of syllable-timed speech. It was reasoned that part of the acceptance of ST speech may have been enhanced if the facilitative effects of fluent ST speech were contrasted with the debilitative effects of increased stuttering. After entering treatment, the members of some groups were required to sustain a criterion amount of speech behavior with double their stuttering base rate.

The data reported by Ingham, Andrews, and Winkler (1972) were collected from assessments made 6 months before treatment, immediately before treatment, partway through the intensive phase, and at the end of the 12 consecutive-day daily treatment program (12 hours per day). On these occasions, subjects provided 1000 syllables in response to the Iowa Job Task (Johnson, Darley & Spriestersbach, 1963), from which percentage of syllables stuttered (%SS) and syllables-per-minute (SPM) data were calculated. The most effective combination of treatments was ST speech and the token economy. This was evident in the data from a group (n=9) which entered with mean scores of 17.4 %SS at 88 SPM (this was virtually identical to their mean scores six months earlier). By the end of the intensive treatment phase, their mean scores were 0.24 %SS at 180.2 SPM. This was compared with the performance of a combination of two groups (n=20) treated by ST speech and group psychotherapy (the Andrews and Harris format). Their preintensive treatment scores were 22.4 %SS at 77 SPM, and after this intensive treatment their scores were 7.4%SS at 109.6 SPM. The pretreatment scores were not significantly different but the postintensive phase scores did differ significantly. Of more relevance, however, was the finding that in the former group, eight of the nine subjects were recorded as not stuttering at the final assessment point, while in the latter group only eight of the 20 subjects were in this category.

Subsequently, the subjects in the groups treated in the Ingham et al. (1972) study were allocated to different postintensive phase schedules. The purpose in these allocations was to compare three different forms of treatment schedules over a 9-month period. Subjects received either weekly or monthly group psychotherapy and ST practice (as per the Andrews and Harris procedure), other subjects received these procedures plus a token system, and still others received no treatment. The results, as reported by Andrews and Ingham (1972), indicated that the subjects treated by the token system during the intensive phase, and who received no follow-up treatment, did just as well at the end of 9 months as did those who received treatment during this period. In other words, there did not appear to be any difference between the performance of the token-system-treated-subjects 9 months after treatment and subjects treated by the Andrews and Harris procedure at the completion of a 9-month follow-up treatment.

Of course, the findings from Ingham and associates' studies do not mean that the groups who received a more intensive treatment might not have done as well (or better) than the token system group at the end of an additional 9-month follow-up. It merely indicated that it was possible to achieve comparable treatment effects in a shorter period of time. Moreover, the clinical significance of these findings is quite questionable. The data were gathered solely from within-clinic conditions and give little indication of either generalization or the quality of speech after treatment. A reassessment of the data from the group treated by the token system reveals that at the completion of the 9-month follow-up period, only 27% of subjects, who were untreated during this period, were recorded as stutter-free and within the target speech rate range.

The less-than-satisfactory findings in the previously mentioned studies led to a further series of experimental treatment studies with a revamped treatment program designed to raise the probability of a more successful outcome (Ingham, 1975). The most significant change was the introduction of a live-in "hospitalized" treatment program which was based on a token economy. The format of the program involved an "establishment" and "transfer" phase. This schedule made it possible to bring almost all of the subject's speech behavior under token control —at least, for the main part of their stay in hospital. The treatment schedule was virtually identical to that used in previously reported "out-patient" programs, except for the speech rate schedule. When the subjects achieved zero stuttering during the establishment phase, they entered a six-step speech rate schedule which required systematic increases from a speed of 30 to 60 syllables per minute to 180 to 220 syllables per minute. Thereafter, the subjects had to demonstrate that they had achieved the target behavior in a hierarchy of transfer situations. The situations were as follows: speaking with patients (male and female) in the hospital, enquiries with department store staff, telephone conversations, job interviews, talking with women in a well-known "red light" district, or conversing with an interviewer on a talk-back radio show. The treatment program ended with a series of rating sessions in which token control conditions were systematically removed. The duration of the treatment varied between 16 and 21 days, depending on when the subjects completed the treatment steps within the criterion range for fluency.

The hospital token-economy program has also been described in a number of places (Ingham, 1975; Ingham & Andrews, 1973a; Martin & Ingham, 1973). Some subjects in this program were treated during the establishment phase by either ST speech or prolonged speech. A 9-month follow-up of the progress of two groups of adult subjects who completed treatment under this program revealed that nine of the 16 subjects (56.2%) treated with ST speech had maintained their target level of fluency during a final 1,000-syllable assessment. Fifteen out of 23 subjects (65.2%) in the Prolonged Speech group, however, achieved the same criterion. The superior findings of the Prolonged Speech group, albeit in within-clinic conditions, was one reason why subsequent developments in this treatment program have involved Prolonged Speech rather than ST speech. Another reason was related to findings in another study (Ingham & Andrews, 1971). In this study samples of speech obtained from both the ST and Prolonged Speech group at the end of the hospitalization phase were analyzed for the "quality of speech." This analysis involved an assessment of the speech rate and types of stuttering moments within both groups of subjects. It was found that the ST group displayed a significantly greater percentage of blocks and prolongations than the Prolonged Speech group. The ST group also had a significantly slower speech rate; the group tended to be restricted to the lower range of the 180-220 SPM rate in order to sustain fluency (Ingham, 1975).

A number of stuttering treatment programs were subsequently introduced using a combination of token reinforcement and syllable-timed speech. These occurred in Australia, mainly, but this token economy system has also been used in conjunction with variations of prolonged speech in England, Canada, and the United States. In Australia, there were reports by Alford and Ingham (1969) and Elliott and Williamson (1971) on the application of the same token system to an ST treatment for children who stutter. These programs were based directly on those reported by Ingham and Andrews (1968) and included only relatively short-term follow-up data. In general, however, this treatment trend has been largely supplemented by a series of variations on the token system treatment program which have used prolonged speech (with and without DAF assistance). These studies will be discussed further in Chapters 9 and 10.

There have been other reports of ST speech in a behavior therapy framework. Some have been reported rather sketchily. Wolpe (1969) reported treating a 25-year-old stutterer using ST speech in an unspecified manner, and claimed it was responsible for a 50% reduction in stuttering. This treatment was supplemented by the use of systematic desensitization. No satisfactory data were reported by Wolpe. This was also the case in a similar report by Lazarus (1969): ST speech was combined with a variety of speech modification procedures (including self-administered shock). This treatment combination was claimed to have achieved improved speech in one subject which was sustained for 1½ years.

Rather more data were provided in a group treatment using ST speech by Helps and Dalton (1979). In an earlier report, Dalton (1977) described an ST treatment program which had been run in London for groups of adolescent and adult stutterers. Helps and Dalton (1979) provided a subsequent report on the results of this program by comparing the performance of subjects treated intensively by ST speech or Prolonged Speech. The ST speech program is not described in any detail (the same is true for the Prolonged Speech program) except that subjects were treated in groups composed of about eight subjects. Treatment lasted about 4 hours per day over four 5-day weeks (a total of 80 hours of therapy). Therapy was then continued on a weekly basis, though the duration is not indicated. There was also a follow-up therapy program used with some other groups. The outcome of treatment, however, was based upon data collected during the 12-month period that followed the intensive 4-week treatment period. In other words, some of the results are unfortunately confounded by the effects of additional treatment.

The results of the Helps and Dalton (1979) study are also of questionable relevance to behavior therapy, since the treatment method is not described in replicable terms and it would appear that the treatment duration was pre-determined. It also contains some other serious deficiencies, including an absence of measurement-reliability data and a serious subject attrition rate (out of an initial 33 subjects, only 17 were assessed at the 1-year follow-up point). Nevertheless, the reported data are of some interest when related to the findings of other ST treatment programs. Measures of percentage of words stuttered and words per minute were obtained from a recording of the subject conversing with a stranger (no details are provided on the amount of data collected). These recordings were made before treatment, after the 4-week treatment, and at "follow-up" intervals of 1 month, 6 months, and 12 months. Personality scores, communication attitude scores, and self-ratings of reactions to speech situations were also obtained on these occasions.

The most meaningful data in the Helps and Dalton (1979) study are those that compare the pretreatment and the 6-month follow-up scores for stuttering and speech rate. These show that the ST treated group failed to achieve a significant reduction in percentage of words stuttered although they showed a slight improvement in speech rate. Only three out of 17 subjects at the 1-year follow-up showed an improvement of more than 60% on words stuttered. Against this background, it seems fair to conclude that the relevance of any of the other measures is rather dubious. In fact, the authors tended to agree with this inference and finally recommended the abandonment of this treatment in favor of one using prolonged speech. The pattern of the study and the conclusions reached are generally similar to those found in the Ingham and Andrews studies.

The general conclusion that can be reached from the "unaided studies" must be tempered by the relatively impoverished nature of the data collected in support of their findings. For the most part, the ST treatment studies have yielded only within-clinic data and have mainly involved rather questionable comparisons between groups of subjects. Few have reported reliability data. For these reasons they give little indication of the clinical validity of the procedure. It is quite clear that many stutterers have shown improvement under ST treatment, but whether these gains are sustained and generalized is very much open to question. To an extent, it appears that some subjects sustained gains over within-clinic assessment that lasted for up to a year. These findings were most apparent in the case of children. In fact, there is some indication in these data that children may have benefited substantially from treatments using ST speech.

Aided Rhythmic Treatments

By most standards, it must be acknowledged that there have been surprisingly few technological developments in past decades that have made a useful contribution to stuttering treatment. One of the more modest contributions has been the use of hearing-aid-style technology to provide rhythmic stimulation for therapy purposes. The advantage that a continuous "treatment condition" may have over a noncontinuous or clinician-directed procedure is ostensibly quite substantial. It creates the possibility of transferring the assistance offered by rhythmic stimulation to *all* speaking situations, while providing a sustained and unvarying treatment condition. But, as will be seen, the manner in which this type of treatment aid has been used exemplifies some of the problems of many behavior-therapy approaches to stuttering—especially when it involves the use of a "speech pattern" procedure.

Meyer and Mair (1963) are credited with introducing the first hearing-aid-style metronome to stuttering treatment. The apparatus they described was relatively cumbersome and limited in its therapeutic possibilities. It used bilateral earpieces wired to a miniature driving unit and provided a fixed rhythmic stimulus. The experimenters reported the use of this apparatus in the treatment of five adult stutterers, one of whom apparently did not respond because of a hearing loss. No data were reported to justify the claim for its effectiveness. Nor was any data provided to support their contention that the gains were less evident when the bpm rate was above 90.

Meyer and Mair's unit was also employed in a subsequent preliminary treatment report by Meyer and Comley (1969). This report described a treatment in which subjects were trained first to speak rhythmically within a clinic setting. Initially, this was accomplished with a metronome and then with either a bilateral or unilateral earpiece apparatus. Subjects used their apparatus in "progressively more stressful situations." Forty-eight subjects (11-58 years) were assessed for treatment and then allocated to either a unilateral apparatus, bilateral apparatus, control, or nonresponder group. The control group was taught ST speech (because they failed to respond to aided rhythmic stimulation) and the nonresponders were those who failed completely to respond to either aided or unaided rhythmic speech. The authors observed that 17 subjects "failed altogether to master rhythmic speech ... [and] about two-thirds of this group exhibited the 'hard blocking' type of stammer" (1969, p.155). The results were reported for 34 subjects at 24 weeks after the end of treatment. At that point, both the experimental groups and control subjects had made sustained gains: "Six patients—equally represented in the experimental groups and control group—achieved complete fluency" (p.156). Yet, absolutely no data were reported in support of these claims.

Following the initial papers by Meyer and colleagues, a number of other reports described slightly different types of electronic metronomes for use in treatment. Horan (1968) and Donovan (1971) described a slightly more sophisticated hearing-aid-style electronic metronome unit, while Wohl (1968) claimed to have evaluated the effects of a portable metronome known as "clinimet." But Wohl provided no information on her treatment, or the method of evaluation which supported the claim that 62% of 146 subjects were either fluent or considerably improved after treatment.

The most widely publicized hearing-aid-style electronic metronome is a unilateral behind-the-ear unit known as the "Pacemaster." This unit was designed by E.R. Libby, following some recommendations by Rothman (1969a) on the features of a unit which would be technically and cosmetically suitable for therapy. Rothman (1969b) outlined a treatment program which required the stutterer to employ the unit over increasingly difficult speaking situations. For some subjects, it was recommended that systematic desensitization procedures (using relaxation) should be used as an adjuvant. The difficulty with this report, like so many, is that it failed to include any data. By contrast, Brady (1971) provided considerable data in his far-better-known account of the use of the Pacemaster in stuttering treatment.

Initially, Brady developed a treatment program (Brady, 1968) which partly involved what was apparently an earlier version of the Pacemaster (it had a smaller bpm range than the unit currently marketed under that name). This three-stage program began with speech habit retraining. The subject was required to speak "in an exaggerated slow and relaxed manner" and then systematically increase speech rate while avoiding excessive tensing of the muscles of phonation, or struggling with a blocked word. If this did not maintain fluency, then slow speech, accompanied by metronome training, was applied. The earpiece metronome was then introduced, and the subject eventually completed a hierarchy of increasingly difficult speech situations. If difficulties were still encountered, then systematic desensitization and relaxation (aided by tranquilizing drugs) was introduced. Six stutterers were reported to have been treated in this program, but only three reached a follow-up assessment. Promising results were claimed, but they were not supported by data of any type.

In 1971, Brady reported on a program that was built exclusively around rhythmic stimulation and is known as Metronome Conditioned Speech Retraining

(MCSR). The MCSR program contains four phases. The first takes place in a clinic, where the subject is taught to speak to the accompaniment of a desk metronome (initially at 40-80 bpm). This is supplemented by home practice. Then follows a phase involving a systematic increase in speech rate. This phase "is completed when the patient is able to speak with the metronome at a rate within the normal range (100-160 words/min.) with no pronounced blocks in speech and a nonfluency rate that is no more than 20% of the nonfluency rate he exhibited before treatment without a metronome" (1971, p.135). In the third phase, the desk metronome is replaced by the Pacemaster, and the subject constructs a hierarchy of difficult speaking situations. The subject then begins to speak in these situations while wearing the unit, and is taught to reduce speech rate if any difficulty is encountered. After the most difficult situation is passed, the subject enters the final phase, at which time the subject systematically discontinues wearing the Pacemaster, first in the least difficult situations, then through to the most difficult situations. At those times, it is recommended that the subject imagine the "beat" is present. It should be noted that no speech performance criteria are mentioned, except for the change between phases two and three. It is quite possible, therefore, that this relatively liberal criterion was used as a target behavior in each of the other phases. Finally, Brady indicated that some subjects may not enter phase four, and may prefer to continue using the Pacemaster at all times.

Brady (1971) reports on 26 stutterers (12-53 years) who entered the MCSR program—although only 23 completed treatment. Their treatment ranged from 5 to 31 hours and they were then reassessed 6 to 44 months later. The assessments were derived from 3 minutes of oral reading and 3 minutes of spontaneous speech, which were obtained before treatment and at follow-up. At the same time, the Iowa Scale for Stuttering Severity, the Stutterer's Self-Rating of Reactions to Speech Situations Scale, the IPAT Anxiety Scale, and two ratings of psychological adjustment were obtained. The data indicate that 90% of the subjects improved and the group as a whole decreased their percentage of nonfluencies by 67.3% (these assessments were obtained while subjects were not wearing the Pacemaster). Twelve subjects were reported to be still wearing the Pacemaster at the time of their follow-up, so, in one sense, they had not freed themselves of the treatment conditons. When their data are deleted, the balance of the group show a 73% reduction in disfluencies. Five of the subjects were reported to have also received "adjuvant psychotherapy" during treatment and another two received systematic desensitization during the third treatment phase. It is not possible to take account of the contribution that these variations in MCSR may have made to the outcome data.

The difficulties in evaluating Brady's study are manifold and serve to highlight a number of problems common to many behavior therapy approaches to stuttering. The more obvious problems are that no measurement reliability data are provided, nor is there information on speech rate or nonclinic data. The absence of speech-rate data in this type of study is especially bothersome, because the treatment procedure depends on the subject speaking at very slow rates: this less-than-normal speech could have been the main factor associated with the reduced nonfluency scores at follow-up. The absence of nonclinic data is also of concern, because there is no clear evidence that the relatively small amount of within-clinic data represented the subject's customary speech performance. This takes on more significance in view of the finding that the subject's self-ratings of their performance outside of treatment only correlated 0.46 with changes in their nonfluency scores. One other factor that may influence the findings is the very large gap in the follow-up range: it is reasonable to expect that a subject's performance 6 months after treatment could be very different from that found in another who was assessed 3 years later. This also points to the need for data collected over post-treatment intervals. This is needed to reveal another important aspect of treatment outcome—stability of performance. Finally, it is relevant to note that not one of the subjects was reported to be free of nonfluencies at the final assessment (of course, it is not at all clear whether these nonfluencies were equivalent to stutterings). The design of the treatment, however, may also be part of the reason for the failure to achieve an absence of nonfluency (stuttering?) at follow-up. It will be recalled that subjects were permitted to pass through the treatment hierarchy while maintaining up to 20% of their nonfluencies. If this liberal criterion was employed at other phases of treatment (and, again, this is not specified), then, arguably, the treatment may have maintained a substantial level of nonfluency. These criticisms of treatment and measurement methodology are not unique to this study. They occur with alarming frequency in behavioral treatments of stuttering and contribute much to the dubious credibility that many clinicians have accorded their findings.

Subsequent reports on Brady's MCSR program have done little more than provide information alluding to the efficacy of this treatment. Brady and Brady (1972) reported a data-less follow-up on 20 subjects from the Brady (1971) report: 17 had "maintained their increased fluency" and "three have had partial relapses." Berman and Brady (1973) surveyed clinicians who had used the Pacemaster, and they reported that 72% of stutterers treated with the unit had "improved."

Adams and Hotchkiss (1973) and Hotchkiss (1974) provided a brief and virtually data-less account of the reactions of three adult stutterers who were treated with MCSR: one failed to respond, another refused to wear the Pacemaster, and a third had responded well to the program. This last subject was followed for over a year, and indicated that he had sustained a low frequency of stutterings even after the unit was withdrawn.

Ost, Gotestam, and Melin (1976) compared three groups of five stutterers (14-46 years) who were treated over a fixed duration (20 sessions of 30-40 minutes over 3 months) by either shadowing or MCSR. The other group formed an untreated control group. Between the treatment sessions, they were given training assignments (45-60 minutes per day) to be carried out "in their natural environments." The subjects were assessed immediately before treatment, immediately after treatment, and 14 months following treatment. The speech performance data were obtained from 3 minutes of oral reading and 3 minutes of spontaneous speech on each occasion. The measures were assessed for reliability. During spontaneous speech the MCSR group reduced their mean percentage of nonfluencies from 16.6

to 9.3 between the first and second assessment. Fourteen months later they were also recorded as having a mean of 9.3% nonfluency. This 44% reduction was accompanied by a nonsignificant change in the word-per-minute scores over all assessment occasions. Intriguingly, the group showed no change in their percentage-of-nonfluency scores and word-per-minute scores on the oral reading task (this was also true for the control group on both speech tasks). From any viewpoint, this is not a very impressive result. But it may be more of a reflection of the limitations of the study than the limitations of the treatment, because the study actually failed to fully assess MCSR: only one subject completed all phases of treatment at the end of 3 months, and the data were collected only from a clinic setting.

Silverman and colleagues have provided an interesting series of reports on the efficacy of the Pacemaster. One of these reports (Silverman & Trotter, 1973) was mentioned previously in connection with the speech quality of metronome-controlled fluency. The other reports have been relatively sketchy, but they give some useful indications on the effects of using the Pacemaster for lengthy periods. Trotter and Silverman (1974) summarized a series of Masters research projects which showed that reductions in the severity and frequency of stuttering could be maintained while the unit is worn continuously or intermittently for up to a month. This report also indicated that when Silverman, himself a stutterer, used the unit (built into his eyeglasses) for 12 to 18 hours a day, he achieved some benefits. Later Silverman (1976) provided some self-report data on the effect of wearing the unit for 3 years: he found the beneficial effects "wore off" almost completely at the end of that time. It is noteworthy that none of the reports from Silverman and colleagues indicated that a therapy schedule (e.g., MCSR) had been used in conjunction with the earpiece metronome.

The only other treatment study involving aided rhythmic stimulation is one conducted by Herscovitch and Le Bow (1973) with twin 12-year-old male stutterers. Their procedure, which actually owes much to Van Dantzig (1940), involved training the speakers to use "private or imaginal beats" to pace their speech. After two base-rate sessions (1 hour per week), the subjects were introduced to metronome-controlled speech (half an hour with metronome stimulation and the rest without stimulation). Initially, the subject was required to speak a syllable to each metronome beat (at a self-directed rate). This procedure was systematically replaced over subsequent treatment sessions by the subject tapping on a table, tapping his thigh, and then imagining the beat. By the eleventh session, each subject was required to speak words rather than syllables to each beat. A useful feature of this procedure was that it utilized a modeling system: each subject often observed the other's treatment. Oral reading and conversational speech data from within the clinic were presented for one subject before, during, and 5 months after treatment. The data indicate that one subject reduced stuttering from about 20 to between three and five words per minute. There was also a substantial improvement in speech rate. Those gains were maintained at follow-up, and parallel findings were reported to occur in the case of the other twin. The only negative feature in this study is that it failed to provide nonclinic data, although feedback from significant others confirmed that their improved speech was not restricted to the clinic.

Conclusions

The overall findings from the rhythmic stimulation studies is not very encouraging. They appear to provide some suggestions that therapy gains can be attributed to the treatment, although there is little, if any, clear evidence that they resulted in generalized normally fluent speech. This is not to say that this effect may not have occurred in the case of some subjects, but the absence of relevant data is at once a weakness and a suggestive aspect in these treatment reports. It is obvious that units such as the Pacemaster may have beneficial effects for some stutterers, and may certainly be a preferred mode of treatment in the case of many. The quality of the treatment reports, however, raises more questions than answers.

The questionable findings in some of these studies take on added significance in a rather intriguing way. This is through the direction that many of the principal proponents of these rhythmic stimulation therapies have taken in recent years. For example, Ingham and Andrews have subsequently replaced the ST speech component of their treatment program with a prolonged speech variant (Ingham, 1975). Similarly, Helps and Dalton (1979) found that prolonged speech provided a more effective basis for their therapy than did ST speech. Azrin, Jones, and Flye (1968) also reported some preliminary effects on the use of rhythmic stimulation in a clinical context; since that time the senior author has proceeded to develop a treatment for stuttering which is based upon a "regulated breathing" technique (Azrin & Nunn, 1974). This technique appears to be related to prolonged speech. There have also been some significant modifications to the program devised by Brady. The MCSR program has now become more problem-oriented rather than technique-oriented. For example, in an overview of this program, Burns and Brady (1980) reported the inclusion of self-management and contingency-management techniques (these techniques will be described in more detail in Chapter 10). Different areas of the treatment program may also be supplemented by assertive training and air-flow techniques: this latter technique appears identical to a prolonged speech method of treatment. Finally, there is a return to the use of pharmocotherapy to provide an assistance in generalization. No data have been provided to describe the results of this approach to treatment. However, there is recognition that metronome conditioning of the speech problem has not been sufficient nor always suitable in the treatment of all subjects in this program.

In general, therefore, it can be seen that there has been a decided drift away from the use of rhythmic stimulation procedures in behavior therapy approaches to stuttering. Perhaps what we have seen in the course of the 20-year period covered by this review is the rise and fall of yet another rhythmic speech era.

References

Adams, M.R., & Hotchkiss, J. Some responses of stutterers to a miniaturized metronome and metronome-conditioning therapy: Three case reports. *Behavior Therapy*, 1973, *4*, 565-569.

Adams, M.R., Lewis, J.I., & Besozzi, T.E. The effect of reduced reading rate on stuttering frequency. *Journal of Speech and Hearing Research*, 1973, *16*, 671-675.

Alford, J., & Ingham, R.J. The application of a token reinforcement system to the treatment of stuttering in children. *Journal of the Australian College of Speech Therapists*, 1969, *19*, 53-57.

Andrews, G., & Harris, M. *The syndrome of stuttering.* Clinics in Developmental Medicine No. 17. London: Heinemann, 1964.

Andrews, G., Holgate, D., Hopper, S., & Ingham, R.J. Current research in stuttering. *Journal of the Australian College of Speech Therapists*, 1967, *17*, 15-19.

Andrews, G., Howie, P.M., Dozsa, M., & Guitar, B.E. Stuttering: Speech pattern characteristics under fluency-inducing conditions. *Journal of Speech Disorders*, 1982, *25*, 208-216.

Andrews, G., & Ingham, R.J. An approach to the evaluation of stuttering therapy. *Journal of Speech and Hearing Research*, 1972, *15*, 296-302.

Ayllon, T., & Azrin, N.H. The measurement and reinforcement of behavior of psychotics. *Journal of the Experimental Analysis of Behavior*, 1965, *8*, 357-383.

Azrin, N., Jones, R.J., & Flye, B. A synchronization effect and its application to stuttering by a portable apparatus. *Journal of Applied Behavior Analysis*, 1968, *1*, 283-295.

Azrin, N.H., & Nunn, R.G. A rapid method of eliminating stuttering by a regulated breathing approach. *Behaviour Research and Therapy*, 1974, *12*, 279-286.

Barber, V. Studies in the psychology of stuttering, XVI. Rhythm as a distraction in stuttering. *Journal of Speech Disorders*, 1940, *5*, 29-42.

Beech, H.R., & Fransella, F. Research and experiment in stuttering. Oxford: Pergamon, 1968.

Berman, P.A., & Brady, J.P. Miniaturized metronomes in the treatment of stuttering: A survey of clinicians' experiences. *Journal of Behavior Therapy and Experimental Psychiatry*, 1973, *4*, 117-119.

Bloodstein, O. A rating scale study of conditions under which stuttering is reduced or absent. *Journal of Speech and Hearing Disorders*, 1950, *15*, 29-36.

Bloodstein,O. *A handbook on stuttering.* (2nd ed.) Chicago: National Easter Seal Society for Children and Adults, 1975.

Brady, J.P. A behavioral approach to the treatment of stuttering. *American Journal of Psychiatry*, 1968, *125*, 843-848.

Brady, J.P. Studies on the metronome effect on stuttering. *Behaviour Research and Therapy*, 1969, *7*, 197-205.

Brady, J.P. Metronome-conditioned speech retraining for stuttering. *Behavior Therapy*, 1971, *2*, 129-150.

Brady, J.P., & Brady, N. Behavior therapy in stuttering. *Folia Phoniatrica*, 1972, *24*, 355-359.

Brandon, S., & Harris, M. Stammering—an experimental treatment programme using syllable-timed speech. *British Journal of Disorders of Communication*, 1967, *2*, 64-86.

Brayton, E.R., & Conture, E.G. Effects of noise and rhythmic stimulation on the speech of stutterers. *Journal of Speech and Hearing Research*, 1978, *21*, 285-294.

Burns, D., & Brady, J.P. The treatment of stuttering. In A. Goldstein & E.B. Foa (Eds.), *Handbook of behavioral interventions.* New York: Wiley, 1980.

Clark, R.M. Our enterprising predecessors and Charles Sydney Bluemel. *Asha*, 1964, *6*, 107-114.

Dalton, P. Research into the effectiveness of intensive group directed treatment for adult stammerers. *Bulletin of the College of Speech Therapists*, 1977, *303*, 8-10.

Donovan, G.E. A new device for the treatment of stammering. *British Journal of Disorders of Communication*, 1971, *6*, 86-88.

Elliott, S., & Williamson, C. An evaluation of a token reward system in the treatment of adolescent stutterers. *Journal of the Australian College of Speech Therapists*, 1971, *21*, 6-13.

Fletcher, J.M. *The problem of stuttering*. New York: Longmans, 1928.

Fransella, F. Rhythm as a distractor in the modification of stuttering. *Behaviour Research and Therapy*, 1967, *5*, 253-255.

Fransella, F. The "rhythm effect" in stuttering as a function of predictability of utterance. *Behaviour Research and Therapy*, 1971, *9*, 265-271.

Fransella, F., & Beech, H.R. An experimental analysis of the effect of rhythm on the speech of stutterers. *Behaviour Research and Therapy*, 1965, *3*, 195-201.

Goldman-Eisler, R. *Psycholinguistics: Experiments in spontaneous speech*. London: Academic Press, 1968.

Greenberg, J.B. The effect of a metronome on the speech of young stutterers. *Behavior Therapy*, 1970, *1*, 240-244.

Hanna, R., & Morris, S. Stuttering, speech rate, and the metronome effect. *Perceptual and Motor Skills*, 1977, *44*, 452-454.

Helps, R., & Dalton, P. The effectiveness of an intensive group speech therapy programme for adult stammerers. *British Journal of Disorders of Communication*, 1979, *14*, 17-30.

Herscovitch, A., & Le Bow, M.D. Imaginal pacing in the treatment of stuttering. *Journal of Behavior Therapy and Experimental Psychiatry*, 1973, *4*, 357-360.

Holgate, D., & Andrews, G. The use of syllable-timed speech and group psychotherapy in the treatment of adult stutterers. *Journal of the Australian College of Speech Therapists*, 1966, *16*, 36-40.

Horan, M.C. An improved device for inducing rhythmic speech in stutterers. *Australian Psychologist*, 1968, *3*, 19-25.

Hotchkiss, J. Some reactions and responses of stutterers to a miniaturized metronome and metronome-conditioning therapy: A follow-up report. *Behavior Therapy*, 1974, *5*, 574-575.

Hutchinson, J.M. A review of rhythmic pacing as a treatment strategy for stuttering. *Rehabilitation Literature*, 1976, *37*, 297-303.

Hutchinson, J.M., & Navarre, B.M. The effect of a metronome pacing on selected aerodynamic patterns of stuttered speech: Some preliminary observations and interpretations. *Journal of Fluency Disorders*, 1977, *2*, 189-204.

Ingham, R.J. The development, application and analysis of a token system for the treatment of adult stutterers. Unpublished doctoral dissertation, University of New South Wales, Aus., 1972.

Ingham, R.J. Operant methodology in stuttering therapy. In J. Eisenson (Ed.), *Stuttering: A second symposium*. New York: Harper & Row, 1975.

Ingham, R.J., & Andrews, G. The control of stuttering: An application of token reinforcement systems in a voluntary setting. Paper read to the Australian Psychological Society Conference, Brisane, Aus., 1968.

Ingham, R.J., & Andrews, G. Stuttering: The quality of fluency after treatment. *Journal of Communication Disorders*, 1971, *4*, 279-288.

Ingham, R.J., & Andrews, G. Details of a token economy stuttering therapy programme for adults. *Australian Journal of Human Communication Disorders*, 1973, *1*, 13-20. (a)

Ingham, R.J. & Andrews, G. Behavior therapy and stuttering: A review. *Journal of Speech and Hearing Disorders*, 1973, *38*, 405-441. (b)

Ingham, R.J., Andrews, G., & Winkler, R. Stuttering: A comparison of the effectiveness of four treatment techniques. *Journal of Communication Disorders*, 1972, *5*, 91-117.

Johnson, W., Darley, F.F., & Spriestersbach, D.C. *Diagnostic methods in speech pathology*. New York: Harper & Row, 1963.

Johnson, W., & Rosen, L. Studies on the psychology of stuttering, VII. Effects of certain changes in speech pattern upon frequency of stuttering. *Journal of Speech Disorders*, 1937, *2*, 105-109.

Jones, R.J., & Azrin, N.H. Behavioral engineering: Stuttering as a function of stimulus duration during speech synchronization. *Journal of Applied Behavior Analysis*, 1969, *2*, 223-229.

Klingbeil, G.M. The historical background of the modern speech clinic. *Journal of Speech Disorders*, 1939, *4*, 115-132.

Lazarus, A.A. Case history of a stutterer treated as an obsessive-compulsive disorder by broad-spectrum behavior therapy. In B.B. Gray & G. England (Eds.), *Stuttering and the conditioning therapies*. Monterey, CA: Monterey Institute of Speech and Hearing, 1969.

Mallard, A.R., & Meyer, L.A. Listener preferences for stuttered and syllable-timed speech production. *Journal of Fluency Disorders*, 1979, *4*, 117-121.

Martin, R., & Haroldson, S.K. Effects of five experimental treatments on stuttering. *Journal of Speech and Hearing Disorders*, 1979, *22*, 132-146.

Martin, R.R. & Ingham, R.J. Stuttering. In B. Lahey (Ed.), *The modification of language behavior*, Springfield, IL: Charles C. Thomas, 1973.

Meyer, V., & Comley, J. A preliminary report on the treatment of stammer by the use of rhythmic stimulation. In B.B. Gray & G. England (Eds.), *Stuttering and the conditioning therapies*, Monterey, CA: Monterey Institute for Speech and Hearing, 1969.

Meyer, V., & Mair, J.M. A new technique to control stammering: A preliminary report. *Behaviour Research and Therapy*, 1963, *1*, 251-254.

Ost, L.G., Gotestam, K.G., & Melin, L. A controlled study of two behavioral methods in the treatment of stuttering. *Behavior Therapy*, 1976, *7*, 587-592.

Perkins, W.H. Articulatory rate in the evaluation of stuttering treatments. *Journal of Speech and Hearing Disorders*, 1975, *40*, 277-278.

Rothman, I. Practical rhythmic desensitization for stuttering with description of a new electronic pacer used for stutterers, insomnia and anxiety. *Journal of the American Osteopathic Association*, 1969, *68*, 573-577. (a)

Rothman, I. Stuttering: Theory and treatment. *Experimental Medicine and Surgery*, 1969, *27*, 336-349. (b)

Silverman, F.H. Long-term impact of a miniature metronome on stuttering: An interim report. *Perceptual and Motor Skills*, 1976, *42*, 1322.

Silverman, H. & Trotter, D. Impact of pacing speech with a miniature electronic metronome upon the manner in which a stutterer is preceived. *Behavior Therapy*, 1973, *4*, 414-419.

Silverman, F.H., & Umberger, F.G. Effect of pacing speech with a miniature electronic metronome on the frequency and duration of selected disfluency behaviors in the spontaneous speech of adult stutterers. *Behavior Therapy*, 1974, *5*, 410-414.

Trotter, W.D., & Silverman, F.H. Does the effect of pacing speech with a miniature metronome on stuttering wear off? *Perceptual and Motor Skills*, 1974, *39*, 429-430.

Van Dantzig, M. Syllable-tapping, a new method for the help of stammerers. *Journal of Speech Disorders*, 1940, *5*, 127-131.

Van Riper, C. The rhythm method. *Western Michigan University Journal of Speech Therapy*, 1971, *8*, 1-2.

Van Riper, C. *The treatment of stuttering*. Englewood Cliffs, NJ: Prentice-Hall, 1973.

Winer, B.J. *Statistical principles in experimental design*. New York: McGraw-Hill, 1971.

Wingate, M.E. Sound and pattern in 'artificial' fluency. *Journal of Speech and Hearing Research*, 1969, *12*, 677-686.

Wingate, M.E. 'Vocalization' ≠ phonation. *Journal of Speech and Hearing Research*, 1979, *22*, 657-658.

Wohl, T. The electronic metronome—An evaluative study. *British Journal of Disorders of Communication*, 1968, *3*, 89-98.

Wolpe, J. Behavior therapy of stuttering: Deconditioning the emotional factor. In B.B. Gray & G. England (Eds.), *Stuttering and the conditioning therapies*, Monterey, CA: Monterey Institute for Speech and Hearing, 1969.

6

Anxiety and Stuttering

Introduction

If stuttering presents difficulties for the definition-seeker, they are miniscule compared with the problems involved in defining anxiety. At best, there exist just a few very broad areas of agreement about the meaning of the term. For example, there is probably general agreement that it refers to a negative and usually undesirable feeling. But can it be distinguished objectively from other negative feelings? For instance, does it produce observable features which differ from those that occur during depression or shame? Undoubtedly, we manage to convey some distinctive images when we refer to these emotions, and we certainly expect depressed and anxious people to behave differently. But, then, there are also different types of anxiety, which may or may not be undesirable. It may be a useful alerting condition as, for example, when a child learns not to step off a sidewalk into a street. But it may also be a fatiguing and debilitative condition, as when a person is obsessed by an unfounded dread of unlikely events. In short, it can be either an adaptive or maladaptive feeling.

Some endeavors have been made to draw distinctions among the many types of anxiety. One useful distinction (at least for research) is Spielberger's (1966) division between "state" anxiety and "trait" anxiety. The former refers to a transitory state of apprehension and tension, while the latter applies to a relatively stable personality construct. This construct is typically identified by paper-and-pencil tests, such as the Taylor Manifest Anxiety Test (Taylor, 1953) or the IPAT General Anxiety Scale (Cattell, 1963), and describes persons who are prone to experience state anxiety under certain conditions. But this division does not help demark the features of the more common type of anxiety, that is, state anxiety.

An obvious starting point for a definition is Webster's Dictionary, which currently describes anxiety as "pain or uneasiness of mind respecting some event, future or uncertain" (Webster, 1975). This two-part description of state anxiety is almost identical to that which has been used by behaviorally oriented researchers. For instance, Estes and Skinner (1941) employed the following frequently cited definition: "[A]nxiety has at least two defining characteristics: (1) it is an emotional state somewhat resembling fear and (2) the disturbing stimulus which is principally responsible does not precede or accompany the state but is anticipated in the future" (p. 390). Common and technical usage, therefore, only leads to the expectation that a person experiencing state anxiety will display certain unusual behaviors that relate to an expected event.

Stuttering has long been regarded as intimately associated in one way or another with anxiety. Surveys have revealed that most clinicians (Turnbaugh, Guitar, & Hoffman, 1979) and parents of stutterers (Fowlie & Cooper, 1978) tend to regard them, as a group, as exceptionally anxious individuals. For some theoreticians (for example, Wischner, 1950), stuttering either originates because of state anxiety, is exacerbated by this condition, or is maintained because of reductions in anxiety. This means that there is supposed to be a learned association between anxiety and stuttering. For other theorists (Brutten & Shoemaker, 1967), stuttering *is* anxiety, and any nonfluent behavior not accopanied by negative affect is simply not stuttering.

The rest of this section will overview the principal theoretical models that have been founded on an assumed direct association between stuttering and anxiety. Consideration will be given to evidence of the effects of anxiety on stuttering, particularly that which suggests that anticipated stimuli and/or related emotional states may modify stuttering.

Theoretical Issues

In earlier chapters, it was argued that stuttering treatments have been much influenced by psychological theories. One of the most powerful influences stemmed from the learning theories that sought to explain the effects of anxiety on learning. During the 1940 to 1960 period, a substantial area of psychology was occupied with attempts to explain the acquisition of behavior within the context of learning-theory models. Two types of learnig theories emerged as influential models of behavior change, and both have been regarded as having heuristic value for stuttering. The first theory derived from the experimental studies of Pavlov during the early part of this century, and eventually resulted in the development of classical or respondent conditioning principles. The second learning theory emerged from the experimental work founded by Thorndike, and led to the development of the concept of instrumental learning. Of course, Skinner ultimately extended the principles of instrumental learning into operant-conditioning principles. Both classical and instrumental learning concepts have had an inestimable influence on normal and abnormal psychology. But, more significantly for stuttering, both regarded anxiety as important in explaining the acquisition of problem behaviors. In short, variations in anxiety were postulated to affect the evocation, maintenance, and reduction of many maladaptive behaviors.

Classical conditioning is based on the proposition that contiguity between an unconditioned stimulus condition and a response may lead to a sustained association between the stimulus and response. A painful or aversive stimulus, such as shock, will produce an identifiable response(s). While an attractive or appetitive stimulus, such as food, will produce a distinguishably different response(s). Both types of stimuli are referred to as unconditioned stimuli. When unconditioned stimuli are repeatedly paired with a neutral stimulus, then that neutral or paired stimulus achieves conditioned properties which, in turn, cause it to produce responses similar to those evoked by the unconditioned stimulus. A conditioned stimulus, which has derived from an aversive unconditioned stimulus, may also evoke so-called avoidant responses. These responses are seemingly "designed" to avoid the occurrence of the unconditioned stimulus. Such conditioning, or learning, may take place in a variety of forms and has been seen as a suitable model for explaining much normal and abnormal behavior. The role of anxiety in the classical conditioning model is inferred. It is usually regarded as equivalent to the response evoked by an unpleasant or aversive stimulus which, in turn, is produced by conditioned stimuli.

Classical, or respondent, conditioning principles point to three different ways in which the conditioned stimulus may cease to evoke a conditioned response. It can be deconditioned by repeated presentation of the conditioned stimulus in the absence of the unconditioned stimulus. This method is termed *habituation.* The second method is *extinction,* and occurs via repeated evocation of the response in the absence of the conditioned stimulus. Finally, pairing the conditioned stimulus with an unconditioned stimulus may evoke a competitive or incompatiable response. This is labeled *counterconditioning.*

Instrumental conditioning is basically a process which occurs when certain stimuli immediately follow a response. The original Law of Effect, as proposed by Thorndike (1933), posited that a response which is followed by a reward strengthens that response, while a response-contingent penalty condition will weaken that response. In recent times, the principle of instrumental conditioning has been largely superseded by the principle of operant conditioning (Skinner, 1938). Operant conditioning occurs when a stimulus, which is made contingent on a response, achieves the effect of altering the frequency of occurrence of that response. In very simple terms, under either of these response-stimulus arrangements the strength or frequency of response of occurrence is altered by either changing or removing the controlling stimulus condition.

During the 1940s and 1950s, two theories of learning based on classical and instrumental conditioning, influenced the conceptual foundations of vast areas of psychology. They were theories developed by Clark Hull (1943) and O.H. Mowrer (1950). Both of these theoriests integrated classical and instrumental conditioning principles in explanations of the acquisition and the maintenance of normal and abnormal behavior, and both gave state anxiety a central role in learning.

Hull introduced the most all-encompassing learning theory explanation of behavior. His theory postulated that virtually all behavior was governed by a combination of drives and habits that were continuously strengthened or weakened by different stimulus-response arrangements, particularly under different drive states. Anxiety was regarded as one drive state which could alter the habit strength of almost all types of responses or behaviors. Thus, anxiety gained the status of a construct which might affect a response, such as stuttering, in the presence of conditioned stimuli.

Mowrer's theory utilized both classical and instrumental conditioning, but with fewer constructs, to explain the learning of problem behaviors. Under his two-factor theory, certain behaviors were regarded as involuntary consequences of classical conditioning, while other more voluntary behaviors were regarded as instrumentally conditioned—mainly (though not always) by being paired with anxiety reduction. As a result, much instrumentally conditioned behavior was conceived of as a consequence of conditioned anxiety which, in turn, was the result of classical conditioning.

Other learning theories were also influential during the same era. These included Guthrie's (1935) contiguity theory, Tolman's (1932) theory of purposive behavior, and Skinner's (1938) atheoretical analysis of operant behavior. Each of these theorists had an immense impact on different aspects of human-learning research. Arguably, operant conditioning has ultimately succeeded in becoming the most influential of all of these theories, particularly with respect to behavior therapy. But this influence was far from evident during the 1940s. A good case may be made for the claim that the widespread influence of both Hull's and Mowrer's theories in abnormal psychology during this time stemmed from the prominent role they gave state anxiety in explaining human behavior. This provided a plausible link between the principles of learning and what many clinicians regarded as the key factor in abnormal behavior—anxiety.

The appeal that Hull's drive-reduction theory and Mowrer's two-factor theory had for those concerned with explaining and treating stuttering was fairly predictable. Here was a behavior which had long been regarded as intimately related to anxiety. Furthermore, the attendant bodily actions that may accompany stuttering had the distinct appearance of responses that had been learned in order to cope with the disorder. This puzzling disorder was therefore ripe for any theory that utilized conditioning principles to explain its variability in the face of environmental conditions. It is not surprising, therefore, that so many derivative theories of stuttering emerged.

One of the first attempts to relate stuttering to a learning theory was offered by George Wischner (1950) with his proposal that stuttering should be viewed as a "learned anxiety reaction system." Wischner's theory utilized Hullian drive-reduction principles which, he considered, offered a suitable explanation for some characteristics of stuttering. He argued that anxiety was integral to stuttering in one of two possible ways. The first was that the anxiety response is learned, but that stuttering was an unlearned response to state anxiety produced by the speech act. The second was that both anxiety and stuttering are learned (interlocked) responses which reinforce anxiety reduction. By either explanation, the act of stuttering was claimed to produce a decrease in the anxiety drive which results in stuttering becoming an instrumentally conditioned response.

Interestingly, Wischner (1952) also regarded stuttering as a behavior which might permit the direct investigation of the anxiety gradient (changes in behavior related to the strength of the anxiety drive). Two forms of anxiety were thought to be expressed by stuttering; general situational anxiety and specific word anxiety. The former was regarded as evident by the effect of different audience sizes on stuttering, and the latter was "presumed to be manifested in the adaptation and expectancy effect."

Two other theories of stuttering emerged during the 1950s, each promulgating stuttering as essentially a fear response. These theories were offered by Joseph Sheehan and Oliver Bloodstein.

Sheehan's Approach-Avoidance Conflict Theory was mainly based on a drive reduction model of problem behavior. It also incorporated Neil Miller's (1944) proposition that when a drive to approach and a drive to avoid are in conflict, they result in oscillating behavior. Sheehan viewed stuttering as a good example of oscillation (mainly in the form of repetitions and prolongations) between the desire to communicate and the desire to avoid stuttering conditions. The act of stuttering was theorized to have the effect of reducing the drive to avoid. Sheehan has described his theory in a number of places (1953; 1958; 1975) and indicated that it contains at least 5 levels of drive avoidance.[1] In later formulations of this theory, Sheehan (1975) has suggested there is a steeper and more accentuated anxiety-motivated avoidance response preceding the speech act. The resulting sharp release from tension would explain the strong reinforcement (and, therefore, maintenance) of the stuttering response.

A related theory has been offered by Bloodstein, (1958; 1972; 1975; 1981). He claimed that stuttering may be profitably viewed as "an anticipatory struggle reaction" in the face of environmental pressures. In effect, the stutterer is judged to be constantly anxious about stuttering. In the process, certain environmental stimuli thereby acquire the property of inducing anxiety about speech behavior as such. It is this fear or anxiety that Bloodstein suggested leads to the production of the tensions and fragmentations that, in essence, form stuttering. But it is mainly the heightened anxiety about speech that Bloodstein judged to be responsible for stuttering.

In recent years, the most behaviorally based learning theory of stuttering has been Brutten and Shoemaker's (1967) two-factor theory. Their theory also borrowed heavily from a more general learning theory, Mowrer's (1950) two-factor theory of learning. Two features of Brutten and Shoemaker's theory tend to distinguish it from those offered by Wischner and Sheehan. The first was that the stuttering moment was not considered a unitary event, but one composed of classically conditioned autonomic responses that are "reflexive and less voluntary." These responses are said to be accompanied by instrumentally conditioned responses, which are usually adaptive and voluntary. Repetitions and prolongations were claimed to be classically conditioned (first factor) responses, while all other types of stuttering behaviors, such as eye blinks and head movements, were viewed as instrumental (second factor) responses. The second distinguishing feature of this theory is that it incorporated an important shift in the definition of stuttering. Stuttering was no longer defined on the basis of its form or frequency, but on the existence of "specific stimulus circumstances and negative emotion that in essence defines stuttering" (Brutten, 1969, p.64). In other words, if a disfluent speaker fails to show evidence of negative emotion (usually in the form of state-anxiety measures such as palmar sweat indices) then the speaker is not regarded as a stutterer—irrespective of any similarities between the speaker's disfluencies and stutterings.

[1] Each may be regarded as in competition with the drive to communicate. These avoidance levels involve conditioned reactions to specific words, reactions to threatening speech situations, guilt and anxiety concerning the emotional content of the speech, anxiety associated with the relationship with the listener, and the threats associated with failure or success.

When these theories are taken together, it becomes evident that the role of anxiety in their explanations of stuttering is either inferred by the presence of stuttering or it is a hypothesized consequence of stimulus conditions, such as audiences or words. Hence, their tenability depends greatly on the methods that are used to independently identify the presence (or absence) of anxiety. The experimental evidence which should support or reject the foundation of these theories will be reviewed in the following sections.

Experimental Studies on Anxiety and Stuttering

Situation Anxiety

It seems logical to expect that chronic stuttering might cause an individual to anticipate speaking situations with some apprehension and, thus, avoid them whenever possible. One obvious reason, especially among adult stutterers, would be the anticipated negative reactions of others. Of course, the stutterer's apprehension may also stem from the fact that the problem is, in reality, more evident in some circumstances. The causal sequence may be open to question, but the discomfort and fear may be equally real.

There are many speaking situations that produce discomfort for most individuals. Some evidence of this was found in a study by Trotter and Bergmann, (1957), which looked at stutterers' (n=50) and nonstutterers' (n=100) responses to the Stutterers' Reactions to Speech Situations Scale (Johnson, Darley, & Spriestersbach, 1963). They found the nonstutterers' mean scores for avoidance and reaction to the situations listed in the scale were significantly lower than the stutterers' mean scores. Intriguingly, the scores that indicate frequency of contact with these situations did not discriminate the groups. But, of most interest was the finding that "a considerable number of nonstutterers were more avoidant of speaking situations and enjoyed speaking in them less than many stutterers" (Trotter & Bergman, 1957, p.45). Furthermore, the ranking of situations by the stutterers and nonstutterers was not essentially different. The only clear exception to this finding were the situations that involved use of the telephone.

There is overwhelming evidence that either changes in speaking situations or certain types of speaking situations are, potentially, related to different frequencies of stuttering. The most commonly mentioned situation factor reported to influence stuttering is audience size. For example, it is often claimed that when stutterers speak alone they lose their problem. The research evidence does not entirely support this claim, but it certainly suggests that stuttering tends to decrease in this situation. Porter (1939) had stutterers (n=13) orally read different 500-word passages under situations that involved reading alone and reading with audiences of one to eight listeners. The group's percentage of words stuttered ranged from 2.8% while reading alone, to 16.7% when reading before eight listeners. Similar effects were reported by Hahn (1940), who had 52 stutterers orally read alone, with an unseen listener, a visible listener, and an audience of between five and 10 listeners. But there was also much evidence of individual differences. In fact, Hahn concluded that "the variation in the number of spasms is significantly more affected by individual differences than by differences in the social complexity of oral reading situations" (Hahn, 1940, p.14).

Audience-size effects have also been reported in group studies by Steer and Johnson (1936), Shulman (1955), Dixon (1955), and Siegel and Haugen (1964). The latter study, for example, measured the effect of increasing and decreasing the size of an audience on the adaptation effect. They reported that stuttering frequency was significantly higher than that found in a control reading for a group which experienced "increasing audience" size conditions. This difference was not evident within another group which orally read throughout "decreasing audience" size conditions. (Unfortunately, their findings were confounded by differences between experimental groups in their frequency of stuttering.) But, among all of these studies, the findings tend to apply to the group rather than to all subjects.

The above-mentioned studies share the characteristic of alerting their subjects to the type of audience or situation they will face during the experiment. This condition was controlled in another audience-size study by Young (1965). When Young's subjects (n=12; 13-16 years) orally read before unanticipated audiences of one to four listeners, no significant differences were found in either severity or frequency of stuttering with respect to audience size. This finding has led to the belief that the audience-size effect is mainly due to the subject's anticipation of a situation, rather than the situation as such.

The deleterious effect of anticipation on stuttering is of course consistent with an "anxiety effect." It is reasonably understandable that some state anxiety could accompany knowledge of a forthcoming unusual event. Lerman and Shames (1965) attempted to isolate this effect by assessing 20 subjects for stuttering and state anxiety before they entered four situations previously rated for "avoidance" in Trotter and Bergmann's (1957) study (half the subjects actually entered the situation and half did not). The subjects' state anxiety was measured by a Discomfort-Relief Quotient (DRQ) (Dollard & Mowrer, 1953), derived from language behavior during interviews that preceded entry into the situation. Lerman and Shames found no significant relationship between the DRQ scores and stuttering frequency within these interviews. In fact, only the least "avoided" situation was associated with a lower (less anxious) DRQ score. The most problematic feature of this study is that the subjects did not individually assess the situations for avoidance reactions, and so the main effects may have been lost because of limited variability in the anxiety measure. A surprising feature of this report is the failure to include data on the stuttering frequencies found in each of the interviews.

It is quite conceivable that the type of listener appearing in an audience may also stimulate different levels of state anxiety. In an early study, which used repeated oral readings, Steer and Johnson (1936) found differing frequencies of "spasms" when stutterers (n=10) spoke before different types of audiences.

They asked subjects to rate the audiences as "friendly or unfriendly," and whether the audience appeared to judge them "as an inferior or a superior individual." Unfortunately, adaptation effects were not controlled, and so Steer and Johnson's conclusion—that these variables were not significantly related to stuttering—is questionable. This is made more likely by the findings from three other studies. Porter (1939) had stutterers (n=13) choose a "hard," "neutral," and "easy" listener and then orally read before each listener. It was found that more than 92% of the readings with "hard" listeners had a higher frequency of stuttering than readings with "easy" listeners. The "neutral" rather than "easy" listeners, however, were associated with least stuttering. A related finding was reported by Berwick (1955) in a study which used photographs that stutterers (n=20) had judged to be of "hard" or "easy" listeners. Each stutterer orally reread a 250-word passage five times, then read to the back of either a "hard" or "easy" listener's photograph. Five further readings were then made to the front of either photograph. A 7.8% increase in frequency of stuttering was obtained between the fifth and seventh reading to "easy" listener photographs but a 20.3% increase occurred during the "hard" listener photograph conditions. A related effect was reported by Sheehan, Hadley, and Gould (1967). They had adult stutterers (n=32) orally reread a passage five times in front of "authority listeners" (males dressed formally and titled "Doctor") or "peer" listeners (males, casually dressed, titled by a customary name). Their data show that reading before an "authority listener" was associated with a significantly higher frequency of stuttering than reading before a "peer" listener—though the differences in stuttering frequency did not exceed 14%.

The findings of these studies suggest that stutterers have a predictable increase in stuttering when faced with different types of audiences. There is also some indication in these studies that this effect might be akin to a self-fulfilling prophecy, that is, expected higher frequencies of stuttering may indeed produce just that result. The contribution of an anxiety factor to such an effect is unclear. In the absence of independent measures of state anxiety, it is impossible to judge whether these expectancies and speaking situations were actually responsible for measurable increases in fear or state anxiety.

Speech Anxiety

The evidence regarding speech-related state anxiety is a little more compelling. Many stutterers certainly appear to expect to stutter on certain words. However, their expectations do not always align with their behavior. For example, Martin and Haroldson (1967) found the relationship between expectancy and stuttering to be less than 50%. Furthermore, as Wingate (1976) has noted, many stutterers also stutter on words they fail to anticipate, so that their expectation is often fulfilled on a relatively random basis. Such randomized and, therefore, unexpected disruption to communication may be a suitable condition for producing anxiety about stuttering.

There is some evidence on the conditioning effects of stuttering expectancies, which is compatible with the notion the stuttering moments might "cue" anxiety.

For example, Johnson and Millsapps (1937) had stutterers (n=26) orally read a passage on three occasions. The experimenters then marked out the words that had been stuttered, and on subsequent passage readings (minus the marked words) found their subjects produced considerably fewer stutterings. They also noted that more stuttering then occurred on words adjacent to the marked-out words, when compared with nonadjacent words. A similar result was reported by Brutten and Gray ((1961). They compared the oral readings of groups of words on cards—which were intermingled with others that contained previously stuttered words (these cards were reversed)—with reading another cluster of word cards which had the previously stuttered word cards removed entirely. These data tended to support the findings of Johnson and Millsapps and suggest that stuttering cues may become conditioned stimuli which also produce stuttering.

Some attempts have been made to obtain independent measures of state anxiety in oral-reading situations. Brutten (1963) used palmar sweat indices (PSI) to compare repeated oral and silent readings by stutterers (n=33) and nonstutterers (n=33). He found that the stutterers' PSI measures tended to decline in concert with stuttering over repeated readings, but a similar trend was not found during silent readings by both groups. These data are not easily interpreted in terms of anxiety effects since the PSI and stuttering scores showed changes that were equally consistent with explanations based on either the reductions in physical effort or the passage of time. Also, rather contrary results were reported by Gray and Brutten (1965) in their assessment of stutterers' PSI indices during the course of repeated readings of a passage—the reductions in PSI scores were not consistent with reductions in stuttering frequency.[2]

The content of certain words, or topics, may provide a more specific source of conditioned stimuli. For example, Adams and Dietze (1965) had stutterers (n=30) and nonstutterers (n=30) write a word that they associated with a presented stimulus word. They found that the stutterers took significantly longer to respond to negative affect words, but did not differ from nonstutterers on neutral or positive affect words. Brutten and Janssen (1979) compared the eye movements of stutterers (n=16) and nonstutterers (n=16) to words which the stutterers indicated they were likely to stutter. On this relatively abstract measure of anxiety, Brutten and Janssen's data revealed more eye fixations on the part of the stutterers. A related effect on stuttering was found by Moore, Soderberg, and

[2] Some studies appear to have wrongly claimed a relationship between anxiety-provoking conditions and changes in stuttering from data obtained within the context of an adaptation effect. For example, Johnson, Larson, and Knott (1937) had stutterers reread a "cue" passage to an audience and then again to an interviewer. This resulted in an increased frequency of stuttering when comparisons were made with stutterings on a control passage not previously read before an audience. Also Gould and Sheehan (1967) had stutterers reread a passage with a 5-minute silent interval between some of the readings, but not for a control passage. They reported a higher frequency of stuttering in the readings which followed the silent interval. In both of these studies, it is possible to attribute the changes during the experimental conditions to alterations in the "rereading conditions," rather than the suggested independent variable. This becomes clear with respect to the latter study, when data obtained by Adams and Brutten (1970) are considered. During an interruption to an adaptation procedure, they had stutterers orally reread some other words, or experience silence conditions. They found no difference in the frequency of stuttering during subsequent oral readings.

Powell (1952); they found that the duration of moments of stuttering were significantly greater when stutterers (n=16; 13-21 years) spoke about their parents, rather than when they spoke of their hopes, misdeeds, fears, aassociates, and good times. These findings point to the possibility that certain topics (not necessarily feared topics) may produce an increased severity of stuttering, and that subjects may react to certain types of stimuli with some hesitancy (though not necessarily in the form of hesitant speech).

Waiting to perform an action, while knowing that it might be performed poorly, could, conceivably, be a situation which is likely to heighten anxiety. Thus, "waiting to speak" under certain conditions could well be an anxiety-provoking circumstance for a stutterer. Some studies on this issue have found that the "wait effect" is variable, though the evidence suggests some interesting trends. Goss (1952) first noted a "U curve" effect when stutterers were required to wait for short intervals between the presentation of a word and its utterance: stuttering tended to be reduced after 1 or 2 seconds elapsed, but after a 5-second interval, stuttering tended to increase to a level comparable with a zero interval. In a later study, Goss (1956) found evidence that stuttering continued to increase over "wait periods" of up to 20 seconds. Another demonstration of this "U curve" effect was obtained by Forte and Schlesinger (1972). They had stutterers wait their turn to orally read within a group of six speakers. It was found that most stuttering occurred when subjects read first, but stuttering declined sharply when the subject was second "in line." When subjects had to wait for five others to read, then their frequency of stuttering tended to resemble that found on the first reading. Presumably, therefore, the expectation of a feared (assumed) situation does not produce altogether predictable consequences. It might be thought that the longer a stutterer had to wait to speak, the more likelihood there would be that state anxiety would increase. Nevertheless, like many of these studies, it is assumed that these "feared" conditions will increase state anxiety and, in turn, will exacerbate stuttering. In the absence of independent measures of anxiety, the link between these variables is very tenuous.

Physiological Factors

There is little dispute that stutterers may experience excessive tension during their speech behavior. But the causal effect of this tension on stuttering is open to question. Snidecor (1955) had stutterers (n=72) identify body areas that were tense during the act of stuttering, and found these were mainly located in the jaws, front of the mouth, and front of the throat. A variety of studies on physiological correlates of stuttering were reviewed by Perkins (1970) and Bloodstein (1981). Both reviewers concluded that most of the more obvious variables, such as heart rate, blood pressure, and muscle tension (particularly around the oral zone), were only likely to be unusual during a moment of stuttering—and at no other time.

Some of the measures of more minute forms of physiological activity have shown interesting relationships to stuttering. For example, Ickes and Pierce (1973) measured vasoconstriction, or blood volume (a presumed correlate of state anxiety), in stutterers and nonstutterers during a 30-second interval preceding and following an utterance. They found that the stutterers displayed a significantly greater increase in vasoconstriction preceding an utterance, and an even greater increase before emitting a stutter. Of most interest was their finding that the stutterers showed a very sharp decrease in vasoconstriction *after* a stutter. This apparent reduction in state anxiety following a stutter was also identified in a study by Dabul and Perkins (1973). They measured systolic blood pressure (which had been increased by shock) before and after high and low stutter conditions and stutter-free conditions while controlling for energy and duration of stuttering (chewing, finger tapping, and time). Their data show that only after the high stuttering condition was there a sharp decrease in systolic blood pressure. In the absence of an independent measure of the physical effort expended during the experimental conditions, however, this result may be attributable to the cessation of this factor following "high stuttering."

Both of the above studies imply that some correlates of state anxiety may increase during very brief intervals preceding a stutter and then decrease following a stutter. This has great relevance for those theories that rely on drive reduction to explain the maintenance of stuttering. The logical step which should follow, in order to determine whether these physiological variables may actually produce stuttering, is to ascertain whether their independent manipulation achieves related effects on stuttering. But there is an additional difficulty in trying to tie these physiological parameters to state anxiety. There is now considerable evidence (Schwartz, 1978) which shows that there may be an asynchronous association between these somatic features of anxiety and the actual experience of anxiety. In other words, physiological evidence of anxiety is not necessarily evidence that the subject actually experiences anxiety.

The Effects of Manipulated State Anxiety or Manipulated Stuttering

The most interesting findings about the effects of anxiety on stuttering have appeared in those studies that have assessed the effect on stutterers of manipulating state anxiety or, conversely, the effect of manipulating stuttering on state anxiety.

For the most part, the former type of study still uses inferential, though reasonably credible, measures of anxiety. For example, Silverman, Zimmer, and Silverman (1974) assessed female stutterers (n=4) during intervals associated with premenstruation and ovulation. They found that spontaneous speech samples (three minutes) recorded at premenstruation had consistently higher levels of stuttering (about 30% higher) than samples recorded at ovulation. Silverman and Zimmer (1975) reported a similar effect with respect to nonfluencies in the speech of nonstuttering females.

Another example of the impact on stuttering of presumed high levels of state anxiety is found in studies that have measured the effects of shock on stuttering.

Van Riper (1937) arranged for stutterers to receive a sample shock and then be told that after the next reading they would receive a shock for each recorded "spasm".[3] The data show that only one of the 16 subjects did not increase stuttering as a result of this procedure. However the effect of shock on stuttering is variable. Martin and Siegel (1966) assessed the effect of a shock which was delivered immediately after each moment of stuttering during spontaneous speech. They found that this arrangement of the shock condition achieved a decrease in stuttering. As will be seen (Chapter 9), this response-contingent arrangement of aversive stimuli forms an integral part of operant-conditioning methodology. Under many similar experimental conditions stuttering has been found to decrease.

While decreased stuttering in response-contingent conditions might reduce the ostensibly anxiety-provoking condition (that is, shock) this cannot occur when shock is delivered noncontingently. Such conditions apply within the Estes-Skinner Conditioned Anxiety Paradigm which Toomey and Sidman (1970) used with four adult stutterers. The paradigm is well illustrated by the design of their study. Each subject orally read under conditions of an irregularly occurring two-minute tone followed by a shock. A comparison between stuttering frequency during a control-tone condition (shock did not follow) and the tone-shock condition revealed that only one stutterer increased stuttering and two subjects actually decreased their stuttering.[4] Such a finding runs counter to expectations, but other information provided by Toomey and Sidman makes it clear why this unusual result was obtained.

> Subject W.J.'s voice pitch rose steadily as he read during buzzer presentation: at the same time he drummed the electrodes on the table top, and after each shock he loudly cursed the experimenter. Subject J.C. increased his voice volume as he read faster and frequently coughed loudly during the shock sessions. Subject G.K. read more rapidly and somewhat more quietly, with longer pauses during the shock condition. He sighed deeply after each shock. Subject R.L. increased reading speed, raised volume and pitch to shouting level, and articulated in a rapid staccato manner during buzzer presentations. (1970, p.128).

[3] In a later report on this study, Van Riper (1971, p.314) indicated that the shocks were not administered at the end of the reading.

[4] There are some disturbing ethical, though somewhat amusing, aspects about Toomey and Sidman's study that testify to the aversive and, presumably, anxiety-provoking features of their experimental procedure. The level of the 250 msec shock was calibrated in the following manner:

> A shock tolerance level was subjectively determined before the first session by increasing the current to the electrodes until the subject reported it so painful that he did not want the current increased further. All shocks in succeeding sessions were administered at double this value of current on the Foringer high scale (1970, p.124).

The effect of this condition on one subject (R.L.) was vividly described in the following quote which should receive a prize for droll commentary in an experiment report:

> A peculiar circumstance occurred during session 20, which was to have been the last session. When the first tone had been on for 1 minute, R.L. shouted, 'I can't take it any more!' He disconnected his electrodes, fled the laboratory without explanation, and the experimenter never heard from him again. This happening suggested that the shock was indeed responsible for the observed changes in his stuttering and reading rates. (1970, p. 127).

In other words, quite dramatic changes occurred in vocal intensity, speech rate, and pitch during the tone-shock condition. This study highlights the interesting possibility that any effects of state anxiety on stuttering might be mollified by induced alterations in the subject's typical manner of speaking. Indeed, under these conditions state anxiety could be justifiably described as having a facilitative, rather than debilitative, effect on stuttering.

The findings of the previous study might also lead us to question whether a reduction in stuttering should be expected to reduce state anxiety. In the context of some theories this should be an anticipated effect. It will be recalled, for example, that Brutten and Shoemaker (1967) have argued that stuttering is a conditioned-anxiety response. It follows, therefore, that decreased stuttering should be accompanied by decreased state anxiety. The data from a number of studies suggests that this is not always the case.

Ingham and Andrews (1971) had stutterers (n=8) assess their "tension state" on a self-rating scale over the course of an intensive treatment program. They found that this group had a 98% reduction in stuttering over the course of treatment, but this was accompanied by a slight increase in self-assessed state anxiety. Also, Adams and Moore (1972) found reduced stuttering occurred while subjects orally read during masking conditions, but this was associated with reductions in palmar sweat indices for only three of their 12 subjects. The challenge offered by these findings to a conditioned-anxiety explanation of stuttering variability is heightened by findings from two well-designed studies by Reed and Lingwall (1976; 1980).

In their 1976 study, Reed and Lingwall measured stuttering and galvanic skin responses (GSR) of 10 stutterers within response-contingent experimental treatment conditions. The subjects were assessed during base rate, treatment, and extinction conditions (an ABA design). In the treatment condition, the subjects heard a second of 95dB SPL white noise contingent on each stuttering. This resulted in more than 50% reductions in stuttering relative to base rate and extinction conditions. The group data show that the mean GSR response was virtually unaffected by changes in stuttering during the experimental conditions. In the 1980 study, they attempted to assess the effect of a conditioned stimulus on GSR responses. Ten stutterers were assessed across three separate ABA experimental runs. In the first run, the B (treatment) condition was paired with a slide showing a face. In the second run, the face slide was presented throughout the B condition and was joined by one second of recorded laughter after each moment of stuttering. The third experimental run was the same as the first. The data show that only the second and third experimental runs affected reduced stuttering during the B condition. This suggested that the face slide had become a conditioned stimulus capable of producing reduced stuttering. But GSR measures made throughout each experimental run again failed to show a consistent relationship with changes in stuttering behavior. Reed and Lingwall aptly concluded that "the position shared by several theories indicating stuttering is acquired and maintained by neutral cues which after association with punishment elicit negative emotionality may be too simplistic" (1980, p.343).

Actually, the data collected in Reed and Lingwall's 1976 and 1980 studies provided an even more direct challenge to Brutten and Shoemaker's (1967) two-factor theory. They collected frequency counts of different types of stuttering behaviors in all experimental conditions and found that in spite of changes in total stutterings the proportion of the different types of stuttering behavior remained virtually stable across all experimental runs. This finding runs counter to Brutten and Shoemaker's hypothesis that repetitions and prolongations are not affected by punishment conditions.

A similar challenge to the foundation of Brutten and Shoemaker's theory occurs in findings from a study by Gray and England (1972). They measured trait and state anxiety during and after a treatment which was specifically designed to decondition state anxiety. As discussed in the next section, the most commonly employed behavioral treatment for anxiety-related behaviors is reciprocal inhibition (Wolpe, 1958). This procedure pairs relaxation (or other anxiety-inhibiting behaviors) with scheduled visualizations of increasingly anxiety-provoking stimuli. Fifteen stutterers were assessed on four occasions over the treatment period via GSR, stuttering, and two trait anxiety scores. Over the course of treatment they found reductions in the state anxiety measure, one trait anxiety measure and also stuttering, but there was "no correspondence between stuttering frequency and anxiety beyond a marginal or coincidental one" (Gray & England, 1972, p.114).

At first glance Gray and England's findings appear to be at odds with findings from a therapy-analogue study conducted by Webster (1970). He had four stutterers read a self-prepared passage that "evoked negative emotion." Across five readings there was a predictable adaptation effect which was then "lost" by an interval introduced before a sixth reading. In a second run of this procedure, the interval after the fifth reading was occupied by systematic desensitization (using relaxation) of the anxiety-evoking content of the passage. The sixth reading then followed, and all subjects showed evidence that their stuttering frequency remained close to the level obtained during the fifth reading. But the difficulty with these data (unlike the Gray and England study) is that they are not accompanied by an independent measure of state anxiety. This leaves open the possibility that the changes in stuttering were not associated with actual reductions in state anxiety.

Some Final Considerations

The overall tenor of the findings from the studies reviewed is that there is little evidence of a clinically significant, or even theoretically palpable, relationship between stuttering and anxiety. In Chapter 11 the effects of biofeedback procedures will be reviewed, and they suggest that more subtle measures of tension may account for some variability in stuttering. But these measures may have a marginal association with the gross forms of tension that typify the anxiety which, allegedly, provokes stuttering.

One dimension of stuttering that may be responsive to changes in state anxiety is the severity, or duration, of methods of stuttering. Aron (1965) conducted an extensive study on the effects of the tranquilizing drug Amylozine on the frequency and severity of stuttering. Across 46 adult stutterers she found a significant reduction in the rated severity of stuttering, but no change in frequency of stuttering. It is noteworthy that Gray and England (1972) also informally observed that their subjects substantially reduced the severity of their moments of stuttering during the course of treatment. It becomes evident, therefore, that the effects of anxiety may be revealed in a variety of ways including, for example, an altered speech pattern and the excessive tension involved in particularly severe moments of stuttering.

As mentioned earlier, there is little doubt that stutterers are generally cast as unusually fearful and anxious, even by clinicians. Turnbaugh et al. (1979) found that clinicians tended to judge stutterers as "more nervous, self-conscious, tense, sensitive, anxious, fearful, afraid, hesitant, insecure, and intelligent than the fluent individual" (Turnbaugh, Guitar, & Hoffman, 1979, p.43). This is a remarkably negative stereotype which, in the case of children, is apparently shared by their parents. Fowlie and Cooper (1978) found that the mothers of stuttering children (6-8 years) perceived them as "more insecure, sensitive, anxious, withdrawn, fearful, and introverted than did mothers of nonstutterers" (Fowlie & Cooper, 1978, p.233). Nevertheless, this image does not appear to have been always transferred into the behavior of stutterers. For example, Trotter and Bergmann (1957) found that stuttering and nonstuttering adults were not distinguishably different in their estimates of the frequency with which they entered speaking situations. Also, Silverman (1970) found that when stuttering children were asked to nominate their "three wishes" only 6.4% made wishes in which either their speech or stuttering was mentioned. In the case of adult stutterers, Knott (1935) found that a request to nominate "pleasant" and "unpleasant" speaking experiences yielded no evidence that these experiences were related to either stuttering or nonstuttering.

The search for a relationship between stuttering and anxiety has not been profitable. Stutterers may appear to be anxious, even fearful, with respect to speaking situations, but it seems unlikely that variations in their speech problem are directly related to this fear or anxiety. Perhaps, like the personality of stutterers (Bloch & Goodstein, 1971; Goodstein, 1958), it is quite surprising that there is not more evidence of abnormalcy from this, ostensibly, fearful affliction. Against this backdrop of relatively unprofitable research, it seems unlikely that treatments directed towards anxiety reduction would prove to have general therapeutic merit. The following review of their application to stuttering will consider whether this is so.

Therapy Procedures

Clinicians of very different persuasions have long regarded the alleviation of anxiety as the primary point of treatment for most of the so-called "functional disorders." It has been a support for a profitable drug industry and a foundation for numerous "talking therapies." The treatment principle used in these therapies is engagingly simple: by reducing the debilitative sensation of fear and/or tension, the disorder will either fade away or be managed more easily. In the light of the previous section, it is not clear that this principle is appropriate to the treatment of stuttering. But it certainly has not deterred its use.

At least four general anxiety-modification techniques have been used to treat stuttering. They are reciprocal inhibition, hypnotherapy, drug therapy, and biofeedback. Stuttering treatments that have mainly employed the first of these types of treatment will be reviewed in the following section. The last three treatment approaches will be reviewed in Chapter 11.

Reciprocal-Inhibition Therapy

Stuttering treatment has had a lengthy association with relaxation methods. During the mental hygiene period of the 1930s and 1940s, it was a recommended component of many treatment programs (Blanton & Blanton, 1936; Gifford, 1940; Hahn, 1941). In fact, Van Riper (1973) argues that "For two decades (1920-1940) relaxation therapy was the dominant form of treatment in this country [USA] and England though it was often combined with other techniques" (p.42-3). But, quite clearly, it was never regarded as a particularly effective method of therapy for either adults or children. Yet, like rhythmic stimulation procedures, it quite suddenly reappeared as a principal treatment agent within a behavior therapy approach to stuttering treatment.

Perhaps no therapy procedure is more closely identified with behavior therapy than Wolpe's (1958) Reciprocal Inhibition Therapy. The essential ingredients of this procedure are systematic desensitization and a behavior which will inhibit anxiety, such as an assertive, sexual, or relaxation response. Both systematic desensitization and relaxation were used to modify problem behaviors long before the advent of behavior therapy. Mary Cover Jones (1924) had adequately demonstrated the desensitizing effects of systematic approximations to a feared subject, while Jacobson (1929) had pioneered "progressive relaxation" as a technique for reducing the handicapping effects of muscle tension. By gradually tensing and relaxing all the major muscle groups, until virtually complete muscular relaxation was achieved, Jacobson (1929; 1970) reported the successful treatment of disorders such as colitis, insomnia, anxiety conditions, and essential hypertension. Wolpe's contribution was to recognize that systematic approximation (or desensitization) and relaxation could combine to form a therapeutic application of the phenomenon known as reciprocal inhibition. This phenomenon, which was described originally by Sherrington (1906), was based upon the general proposition that, "if a response inhibiting to anxiety can be made to occur in the presence of anxiety-evoking stimuli so that it is accompanied by a complete or partial suppression of the anxiety response, the bond between these stimuli and the anxiety response will be weakened" (Wolpe, 1961, p.189). In the context of treating neurotic human behavior, Wolpe (1958) recommended instigating anxiety-inhibiting behaviors in the stimulus conditions that provoke this behavior. The repeated exercise of these behaviors was designed to weaken the anxiety-response habit. By systematically instigating this anxiety-inhibiting behavior to successively more anxiety-stimulating conditions, it was theorized that the problem response would eventually disappear.

Wolpe (1958) carefully outlined a procedure that should be followed for reciprocal inhibition therapy. In the first place, the inhibiting response should be chosen carefully so that it effectively inhibits autonomic over-reactivity. This may be achieved by assertive responses, sexual responses, or even mild non-aversive shock. But the most common method was via muscle relaxation. The means of achieving this include hypnosis and drug therapy, though greatest use has been made of an abbreviated version of Jacobson's progressive relaxation. The relaxation procedure is now well known and widely used. It usually involves about five to six sessions in which the subject learns to relax the major muscle groups by tensing and relaxing them, usually to the accompaniment of a covertly uttered cue word. The relaxation procedure may also use deep breathing to accompany the relaxing operation. This procedure is combined with home practice until, ideally, the subject is able to rapidly "turn on" relaxation via the cue word. The clinician and subject then carefully construct a hierarchy of increasingly anxiety-provoking situations. At about the same time, the subject is also taught to visualize either neutral or pleasant scenes. The systematic desensitization sessions begin by asking the subject to visualize the lowest situation on the hierearchy, while totally relaxed. When this 10- to 20-second visualization succeeds in not producing anxiety on two or three successive occasions, the next highest item is then visualized. If an item is failed, then either shorter intervals of item visualization are introduced, or the subject returns to the previous item in the hierarchy. This procedure continues until each of the hierarchy items is passed. The subject may also be required to actually enter hierarchy situations while practicing the cue-controlled relaxation.

It will be obvious that this procedure presents some intriguing issues for behavior therapy. To begin with, most aspects of the procedure are not immediately available to empirical analysis. For instance, the criteria for muscle relaxation may never be anchored to observable behavior (other than via the subject's report). Another issue is the indirect nature of the therapy approach with respect to certain disorders. Treatment is usually directed at anxiety-provoking situations and the behavior, as such, is expected to yield to the effects of this process. It is noteworthy that this approach shares much in common with some aspects of a medical-model approach to treatment. The theoretical foundations of this procedure are also shaky, especially since similar treatment effects have been obtained with radical variations of Wolpe's strictly prescribed therapy strategy (Yates, 1975). At the same time, it remains as one of the most useful and effective treatment techniques for many disorders (Kazdin & Wilcoxon, 1976).

During behavior therapy's infancy, reciprocal inhibition was reported to achieve almost (if not entirely) unbelievable levels of success in treating a wide range of neurotic disorders. In the light of present standards for treatment evaluation, the claims for success made by Wolpe (1961) and Lazarus (1963) are almost ludicrous. With only limited reference to follow-up assessment, and no data-based evaluation of the problem behavior, it was claimed that between 89%

(Wolpe, 1958) and 78% (Lazarus, 1963) of neurotic individuals had achieved lasting benefits as a result of this therapy. This was a dubious claim that did little to advance the credibility of behavior therapy.

The questionable methodology used to support the therapy success of reciprocal inhibition, and its attack on the nonbehavioral paradigm during this era, actually set a pattern for treatment evaluation. One of the cornerstone beliefs of the nonbehavioral approach to the treatment of many problem behaviors was that these were merely symptomatic of more serious problems, and their removal would lead inevitably to symptom substitution. Consequently, one of the initial concerns of behavior therapists was to demonstrate that successful treatment of a problem behavior did not have this dire effect. During this early period, this concern appeared to take priority over a systematic evaluation of posttreatment results.

Reciprocal Inhibition and Stuttering

Wolpe, like many of the early behavior therapists, conceived of stuttering as a habit response to conditioned anxiety which, therefore, made it an obvious contender for reciprocal inhibition therapy. Both Wolpe and Lazarus actually provided some cursory accounts of stuttering treatment with this therapy. Wolpe (1958) reported that two adult stutterers and one 14-year-old stutterer had been treated with mixed success. In a later publication (Wolpe, 1969), it was revealed that one adult was treated mainly by assertive training, and when "seen two years later [he] spoke without any suggestion of stutter" (p.23). The other was reported to be "much improved," but the 14-year-old showed marked relapse shortly after treatment ceased.

Lazarus and Rachman (1957) and Lazarus (1964) provided similar vague information on the treatment of three late adolescent and two adult stutterers. Follow-up evaluation (nine months to four years) for three of these subjects indicated "improvement" and "some gains" had resulted. The treatment of one of these subjects (an 18-year-old male) closely resembled a therapy procedure later recommended by Brutten and Shoemaker (1967), in that he received a combination of systematic desensitization and massed practice. In Lazarus's (1963) well-known report on the effects of treating 126 severe neurotics by reciprocal inhibition, these five subjects reappear, and four were there rated as "unimproved" by treatment. It is interesting to observe that the treatment outcome of the stuttering group in Lazarus's report was the least successful of all the differentially diagnosed groups.

The questionable success of reciprocal inhibition with stuttering was also recognized by Rachman (1962), who recommended that other methods might be more suitable for this disorder. This point was also mentioned in later brief reports by Wolpe and Lazarus. In a 1969 report, Wolpe redescribed his, allegedly, successful treatment of a 31-year-old stutterer using assertive training (see Wolpe, 1958) and added a description of the treatment of a 25-year-old male. This subject was treated with rhythmic speech followed by systematic desensitization and relaxation. It was claimed that his speech improved by 90 to 95%, and remained that way a year later "as judged by me and as reported by his wife" (Wolpe, 1969, p.24). Lazarus (1969) also acknowledged that anxiety deconditioning may not be suitable for stuttering and backed this with a report of a multimodel treatment for a 22-year-old male stutterer. His therapy involved systematic desensitization, relaxation, assertive training, shadowing, choral reading, solitary reading, and rhythmic speaking. Six months after treatment, the subject was still reported to have "one or two blocks per minute of less than 2 seconds duration." No other stuttering frequency data were given and claims for the effectiveness of the treatment, while vaguely described, appear to rest with an apparent reduction in stuttering severity. Many later reports of reciprocal inhibition therapy also included little speech behavior data. For example, Kraft (1970) used relaxation supplemented by "hypnosis or. . .intraveneous injections of Methohexitone Sodium" in the treatment of a group of neurotic patients, one of whom was a stutterer. This subject was reported to show "marked improvement" at a 12-month follow-up. Kuchner (1970) provided an equally abbreviated account of the "successful" treatment of a female stutterer. Rosenthal (1968) went to the trouble of treating a 26-year-old stutterer with the longest hierarchy yet reported in the reciprocal inhibition therapy literature—215 items! The only information on the subject's speech behavior was that he began treatment with blocks of beyond 3 minutes duration and ended treatment with socially acceptable speech; though 7½ months later there was "some slight worsening of speech."

Walton and Mather (1963) reported the treatment of two adult stutterers, one with assertive training and the other with relaxation. In their data-free report, both subjects were reported to have markedly improved as a result of treatment, and this improvement was said to be maintained 6 to 12 months later. A noteworthy feature of the relaxation procedure used in this study was the inclusion of deep breathing to induce relaxation. This method of relaxation is often used in reciprocal inhibition (Paul, 1966). It is also a procedure which may have special relevance for stuttering treatment, but, unfortunately, it is often unclear as to whether it has been used in this context. The significance of this technique will be evident in Chapter 10, where stuttering treatments that employ "breathstream management" are described.

The combining of reciprocal inhibition with other therapy techniques was also used in some stuttering treatments reported during the 1960s. Damste, Zwaan, and Shoemaker (1968) outlined a method which used a form of breathstream management along with systematic desensitization and relaxation. Subjects were first taught "stopping" before the stuttering response, then to relax and control breathing before continuing to speak. Also, during relaxation training the subject was taught to "wait till the breathing movement has reached its top [and] only then. . .to start speaking" (1968, p.333). Thereafter, systematic desensitization procedures were used to the accompaniment of positive comments about speaking situations. Forty-four subjects treated "in the last 3 years," as well as close relatives of most subjects, responded to a questionnaire designed to self-rate improvement. More than 90% of subjects were assessed as "improved or much improved," but no supportive speech performance data were presented.

Browning (1967) provided the first report of a reciprocal inhibition treatment that included daily speech performance data. This treatment, which also combined reciprocal inhibition and other therapy methods, was for a 12-year-old mildly schizophrenic boy who stuttered. The 5-month treatment in a hospital setting began with systematic desensitization and relaxation procedures, which were then blended with a system of token and social reinforcement. Daily oral reading and conversational data revealed that the subject's stuttering declined during oral reading, but actually increased during conversational speech. This may be due to a procedure introduced during the desensitization phase: the subject was token-rewarded for ceasing to speak at a block, relaxing, and then saying the word fluently. Actually, the main benefits of treatment appear to be due to the subsequent reinforcement procedures rather than reciprocal inhibition. But, unfortunately, it is impossible to identify the potency of any treatment agent from the reported data trend.

Brutten and Shoemaker's (1967) Two-Factor Theory of stuttering claimed important therapy implications. If, as they theorized, stuttering was composed of classically conditioned and instrumentally conditioned behaviors then a treatment package was needed to cope with those different behaviors. Essentially, their procedure (Brutten, 1969; Shoemaker & Brutten, 1969) was "two-factored": reciprocal inhibition for treating first-factor behaviors, and massed practice to inhibit second-factor behaviors. This treatment is also based on a detailed diagnostic procedure (Brutten, 1973; 1975) for identifying suitable "Inhibition Therapy" candidates. But, in spite of its carefully formulated theoretical foundations, it does not appear to have been an especially beneficial therapy. The only information on therapy benefits that Brutten and/or Shoemaker have ever provided is a brief and intriguing comment on 30 subjects: "clinical experience with these stutterers does not permit the proclamation that inhibition therapy has been universally effective; some of the stutterers have showed dramatic improvement and some have failed to evidence more than a limited degree of behavior change" (Brutten, 1969, p.81). This finding is also underscored by a subsequent treatment study by Adams (1972).

Adams's (1972) report is perhaps the only documented account of an attempt to assess the effect of much of Brutten and Shoemaker's therapy procedure. From a pool of 67 subjects, 39 were apparently diagnosed as stutterers according to criteria identical to those specified by Brutten and Shoemaker.[5] Eighteen (7-28 years) of the 39 subjects were treated by reciprocal inhibition using relaxation sessions (one hour per week) over a 10- to 70-week period. Six subjects left treatment (three failed to achieve the relaxation criteria) and four of the remaining 12 were still in therapy at the time of the report. Three of these four subjects were reported to have "demonstrated no stuttering behavior change whatsoever." Five of the remaining eight subjects were assessed at least 18 months after their treatment ceased, and were apparently "free of stuttering in every one of the circumstances that had previously been listed on their hierarchy

[5]This could be one estimate of the extent to which these criteria might distinguish "stutterers" from "disfluents." From Adams's (1970) report it can only be assumed that the other 28 subjects also displayed stuttering behavior, but theirs did not fit Brutten and Shoemaker's definition of stuttering.

of feared speech situations" (Adams, 1972, p.67). This finding was confirmed by personal interviews and independent reports, but absolutely no speech behaviors were collected to add credence to this claim. This may be a reasonably promising report on the efficacy of at least part of Brutten and Shoemaker's therapy procedure, but the absence of one of the essential ingredients of behavior therapy, objectively recorded data, is disappointing.

A number of more recent group treatment studies have endeavored to isolate treatment effects during reciprocal inhibition with stuttering. Most have included speech-behavior data, which helps to give some indication of the general efficacy of this treatment. The previously mentioned study by Gray and England (1972) gives some idea of treatment gains, but it also illustrates the difficulty in evaluating treatment via a group study. Their 15 stutterers (14-45 years) were treated by reciprocal inhibition (using relaxation) over a fixed schedule of sessions: for 8 weeks they received a decreasing number of weekly sessions (30 minutes), then one session every 2 weeks over 3 months, and a final session 6 months later. Thus, each subject received a total of 13.5 hours treatment, seemingly without reference to the time required for each individual's hierarchy. Oral-reading data, obtained before, during, and at the 6-month assessment point, showed a "significant reduction in fluency failures" by the end of treatment. The clinicians judged six subjects as "cured" or "greatly improved," but in the absence of supportive data. There was some evidence of reduced speech-related anxiety, although "in real life there was little effect of the anxiety reduction upon the frequency [of stuttering]. However, there were noticeable changes, informally noted, in the degree of severity of the stuttering" (1972, p.121). This suggests that the clinical benefits of treatment were not substantial.

Rather more speech data were reported in a study by Boudreau and Jeffrey (1973) on 12 stutterers (16-22 years). These subjects were divided into a treatment (n=8) and control group (n=4), with the treatment group receiving a fixed number of treatment sessions. These sessions were also accompanied by home practice. Data were collected from four 10-minute oral reading and spontaneous speech tasks given before and after treatment and then again 20 months later. The interesting feature of this treatment was that it also incorporated speech behavior: the subject had to talk about the anxiety-provoking scene after it had been imagined. Unfortunately, it is not clear whether the subject's speech performance was also used as a criterion for passage through the hierarchy. The data show that the treatment group's percentage of words stuttered was reduced by a mean of 58.9% on the oral reading tasks and 63.5% on spontaneous speaking tasks. The control group showed a nonsignificant change over this period. But the clinical meaningfulness of the posttreatment data are questionable. For example, no subject was reported stutter-free (the lowest percentage of words stuttered on the spontaneous speech task was 3%) and no speech rate or reliability data were included. Furthermore, during the following 20 months, five of the eight subjects were actually continued in treatment. For instance, two subjects were given 10 1-hour sessions of metronome training and another received six 1-hour sessions of masking treatment. The experimenters report that the follow-up data "indicated stability of results," but it is difficult to understand how this stability could be attributed to the original treatment.

Burgraff (1974) compared systematic desensitization treatment and Van Riper's treatment procedures via a group of 18 stutterers (19-51 years) who were split into two groups of nine after receiving relaxation training. A significant reduction in disfluencies (35-40%) and "block duration" was reported for both groups on the basis of spontaneous speech data collected within the clinic before and after treatment. And although no significant differences were found between the groups, the findings are confounded because the group treated by Van Riper's procedure also systematically worked through a desensitization hierarchy. In other words, the experience of "passing through the hierarchy" (albeit by discussion) might have been the crucial treatment agent for both the Van Riper-treated group and the systematic desensitization group.

A confounding of treatment agents may have also occurred in a reciprocal inhibition study by Dalali and Sheehan (1974). They attempted to ascertain whether "assertion training would add to the effectiveness of current therapy for stuttering" (p.98). The "current therapy" was a program devised by Sheehan (1975). Twenty-four stutterers, already involved in therapy, were divided into three groups, and treated for 6 hours over 3 weekends. Each group recieved a different treatment schedule. One was trained in "active assertion," another received "feeling clarification," and the third formed a control group. No differences were found before or after treatment between each group's frequency and severity of stuttering, or their responses to an Assertion Inventory and a projective test. Although this finding suggests that assertion training was ineffective, it is difficult to bypass the possibility that the "current therapy" might have exerted far more control over the subjects' speech behavior than the experimental treatments. It is also possible that the assertion training was not given adequate time to take effect. Dalali and Sheehan claim that 6 hours of treatment were sufficient because this resembled the time used for reciprocal inhibition in a study by Paul (1966). However, Paul's study actually involved relaxation rather than assertion training.

The preceding group studies have yielded some evidence that reciprocal inhibition may produce some reductions in stuttering, but the clinical meaningfulness of these reductions, and the extent to which anxiety modification may have contributed to this effect, is far from clear. Data from a study by Moleski and Tosi (1976) suggest the possibility that other procedures, involving modification of reactions to speaking situations, might be even more effective than reciprocal inhibition with relaxation. They assigned 20 stutterers (mean age 28 years) to groups that received either Rational-Emotive Therapy (Ellis, 1971), systematic desensitization and relaxation (these groups were subdivided into those who were treated with in vivo tasks and those who were not), or no treatment. All treated subjects received eight 45-minute sessions and were assessed before and after these sessions on oral reading and spontaneous speech tasks, plus a trait anxiety and attitude-to-stuttering scale. The findings show that Rational-Emotive Therapy was significantly more effective than reciprocal inhibition therapy in reducing stuttering, anxiety, and negative attitudes. However, no data were provided which would indicate the magnitude of these changes or, more importantly, the treatment's effects on task-relevant speech behavior. For example, both treatments were directed towards improving speech behavior with strangers and on the telephone, yet no assessment was made of speech behavior on either task.[6] The findings of this study provide the interesting suggestion that reciprocal inhibition may not be a preferred treatment for those stutterers who have debilitating anxiety reactions to speech situations.

Finally, a study by Janssen and Damste (1976) provides some further evidence that reciprocal inhibition may have variable effects on speech-related anxiety. They reported treating 100 stutterers, in groups of around 20, for four 6-day periods over a period of 6 months. Their treatment included systematic desensitization and relaxation for deconditioning speech-related anxiety, plus a mixture of psychotherapy and "speech modification techniques [unspecified] for obtaining fluent speech." Pre- and posttreatment data were collected from counting and spontaneous speech (1 minute of each) within the clinic, physiological measures of heart and respiration rates, and questionnaire ratings of state anxiety, stuttering severity, neuroticism, and failure anxiety. The principal findings were that stuttering decreased by a mean of about 58% on the spontaneous speaking task, with no change in speech rate. There was also a significant decline in both the self-rated state anxiety measures, plus most of the counterpart physiological measures. The intercorrelations between these measures were of most interest, however. These indicated there were:

> significant negative correlations between improvement and heart rate, and between improvement and anxiety rating while speaking. These findings suggest that stutterers characterized by relatively high levels of speech-related anxiety were likely to be the least responsive to the type of treatment evaluated in this study. This is the more surprising since anxiety reduction is one of the principal therapeutic agents of this therapy (p.239).

The only problem with this conclusion is that it is based on two dubious premises. The first is that the data measures were not accompanied by estimates of their reliability. And the second is that the mixture of treatment procedures may have produced interactions within and between some of the pertinent variables. For example, it is impossible to ignore the possibility that the relationship between the anxiety measures and changes in stuttering may have been affected by the "speech modification" treatment procedures.

In the main, the findings from these group studies are rather disappointing. All fail to provide sufficient data to estimate the effects of reciprocal inhibition in clinically meaningful speaking situations. On the other hand, they do show a relatively consistent pattern; stuttering appears to be reduced during this treatment, but not always in association with predicted amounts of anxiety. At best, it appears that this treatment has some effect on speech-related anxiety and it reduces stuttering, though not enough to justify its use as a primary treatment

[6] Of course, this criticism applies to all the reciprocal inhibition studies which have failed to report this type of data.

agent. This is also borne out by some other reports of reciprocal inhibition treatment.

Lanyon (1969) treated a 25-year-old male stutterer with systematic desensitization and relaxation over a 3-month period. Oral reading and spontaneous speech samples, plus severity ratings were obtained before treatment, immediately after treatment, and 9 months later. The data show that by the end of treatment, there was a 56% reduction in "nonfluencies" on the spontaneous speech task, along with a 6% reduction in speech rate. As this writer has noted (Ingham & Andrews, 1971), this raises the possibility that the treatment benefits may have derived, in part, from a reduction in speech rate. (Although the oral reading task did show a 40% reduction in nonfluencies and a 35% increase in speech rate.) There are also additional problems with this study. For example, it is not supported by reliability data, or by speech performance data at the 9 month follow-up assessment.

Tyre, Maisto, and Companik (1973) reported an identical treatment study with a 23-year-old stutterer. In fact, their subject also received 16 treatment sessions, but over 2 (rather than 3) months. Pretreatment, posttreatment and 6 months after treatment assessments were made using Lanyon's (1967) Scale for Severity of Stuttering and 10 minutes of conversational speech. Quite surprisingly, only the rating scale data were reported.[7] These data reveal improvement, but certainly not fluency.

Porter (1976) reported treating a 20-year-old stutterer over five weekly sessions of systematic desensitization and relaxation. She reported about an 80% reduction in stuttering and some evidence of an increase in speech rate by the end of treatment. It was also claimed that follow-up contacts, 11 months and 2 years after treatment, found the subject had maintained his "nonstuttered speech." Unhappily, this report also failed to report supporting follow-up data or estimates of measurement reliabililty.

There have also been some interesting variations on reciprocal inhibition procedures in stuttering treatments. Yonovitz, Shepherd, and Garrett (1977) used colored slides, or video, to depict speech situation scenes for the systematic desensitization phase in the treatment of two stutterers (13 and 5 years). The 13-year-old was treated with relaxation procedures in order to control anxiety reactions to the classroom situation. (The level of relaxation was checked from the subject's GSR responses transmitted to the experimenters.) The 5-year-old was treated with an assertive muscular response induced by pedaling a stationary exercise bicycle while watching a video scene of a classroom. Both subjects were reported to have reduced stuttering in these situations, but the data are not sufficient to show that the outcome was necessarily associated with the introduction of treatment.

Another inventive application of reciprocal inhibition is Lee, McGough, and Peins's (1976) automated desensitiztion procedure for the telephone difficulties of

[7] Actually a significant reduction in stuttering frequency was reported to have been obtained. This was based on an analysis of variance procedure. But this finding is clouded because of the inappropriateness of this statistical procedure on single-subject data.

stutterers. A 15-minute tape recording of relaxation instructions and scene visualization was used to precede a standardized hierarchy of in vivo activities with the telephone. This was accompanied by programmed home practice and therapist-directed procedures every 2 weeks. Abbreviated information is reported on the treatment of three stutterers who were all said to have responded favorably to treatment.

Finally, Adams (1982) has recently reported using flooding within a reciprocal inhibition therapy framework with a 27-year-old stutterer. The subject's stuttering was quite problematic for his work as a fireman; he was obliged to make "short but important announcements to the on duty fireman" via an intercom and shortwave radio. Following an abbreviated version of Perkins's (1973) breathstream management program, the subject was reported to be much improved except in the broadcasting task "where his strong anxiety got the best of him so that he could not concentrate on and effectively use his newly acquired, fluency enhancing behaviors" (Adams, 1982, p.348). A relaxation program proved ineffective in solving this problem and was replaced by a flooding technique similar to that described by Stampfl and Levis (1967). In this technique, the subject visualizes anxiety-provoking scenes over a series of sessions until self-rated anxiety reactions are reduced. Unfortunately, no speech performance data were collected to accompany the subjectively reported benefits of this procedure.

Other alternative relaxation procedures have been suggested for aiding stuttering treatment. These include biofeedback, hypnosis, and drugs (these three methods are reviewed in Chapter 11), metronomic stimulation (Brady & Brady, 1972), self-relaxation or "autogenic training" (Schilling, 1966) and transcendental meditation. In the case of the latter procedure, McIntyre, Silverman and Trotter (1974) reported that six male stutterers had engaged in this relaxation procedure for between 2 weeks and 3½ years. All claimed that it benefited their fluency. But, like metronomic relaxation and autogenic training, there is, as yet, no worthwhile data that would lead one to advocate these procedures in stuttering treatment.

Conclusions

It is difficult not to conclude this review on a pessimistic note. The reasons are not because of a lack of positive treatment reports, but because of what those reports lack. It is quite remarkable that a treatment procedure, which is so closely identified with behavior therapy, has been used with so little regard for systematic evaluation. For example, among all these treatment reports not one has demonstrated that the treatment of speech-related or situation-related anxiety produced reduced stuttering in relevant situations. A more clinically important result is that in none of the reports, where speech behavior data are reported, is there evidence of stutter-free speech following treatment. There is some evidence that the treatment improved the speech of some subjects, but it is not clear that the effects have been sustained. This is underscored by some evidence that additional therapy intruded between the cessation of relaxation treatment and subsequent assessment. This generally poor finding may have been a necessary consequence of a treatment which may only train the subject to use certain methods in the face of difficult speaking situations.

There are two aspects of reciprocal-inhibition therapy which suggests reasons why its benefits for stuttering treatment have been relatively mediocre. The first is that the treatment is more accurately described as a "train and hope" technique (Stokes & Baer, 1977). The duration of treatment is normally governed by the number of items on the desensitization hierarchy. When the items are completed (either in vivo or in situ), then, presumably, it is "hoped" that there will be a related improvement in the subject's speech. None of the treatment studies indicated that progress through a hierarchy was yoked to the subject's speaking behavior, either within the treatment setting or, more logically, in the setttings for which the treatment is designed (the 1976 Lee, McGough, and Peins study may be a notable exception). The second aspect concerns a procedure which seemingly demands that the speaker should always be physically relaxed before speaking in certain speaking situations. These reports do not indicate whether this should always be the case. Indeed it would be almost unusual if it were, since it is manifestly obvious that certain speaking situations provoke an above-average level of anxiety (for example, speaking before a large audience). Under such circumstances certain skills often benefit from some measure of anxiety. There is, for example, a substantial literature that shows state anxiety may be quite facilitative for certain types of human performance (Alpert & Haber, 1960).

The current general status of reciprocal inhibition in behavior therapy is quite relevant to its contribution to stuttering therapy. In a number of studies it has been shown that components of the treatment can be radically changed without damaging its efficacy (Yates, 1975). The true source of its treatment effects are certainly unclear (Kazdin & Wilcoxon, 1976), nevertheless, the treatment appears to "work." Bandura (1977) has argued that perhaps relaxation may only have a beneficial, rather than necessary, role in desensitization. Possibly the only necessary condition that remains as intrinsic to this therapy method is pairing anxiety-provoking stimuli with a different response.

These issues may be especially pertinent in explaining the treatment's limited success with stuttering. For instance, while anxiety appears not to be specifically related to stuttering variability, the modification of anxiety may certainly have facilitative effects. Also, since the systematic exposure of a patient to increasingly difficult speaking situations is integral to many treatment methods, it may mean that their utility—even their success—depends upon desensitization. But all of this is not to deny the beneficial effects that anxiety reduction may provide, particularly for specific situational difficulties, and for stutterers who also have quite debilitative anxiety. It may be that its best application is as an aid rather than as an essential treatment agent in stuttering treatment. However, more specific modifications of tension may achieve different effects. This occurs within treatments such as hypnosis, drug therapy, and biofeedback. The contribution of these treatments to stuttering therapy will be considered in Chapter 11.

References

Adams, M.R. The use of reciprocal inhibition procedures in the treatment of stuttering. *Journal of Communication Disorders,* 1972, *5,* 59-66.

Adams, M.R. A case report on the use of flooding in stuttering therapy. *Journal of Fluency Disorders,* 1982, *7,* 343-353.

Adams, M.R., & Brutten, G.J. An exploratory study of some learning-based procedures for modifying stuttering. *Journal of Communication Disorders,* 1970, *3,* 123-132.

Adams, M.R., & Dietze, D.A. A comparison of the reaction times of stutterers and nonstutterers to items on a word association test. *Journal of Speech and Hearing Research,* 1965, *8,* 195-202.

Adams, M.R., & Moore, Jr., W.H. The effect of auditory masking on the anxiety level, frequency of disfluency, and selected vocal characteristics of stutterers. *Journal of Speech and Hearing Research,* 1972, *15,* 572-578.

Alpert, R., & Haber, R.N. Anxiety in academic achievement situations. *Journal of Abnormal and Social Psychology,* 1960, *61,* 207-215.

Aron, M.L. The effects of the combination of trifluoperazine and amylobarbitone on adult stutterers. *Medical Proceedings, South African Journal for the Advancement of Medical Science,* 1965, *11,* 227-233.

Bandura, A. Self-efficacy: Toward a unifying theory of behavioral change. *Psychological Review,* 1977, *84,* 191-215.

Berwick, N.H. Stuttering in response to photographs of selected listeners. In W. Johnson & R.R. Leutenegger (Eds.), *Stuttering in children and adults.* Minneapolis: University of Minnesota Press, 1955.

Blanton, S., & Blanton, M.G. *For stutterers.* New York: Appleton-Century-Crofts, 1936.

Bloch, E.L., & Goodstein, L.D. Functional speech disorders and personality: a decade of research. *Journal of Speech and Hearing Disorders,* 1971, *36,* 295-314.

Bloodstein, O. Stuttering as an anticipatory struggle reaction. In J. Eisenson (Ed.), *Stuttering: A symposium.* New York: Harper & Row, 1958.

Bloodstein, O. The anticipatory struggle hypothesis: Implications of research on the variability of stuttering. *Journal of Speech and Hearing Research,* 1972, *15,* 487-499.

Bloodstein, O. *A handbook on stuttering.* (2nd ed.) Chicago: National Easter Seal Society, 1975.

Bloodstein, O. *A handbook on stuttering.* (3rd ed.) Chicago: National Easter Seal Society, 1981.

Boudreau, L.A., & Jeffrey, C.J. Stuttering treated by desensitization. *Journal of Behavior Therapy and Experimental Psychiatry.* 1973, *4,* 209-212.

Brady, J.P., & Brady, C.N. Behavior therapy of stuttering. *Folia Phoniatrica,* 1972, *24,* 355-359.

Browning, R.M. Behavior therapy for stuttering in a schizophrenic child. *Behaviour Research and Therapy.* 1967, *5,* 27-35.

Brutten, G.J. Palmar sweat investigation of disfluency and expectancy adaptation. *Journal of Speech and Hearing Research,* 1963, *6,* 40-48.

Brutten, G.J. Stuttering: Reflections on a two factor approach to behavior modifications. In B.B. Gray & G. England (Eds.), *Stuttering and the conditioning therapies,* Monterey, CA: Monterey Institute for Speech and Hearing, 1969.

Brutten, G.J. Behavior assessment and the strategy of therapy. In Y. Lebrun & R. Hoops (Eds.), *Neurolinguistic approaches to stuttering,* The Hague: Mouton, 1973.

Brutten, G.J. Stuttering: Topography, assessment, and behavior-change strategies. In J. Eisenson (Ed.), *Stuttering: A second symposium*. New York: Harper & Row, 1975.

Brutten, G.J., & Gray, B.B. Effect of word cue and removal on adaptation and adjacency: A clinical paradigm. *Journal of Speech and Hearing Disorders*, 1961, *26*, 385-389.

Brutten, G.J., & Janssen, P. An eye-marking investigation of anticipated and observed stuttering. *Journal of Speech and Hearing Research*, 1979, *22*, 20-28.

Brutten, G.J., & Shoemaker, D.J. *The modification of stuttering*, Englewood Cliffs, NJ: Prentice-Hall, 1967.

Burgraff, R.I. The efficacy of systematic desensitization via imagry as a therapeutic technique with stutterers. *British Journal of Disorders of Communication*, 1974, *9*, 134-139.

Cattell, R.B. *I.P.A.T. Self Analysis Scale*. Champagne, IL: Institute for Personality & Ability Testing, 1963.

Dabul, B., & Perkins, W.H. The effects of stuttering on systolic blood pressure. *Journal of Speech and Hearing Research*, 1973. *16*, 586-591.

Dalali, I.D., & Sheehan, J.G. Stuttering and assertion training. *Journal of Communication Disorders*, 1974, *7*, 97-111.

Damste, P.H., Zwaan, E.J., & Schoenaker, T.J. Learning principles applied to the stuttering problem. *Folia Phoniatricia*, 1968, *20*, 327-341.

Dixon, C.C. Stuttering adaptation in relation to assumed level of anxiety. In W. Johnson & R.R. Leutenegger (Eds.), *Stuttering in children and adults*. Minneapolis: University of Minnesota Press, 1955.

Dollard,J., & Mowrer, O.H. A method of measuring tension in written documents. In O.H. Mowrer (Ed.), *Psychotherapy and research*, New York: Ronald Press, 1953.

Ellis, A. *Growth through reason: Verbatim cases in rational-emotive therapy*, Palo Alto, CA: Science & Behavior Books, 1971.

Estes, W.K., & Skinner, B.F. Some quantitative properties of anxiety. *Journal of Experimental Psychology*, 1941, *21*, 390-400.

Forte, M., & Schlesinger, I.M. Stuttering as a function of time of expectation. *Journal of Communication Disorders*, 1972, *5*, 347-358.

Fowlie, G.M., & Cooper, E.B. Traits attributed to stuttering and nonstuttering children by their mothers. *Journal of Fluency Disorders*, 1978, *3*, 233-246.

Gifford, M.F. *How to overcome stammering*. Englewood Cliffs, NJ: Prentice-Hall, 1940.

Goodstein,L.D. Functional speech disorders and personality: A survey of the research. *Journal of Speech and Hearing Research*, 1958, *1*, 359-376.

Goss, A.E. Stuttering behavior and anxiety as a function of the duration of stimulus words. *Journal of Abnormal and Social Psychology*, 1952, *47*, 38-50.

Goss, A.E. Stuttering behavior and anxiety as a function of experimental training. *Journal of Speech and Hearing Disorders*, 1956, *21*, 343-351.

Gould, E., & Sheehan, J. Effect of silence on stuttering. *Journal of Abnormal Psychology*, 1967, *72*, 441-445.

Gray, B.B, & Brutten, E.J. The relationship between anxiety, fatigue and spontaneous recovery in stuttering. *Behaviour Research and Therapy*, 1965, *2*, 251-259.

Gray, B.B., & England, G. Some effects of anxiety deconditioning upon stuttering frequency. *Journal of Speech and Hearing Research*, 1972, *15*, 114-122.

Guthrie, E.R. *The psychology of learning*. New York: Harper & Brothers, 1935.

Hahn, E.F. A study of the relationship between the social complexity of the oral reading situation and the severity of stuttering. *Journal of Speech Disorders*, 1940, *5*, 5-14.

Hahn, E.F. A study of the effect of remedial treatment on the frequency of stuttering in oral reading. *Journal of Speech Disorders*, 1941, *6*, 29-38.

Hull, C.L. *Principles of behavior*. New York: Appleton-Century-Crofts, 1943.

Ickes, W.K., & Pierce, S. The stuttering moment: A plethysmographic study. *Journal of Communication Disorders*, 1973, *6*, 155-164.

Ingham, R.J., & Andrews, G. The relation between anxiety reduction and treatment. *Journal of Communication Disorders*, 1971, *4*, 289-301.

Jacobson, E. *Progressive relaxation*, Chicago: University of Chicago Press, 1929.

Jacobson, E. (Ed.), *Modern treatment of tense patients*. Springfield, IL: Charles C. Thomas, 1970.

Janssen, P., & Damste, P.H. Behavioral assessment procedures for stutterers. *Proceedings of the XVIth International Congress on Logopedics and Phoniatrics, Interlaken, 1974*. Basel: Karger, 1976.

Johnson, W., Darley, F.L., & Spriestersbach, D.C. *Diagnostic methods in speech pathology*. New York: Harper & Row, 1963.

Johnson, W., Larson, R.P., & Knott, J.R. Studies in the psychology of stuttering: III. Certain objective cues related to the precipitation of the moment of stuttering. *Journal of Speech Disorders*, 1937, *2*, 23-25.

Johnson, W., & Millsapps, L.S. Studies in the psychology of stuttering: VI. The role of cues representative of past stuttering in the distribution of stuttering moments during oral reading. *Journal of Speech Disorders*, 1937, *2*. 101-104.

Jones, M.C. A laboratory study of fear. The case of Peter. *Journal of Genetic Psychology*, 1924, *31*, 308-315.

Kazdin, A.E., & Wilcoxon, L.A. Systematic desensitization and nonspecific treatment effects: A methodological evaluation. *Psychololgical Bulletin*, 1976, *83*, 729-758.

Knott, J.R. A study of stutterers' stuttering and non-stuttering experiences on the basis of pleasantness and unpleasantness. *Quarterly Journal of Speech*, 1935, *21*, 328-331.

Kraft, T. A short note on forty patients treated by systematic desensitization. *Behaviour Research and Therapy*, 1970, *8*, 219-220.

Kuchner, S. Stotterbehandlung aus verhaltenstherapeutischer sicht. *Sprachheilarbeit*, 1970, *15*, 103-109.

Lanyon, R.I. The measurement of stuttering severity. *Journal of Speech and Hearing Research*, 1967, *10*, 836-843.

Lanyon, R.I. Behavior change in stuttering through systematic desensitization. *Journal of Speech and Hearing Disorders*, 1969, *34*, 253-260.

Lazarus, A.A. The results of behaviour therapy in 126 cases of severe neurosis. *Behaviour Research and Therapy*, 1963, *1*, 69-79.

Lazarus, A.A. Objective psychotherapy in the treatment of dysphemia. In H.J. Eysenck (Ed.), *Experiments in behaviour therapy*. Oxford: Pergamon, 1964.

Lazarus, A.A. The case history of a stutterer treated as an obsessive-compulsive disorder by broad-spectrum behavior therapy. In B.B.Gray & G. England (Eds.), *Stuttering and the conditioning therapies*, Monterey, CA: Monterey Institute for Speech and Hearing, 1969.

Lazarus, A.A. & Rachman, S. The use of systematic desensitization in psychotherapy. *South African Medical Journal*, 1957, *31*, 934-937.

Lee, B.S., McGough, W.E., & Peins, M. Automated desensitization of stutterers to use of the telephone. *Behavior Therapy*, 1976, *7*, 110-112.

Lerman, J.W., & Shames, G.H. The effect of situational difficulty on stuttering, *Journal of Speech and Hearing Disorders*, 1965, *8*, 271-280.

Martin, R.R., & Haroldson, S.K. The relationship between anticipation and consistency of stuttered words. *Journal of Speech and Hearing Research*, 1967, *10*, 323-327.

Martin, R.R., & Siegel, G.M. The effects of response contingent shock on stuttering. *Journal of Speech and Hearing Research*, 1966, *9*, 340-352.

McIntyre, M.E., Silverman, F.H., & Trotter, W.D. Transcendental meditation and stuttering: A preliminary report. *Perceptual and Motor Skills,* 1974, *39,* 294.

Miller, N.E. Experimental studies of conflict. In J. McV. Hunt (Ed.), *Personality and the behavior disorders* (Vol. I.) New York: Ronald Press, 1944.

Moleski, R., & Tosi, D.J. Comparative psychotherapy: Rational-emotive therapy versus systematic desensitization in the treatment of stuttering. *Journal of Consulting and Clinical Psychology,* 1976, *44,* 309-311.

Moore, W.E., Soderberg, G.A., & Powell, D. Relations of stuttering in spontaneous speech to speech content and verbal output. *Journal of Speech and Hearing Disorders,* 1952, *17,* 371-376.

Mowrer, O.H. *Learning theory and personality dynamics,* New York: Ronald Press, 1950.

Paul, G.L. *Insight vs. desensitization in psychotherapy,* Palo Alto, CA: Stanford University Press, 1966.

Perkins, W.H. Physiological studies. In J.G. Sheehan (Ed.), *Stuttering: Research and therapy,* New York: Harper & Row, 1970.

Perkins, W.H. Replacement of stuttering with normal speech: II Clinical procedures. *Journal of Speech and Hearing Disorders,* 1973, *38,* 295-303.

Porter, H.K. Studies in the psychology of stuttering: XIV. Stuttering phenomena in relation to size and personnel of evidence. *Journal of Speech Disorders,*, 1939, *4,* 323-333.

Porter, J.F. Homosexuality treated adventitiously in a stuttering therapy program: A case report presenting a heterophobic orientation. *Australian and New Zealand Journal of Psychiatry,* 1976, *10,* 185-189.

Rachman, S. Learning therapy and child psychology: Therapeutic possibilities. *Journal of Child Psychology and Psychiatry,* 1962, *3,* 149-163.

Reed, C.G., & Lingwall, J. Some relationships between punishment, stuttering, and galvanic skin responses. *Journal of Speech and Hearing Research,* 1976, *19,* 197-205.

Reed, C.G., & Lingwall, J.B. Conditioned stimulus effects on stuttering and GSR's. *Journal of Speech and Hearing Research,* 1980, *23,* 336-343.

Rosenthal, T.L. Severe stuttering and maladjustment treated by desensitization and social influence. *Behaviour Research and Therapy,* 1968, *6,* 125-130.

Schilling, A. Speech pathology in Germany. In R.W. Rieber & R.S. Brubaker (Eds.), *Speech pathology,* Amsterdam: North-Holland, 1966.

Schwartz, G.E. Psychobiological foundations of psychotherapy and behavior change. In S.L. Garfield & A.E. Bergin (Eds.), *Handbook of psychotherapy and behavior change: An empirical analysis.* New York: Wiley, 1978.

Sheehan, J.G. Theory and treatment of stuttering as an approach-avoidance conflict. *Journal of Psychology,* 1953, *36,* 27-49.

Sheehan, J.G. Conflict theory of stuttering. In J. Eisenson (Ed.), *Stuttering: A symposium,* New York: Harper & Row, 1958.

Sheehan J.G. Conflict theory and avoidance-reduction therapy. In J. Eisenson (Ed.), *Stuttering: A second symposium,* New York: Harper & Row, 1975.

Sheehan, J.G., Hadley, R., & Gould, E. Impact of authority on stuttering. *Journal of Abnormal Psychology,* 1967, *72,* 290-293.

Sherrington, C.S. *Integrative action of the nervous system.* New Haven, CN: Yale University Press, 1906.

Shoemaker, D.J., & Brutten, G.J. A two-factor approach to the modification of stuttering and related behaviors. In B.B. Gray & G. England (Eds.), *Stuttering and the conditioning therapies.* Monterey, CA: Monterey Institute for Speech and Hearing, 1969.

Shulman, E. Factors influencing the varibility of stuttering. In W. Johnson & R.R. Leutenegger (Eds.), *Stuttering in children and adults,* Minneapolis: University of Minnesota Press, 1955.

Siegel, G.M., & Haugen, D. Audience size and variations in stuttering behavior. *Journal of Speech and Hearing Research,* 1964, *7,* 381-388.

Silverman, E.M., & Zimmer, C.H. Speech fluency fluctuations during the menstrual cycle. *Journal of Speech and Hearing Research,* 1975, *18,* 202-206.

Silverman, E.M., Zimmer, C.H., & Silverman, F.H. Variability of stutterers' speech disfluency: The menstrual cycle. *Perceptual and Motor Skills,* 1974, *38,* 1037-1038.

Silverman, F.H. Concern of elementary school stutterers about their stuttering. *Journal of Speech and Hearing Disorders,* 1970, *35,* 361-363.

Skinner, B.F. *The behavior of organisms.* New York: Appleton-Century-Crofts, 1938.

Snidecor, J.C. Tension and facial appearance in stuttering. In W. Johnson & R.R. Leutenegger (Eds.), *Stuttering in children and adults,* Minneapolis: University of Minnesota Press, 1955.

Spielberger, C.D. Theory and research on anxiety, In C.D. Spielberger (Ed.), *Anxiety and behavior,* New York: Academic Press, 1966.

Stampfl, T., & Levis, D. Essentials of implosive therapy. *Journal of Abnormal Psychology,* 1967, *72,* 496-503.

Steer, M.D., & Johnson, W. An objective study of the relationship between psychological factors and the severity of stuttering. *Journal of Abnormal and Social Psychology,* 1936, *31,* 36-46.

Stokes, T.F., & Baer, D.M. An implicit technology of generalization. *Journal of Applied Behavior Analysis,* 1977, *10,* 349-367.

Taylor, J.A. A personality scale of manifest anxiety. *Journal of Abnormal and Social Psychology,* 1953, *48,* 285-290.

Thorndike, E.L. A proof of the law of effect. *Science,* 1933, *77,* 173-175.

Tolman, E.C. *Purposive behavior in animals and men.* New York: Appleton-Century-Crofts, 1932.

Toomey, G.L., & Sidman, M. A experimental analogue of the anxiety-stuttering relationship. *Journal of Speech and Hearing Research,* 1970, *13,* 122-129.

Trotter, W.D., & Bergmann, M.F. Stutterers' and nonstutterers' reactions to speech situations. *Journal of Speech and Hearing Disorders,* 1957, *22,* 40-45.

Turnbaugh, K.R., Guitar, B.E., & Hoffman, P.R. Speech clinicians' attribution of personality traits as a function of stuttering severity. *Journal of Speech and Hearing Research,* 1979, *22,* 37-45.

Tyre, T.E., Maisto, S.A., & Companik, P.J. The use of systematic desensitization in the treatment of chronic stuttering behavior. *Journal of Speech and Hearing Disorders,* 1973, *38,* 514-519.

Van Riper, C. The effect of penalty upon frequency of stuttering spasms. *Journal of Genetic Psychology,* 1937, *50,* 193-195.

Van Riper, C. *The treatment of stuttering.* Englewood Cliffs, NJ: Prentice-Hall, 1973.

Walton, D., & Mather, M.D. The relevance of generalization techniques to the treatment of stammering and phobic symptoms. *Behaviour Research and Therapy* 1963, *1,* 121-125.

Webster, L.M. A clinical report on the measured effectiveness of certain desensitization techniques with stutterers. *Journal of Speech and Hearing Disorders,* 1970, *35,* 369-376.

Webster, N. *The living Webster encyclopedic dictionary of the English language.* Chicago: The English Language Institute of America, 1975.

Wingate, M.E. *Stuttering: Theory and treatment.* New York: Irvington, 1976.

Wischner, G.J. Stuttering behavior and learning: A preliminary theoretical formulation. *Journal of Speech and Hearing Disorders,* 1950, *15,* 324-335.

Wischner, G.J. Anxiety-reduction as reinforcement in maladaptive behavior: Evidence in stutterers' representations of the moment of difficulty. *Journal of Abnormal and Social Psychology,* 1952, *47,* 566-571.

Wolpe, J. *Psychotherapy by reciprocal inhibition*. Palo Alto, CA: Stanford University Press, 1958.

Wolpe, J. The systematic desensitization treatment of neuroses. *Journal of Nervous and Mental Disease*, 1961, *132*, 189-203.

Wolpe, J. Behavior therapy of stuttering: Deconditioning the emotional factor. In B.B. Gray & G. England (Eds.), *Stuttering and the conditioning therapies*, Monterey, CA: Monterey Institute for Speech and Hearing, 1969.

Yates, A.J. *Theory and practice in behavior therapy*, New York: Wiley, 1975.

Yonovitz, A., Shepherd, W.T., & Garrett, S. Hierarchial simulation: Two case studies of stuttering modification using systematic desensitization. *Journal of Fluency Disorders*, 1977, *2*, 21-28.

Young, M.A. Audience size, perceived situational difficulty, and stuttering frequency. *Journal of Speech and Hearing Research*, 1965, *8*, 401-407.

7

Auditory Masking and Stuttering

Introduction

The relationship between audition and stuttering has been fertile for both theory and research. This has stemmed from observations about four main aspects of this relationship: the association between hearing loss and stuttering, the effects of noise on stuttering, differences between stutterers and normals on certain auditory-processing tasks, and the intriguing effects of delayed auditory feedback on stutterers and nonstutterers. The evidence from research in most of these areas has spawned at least six theoretical models (Butler & Stanley, 1966; Cherry & Sayers, 1956; Martin, 1970; Mysak, 1960; Webster & Lubker, 1968b Yates, 1963) which claim that stuttering is related to an unusual auditory-feedback system. These models have been constructed with different levels of explanatory strength, but they have a common claim; in some way or other, the stutterer's speech is disrupted by feedback from the voice signal. It is this disruption which is postulated to either mediate or cause stuttering.

There exist a number of reviews on the role of audition in stuttering which have integrated and critically appraised the research in this area (Bloodstein, 1981; Garber & Siegel, 1982; Siegel, 1978; Timmons & Boudreau, 1972; Van Riper, 1971; Webster & Lubker, 1968b; Wingate, 1970; 1976). These show, increasingly, that there may be a profit in a closer examination of the motoric and, thereby, physiological concomitants of stuttering's variability during auditory modification. This means that any review of the role of audition in stuttering demands a wider and wider ambit. It really requires consideration of the effects of delayed auditory feedback, shadowing, chorus reading, and altered vocalization on stuttering, which is well beyond the aims of an introduction to masking treatment. For this reason, this chapter will review only some of the research relevant to the above-mentioned theory models. The rest of this research will be considered in Chapter 10.

Hearing Loss and Stuttering

Wingate (1970) has pointed out that Bluemel (1912) was probably the first to highlight the possibility that stuttering could be linked to audition because of its apparent absence among the deaf. Some years later, surveys by Backus (1938) and Harms and Malone (1939) on hearing-impaired populations lent some weight to Bluemel's observation. They showed that while stuttering was not completely unknown among the deaf and hard-of-hearing, it did not occur as frequently as in the general population. Backus (1938) sent questionnaires to schools for the deaf or hard-of-hearing requesting information about stutterers and found 55 cases among a population of 13,691, or 0.40%. At least eight of the 55 cases could be considered profoundly deaf, and three had been diagnosed as such from birth. In a similar study, Harms and Malone (1939) found a total of 42 stutterers among 14,458 persons who had a hearing loss of 22% or greater. This represents about 0.29% which, like Backus's finding, is much less than the 1% figure usually reported for the general population (Bloodstein, 1981).

The intriguing feature in both surveys is that their findings also present some difficulties for the claim that reduced hearing may have a crucial link with reduced stuttering. The Harms and Malone (1939) study illustrates this point via some additional data they collected. They described three children who had acquired a hearing loss as a result of either scarlet fever or chicken pox, and shortly afterwards began to stutter. They also made audiometric assessments on 62 stutterers and found that *all* had "hearing losses for the better ears [of]from 10 to 22%." This leads to the paradoxical conclusion that fewer stutteres are to be found among the hard-of-hearing, and yet *all* stutterers are purported to have some hearing loss. The confusing implications of this study do not end there. There is also a conceptual problem. If audition is supposed to be essential for stuttering, then it surely follows that stuttering should not occur at all among the deaf. Its very presence among individuals who have been totally deaf since birth surely embarrasses the claim that audition is a necessary condition for stuttering. Of course, even if audition is not essential, it does not exclude the possibility that reduced audition may also suppress stuttering.

Harms and Malone's (1939) finding of a general hearing-loss factor among stutterers has never been replicated. In fact, later studies by Gregory (1964) and Brown, Sambrooks, and MacCulloch (1975) have shown that stutterers are definitely not characterized by impaired hearing. The explanation for Harms and Malone's finding probably relates to the very high incidence of severe childhood diseases prevalent during the era of their study. Actually 93.5% of their 62 stutterers had had childhood diseases that could have caused hearing loss. Again, this is not to suggest that other aspects of audition are not significant in stuttering. In fact, some evidence will be reviewed which shows that the auditory-processing system of stutterers (as a group) does have some unusual characteristics.

The location of relatively small numbers of stutterers among the deaf or hard-of-hearing population has been explained in different ways. Some argue that this is related to the improved fluency that occurs when a stutterer's perception of the air-conducted voice signal is attenuated by experimental procedures such as masking (Webster & Lubker, 1968b). Others, especially Wingate (1970; 1976), speculate that the factors responsible for fewer stutterers among the hard-of-hearing, and the ameliorative effects of masking, share another characteristic—

they modify the speech pattern in ways known to reduce stuttering. Wingate (1976), for example, has drawn attention to the "scanning" quality of speech among the hard-of-hearing, the evidence that their speech is slower (Voelker, 1937), and that it is typified by extended phonation (Hood & Dixon, 1969).To summarize, the beneficial effects of hearing impairment on stuttering are generally attributed to either a perceptual change (the speaker being unable to perceive disruptive aspects of the voice signal), or changes in the speaker's usual way of speaking. Both have been used to explain the effects found when noise masks a stutterer's perception of part or all of the voice signal.

The Effects of Noise on Stuttering

The experimental modification of a stutterer's hearing was reported first in a study by Kern (1932). He used a Barany drum to partially deafen stutterers while they orally read. The results were described informally, but they were apparently quite impressive.The first study to provide some measure of the effect of auditory masking on stuttering was Shane's (1955) report of an experiment actually conducted in 1946. She had 25 stutterers (15-25 years) orally read during the presence and absence of a 95dB binaurally presented noise (unspecified). During the control reading of 250 words, the group had a mean of 18.7% words stuttered. This was reduced to 4.5% words stuttered when they read another 250-word passage in the noise condition. Ten of these subjects then reread the same passages with a 25dB noise level, but they showed no significant improvement in fluency relative to their control passage reading.

The effect of different levels of noise intensity was also assessed in a study by Maraist and Hutton (1957). They had 15 stutterers (mean age 20 years) orally read five different 75-word passages during conditions in which binaurally presented white noise was delivered at 0, 30, 50, 70 and 90dB's above the noise-detection threshold. The mean number of speech errors and words-per-minute rate found during each of the noise conditions are shown in Table 7-1. The results indicate a decrease in errors correlated with an increase in the noise-intensity level. The decrease in errors also appears to be generally associated with an increase in oral

TABLE 7-1
Mean number of errors and oral reading rate of stutterers (n=15) as reported by Maraist & Hutton (1957).*

Masking in dB	*Number of Errors*	*Rate in WPM*
0	26	78
30	22	90
50	18	138
70	11	126
90	6	144

*From Maraist & Hutton (1957, p.386).

reading rate. One interesting finding was the very substantial decrease in the number of errors found during the 50dB condition, a noise level which is unlikely to prevent the speaker from hearing most of his voice.

Part of the "treatment effect" in Maraist and Hutton's (1957) study may have been due to their "error" measure. This appeared to include the duration of an interval of stuttering. For, in addition to the usual categories of stuttering (Wingate, 1964), they had "each component of multiple repetition counting as one error" (Maraist & Hutton, 1957, p.387). This means, for example, that 'g..g..g..girl" would count as three or even four, errors. Quite possibly this explains the relatively large reduction in errors they found. This measurement method might also explain an equally substantial masking effect reported by Cherry and Sayers (1956). They had 54 stutterers orally read a 120-word passage to the accompaniment of a 120Hz tone set at a level "close to the threshold of pain." The mean "duration of breakdown" (the total duration due to hesitations, blockages, and repetitions) for the group was graphically depicted to be dramatically less during masking than during nonmasking conditions.

There are, however, quite unambiguous demonstrations of masking's inhibiting effects on stuttering. This is particularly evident in studies that have masked different intervals of oral reading. Burke (1969) assessed the effect of 100dB SPL white noise for 100, 75, 50, and 25% of oral reading time with 12 male stutterers. He reported a progressive decrease in the percentage of words stuttered as masking time increased. This was also associated with a concomitant increase in words read during the 120-second reading time. A comparison between masked and nonmasked readings showed that masking produced a 58% decrease in words stuttered and 32% increase in words read.

Murray (1969) also compared continuous and intermittent white noise masking at a level sufficient to prevent the subject hearing his own voice during oral reading. The stutterers' (n=30) oral reading during the intermittant masking conditions involved either random 1-second noise bursts, at intervals of up to 9 seconds between each burst, or 1-second bursts applied by subject or experimenter after, and during, a stuttering moment. It was found that continuous masking produced less frequent stuttering than intermittent masking, but the subject- and experimenter-administered noise bursts failed to achieve reduced stuttering.

Voice-Signal Masking

The findings from some masking studies, most notably those obtained by Maraist and Hutton (1957), have shown that not all of the subject's voice signal must be attenuated to produce a beneficial "masking effect" on stuttering. This suggests that the necessary conditions for this effect involve masking only certain components of the voice signal. This hypothesis received the most impetus from a series of experiments reported by Cherry and Sayers (1956) which, in turn, have caused much speculation about the role of auditory feedback on stuttering.

The most influential of Cherry & Sayers's (1956) experiments was one that compared the effect of two different types of masking. They had 14 stutterers orally read a 120-word passage during three different conditions: no masking, white noise low-pass filtered to 500Hz, and white noise high-pass filtered to 500Hz. The noise level was not specified but probably "approached pain level." During the low-pass condition it was assumed that most low frequency bone-conducted voice signals would be masked, and during the high-pass conditions most of the air-conducted (high frequency) portions of the voice signal would be masked. In other words, during the high-pass condition the subject would hear only the lower frequencies of his voice. The results were presented in terms of the "total breakdown time" each subject experienced while reading the passage. They showed that when subjects experienced the low-pass condition there was a mean 94% reduction in breakdown duration (compared with nonmasked reading), while the high-pass condition produced only a 35% reduction in breakdown duration. The findings of this study led Cherry and Sayers to conclude "that stammering is mediated by (note: not caused by) the subject's perceptions of his low-frequency-voice sounds" (1956, p.243).

Cherry and Sayers's findings were taken up by Yates (1963) and Webster and Lubker (1968b) as cornerstones for their independently produced auditory-perception theories of stuttering. But it is a very fragile cornerstone for many reasons. To begin with, the Cherry and Sayers's study contains some very suspect features. For example, no information was provided on the reliability with which the "duration of breakdown" measures were made and, remarkably enough, there is no indication that adaptation effects were controlled. The subjects appear to have read the same text in each condition, but no details were given on the sequence of these conditions. There is also no indication that the intensity of the noise signal in the low- and high-pass conditions was matched. Far more significantly, the findings were not replicated in two similar studies by May and Hackwood (1968) and Conture (1974).

May and Hackwood (1968) had 10 stutterers (16-33 years) orally read different 100-word passages under the masking conditions used by Cherry and Sayers (1956). The only difference in their study was that total reading time, rather than duration of breakdown, was the dependent variable. On this measure they found no significant difference between the low-pass and high-pass masking noise conditions. Conture's (1974) experiment was more elaborate. He used nine adult stutterers and obtained measures of stuttering frequency during 5-minute oral readings performed under conditions in which white noise was either low-pass or high-pass filtered to a 500Hz cut-off point. In addition, the noise level was set at a low and high dB SPL point under each condition. Thus, subjects experienced the low-pass filtered white noise at either 76.5 or 96.5 dB SPL, and the high-pass filtered white noise at either 70.2 or 89.5 dB SPL. They also experienced broadband (or unfiltered) white noise under two different intensity levels (75.5 and 95 dB SPL). Conture's most pertinent finding, vis-á-vis Cherry and Sayers's (1956) study, was that there was no difference among the stuttering frequency levels in the broadband, high-pass or low-pass filtered conditions. Another interesting finding was that significantly less stuttering occurred in all the high-noise level conditions when compared with the low-noise level conditions (these differences were not associated with changes in reading rate). Finally, high-level noise produced an increase in the speaker's vocal level when compared with levels found during the low-level noise conditions. This was also true for broadband noise when compared with the low- and high-pass filtered-noise conditions. In short, the findings of May and Hackwood (1968) and Conture (1974) effectively demolished the notion that the low frequency elements of the voice signal were critical to stuttering.

These findings do not exclude the possibility that different types of masking noise, irrespective of their intensity levels, may produce different effects on stuttering. This is suggested in some data reported by Barr and Carmel (1969). They used the Carhart tone test to identify their stutterers' (n=10) responsiveness to either 4,000 or 6,000Hz narrow band noise. These noise frequencies were then presented (to the most responsive ear) at 50dB SPL during oral reading conditions. A comparison between the number of stutterings during these conditions, and a control reading, showed that the most responsive frequencies (that is, the one that produced most tone decay for each subject) was associated with the least number of stutterings. Both masking conditions also produced significantly less stuttering than the control condition.

Voice and Non-Voice Masking

Another premise of the theories which placed store on the role of audition in stuttering (Mysak, 1960; Webster & Lubker, 1968b) was that the masking effect depended on partial or complete suppression of the voice signal. This premise came under challenge with a brief letter to the editor of *Journal of Speech and Hearing Research* by Sutton and Chase in 1961. They used a voice-activated relay system to deliver binaural white noise (level unspecified) during either phonation or nonphonation intervals of oral reading by nine stutterers. This meant that the masking noise either masked the subject's voice or masked the silent intervals between voicing. Oral reading during these two conditions was compared with continuous masking and two control conditions (reading with and without headphones). The mean "correct word rates" (CWR) during oral readings under

TABLE 7-2
Mean correct word rate (CWR) for nine stutterers during oral reading under five conditions as reported by Sutton & Chase (1961)*.

	No Headphones	*Headphones*	*Noise During Silence*	*Noise During Phonation*	*Continuous Noise*
Mean	1.09	1.31	1.90	1.74	1.89

* Adapted from Sutton & Chase (1961, p. 72).

each of the five conditions are shown in Table 7-2. Their data revealed that all masking conditions increased the mean CWR scores. Of most interest, however, was the finding that the condition in which the noise did not mask the speaker's voice (noise during silence) was just as effective in improving CWR scores as the other two masking conditions!

Sutton and Chase's (1961) findings were later challenged by Webster and Lubker (1968a) on the grounds that the voice-activated relay system has a built-in lag-time, which meant that the "noise during silence" condition would cause noise to mask the initial brief part of the voice signal. Webster and Lubker (1968a) claimed that Sutton and Chase's data merely demonstrated that ameliorative effects occur when *initial* auditory feedback of the voice signal is masked. But, as Chase and Sutton (1968) perceptively noted, the same claim should apply to the masking-during-phonation condition when noise could not hide what Webster and Lubker (1968a) claimed to be "the critical portion of auditory feedback in stuttered speech." As can be seen in Table 7-2 the noise-during-phonation condition was almost as effective in improving fluency as the continuous-noise condition, that is, when that "critical portion" was definitely masked.

Webster and Dorman (1970) conducted an experiment which, they claimed, obviated some problems involved in Sutton and Chase's (1961) study. They had nine stutterers (16-50 years) orally read with a one-second pause between each word.[1] This was introduced to control for the possibility that in continuous oral reading more initial parts of a word could be masked in the noise-during-phonation condition. This might occur if the shut-off speed of the voice-activated relay was not quick enough to produce a silence during all nonphonated intervals.[2] The results are shown in Table 7-3 and reveal that, once again, there was no significant difference between each of the noise conditions. Their finding was

TABLE 7-3
Mean number of disfluent words produced by stutterers (n=9) during oral reading under four conditions reported in an experiment by Webster & Dorman (1970).*

	No Noise	*Continuous Noise*	*Noise During Phonation*	*Noise During Silence*
Mean No. of Disfluent Words	76.9	34.2	36.8	36.0

*Adapted from Webster & Dorman (1970, p.84).

therefore consistent with that reported by Sutton and Chase (1961). Webster and Dorman (1970) did offer themselves a saving hypothesis. They speculated that middle-ear contractions, which may occur briefly before vocal emission, could have been stimulated enough by the white noise in order to mask the initial part of the voice signal.

[1] It should be noted that this procedure may also produce rhythmic speech. But since this procedure was common to all experimental conditions, it cannot be invoked as the sole source of treatment effects.

[2] Of course this "solution" ignores the reverse effect, that is, the noise-during-silence condition would be equally likely to mask as many voice-onset intervals.

Another attempt to resolve the Sutton and Chase/Webster and Lubker argument was offered by Altrows and Bryden (1977). They conducted a similar experiment, but one in which the interval between sentences (rather than words) was varied, and periods without noise were common to all treatment conditions. They had 17 stutterers (13-43 years) read orally during a 95dB SPL masking condition that was presented in three different conditions: (1) experimenter-activated noise during six- to 10-word sentences, (2) experimenter-activated noise during silent intervals preceding a sentence (but not for 5 seconds after completing a sentence—there was a 5- to 10-second interval between each sentence), and (3) almost continuously (except for 5 seconds following the completion of the sentence). The findings from this study are difficult, if not impossible, to relate to those obtained by either Sutton and Chase or Webster and Dorman, since the procedural differences are immense. For example, Altrows and Bryden used a hazardous method of activating the masking signal (experimenter judgment), and failed to provide a condition in which noise was present during all silent intervals (that is, intervals between the words within a sentence). This may explain why the noise-during-silence condition resulted in the same number of disfluent words as the control-reading condition. Their finding that the noise-during-reading and continuous-noise conditions produced significantly less disfluent words (and faster reading rate) than the noise-during-silence conditions is rather simply explained by their failure to provide noise during *all* silent intervals. It is therefore difficult to accept their claim that these data confirm that auditory feedback control of speech partly mediates stuttering.

At present, the issue about the essentialness of voice-signal masking in the masking effect remains unresolved. The weight of evidence tends to suggest that this is not a necessary ingredient.

The Role of Changed Vocal Characteristics in the Masking Effect

To this point, the evidence from masking studies suggests that its moderating effect on stuttering is related to the level of masking. Yet it does not appear to depend on the subject being unable to hear either part or virtually all of the voice signal. It almost seems that the noise condition induces some other sort of activity which is much more responsible for any reduced stuttering during this condition. One possibility is that it causes an alteration in the subject's manner of speaking—a well-known modifier of stuttering.

Since the early part of this century, it has been known that talking in noise conditions can induce a speaker to talk more loudly. The effect was first investigated, in some detail, by Etienne Lombard (see Lane & Tranel,1971) in 1909. He noted that when an intense noise was presented monaurally to a normal-hearing speaker there was an increase in vocal level. Lombard found an even greater increase when the noise was presented binaurally. Significantly, the effect was not found with speakers who had a substantial hearing loss. For the most part, the Lombard effect is now generally regarded as a change in speech behavior that the speaker "would make if he were trying to maintain constant intelligibility of his speech for an active listener" (Lane & Tranel, 1971, p.701).

In recent years a number of experiments on the effects of masking noise on the speech of normal speakers have identified some of the changes that may transpire within different parameters of the voice signal. What follows is a brief account of their findings. Atkinson (1952) found that different combinations of frequency and dB level of pure tones during oral reading resulted in evidence that the loudness of the tone (up to 100dB's) was correlated with increased intensity and fundamental frequency in the voice signal. Hanley and Steer (1949) showed that an increase in dB level during oral reading produced an increase in syllable duration. A similar finding was reported in Ringel and Steer's (1963) assessment of the comparative and combined effects of anaesthesia and 94dB level binaural white noise. They found that phonation time and fundamental frequency were increased, but masking was not associated with any change in speech rate. Winchester and Gibbons (1958) also found that oral-reading rate was unaffected by the imposition of a binaural 80dB SL "saw-tooth masking noise." On the other hand, Black (1961) found that when vocal levels were manipulated (not in the presence of masking), this produced an increase in fundamental frequency and speech rate. A study by Garber, Siegel, Pick, and Alcorn (1976) found that vocal intensity tended to increase according to the relationship between the frequency band of masking and the frequency range of the voice signal. There was also a concomitant decrease in the intelligibility of the speaker's utterances. In a related study, Garber, Siegel, and Pick (1980) compared high- and low-pass filtering of sidetones (the subject's own voice signal amplified via headphones) and found that only low-pass conditions increased vocal intensity and intelligibility. But their subjects' intelligibility was unchanged when vocal intensity was controlled.

When these studies are considered together, it is quite evident that altering a normal-speaker's audition probably affects a change in the loudness, pitch, duration, and intelligibility of the speech. Of course, the critical issue, as far as stuttering is concerned, is whether these changes are also sufficient to cause reductions in this behavior.

Among some of the earlier studies on masking and stuttering, there was obvious awareness of the Lombard effect. Shane (1955) offered one control over this variable by instructing the subject "not to try to hear himself. The experimenter explained that she would signal with her hand for him to lower his voice if he were talking too loudly" (Shane, 1955, p.289). She reported that during the 95dB noise condition "all subjects appeared to show definitely decreased control of articulation and voice" (p.292). Cherry and Sayers (1956) were also concerned that speaking loudly might have confounded the effects that they obtained in their nonfiltered masking study. They offered the following control for this factor:

> Each of the last 30 subjects in our series was instructed ... to speak very quietly for a 30-second period while the masking tone was applied. We have

> found no deterioration of the subject's performance, whilst reading, due to quiet speaking (at or below normal levels) in any case. Under the influence of the masking noise, some subjects spontaneously spoke at normal or less than normal levels. It is therefore evident that the loudness of speaking was not a significant factor in these experiments. (p.241).

These observations are rather prophetic, but they are based on uncontrolled attempts to offset the Lombard effect. They certainly did not necessarily eliminate its contribution to their findings.

Some indication of the relationship between altered speech behavior, masking, and stuttering have been reported in a number of places. Possibly the first was in a technical report by Stromsta in 1967 (see Wingate, 1976). In summary, Stromsta's data show that when masking frequencies were systematically decreased below 500Hz, there was a concomitant increase in voice signal fundamental frequency, and a decrease in stuttering. More readily available data are contained in a study by Adams and Moore (1972). They assessed the effect of binaural 90dB SL white noise on the oral reading of a 176-word passage by 12 stutterers (15-30 years). Measures made of vocal intensity, frequency of stuttering, and palmar sweat indices (PSI) showed that masking was associated with a significant increase in vocal intensity and a 79% decrease in the median frequency of stuttering. (The PSI measures showed a nonsignificant change between the masking and nonmasking conditions.) Conture (1974) also found that vocal intensity increased during masking conditions, and there was some correlation between increased vocal intensity and reductions in stuttering frequency. Yairi (1976) also observed that binaural masking (90dB SPL) of oral reading by six adult stutterers was generally associated with decreased stuttering and increased vocal level, Finally, there is a report by Adams and Hutchinson (1974) on the effects of 10, 50, and 90dB SL white noise masking, plus quiet, on the vocal characteristics of 16 stutterers (18-30 years) while orally reading a 114-word passage. Their data show that vocal intensity systematically increased across each of the four noise conditions, while stuttering frequency showed a related decrease. The oral reading rate did not show a similar expected pattern. One exceedingly interesting finding from this study was that the 10dB condition was associated with significantly less stuttering than the quiet condition.

Three other studies in this research stream obtained slightly unexpected results. Brayton and Conture (1978) found that binaural white noise at 95dB SL produced a significant increase in the mean fundamental frequency and vocal level of nine adult stutterers during oral reading conditions. But, intriguingly, the duration of their vowel sounds did not significantly increase during these conditions. Lechner (1979) also found an increase in the fundamental frequency of the voice signal of stutterers and nonstutterers while orally reading during 90dB SPL white noise. Once again, however, the duration of voicing was not found to increase during masking (this was so for nonstutterers as well as stutterers). Andrews, Howie, Dozsa, and Guitar (1982) illustrated some of the pitfalls involved in reaching conclusions from group data. They assessed the spontaneous speech of three adult male stutterers under "wide-band 80-dB" masking and reported that there was generally no evidence of change in mean phonation durations. An examination of their subjects' data, however, show that the subject whose stuttering decreased most under masking markedly increased his mean phonation durations.

The tenor among these studies is that noise does tend to alter a stutterer's vocal characteristics, and mainly in ways that resemble those found in the speech of the normal speakers. They appear to suggest that changes in vocal level and fundamental frequency are principally responsible for reduced stuttering during noise conditions. But the similarity between the effects of noise on stutterers and normal speakers is not complete. There are at least two notable differences. The first is that the speech rate of normal speakers was usually unchanged, but there was an increase in the stutterers' rate. This difference can probably be explained by the influence of reduced stuttering moments on speech rate. But this explanation does easily lend itself to the second difference—the failure to find general increases in vowel or phonation durations within stutterers' speech during masking conditions. It may be an explanation if the reduced stutterings during masking are mainly prolongations, or if increased speech rate actually produced reduced vowel durations. But if either explanation fails, then the difference between stutterers and nonstutterers on this variable is intriguing. At least, it would remove one of the suggested causes of masking's beneficial effects on stuttering—vowel extension.

In most of the foregoing studies, and in reviews by Wingate (1970, 1976), the fluency-inducing effects of masking are virtually "explained away" by the changes it causes in vocal characteristics. For instance, after reviewing many of these studies, Wingate concluded that, "One might also deduce that it may be such changes in manner of speaking, rather than altered auditory stimulation, that are responsible for the reduction in stuttering" (Wingate, 1976, p.226). But none of these studies had compared the effect on stuttering of manipulating vocal characteristics during the presence and absence of masking. The findings of an experiment reported by Garber and Martin (1977) appear to demonstrate that this has been a most significant omission.

Garber and Martin (1977) had eight stutterers speak spontaneously in four different treatment conditions: speaking in quiet conditions at a normal vocal level (quiet-normal), speaking in quiet conditions at 12dB's above normal vocal level (quiet-loud), speaking in the presence of 100dB SPL white noise at normal vocal level (noise-normal), and speaking in the presence of the 100dB SPL white noise at 12dB's above normal vocal level (noise-loud). The subjects were trained, during a 10-minute "warm-up" period, to monitor a VU meter so that they could sustain their vocal level during each following 14-minute treatment session. The results of this study, with respect to stuttering frequency, are summarized in Table 7-4. After appropriate data analysis it was found that their subjects significantly reduced stuttering in noise, when compared with quiet conditions, but there was no difference in stuttering when subjects spoke in either a loud or a normal voice. They also found no significant differences between the word rate in each of these conditions. Quite clearly this finding is in conflict with any claim that masking's effect on stuttering can be attributed to increased vocal intensity. It is still possible that changes in other characteristics, especially fundamental frequency, may be implicated in the masking effect. But it is obvious that the gains from masking cannot be dismissed as expected byproducts of the Lombard effect.

TABLE 7-4
The mean percentage words stuttered during warm-up (W) and treatment (T) periods for four experimental conditions as reported by Garber & Martin (1979)*. ("Quiet"=no noise; "Noise"=100dB SPL white noise; "Normal"=normal vocal level; "Loud"=12dB's above normal vocal level).

	Quiet-Normal		*Quiet-Loud*		*Noise-Normal*		*Noise-Loud*	
	W	T	W	T	W	T	W	T
Mean Percentage Words Stuttered	8.0	6.9	8.0	7.5	8.6	4.6	7.7	6.1

*Adapted from Garber & Martin (1977, p.236).

The Stutterers' Auditory System As a Relevant Variable

The suggestion that stutterers may react in unusual ways to masking should not be surprising. There are now quite a few studies which have shown that the auditory system of many stutterers may be unusual. They merit consideration in this context. Lane and Tranel (1971) cite a study by Panconcelli-Calzia (1955) which showed that only 27% of stutterers tested showed the Lombard sign, compared with 70% of those with other speech disorders, and 80% of normals. Brown, Sambrooks, and MacCulloch (1975) found that, although stuttering and nonstuttering children did not differ on hearing threshold tests, the stutterers did show significantly lower thresholds for auditory discomfort. Another puzzling difference was found in Horovitz, Johnson, Pearlman, Schaffer, and Hedin's (1978) assessment of stutterers' (n=9) and nonstutterers' (n=9) stapedial reflexes. They found that when both groups imagined a stressful scene, which produced a related GSR change, only the stutterers showed a significantly different mean stapedial reflex.

One of the most significant findings, with respect to feedback theory, was obtained in a study by Stromsta (1972). A bone-conducted tone was presented to stutterers (n=25) and nonstutterers (n=25) who were required to cancel the auditory sensation of the signal by phase and amplitude adjustments of a bilaterally presented air-conducted signal of the same frequency. The point at which the subject can no longer hear the tone provides a measure of interaural phase disparity. The time-equivalent values of the mean interaural phase differences for stutterers were approximtely twice as great as for nonstutterers at 150, 300, and 1,200Hz. The implications of this finding are not altogether clear, but the magnitude of the phase shift in stutterers, particularly at 150Hz, may be closely related to that which is sufficient for normal delayed air-conducted feedback to induce phonation blockage (Stromsta, 1959).

Hall and Jerger (1978) assessed stutterers and nonstutterers on tests designed to assess central auditory function and found differences between the groups on some of these tasks, through the differences were not substantial. Moreover, Wynne and Boehmler (1982) failed to replicate the substance of this effect by using a control group containing disfluent nonstutterers. Finally, there have been a variety of studies that have assessed stutterers' reaction times to various types of stimuli, including auditory signals. In some pertinent studies (Adams & Hayden, 1976; Cross & Luper, 1979; McFarlane & Prins, 1978), which will be reviewed in a later chapter, the stutterers have consistently shown a slower reaction time to these stimuli.

The findings from these studies are certainly suggestive, though it should be mentioned that they mainly emerge from comparisons between groups of stutterers and nonstutterers and do not follow from a test of a particular theoretical issue. There are also many studies that have shown no differences between these groups. Nevertheless, they do point to the need to take account of the possibility that stutterers may be affected by an unusual auditory system.

Clinical Implications of Masking Studies

The clinical significance of the masking studies are, at best, inferential. They show that stuttering is likely to be reduced during different levels of masking noise, mainly above 50dB SPL. But these data have been obtained mostly from group studies, usually with relatively brief exposure to masking, and generally during the least customary speaking situation—oral reading.

The universality and magnitude of the masking effect also has clinical implications. To begin with, not all stutterers respond positively to masking. Conture and Brayton (1975) found that three out of 17 adult stutterers failed to reduce their disfluencies while oral reading with 95dB SPL white noise. Similarly, Martin and Haroldson (1979) found two of their 20 adult stutterers did not decrease stuttering while speaking spontaneously in 100dB white noise conditions (5 minutes "on" and 5 minutes "off") for 30 minutes. The masking effect may also be variable and comparatively modest. Conture and Brayton (1975) found that the only disfluency class within the stutterers' (n=17) speech that decreased significantly during masking was part-word repetitions.[3] Also, some studies have reported less than a 50% reduction in stuttering, particularly those which have used spontaneous speech. Garber and Martin (1977), for instance, found a mean 46% reduction in percentage of stuttering during 14 minutes of masking. And Martin and Haroldson (1979) found a mean 40% reduction in percentage of words stuttered during 30-minute masking of spontaneous speech. More intriguingly,

[3]It is noteworthy that Silverman and Goodban (1972) found that 95dB SPL white noise masking with nonstutterers (n=20) also reduced their disfluent speech, and only via two classes; part-word repetitions and revisions.

Mallard and Webb (1980) found that 90dB SPL white noise masking actually produced no significant reductions in stuttering over 2 minutes of spontaneous speech by 10 adult stutterers.

A study by Garber and Martin (1974) has important theoretical and clinial implications for masking with stutterers. They assessed the long-term effects of masking during single-subject experiments on three stutterers (28, 55, and 30 years). Each subject spoke spontaneously for 100 minutes in base-rate conditions and then continued in treatment conditions, initially with 100dB SPL binaural white noise (alternating 5 minutes with and 5 minutes without masking to offset any temporary threshold shift), until a 50% reduction in stuttering was achieved. Following subsequent extinction sessions, the subject was run in 80dB SPL masking sessions until the 50%-reduced-stuttering criterion was reached. After further extinction sessions, 60dB SPL sessions were introduced, again with the 50%-reduced-stuttering criterion, and again followed by extinction sessions.

Only one subject was run through all the experimental conditions, because two failed to respond to the 100dB SPL condition. The first subject decreased stuttering during 100dB SPL masking, but showed no clear masking effect during the 80 and 60dB SPL conditions. The most interesting finding was the difference between the reductions in stuttering that each subject achieved after a minimum of 100 minutes of the 100dB masking conditions. Subjects 1, 2, and 3 decreased their stuttering frequencies by 82, 15, and 38%, respectively, during the first 5 minutes. But, by the end of the 100dB masking sessions, Subject 1 appeared to average only 50% less stuttering, Subject 2 actually increased stuttering, and Subject 3 showed only a slight decrease in stuttering (all relative to base rate). In other words, the intervals of masking time that have been used in almost all the previously reviewed experiments produced treatment effects that bore little relationship to those found over much longer and more clinically meaningful periods. The implication of this finding is both self-evident and considerable for the experimental and clinical literature on masking with stutterers.

Conclusions on Masking Research

It is almost impossible to extract any general conclusions from this review of masking and stuttering. At the time of writing, it almost appears as though *any* implication drawn from research in this area is likely to be premature. It is quite apparent, for example, that different levels of masking, even as low as 10dB SL (Adams & Hutchinson, 1974), might reduce stuttering. Probably the most substantial reductions are achieved under masking conditions that occlude most of the voice signal. The evidence that masking the intervals between phonation achieves almost the same reductions as masking phonation, however, appears to implicate auditory factors, rather than the voice signal, in masking's effects.

The possibility that masking may modify various vocal characteristics which, in turn, cause reduced stuttering is an appealing theory. But its validity is now under fire, following the Garber and Martin (1974) study. This is the only study of its type (thus far), and similar studies need to be conducted in order to test the role of other vocal parameters within masking's effect on stuttering. Ironically, the search for an explanation for this effect may turn yet again to audition. This is increasingly likely in view of evidence that the auditory system of many stutterers may be unusual, and in ways that seem important to this speech problem.

The clinical pertinence of most masking studies is also confused because the effects may only be short-term, and even inconsequential, when they involve spontaneous speech. No study has reported an experimental assessment of masking during conversational speech (the very condition in which the Lombard effect is expected to be most evident). Such a study would add much to an understanding of clinical aspects of masking.

It is almost predictable to read at the end of this type of review that "there is a need for much more systematic investigation." But in this instance it is especially apposite. The area is in such confusion that almost all the previous research needs replication with more appropriate methodology. Single-subject investigations, especially those involving analyses of vocal parameters during lengthy intervals of spontaneous speech, might be a most useful direction for research in this area. Another might be long-term analyses of the effects identified by Sutton and Chase (1961). These studies would go some distance towards resolving yet another enigmatic feature of this enigmatic disorder.

Therapy Procedures Using Masking

Introduction

The potential value of masking to stuttering treatment appears restricted. It is restricted in a relative sense because it is rarely reported to entirely remove stuttering—a feature overlooked in most reviews of masking and stuttering. Another restriction is that masking can be both uncomfortable and limiting, particularly for conversational speech—although this difficulty has been partly offset by the development of a portable voice-operated system which permits the wearer to hear other speakers. Such impediments may be inconsequential, however, if this procedure yields therapeutic benefits that are not available through other methods.

The history of the clinical use of masking is obscure. This is partly due to the inaccessability of non-English-written reports on stuttering (and perhaps the unwillingness of reviewers to seek and translate these reports). Apparently, masking has been used clinically for some time in European (Froeschels, 1962) and South American (Gorin, 1980) countries. Froeschels provided an enlightening general review of the European literature in 1962, and noted that Imhofer had used "deafening (delayed feedback)" to treat speech and voice disorders as early as 1917.[4]

[4] Froeschels's reference to "delayed feedback" probably means masking rather than DAF.

Continuous Masking Treatments

The earliest use of electronic masking in stuttering treatment occurred in 1939, according to a report from a Russian clinician, Derazne (1966). In that year he invented a unit known as the Derazne Correctophone, which delivers a binaural 50Hz tone at 50 to 60dB's. He also reported that it had been used with considerable success in the treatment of children. The unit could be made portable (the size of a hearing-aid), but was found to be just as effective when used within a clinic setting. Derazne claimed that stuttering was removed "in the majority of our cases" (number not stated) as a result of 1.5 to 2 months of daily practice with the Correctophone, plus exercises and increased sleeping time ("not less than 11 or 12 hours a day"). Additional masking practice (2 or 3 weeks) was given to those who relapsed, though the procedure "did not give positive results in stuttering which was of an organic nature." No other qualifications (or data) are provided on the overriding success of this treatment. One interesting side effect of the Correctophone was Derazne's report that the heartbeat rate of stutterers decreased by 50% whenever the unit was active. The same effect was not found with normal speakers.

Later reports on the use of the Correctophone in Eastern bloc countries are not as glowing. Razdol'skii (1965) found the improvements in fluency did not always extend to conversational speech, while Petkov and Iosifov (1960) found it useful only in the case of severe stuttering. Guttman (1960) reported that during a visit to Leningrad in 1958, he was shown "a hearing-aid-like, noise-generating device to be worn by stutterers," but he was informed that it was no longer used "because stutterers did not experience lasting improvement and found it cumbersome." Nevertheless, in a later Russian report, Neimark (1968) described the apparently successful use of a nonportable "correctophone" with 25 stutterers (8 to 32 years). The treatment procedures and treatment format closely resembled that described by Derazne, except that a 100Hz tone was used, and the intensity of the tone was reduced as the subject's speech improved. The treatment was said to be less successful with children (8 to 9 years); they complained about the noise and headaches. No data were provided to support Niemark's claim to be "able to achieve a significant improvement of speech if the patients regularly visited (daily) the mobile clinic for a period of 1-1.5 months" (Niemark,1968, p.334).

In the Western world, 1963 appears to have been the year for developing hearing-aid treatment devices for stutterers. In that year, Meyer and Mair (1963) described the preliminary use of an earpiece metronome unit in stuttering treatment. In the same year, Parker and Christopherson (1963) described and used a miniaturized masking unit, which the subject activated to deliver binaural 150 to 300Hz tone at 27dB above hearing threshold. Other units of this type were described by Trotter and Lesch (1967) and Donovan (1971). (Donovan's unit also incorporated a facility for using either masking or metronomic stimulation.) Like the portable metronome unit, this type of system also offers the possibility of treatment control under the most clinically meaningful conditions, though it depends on the subject's skill in using the unit and willingness to advertise a defect—perhaps a small price to pay in the case of severe stutterers.

Parker and Christopherson (1963) briefly outlined some clinical applications of their masking unit. These required subjects to use it in the clinic, then at home, and to finally reduce the tone's intensity. Subjects tended to shout while using the unit, but this was reported to be solved by clinician instructions. Three subjects (10, 17, and 26 years) were treated "with great success," according to this dataless report. Unfortunately, it is not clear whether this assessment was made when subjects had actually ceased using the unit.

Van Riper (1965) reported some general observations on the use of a "portable masking device" with 25 stutterers. He noted that the use of intermittent white noise masking was most effective when applied "at the moment of stuttering rather than during the period prior to speech attempt" (p.381). The clinical benefits were stated to be reduced severity of stuttering, rather than frequency of stuttering, though no data accompanied this brief abstract report. In a later report, Van Riper (1973) indicates that he mainly uses masking to assist stutterers in stabilizing the gains of treatment.

Trotter and Lesch (1967) also described the development of a couple of portable subject-controlled masking units, plus the senior author's experience—as a stutterer—in using these aids over a 2½ year period. One unit had a 50 to 500Hz and 70 to 100dB SPL range, and the other a 35 to 770Hz and 97 to 119dB SPL range. The subject could control the frequency, loudness, and presence of the signal, which was binaurally delivered through stethoscope headsets. Trotter used the noise when he "felt [he] was going to stutter or was in the middle of a block." The unit was worn approximately 15 minutes a day on about 360 of 800 days, mainly during the course of 50-minute lectures. He normally experienced about 80 blocks during a lecture, but with noise assistance these were reduced in severity, and by about 75% in frequency. Trotter also observed that there was a 15dB hearing loss while the earpiece was worn. He concluded, however, that while there was a "reduction in both the frequency and duration of my stuttering, it has never been entirely eliminated" (1967, p.271).

Virtually the same conclusions were reached in a brief clinical report by Perkins and Curlee (1969). Three adult stutterers used one of the units built for Trotter over a 3-to-5-day period. These subjects were in the final phase of Conversational Rate Control Therapy (Curlee & Perkins, 1969). All said the unit was beneficial in some ways, but the effect was most advantageous when the subject "concentrated on maintaining a relatively slow easy flow of speech." Unfortunately, it is not clear whether this speech was induced by their therapy or the masking unit. No data were reported and each subject objected to the unit's inconvenience, hearing loss, and the ear plugs advertising their disability.

Gruber (1971) used Trotter's portable masking unit as a adjunct to Van Riper's (1963) therapy, with eight high school and three adult stutterers. The masker was used initially within clinic conditions where subjects were trained to activate the signal "only after the block had occurred and when they felt themselves struggling to utter the beginning sound of a word" (Gruber, 1971, p.288). Thereafter, the subjects used the unit outside the clinic. Because the unit was activated *after* stuttering began, their finding is not surprising: "while using the masker, none of the stutterers obtained stutter-free speech. The frequency of their stuttering remained approximately the same; however there was a significant reduction in the severity of the block'' (p.288).

It becomes clear, after reviewing these reports, that masking has been used clinically with different purposes. It is used as a means of either suppressing stuttering or modifying the severity of moments of stuttering. It may also be used to modify other extraneous features of stuttering behavior. Barr and Carmel (1970), for instance, noted that monaural 50dB SL narrow-band noise, when used with five stutterers, had the effect of removing their ''facial contortions, tics and gross body movements.'' A similar effect was also noted by Dewar, Dewar, and Anthony (1976), using a voice-activated masking unit.

Only one masking study has reported systematically gathered data across the course of a therapy program. That study was conducted by MacCulloch, Eaton, and Long (1970) with eight stutterers (drawn from 20 who had a mean age of 11.9 years) who were treated in 24 ½-hour sessions once weekly. All these subjects had received ''conventional therapy for periods ranging from a few months to several years.'' The sessions involved oral reading or conversation with continuous 300Hz tone delivered at a level sufficient to ''prevent self-monitoring of speech.'' The tone was activated by the clinician or subject immediately before the subject began to speak (two subjects used a portable unit at home as well as in the clinic). The treatment was assessed via a 263-word passage which was orally read (without masking) at the first, 12th and 24th sessions. The mean vocal errors (of any kind) and reading time are summarized in Table 7-5. They show that the group's scores did not improve beyond the 12th treatment session; indeed, if anything, their speech performance tended to deteriorate. The individual data are especially revealing. They show that not one subject was ''error free'' at any time throughout treatment and some actually became more severe, that is, if reading time is used as a measure of severity. One subject began treatment with 95 errors and took 425 seconds to read the 263-word passage. By the 24th session, this subject had 55 errors, but took 701 seconds to read the same passage! Moreover, since four subjects increased their errors and reading time between the 12th and 24th sessions, therapy gains from the procedure were neither substantial nor consistent.

Table 7-5

Mean errors and time to orally read a 263-word passage by stutterers (n=8) in an auditory masking study by MacCulloch, Eaton, & Long (1970).*

		Week 1	*Week 12*	*Week 24*
Mean Scores	Errors	41.6	15.5	15.0
	Time	201.0	151.1	203.6

*Adapted from MacCulloch, Eaton & Long (1970, p.71).

Voice-Activated Masking Treatments

The most obvious problem with many masking treatments is that they rely on clinician- or subject-controlled auditory masking units. This means the operator's skill may have influenced the potential effectiveness of treatment. With the developments in transistor technology, a solution to this problem was in the offing. It was inevitable that a transistorized voice-operated unit would be produced—especially in the light of the voice-activated masking effects identified by Sutton and Chase. The clinical utility of such a unit is obvious. At the very least, it makes consistent treatment available in nonclinic conditions.

The first reported voice-activated clinical unit was the "Speech Rectifier," which was invented and patented by Marvin Klein in 1967 (see Katz, 1977). This compact portable unit delivered a random noise below 500Hz through binaural (vented) earpieces. The noise signal was activated by voice-detection through a miniature microphone worn over the layrnx (see *Asha*, 1970, p.469). The unit could also be mounted within spectacle frames. Much publicity surrounded the introduction of this unit *(Time*, August 24, 1970), but no data ever emerged to justify this publicity.

Other portable units, remarkably similar to Klein's unit, were apparently developed by Barnes in 1970 (see Dewar, Dewar & Barnes, 1976) and Birtles and Dixon (1973). Barnes's unit was developed further and ultimately manufactured under the brand name "Edinburgh Masker." This unit, which provides a masking tone around 150Hz, has received extensive world-wide publicity, mainly on the basis of three papers by Dewar and colleagues (Dewar, Dewar, & Anthony, 1976; Dewar, Dewar, Austin, & Brash, 1979; Dewar, Dewar, & Barnes, 1976). Since these papers purport to provide evidence for the efficacy of this unit, the claims for its success are open to scrutiny.

In the light of the foregoing, it is clearly improper for Dewar, Dewar, and Barnes (1976) to claim that the Edinburgh Masker differs from all previous devices in that "all devices [masking units] so far have been under the conscious control of the subject" (p.19). But they may have some justification for claiming that it is the first to be assessed. They reported data from 52 stutterers (9-56 years) who were assessed while using the Edinburgh Masker under masking and nonmasking conditions during three speaking tasks: oral reading, reciting a rhyme, and describing a drawing. The group data indicate that masking produced a mean 93% to 95% reduction in "vocal errors," and approximately 54% less time to complete the speaking tasks. This data trend was also reflected in findings from an additional subject who completed the oral reading task on 11 occasions over 22 weeks—again, with and without masking on each occasion. This subject almost completely eliminated "vocal errors" during masking, but had substantially more when masking was absent.

The most striking feature of Dewar, Dewar, and Barnes's report is that it has little relevance to the clinical use of the Edinburgh Masker. This is because of four main limitations. The first is their failure to provide any information on the reliability of their speech measures. Second, the "vocal error" measure may have incorporated much more than stuttering, as the experimenters' state, "all articulatory errors were scored as well as disfluency of stammering" (Dewar, Dewar, & Barnes, 1976, p.21). In other words, it is not clear that masking effects were as evident with stuttering as they were with disfluent speech. The third limitation is the brevity of their data: the mean total speaking time for the group data was just over 6 minutes, and this included less than 2 minutes of masking conditions! No speaking-time data are provided for the single subject's oral-reading task, but if the group's data are used as a guide, then, over the 11 assessments, the subject orally read under masking conditions for just over 7 minutes. The brevity of these data becomes a very important source of concern in view of Garber and Martin's (1974) finding that improved fluency during similar brief intervals of continuous masking may not resemble long-term performance under this condition. Finally, the most significant limitation is that Dewar and colleagues' data were gathered only in clinic conditions and did not involve conversational speech.

Dewar, Dewar, and Anthony's (1976) study does not provide any further data of substantial clinic relevance. This study on six stutterers, two "ex-stammerers," and three nonstutterers, found that the active masking unit reduced abnormal obicularis oculi muscle activity in all stutterers. They also found that the automatic masking signal was activated more rapidly than when it was self-operated by the stutterers.

The Dewar, Dewar, Austin, and Brash (1979) report included a description of a treatment procedure for using the Edinburgh Masker, and the results of a survey of treated subjects. Their treatment format involves four steps: assessment during conversation and oral reading, continuous masking to train the subject to control vocal level, fitting the portable unit, and instructions on using the unit to best advantage. Their assessment identified 174 out of 195 stutterers (89%) who "reponded well to the device." No criteria for responsiveness were provided, but the 21 nonresponders were said to be characterized by glottal blocks, reservations about using the masking, hearing-loss, or an additional speech disorder. Sixty-seven subjects who had used the Edinburgh Masker for between 6 and 28 months were followed up, mostly by questionnaire, and occasionally via telephone, relatives, or observation. They found that 42% claimed "great" benefit from the unit, 40% received "considerable" benefit, and 18% obtained only "slight" benefit. Forty-six percent said, "their unaided speech had improved," and five subjects said they had become fully fluent. Although the majority of respondents were hesitant about wearing the unit in public, 88% thought the advantages of the unit outweighted this and other disadvantages. Some evidence was also presented to show that the masking unit's effect on hearing was minimal, even though some subjects had worn the unit for as long as 8 hours each day.

These are the only reports by Dewar and colleagues on the clinical benefits of the Edinburgh Masker. By any standard they must be regarded as exceedingly suspect indicators of the unit's effect on speech behavior. Code and Muller (1980) have criticized the Dewar et al. (1979) paper on the grounds that it failed to include objective data, provided no details on the assessment of subject responsiveness, used mainly self-report data, and showed a lack of concern for treatment evaluation methodology. In a quite revealing reply, Dewar and Dewar (1980) disavowed the need for objective speech performance data and professed a preference for essentially subjective assessments.

Despite these shortcomings, the Dewars's confidence in the Edinburgh Masker is generally supported by scattered reports from users of the device. For example, Tinklin (1980), an adult female stutterer, described the benefits she obtained while using the unit over a 6-month period. Also, Walle (1980) reported using the masker with some success in treating an important figure in a disguised country, plus a 64-year-old prisoner. Walle, however, attributed half the treatment's success to the addition of Van Riper's procedures. Another interesting assessment of the masker was Perry's (1979) account of a survey of British clinicians who had issued the unit to stutterers. The unit's sales are apparently going well; by 1979, between 300 and 400 were issued to stutterers in the British health system. Perry's report is difficult to evaluate, since it is not clear how many stutterers were actually included in the survey. The 40 clinicians who returned Perry's questionnaire indicated that only 52% of assessed subjects responded to the unit. This is far less than the 89% mentioned by Dewar et al. (1979). Eight clinicians reported that some patients were able to speak fluently without the unit after they had used it for some time, but a substantial number of clinicians found it presented some problems for their patients. The most prominent of these were that the noise was intolerable, the unit was too conspicuous, and the signal impeded concentration. These reports tend to lend some credence to the claims made for the benefits of the unit; however, the absence of pertinent speech behavior data still makes it difficult to decide whether the claims refer to normally fluent speech behavior (obtained with or without the unit).

One limited attempt to assess the efficacy of the Edinburgh Masker on the basis of speech performance data was reported in a study directed by this writer (Ingham, Southwood, & Horsburgh, 1981). Four stutterers (12-19 years) were assessed during oral reading and spontaneous speech.They spoke for 30-minute intervals while wearing the unit without masking (A), and 30-minute intervals with masking (B). The results showed that only one stutterer reduced stuttering almost completely during all B conditions. Two subjects showed either marginal or temporary reductions during only one of the speaking tasks, and the other subject reduced stuttering while using spontaneous speech only. None of the reductions in stuttering were associated with reduced speech rate. One additional finding was that two of the subjects showed evidence of a perceptual change in their speech quality during the masking conditions. These results are far less impressive than those reported by Dewar et al. (1976). The principal reason for the findings in this study appear related to the longer time that subjects experienced the masking conditions. Another possibility is that the four subjects were assessed for stuttering frequency by measures that were demonstrated to be reliable. None of these factors were present in Dewar, Dewar, and Barnes' (1976) study.

In spite of the disappointing findings in Ingham, Southwood, and Horsburgh's (1981) study, at least one of their subjects did show a worthwhile response to the Edinburgh Masker. It is quite possible, therefore, that many similar subjects could find that the unit offered some therapeutic benefits. Incidentally, it was noteworthy that the four subjects in this study found the masking signal to be extremely annoying. Nevertheless, as mentioned before, some subjects might be prepared to balance this problem against the unit's benefits. In fairness, it should be mentioned that Dewar and colleagues have always regarded the Edinburgh Masker as a prosthesis, rather than a treatment for stuttering. Possibly, the unit's main benefit, therefore, is to assist some stutterers who fail to respond to other therapy procedures. For this reason alone it merits consideration in a clinical setting.

Conclusions from Therapy Studies

What final conclusions can be reached in surveying the clinical applications of masking? The available crop of studies does not provide much confidence in the general utility of auditory masking in a therapy setting. It appears to have been a useful adjunct to some therapy procedures, but the data that support this tentative proposal are relatively weak. Perhaps there is some promise in this method via units such as the Edinburgh Masker. At present, however, there are absolutely no speech behavior data that support the claim by Dewar et al. (1979) that this unit is "effective in abolishing or greatly reducing stammering" (1979, p.219) in nonclinic conditions. This is not necessarily the fault of the procedure, but rather, the weaknesses of studies which claim to have assessed its efficacy. It will be most interesting to learn the results of future research with units such as the Edinburgh Masker. In the meantime, it is clear that masking has very limited clinical value in stuttering therapy.

References

Adams, M.R., & Hayden, P. The ability of stutterers and nonstutterers to initiate and terminate phonation during production of an isolated vowel. *Journal of Speech and Hearing Research,* 1976, *19,* 290-296.

Adams, M.R., & Hutchinson, J. The effects of three levels of auditory masking on selected vocal characteristics and the frequency of dysfluency of adult stutterers. *Journal of Speech and Hearing Research,* 1974, *17,* 682-688.

Adams, M.R., & Moore, W.H., Jr. The effects of auditory masking on the anxiety level, frequency of dysfluency, and selected vocal characteristics of stutterers. *Journal of Speech and Hearing Research,* 1972, *15,* 572-578.

Altrows, I.F., & Bryden, M.P. Temporal factors in the effects of masking noise on fluency of stutterers. *Journal of Communication Disorders,* 1977 *10,* 315-329.

Andrews, G., Howie, P.M., Dozsa, M., & Guitar, B.E. Stuttering: Speech pattern characteristics under fluency-inducing conditions. *Journal of Speech and Hearing Research,* 1982, *25,* 208-216.

ASHA equipment. The speech rectifier, *Asha,* 1970, *12,* 169.

Atkinson, C.J. Vocal responses during controlled aural stimulation. *Journal of Speech and Hearing Disorders,* 1952, *17,* 419-426.

Backus, O. Incidence of stuttering among the deaf. *Annals of Otology, Rhinology, and Laryngology* 1938, *47,* 632-635.

Barr, D.F., & Carmel, N.R. Stuttering inhibition with high frequency narrow band masking noise. *Journal of Auditory Research,* 1969, *9,* 40-44.

Barr, D.F., & Carmel, N.R. Stuttering inhibition with live voice interventions and masking noise. *Journal of Auditory Research*, 1970, *10*, 59-61.

Birtles, C.J., & Dixon, K.L. Simple dual-purpose device for the treatment of stutter. *Medical and Biological Engineering*, 1973, September, 651-653.

Black,. J.W. Relationship among fundamental frequency, vocal sound pressure, and rate of speaking. *Language and Speech*, 1961, *4*, 196-199.

Bloodstein, O. *A handbook on stuttering* (3rd ed.), Chicago: National Easter Seal Society, 1981.

Bluemel, C.S. *Stammering and cognate defects of speech*. New York: G.E. Stechert, 1912.

Brayton, E.R. & Conture, E.G. Effects of noise and rhythmic stimulation on the speech of stutterers. *Journal of Speech and Hearing Research*, 1978, *21*, 285-294.

Brown, T., Sambrooks, J.E., & MacCulloch, M.J. Auditory thresholds and the effect of reduced auditory feedback on stuttering. *Acta Psychiatrica Scandinavia*, 1975, *51*, 297-311.

Burke, B.D. Reduced auditory feedback and stuttering. *Behaviour Research and Therapy*, 1969, *7*, 303-308.

Butler, R.R., Jr., & Stanley, P.E. The stuttering problem considered from an automatic control point of view. *Folia Phoniatrica*, 1966, *18*, 33-44.

Chase, R.A. & Sutton, S. Reply to "Masking of auditory feedback in stutterers' speech." *Journal of Speech and Hearing Research*, 1968, *11*, 219-223.

Cherry, C., & Sayers, B. McA. Experiments upon the total inhibition of stamering by external control, and some clinical results. *Journal of Psychosomatic Research*, 1956, *1*, 233-246.

Code, C., & Muller, D. Comments on paper "The long-term use of an automatically triggered masking device in the treatment of stammering." *British Journal of Disorders of Communication*, 1980, *15*, 141-142.

Conture, E.G. Some effects of noise on the speaking behavior of stutterers. *Journal of Speech and Hearing Research*, 1974, *17*, 714-723.

Conture, E.G., & Brayton, E.R. The influence of noise on stutterers' different dysfluency types. *Journal of Speech and Hearing Research*, 1975, *18*, 381-384.

Cross, D., & Luper, H. Voice reaction time of stuttering and non-stuttering children and adults. *Journal of Fluency Disorders*, 1979, *4*, 59-77.

Curlee, R.F., & Perkins, W.H. Conversational rate control therapy for stuttering. *Journal of Speech and Hearing Disorders*, 1969, *34*, 245-250.

Derazne, J. Speech pathology in the U.S.S.R. In R.W. Rieber & R.S. Brubaker (Eds.), *Speech pathology*. Amsterdam: North-Holland, 1966.

Dewar, A., & Dewar, A.D. Comments on comments of Muller and Code on Dewar et al. (1979). *British Journal of Disorders of Communication*. 1980, *15*, 142.

Dewar, A., Dewar, A.D., & Anthony, J.F.K. The effect of auditory feedback masking on concomitant movements of stammering. *British Journal of Disorders of Communication*, 1976, *11*, 95-102.

Dewar, A., Dewar, A.D., Austin, W.T.S., & Brash, H.M. The longterm use of an automatically triggered auditory feedback masking device in the treatment of stammering. *British Journal of Disorders of Communication*, 1979, *14*, 219-229.

Dewar, A., Dewar, A.D., & Barnes, H.E. Automatic triggering of auditory feedback masking in stammering and cluttering. *British Journal of Disorders of Communication*, 1976, *11*, 19-26.

Donovan, G.E. A new device for the treatment of stammering. *British Journal of Disorders of Communication*, 1971, *6*, 86-88.

Froeschels, E. A survey of European literature in speech and voice pathology. *Asha*, 1962, *4*, 172-181.

Garber, S.F., & Martin, R.R. The effects of white noise on the frequency of stuttering. *Journal of Speech and Hearing Research,* 1974, *17,* 73-79.

Garber, S.F., & Martin, R.R. Effects of noise and increased vocal intensity on stuttering. *Journal of Speech and Hearing Research,* 1977, *20,*, 233-240.

Garber, S.R. & Siegel, G.M. Feedback and motor control in stuttering. In D.K. Routh (Ed.), *Learning, speech and the complex effects of punishment: Essays honoring George J. Wischner.* New York: Plenum, 1982.

Garber, S.R., Siegel, G.M., & Pick, H.L., Jr. Effects of feedback filtering on speaking intelligibility. *Journal of Communication Disorders,* 1980, *13,* 289-294.

Garber, S.F., Siegel, G.M., Pick, H.L., Jr., & Alcorn, S.R. The influence of selected masking noises on Lombard and sidetone amplification effects. *Journal of Speech and Hearing Research,* 1976, *19,* 523-535.

Gorin, L.C. Stuttering in Lima, Peru: a qualitative case study of current concepts, theories, and treatment facilities. *Journal of Communication Disorders,* 1980, *13,* 263-376.

Gregory, H.H. Stuttering and auditory central nervous system disorder. *Journal of Speech and Hearing Research,* 1964, *7,* 335-341.

Gruber, L. The use of the portable voice masker in stuttering therapy. *Journal of Speech and Hearing Disorders,* 1971, *36,* 287-289.

Guttman, N. Speech correction in the U.S.S.R. *Journal of Speech and Hearing Disorders,* 1960, *25,* 306.

Hall, J., & Jerger, J. Central auditory function in stutterers. *Journal of Speech and Hearing Research,* 1978, *21,* 324-337.

Hanley, T.D., & Steer, M.D. Effect of level of distracting noise on speaking rate, duration and intensity. *Journal of Speech and Hearing Disorders,* 1949, *14,* 363-368.

Harms, M.A., & Malone, J.Y. The relationship of hearing acuity to stammering. *Journal of Speech Disorders,* 1939, *4,* 363-370.

Hood, R.B., & Dixon, R.F. Physical characteristics of speech rhythm of deaf and normal-hearing speakers. *Journal of Communication Disorders,* 1969, *2,* 20-28.

Horovitz, L., Johnson, S., Pearlman, R., Schaffer, E., & Hedin, A. Stapedial reflex and anxiety in fluent and disfluent speakers. *Journal of Speech and Hearing Research,* 1978, *21,* 762-767.

Ingham, R.J., Southwood, H., & Horsburgh, G. Some effects of the "Edinburgh Masker" on stuttering during oral reading and spontaneous speech. *Journal of Fluency Disorders,* 1981, *6,* 135-154.

Katz, M. Survey of patented anti-stuttering devices. *Journal of Communication Disorders,* 1977, *10,* 181-206.

Kern, A. Der Einfluss des Horens auf das Stottern. *Archives of Psychiatry,* 1932, *97,* 429-449.

Lane, H., & Tranel, B. The Lombard sign and the role of hearing in speech. *Journal of Speech and Hearing Research,* 1971, *14,* 677-709.

Lechner, B.N. The effects of delayed auditory feedback and masking fundamental frequency of stutterers and nonstutterers. *Journal of Speech and Hearing Research,* 1979, *22,* 343-353.

MacCulloch, M.J., Eaton, R., & Long, E. The long term effect of auditory masking on young stutterers. *British Journal of Disorders of Communication,* 1970, *5,* 165-173.

Mallard, A.R., & Webb, W.G. The effect of auditory and visual "distractors" on the frequency of stuttering. *Journal of Communication Disorders,* 1980, *13,* 207-212.

Maraist, J.A., & Hutton, C. Effect of auditory masking upon the speech of stutterers. *Journal of Speech and Hearing Disorders,* 1957, *22,* 385-389.

Martin, J.E. The signal detection hypothesis and perceptual defect theory of stuttering. *Journal of Speech and Hearing Disorders,* 1970, *35,* 252-255.

Martin, R., & Haroldson, S.K. Effects of five experimental treatments on stuttering.

Journal of Speech and Hearing Research, 1979, *22,* 132-145.

May, A.E., & Hackwood, A. Some effects of masking and eliminating low frequency feedback on the speech of stammerers. *Behaviour Research and Therapy,* 1968, *6,* 219-223.

McFarlane, S., & Prins, D. Neural response time of stutterers and nonstutters in selected oral motor tasks. *Journal of Speech and Hearing Research,* 1978, *21,* 768-778.

Meyer, V., & Mair, J.M. A new technique to control stammering: A preliminary report. *Behaviour Research and Therapy,* 1963, *1,* 251-254.

Murray, F.P. An investigation of variably induced white noise upon moments of stuttering. *Journal of Communication Disorders,* 1969, *2,* 109-114.

Mysak, E.D. Servo-theory and stuttering. *Journal of Speech and Hearing Disorders,* 1960, *25,* 188-195.

Niemark, E.Z. The treatment of the stuttering neurosis on the basis of the physiological interpretation of its mechanisms. In R.E. West (Ed.), *Russian translations in speech and hearing.* Washington, DC: American Speech & Hearing Association, 1968.

Panconcelli-Calzia, G. Die Bedingtheit des Lombardschen Versuches in der Stimm-und-Sprachheilkunde. *Acta Otolaryngology,* 1955, *45,* 244-251.

Parker, C.S., & Christopherson, F. Electronic aid in the treatment of stammer. *Medical Electronic and Biological Engineering,* 1963, *1,* 121-125.

Perkins, W.H., & Curlee, R.F. Clinical impressions of portable masking unit effects in stuttering. *Journal of Speech and Hearing Disorders,* 1969, *34,* 360-362.

Perry, A. Results of a national survey on the use of the Edinburgh Masker Clinical Bench Model and issuing of portable models. *Bulletin of College of Speech Therapists,* 1979, *332,* 9-12.

Petkov, D., & Iosifov, I. Our experience in the treatment of stuttering in a speech rehabilitation colony. *Zhurnal Nervopatologii i Psikhiatrii imeni S.S. Korsakova* 1960, *60,* 903-904.

Razdol'skii, V.A. State of speech of stammerers when alone. *Zhurnal Nevropatologii: i Psikhiatrii imeni S.S. Korsakova,* 1965, *65,* 1717-1720.

Relief for the stutterer. *Time,* August 24, 1970, p.35.

Ringel, R.L., & Steer, M.D. Some effects of tactile and auditory alterations on speech output. *Journal of Speech and Hearing Research,* 1963, *6,* 369-378.

Shane, M.L. Effect on stuttering alteration in auditory feedback. In W. Johnson & R.R. Leutenegger (Eds.), *Stuttering in children and adults,* Minneapolis: University of Minnesota Press, 1955.

Siegel, G.M. Auditory feedback and speech development. Unpublished manuscript, 1978.

Silverman, F.H., & Goodban, M.T. The effect of auditory masking on the fluency of normal speakers. *Journal of Speech and Hearing Research,* 1972, *15,* 543-546.

Stromsta, C. Experimental blockage of phonation by distorted side-tone. *Journal of Speech and Hearing Research,* 1959, *2,* 286-301.

Stromsta, C. The effects of altering the fundamental frequency of auditory masking on the speech performance of stutterers. *Technical Report of Public Service Grant No. B-1331,* Ohio State University, 1967.

Stromsta, C. Interaural phase disparity of stutterers and nonstutterers. *Journal of Speech and Hearing Research,* 1972, *15,* 771-780.

Sutton, S., & Chase, R.A. White noise and stuttering. *Journal of Speech and Hearing Research,* 1961, *4,* 72.

Timmons, B.A., & Boudreau, J.P. Auditory feedback as a major factor in stuttering. *Journal of Speech and Hearing Disorders,* 1972, *37,* 476-484.

Tinklin, I.G. The Edinburgh Masker. *Bulletin of College of Speech Therapists,* 1980, *340,* 7-10.

Trotter, W.D., & Lesch, M.M. Personal experiences with a stutter-aid. *Journal of Speech and Hearing Disorders*, 1967, *32*, 270-272.

Van Riper, C. *Speech correction: Principles and methods*, Englewood Cliffs, NJ: Prentice-Hall, 1963.

Van Riper, C. Clinical use of intermittent masking in stuttering therapy. *Asha*, (Abstract), 1965, 7, 381.

Van Riper, C. *The nature of stuttering*, Englewood Cliffs, NJ: Prentice-Hall, 1971.

Van Riper, C. *The treatment of stuttering*, Englewood Cliffs, NJ: Prentice-Hall, 1973.

Voelker, C.H. An objective study of the comparative number of speech sounds spoken per minute by the deaf and the normal. *Annals of Otology, Rhinology, and Laryngology*, 1937, *46*, 471-476.

Walle, E.L. Masking devices and the Edinburgh Masker—Clinical applications within a prison setting. *Journal of Fluency Disorders*, 1980, *5*, 69-74.

Webster, R.L., & Dorman, M.F. Decreases in stuttering frequency as a function of continuous and contingent forms of auditory masking. *Journal of Speech and Hearing Research*, 1970, *13*, 82-86.

Webster, R.L., & Lubker, B. Masking of auditory feedback in stutterers' speech. *Journal of Speech and Hearing Research*, 1968, *11*, 221-223. (a)

Webster, R.L., & Lubker, B.B. Interrelationships among fluency producing variables in stuttered speech. *Journal of Speech and Hearing Research*, 1968, *11*, 754-766. (b)

Winchester, R.A., & Gibbons, E.W. The effect of auditory masking upon oral reading rate. *Journal of Speech and Hearing Disorders*, 1958, *23*, 250-252.

Wingate, M.E. A standard definition of stuttering. *Journal of Speech and Hearing Disorders*, 1964, *29*, 484-489.

Wingate, M.E. Effect on stuttering of changes in audition. *Journal of Speech and Hearing Research*, 1970, *13*, 861-873.

Wingate, M.E. *Stuttering: Theory and treatment*, New York: Irvington, 1976.

Wynne, M.K., & Boehmler, R.M. Central auditory function in fluent and disfluent normal speakers. *Journal of Speech and Hearing Research*, 1982, *25*, 54-57.

Yairi, E. Effects of binaural and monaural noise on stuttering. *Journal of Auditory Research*, 1976, *16*, 114-119.

Yates, A.J. Recent empirical and theoretical approaches to the experimental manipulation of speech in normal subjects and in stammerers. *Behaviour Research and Therapy*, 1963, *1*, 95-119.

8

Chorus Reading/Shadowing Effects on Stuttering

Introduction

One of the most fascinating features of stuttering is the immediacy with which it seems to disappear when a stutterer amd accompanist read aloud identical material.This is known as the chorus-reading effect. It is also evident, though to a lesser extent, when the stutterer and accompanist read different material or when the stutterer accompanies a recorded reading. A related form of this phenomenon occurs when the stutterer repeats or "shadows" the words of another speaker. As Wingate (1969) has observed, the effect is an impressive universal characteristic in a disorder noted for variability and inconsistency. Equally impressive, though, is the limited amount of research this characteristic has provoked. It has been virtually regarded as a puzzling oddity with limited theoretical or clinical value, even to the extent of seeming to have more interest for television audiences than for clinical researchers. Sheehan (1975), for example, reports giving numerous graphic displays of the chorus reading effect on national television in order to show features of stuttering. In one sense, this not only highlights the dramatic nature of the effect, it also testifies to the reliability with which it can be demonstrated.

The chorus reading effect was certainly well know before the advent of television, although it received only limited attention from earlier clinicians. Klingbeil's (1939) review of the practices of some of these clinicians includes only one definite reference to it. That was by Comstock, a Philadelphian physician of the 1880s, whose treatment of speech defects "consisted in exercising the voice daily by reading aloud in unison with others." The French elocutionist Chervin, who practiced in the same decade, probably used a procedure resembling shadowing, since his stuttering treatment involved imitating the instructor's pronunciation. By the beginning of this century, it was evident that most of the prominent clinicians were not only familiar with chorus reading, but also had explanations for its effectiveness. Fletcher (1928) felt that stutterers judged it to be of assistance becasue "in reading with someone they did not have the feeling that the sole responsibility was resting upon them, and if they 'got stuck' the other person would keep going"(p. 239). Bluemel (1935) regarded its effect as a conditioned response to the stimulus effects of the fluent accompanist. He claimed that when others "speak in unison with the stammerer their words furnish the conditioned stimulus for which his speech is the conditioned response''(p. 86). Wendell Johnson apparently regarded chorus reading in a related way. He saw it as an example of a ''speech pattern'' which altered the stimulus value of words, and other cues, with respect to stuttering (Johnson & Rosen, 1937). At the same time, by describing it is as a ''speech pattern,'' he implied that it also produced a distinctive manner of speaking.

Stutterers also sppear to be quite familiar with the benefits of chorus reading. In Bloodstein's (1950) survey of conditions under which stuttering is reduced or absent, 50 stutterers said they had experienced unison reading. All reported that it produced hardly any stuttering, or no stuttering at all. It is also interesting to note that Bloodstein (1949) regarded its effects as likely to be due to either reduced communicative responsibility or an altered speech pattern.

Experimental Investigations of Chorus Reading and Shadowing

The first serious investigation on the chorus reading effect was conducted by Johnson and Rosen (1937). They had 18 adult stutterers orally read the same 500-word passage with a variety of ''speech patterns'' that included reading in chorus with a stutterer and also with a normal speaker. Under both conditions, the group recorded only one stuttering, but at least 316 stutterings occurred during a control reading. Actually, this is one of the most substantial reductions in stuttering mentioned in any chorus reading study, though part of this considerable effect may have been because subjects were required to reread the same passage in all conditions.

In a subsequent study, Barber (1939) investigated many parameters of chorus reading. She had 18 stutterers (15-33 years) read 14 different 500-word passages under 14 different situations. These included orally reading alone, with stutterers or normal speakers, using similar or different reading material, nonsense syllables, the accompanist phonating ''ah,'' or unpatterned mechanical noise. The data show that the situations in which the stutterer and accompanist(s) read identical material produced significantly less stuttering than all other situations. Within the identical-reading situations, the mean number of stuttered words was reduced from, at least, 86.4 to, at least, 1.4. By contrast, most of the situations that required subjects and accompanists to use different reading material produced only about 50% reductions in stuttering. Generally speaking, greater reductions in stuttering occurred when the subject was accompanied by more than one reader, and regardless of whether the accompanists were stutterers or nonstutterers.

Barber's (1939) findings seemed to spell the end to one explanation of the chorus reading effect—that it was due to distraction. Because the effect differed according to the reading material and size of the reading audience, it made more sense to seek causal variables within situational characteristics, rather than describe them as ''more or less distracting.'' Barber recognized that there might be a number of causes, including the subject's speech pattern, the meaning of the material, personal factors, and the amount of "support" in the situation. Her data certainly show considerable individual differences as well as the significance of reading material and chorus size variables. But they give no clue about the role of speech pattern features. Her final conclusion was that chorus reading benefits stutterers because they are placed in conditions where speech performance is not likely to be evaluated. In other words, when the responsibility to communicate well is increased (that is by using different material, or fewer accompanists) then the effect should be diminished.

Eisenson and Wells (1942) also hypothesized that the chorus-reading effect is due to the speaker experiencing reduced "communicative responsibility." Accordingly, they had 19 male stutterers chorus read in two situations; reading with a normal-speaking accompanist, then again with the accompanist after being induced to believe they would be heard (via microphone) by students who were to answer questions based on the reading. No significant differences were found, however, between the number of their "errors" in either reading condition. Pattie and Knight (1944) also pursued this hypothesis. They assessed 12 stutterers (adults and children) during chorus-reading conditions in which the stutterer's and accompanist's reading material was the same or different, and the accompanist was either in the same room or heard via telephone. The burden of communicative responsibility was presumed to increase because the subject orally read to an audience of four or five persons, with the accompanist heard only by the stutterer over the telephone. Four different 550-word passages (same words rearranged) were used in six conditions that included reading alone, with, and without the audience. Once again the findings failed to support the reduced communicative responsibility hypothesis, but they did indicate the strength of the effects produced by similarity of reading material; the mean percentages on blocks was reduced by around 85 to 90% in the matched reading material condition, and by approximately 50% when different material was used. The next hypothesis to emerge as an explanation for the chorus-reading effect stemmed from the servosystem theory of speech behavior (see Chapter 10). Lee's (1951) studies on the disruptive effects of delayed auditory feedback promoted much speculation about the role of auditory feedback in controlling speech and in producing stuttering. Lee suggested that the chorus-reading effect may be due to the correct feedback supplied by the accompanist(s). It should have been immediately obvious, however, that this explanation is inadequate, for it fails to account for the benefits that occur when different reading material is employed.

Another auditory feedback explanation was promoted by Cherry and Sayers (1956) on the basis of some experiments with chorus reading and shadowing. They first observed that their stutterers could achieve fluency while accompanied by similar material. But then the control reader could shift to different material, even gibberish, and "stammering [remained] completely inhibited in all cases, on all occasions" (p. 236). They also reported that similar results were obtained when the stutterer accompanied a recording of reversed speech. This led them to conclude that the effect is due not so much to correct feedback, but to speakers being compelled to transfer their perception to a source of sound other than their own speech. Unhappily, Cherry and Sayers's explanation has just as many problems as Lee's explanation. It also fails to explain the results of other studies which show differences between the effects obtained with identical and nonidentical reading material. It does point to a possible connection between the processes that occur within chorus reading and masking conditions, however. It may well be, for example, that a portion of the effect is attributable to the variables responsible for reductions caused by masking—whatever they might be.

One of the differences between Cherry and Sayers's (1956) procedure for observing the chorus-reading effect and that used by others is that they systematically altered the control reading conditions *after* stuttering had been reduced during unison reading. Wingate (1976) has speculated that this may have introduced another variable which sustained the benefits caused by unison reading; the speaker was induced to continue using an unusual speech pattern. The notion that chorus reading is implicated with an altered speech pattern was referred to by Johnson and Rosen (1937), Barber (1939), and Bloodstein (1949; 1950). It was substantially revitalized by Wingate (1969; 1976), however, with his observation that many of the conditions that produce fluent speech behavior may depend for their effects on the speaker doing "something with his voice that he does not ordinarily do."

Wingate's (1969;1976) speculations about the role of speech pattern changes during chorus reading and shadowing merit special consideration because they have fueled further research on these procedures (and other stuttering modification methods). In his 1969 seminal paper, Wingate argued that both chorus reading and shadowing share one distinctive element, they induce "some kind of pacing or patterning." He noted, especially, the observations of Cherry (1953), who was the first to describe the impact of the shadowing procedure on normal speakers. Cherry conducted some speech recognition experiments which required the listener to repeat one of two messages heard concurrently in each headphone. He found that a speaker could perform this task with surprising skill, but that "one marked characteristic of his speaking voice is its monotony. Very little emotional content or stressing of the words occurs at all" (p. 988).

Experimental Investigations of Shadowing

The effects of shadowing on stuttering have usually been linked to chorus reading, and so the variables that are implicated in chorus readng are usually related to shadowing. The uncritical acceptance of this connection may explain the puzzling absence of research on shadowing. In shadowing, the stutterer copies immediately what the other speaker says or reads, but—unlike chorus reading—may have no idea of the words required to be spoken.

The skill with which normal speakers can shadow was investigated by Sergeant (1961) and found to be affected by the rate and intensity of the message. When the words were heard at a rate of 70 wpm, 69% of the followers' utterances were rated intelligible, but this dropped to 42% when the rate was 180 wpm. With practice, 10 out of 12 speakers were found to achieve above 70% intelligibility ratings at different wpm rates. This is not particularly high, which tends to suggest that shadowing may very well produce unusual sounding speech—almost certainly error-ridden speech.

The effect of shadowing on stuttering has not been carefully investigated. Cherry and Sayers (1956) claimed to have assessed the results of shadowing in a study with 51 stutterers. The subjects shadowed a 150-word message which was read at 50-100 wpm. It was reported that 39 cases had "relatively few breakdowns. . . the total duration of breakdown for the worst case, whilst shadowing, was 4 seconds" (p. 240). But this investigation failed to provide a comparison between shadowed and nonshadowed reading, nor any indication of their procedure, or the reliability of their data. The only reference that Cherry and Sayers make to an altered speech pattern during shadowing is that when the control speaker was English and the subject was American, the subject did not always imitate the control: "It has been found that the latter [the subject] lapses into common Americanism (like gotten, rail-road, etc), those being his own speech habits." (p. 234). This indicates that the shadowing effect is not simply caused by the stutterer imitating the control reader's speech pattern.

The only other investigation is a report by Andrews, Howie, Dosza and Guitar (1982) on the effects of shadowing a recording of oral reading. They found that three adult male stutterers reduced their base rate frequency of stuttering by a mean of 95%.

Evaluating Wingate's Explanation for Chorus Reading and Shadowing Effects

Wingate's (1969; 1976) observations on both choral speaking (chorus reading) and shadowing led him first to conclude that, "careful attention to the performance of the 'follower' reveals that the salient feature of the speech is that it has an 'intoning' character. This means that speaking under such circumstances encourages accentuation of 'melody' " (1969, p. 682). In a later review of the literature (Wingate, 1976), he argued that at least three fluency-inducing variables are involved in the subject's changed manner of speaking during these conditions: "They are: (1) reduced rate, (2) emphasis on phonation, with reduction of stress contrasts and (3) subordination of consonant articulatory gestures" (1976, p. 209).

The role of reduced speech rate partly stemmed from Cherry and Sayers's (1956) report that their shadowing procedure required the lead reader to use a rate of between 50 and 100 words per minute. The other was information derived from an unpublished study in which Wingate (1973) found that during unison reading each reader showed "an average decrease of 20 percent below his solo reading rate." Wingate acknowledged, however, that this factor may not be as fundamental to the effect as is the stutterer's altered speech quality. This led him to argue that the "predominant change is in phonation, expressed on the one hand through increased duration—primarily of vowels—and on the other by modulation of stress contrasts and some increases in volume" (Wingate, 1976, p. 203).

Wingate's (1969; 1976) speculations are an excellent example of the effect on research of a plausible and testable proposition. It will be seen in later chapters that the speculation about the role of an altered speech pattern on stuttering has sent many researchers scurrying to investigate many well-worn areas. It has certainly had the effect of shifting attention away from environmental factors and back to motoric variables. Like the search for "explanations" of the rhythm effect, the aim has been to seek commonalities that relate chorus reading and shadowing to other fluency-inducing variables. This presents some interesting problems; perhaps the most prominent is the need to explain the consistent finding that chorus reading with similar material produces less stuttering than does reading with different material. If the motoric theory is viable, it must mean that "different reading" produces either less consistent change, or simply less change among some of these fluency-inducing variables.

Four studies have been conducted in order to test Wingate's hypotheses regarding chorus reading, and all have involved unison reading. The first two studies were conducted by this writer and colleagues (Ingham & Carroll, 1977; Ingham & Packman, 1979). Both studies used recorded oral reading as the accompanist for the stutterer, plus perceptual analysis procedures to assess whether listeners could discern differences between stutterers' speech during chorus- and nonchorus-reading conditions. Ingham and Carroll (1977) found that the chorus reading conditions produced a mean 82.5% reduction in stuttering across nine stutterers (8-18 years). (This is comparable to the reductions that are reported when the accompanist is present during chorus reading.) There was also a mean increase in their subjects' speech rate during the chorus-reading conditions. Stutter-free samples, of identical prose content, were obtained from oral readings made between and within both conditions. When observers had to judge whether the pairs of samples from each stutterer were drawn from different or similar reading situations, their answers only partially supported Wingate's hypothesis: they correctly identified the samples made under different speaking conditions from only four of the nine stutterers.

The Ingham and Carroll (1977) study had two important limitations; it used only two relatively short (10-second) pairs of samples and failed to control for each individual's speech rate during the chorus-reading conditions. These problems were addressed in a study by Ingham and Packman (1979). They used much the same methods as those employed by Ingham and Carroll (1977), but with only three stutterers (18, 28, and 20 years). Each subject's fluent oral reading rate was obtained prior to the experiment, then a control reader tape was constructed using that oral reading rate. Also, 20 pairs (that is, 10 "same" and 10 "different") of samples (15 words per sample) were obtained for one subject and 24 sample pairs for the other two subjects (15 and 20 words per sample). The chorus-reading condition produced more than a 90% reduction in stuttering with two subjects, and a 56% reduction for the other subject. For all but one of the 12 oral readings, the chorus-reading rate of speaking was substantially greater than the nonchorus-reading rate. Again, the results were only partially supportive of Wingate's hypothesis. The judges definitely distinguished between the chorus- and non-chorus-reading samples for two stutterers (including the subject who showed the least chorus-reading effect), but did not distinguish between the samples from the third stutterer.

Taken together, the findings from the Ingham and Carroll (1977) and Ingham and Packman (1979) studies suggest that some stutterers may exhibit perceptual differences between their speech in chorus and nonchorus reading, although this is not true for all stutterers. Their findings also showed that the chorus-reading effect does not depend upon the stutterer using a slower-than-usual oral reading rate. This finding is also supported by data from May and Hackwood (1968). In one condition in their study, they had stutterers (n=10) orally read to the accompaniment of the experimenter who was reading different material. Their data also show that this condition resulted in a significant increase in the subjects' mean oral reading rate when compared with reading alone.

Adams and Ramig (1980) investigated Wingate's proposition that the chorus-reading effect is associated with increased duration of phonation, mainly vowels, and increased volume. They also assessed the chorus-reading effect using a recorded normal speaker as an accompanist for oral reading by 10 stutterers (15-40 years) and 10 nonstutterers.[1] A 51-syllable passage was orally read during widely separated chorus- and nonchorus-reading conditions, then measures were made of vowel duration, peak vocal SPL, and continuity of phonation. The chorus-reading effect was obviously evident since there was a 91% decrease in all disfluencies, 66% of which were stutterings, during the chorus reading conditions. They found no significant differences in peak vocal SPL or continuity of phonation scores on samples obtained in the chorus- and nonchorus-reading conditions. This was true for both the stutterers and nonstutterers. Of further interest was their finding that there were indeed changes in vowel duration scores, but not in the expected direction: relative to nonchorus reading conditions, the stutterers significantly *shortened* their vowels and the nonstutterers tended to lengthen theirs (though not significantly).

In contrast to Adams and Ramig (1980), are findings reported by Andrews, Howie, Dozsa, and Guitar (1982) who used a "live" chorus-reading condition; that is, the subjects (three adult male stutterers) read " from a newspaper in unison with two fluent speakers." Their results also showed that the chorus-reading effect (a 100% reduction in stuttering in all three subjects) was not associated with an obvious increase in mean phonation duration. As previously mentioned, this study also investigated shadowing conditions and reported increases in mean phonation duration similar to those reported during chorus reading.

The findings from the previous studies clearly produce problems for the explanation proposed by Wingate. Quite obviously, the chorus-reading effect does

[1] For some reason, Adams and Ramig (1980) claim that "Wingate was careful to limit this explanation [alterations in vocalization] to only those choral reading conditions wherein the stutterer and his companion speaker are reading or speaking in each other's physical presence" (p. 458). Careful reading of Wingate's (1969; 1976) papers reveals that this is not necessarily true. In fact, Wingate (1976) noted that the data obtained by Pattie and Knight (1944) indicated "the effect was the same whether the accompanying speaker was physically present or speaking from another room" (p. 200).

not depend on either reduced reading rate, increased vowel durations, phonation continuity, or vocal level. In some ways this finding is also related to effects produced by masking. It will be recalled from Chapter 7 that at least two studies on masking and stuttering have shown that masking may not affect vowel duration in stuttering. There is evidence, however, that many speakers definitely do change their speech pattern during chorus reading, while others appear not to. Of course it may be that these studies have not measured the most relevant vocal characteristics for this issue. Nevertheless, this first skirmish between the modified vocalization hypothesis and the experimental method has not left the hypothesis unscathed. It may have explanatory strength, but its survival probably depends on measures of more subtle parts of speech behavior, or the concession that it applies only to some subjects.

Conclusions from Experimental Studies

Many aspects of the chorus reading and shadowing effect should attract investigation. These include the influence of different speech rates by the accompanist, the relationship between the speech quality during different types of chorus reading (similar and different material), and the control reader's speech rate. Adams and Ramig (1980) suggest that one explanation for the trends in their data, especially with respect to vowel durations, is that the mean scores of both groups during chorus reading tended towards the scores obtained from samples of the recorded accompanist's speech. This imitative aspect of the chorus-reading effect has not been seriously investigated and may prove a profitable source of enquiry. This point is made more cogent by findings from a study by Adamczyk, Kuniszyk-Joskowiak and Sadowska (1976). They compared different combinations of stutterers and nonstutterers as accompanists for oral readings by 30 stutterers and found significantly less stuttering when a nonstutterer was included in the audience.

At present the source of benefits from chorus reading and shadowing remain open to conjecture. It is quite possible that part of the chorus-reading effect may be associated with variables responsible for masking's benefits. But, then, it is not at all clear what those variables are—at least, both the masking and chorus reading share some difficulties with the modified vocalization hypothesis. Furthermore, the contribution of auditory stimulation factors to an explanation for benefits from both methods may have been cast aside a little prematurely.

Therapy Applications of Chorus Reading and Shadowing

Introduction

Up until this point, the stuttering therapy techniques that have been mentioned within the behavioral preparadigm share at least one common feature—the technique can be "used" by the stutterer in natural or nonclinic conditions. For example, rhythmic speech and relaxation (or assertion) can be practised either regularly or continuously in almost all speaking circumstances. Similarly, with the assistance of hearing-aid technology, it is possible to extend and sustain the essential treatment elements of rhythm and masking. These possibilities do not obviously apply in the case of chorus reading and shadowing. Both methods need the subject to follow or accompany another speaker in order to achieve treatment benefits, a restriction which has probably led to their relatively limited use in therapy.

Many clinicians have opted to use chorus reading as either a treatment adjunct, as a means to demonstrate that the speaker is able to achieve fluency, or even as a diagnostic indicator for other treatment methods. Some earlier clinicians, such as Kingdon-Ward (1941), used communal verse-speaking to desensitize the speaker's fears about speaking socially. Van Riper (1959; 1963) recommended "stuttering in unison" as a means of teaching the modification of severe stutterings. He suggested that the clinician should first accompany and mimic the stuttering, then do so with less "severity" until the gross features of the subject's blocks are removed. And Cooper (1979) has recommended that unison reading and shadowing (as well as other techniques) should be used to identify "fluency-initiating gestures" that could then be used as part of other therapy procedures.

The Cherry and Sayers Therapy Initiative

Both chorus reading and shadowing have been employed as principal treatment techniques within some behaviorally oriented stuttering therapies. Their use in this context began with a report by Marland, which was appended to Cherry and Sayers's (1956) research paper. This described a series of "preliminary clinical trials" on the use of shadowing with 10 stutterers (5-59 years). The treatment was not evidently systematic, and its assessment amounted to sketchy descriptions of outcome. The children were treated by a combination of recordings and parent-directed practice, though some treatment descriptions indicated that more than shadowing may have been involved. For instance, those who had difficulty in mastering shadowing were said to have improved when they were reminded "to attend to the rhythm," whisper, or, in the case of adults, shadow a slow rate of speech. It was also mentioned that "psychological help" was needed with most cases. The case descriptions indicate that seven of the 10 subjects responded to this treatment, though most showed signs of improvement rather than stutter-free speech. This is virtually impossible to establish clearly in the absence of data, however. It was also observed that the 5- and 6-year-old children benefited most from this treatment.

Further descriptions of Cherry and Sayers's (1956) shadowing therapy procedure occur in articles by Marland (1957) and Maclaren (1960). The Marland article virtually overviewed the continued use of this procedure in a program which she and Maclaren directed, mainly for 3- and 4-year-old stutterers. Their treatment for older stutterers included a variety of methods in addition to shadowing. These were usually chorus reading with different texts, plus procedures advocated by Van Riper (1959). Maclaren (1960) reviewed the results of this therapy in a very cursory fashion, claiming particularly good outcome with children. But, again, absolutely no data were presented to support this claim. She did infer, however, that this procedure was not very successful with older subjects: "With the older patient the anxiety attached to the speech situation itself often spreads its tentacles through the whole pattern of life. It would be absurd to expect that auditory retraining alone could bring any real relief to such patients." (p. 460).

The degree of enthusiasm for this treatment, especially with adults, appeared to decline further in later reports. Jones (1969; 1970) reported the experiences of a colleague (Krikler) who had used a shadowing treatment program with 50 adult or adolescent stutterers (mainly 20 to 30 years). She conducted once-weekly therapy sessions for 8 weeks, using daily home shadowing practice via recordings of graded difficulty. Jones (1969) described the results in the following way: "a few patients improved dramatically, the overall success of the therapy is unlikely to be greater than when more traditional methods are employed over the same period. Enquiries Mrs. Krikler has made at other clinics also indicate a disappointing outcome although there are indications that the technique is more effective with young children" (p. 192). Clearly, Cherry and Sayers's shadowing treatment had fairly limited success, mostly with children, and its clinical usefulness probably depends on its amalgamation with other therapy techniques. Of course, this could be the main reason why it showed promise in the treatment of children.

Data-based Treatment Studies

The limitations that shadowing, as such, has in producing sustained reductions in stuttering present some obvious difficulties for its use in therapy. A striking illustration of this limitation occurs in a report by Frank and Bloodstein (1971) on the effects of unison reading on the adaptation effect. They had 15 stutterers (13-29 years) orally reread a 200-word passage on six successive occasions. The first five readings were in unison with the experimenter, and the last was unaccompanied. Their mean stuttering frequency went from around eight to five over the course of the first five readings, but leapt to about 27 during the sixth reading. (This was not significantly different from the sixth reading of these passages when all were made alone.) In effect, whatever benefits accrued from repeated unison reading were immediately lost the instant these subjects orally read alone—hardly a promising indicator for treatment carry-over.

The first clinical use of shadowing in treatments that included some evidence of systematically gathered speech behavior data occurred in a series of reports by Walton and colleagues. Walton (1958) first provided a general description of shadowing in treating stuttering during telephone conversations for one adult stutterer, and for stuttering in all circumstances in the case of another adult stutterer. A more detailed report of the same (presumably) adult stutterer's treatment for telephone conversation difficulty was provided by Walton and

Black (1958). This 32-year-old male's treatment was conducted in two phases. The first phase combined shadowing and "graded re-education" over 49 sessions of shadowed oral reading. Initially, the subject spoke on the phone, with the control reader in the same room or in another room. In either case, the subject was heard by another person. In later sessions, the listening audience was gradually increased with decreasingly familiar members. The graphed data show that in the first four shadowing trials, without the telephone, the subject averaged around 20 "errors" per page and this decreased to around four per page during the last sessions. In the second phase, the subject spoke for 20 10-minute sessions without shadowing assistance. The number of stutterings recorded during these conversations declined from approximately 80 to 15. The problem with these findings is that they cannot be regarded as byproducts of shadowing alone. To begin with, no reliability or speech rate data are included: moreover, there is every possibility that the changes during either phase of the treatment were simply the result of extended practice in using the telephone. In fact, the subject's observations on his treatment were astute: "The shadowing may have been responsible for maintaining this high level (of fluency) but I have responded most I feel to the use of, and length of time using, the telephone" (p. 176). Further limitations with shadowing were evident in a report by Walton and Mather (1963). Initially, they treated a 40-year-old male stutterer with 48 sessions of shadowing practice over four months, but they found that his improved performance failed to extend beyond the clinic. Thereafter the subject was treated by systematic desensitization and relaxation. Unfortunately, this report failed to provide any data which would point to the gains that shadowing produced, even in clinic conditions.

Another report, which gave some evidence of the effects of a shadowing treatment, was provided by Kondas (1967). He treated 20 stutterers (16 who were 16-18 years; three 5-6 years; one 20-year-old) by a two- or three-stage procedure, then followed their progress for three to five years after therapy. The treatment began with relaxed breathing exercises followed by a combined clinic- and home-based program of shadowing practice. After shadowing was mastered within the clinic (using oral reading or a puppet show for children), a parent-directed home program was instituted. Decreasing clinic contact was used in a treatment schedule which lasted between two and nine months. Four subjects failed to improve after 10-15 sessions, so they were treated by desensitization methods. The treatment results were based upon four assessment categories (no effect, little improved, much improved and "cured," that is, when "people cannot tell that the child was a stammerer"). It was also indicated that "at the termination of therapy, or 1 month later, the frequency of stammers and hesitations decreased from 12.2 to 2.2." No other details are provided and this is the only evidence that stuttering was measured. At follow-up, only five cases were assessed by the therapists; the others had their performance described by parents and school teachers. From these assessments, it was concluded that 70.6% of the cases were "cured" or "much improved" at the end of treatment, with 58.8% in these categories at follow-up. Twenty-five percent of the subjects were reported unimproved at follow-up.[2] Perhaps the most interesting finding was that the children responded well: the three young children (5-6 years) were "much improved" or "cured" after only three to five clinic sessions, and 3 to 6 weeks of home exercises. Their improved speech was reported to have remained unchanged 1 to 3 years later. The unfortunate feature of the Kondas study is that these promising results are not supported by speech performance data, let alone the refinements of assessment reliability or repeated measurement. Furthermore, with the use of such a long follow-up with children, and no intervening measures of performance, it is possible that some findings could be ascribed to spontaneous remission (although this needs more consideration, in the light of factors mentioned in Chapter 4.)

Another group-subject treatment report was provided by Kelham and McHale (1966). They treated 38 stutterers (4 to 43 years) over 5 to 70 sessions. These sessions involved 2 to 10 minutes of shadowed oral reading and included instructions "to concentrate on and imitate the rhythm of speech used by the therapist." These sessions also included the systematic introduction of an increasingly "difficult" audience, and telephone situations. The treatment ceased

> When it was certain that the patient had ceased to stammer in any of the situations described, or when it became clear that there was no improvement or no further improvement in speech. Each case was then rated by the therapist on a three point scale as "much improved," "improved," or "not improved" (1966, p. 116).

No follow-up assessment was included, and on the basis of this very crude assessment, 74% of the subjects were rated a "success". (A subject was a "success" if the rating was "much improved" or "improved.") To make matters worse, there was no evidence that these assessments were made independently of shadowing.

Only two shadowing treatment studies have reported using an assessment format which might make it possible to determine the effects of therapy intervention. These studies were reported by Ottoni (1974) and Ost, Gotestam, and Melin (1976).

Ottoni (1974) used a single-subject therapy evaluation design to describe the treatment of a 9-year-old male stutterer and a 13-year-old female stutterer. Each received 4-minute assessments of oral reading and drawing descriptions for 5 days per week. The first five assessment sessions established a base rate of the number of 5-second intervals in 4 minutes of speech that contained stutterings. For both stutterers, close to 100% of these speaking intervals contained stutterings. In the treatment sessions, the subjects shadowed oral readings and drawing descriptions by the clinician, with increasingly more words between the clinician's and subject's utterances. This gap in the "shadowing interval" ranged from one to five words contingent on a criterion of reduced stuttering. The subjects ultimately achieved a stable level of stutterings in approximately 2-5%

[2] It is noteworthy that one of the unimproved cases was reported to be "feeble-minded," with an IQ of 58.

of their 5-second speaking intervals per session. This low level of stuttering was also maintained during five daily sessions that were conducted 15 and 30 days after they ceased the treatment sessions (totaling 48 for the male subject and 34 for the female subject). The reassuring feature of these data is that they are supported by similar scores from another observer (95% agreement). The absence of speech-rate data, conversational speech, or a nonclinic assessment means that the findings have fairly limited clinical value, however.

The Ost, Gotestam, and Melin (1976) study also contains a well-conceived treatment evaluation design. It will be recalled from Chapter 5 that this group study compared the effects of Metronome Conditioned Speech Retraining (MCSR) with shadowing treatment and no treatment. In the course of this comparison, five stutterers (part of a group whose ages ranged from 14 to 46 years) recieved 20 sessions (30-40 minutes) spaced over a 3-month period. The "shadowing treatment" actually involved a sequence of procedures, beginning with chorus reading and followed by shadowing, "copying" (the subjects responded after the control reader had spoken two words or half a sentence), and "whispering" (subjects learned to whisper fluently and then increased their vocal level). These clinic sessions were supplemented by daily training assignments outside the clinic. The subjects were assessed before and after treatment, and again 14 months later via oral reading and spontaneous speech tasks (3 minutes each). The results showed no significant change in the group's percentage of "nonfluency" on either task. The only change was an increase in word-per-minute rate on the oral reading task. In other words, the treatment was demonstrated to be almost completely ineffectual—at least, for these five subjects. While this study has the advantage of being one of few shadowing treatment reports (in the Western literature) that demonstrated its trend of evaluation was independent of clinician assessment, it also suffers some disadvantages as an assessment of a treatment. Like the MCSR-treated subjects, the subjects in the shadowing treatment program received a "fixed amount" of therapy. And without "trend data," it is impossible to decide whether some may have benefited from a much longer period of treatment. But, more importantly, it is not clear which part(s) of this treatment were ineffective or even counterproductive. The subjects received a veritable treatment pot pourri, so that some techniques could have cancelled the benefits of others. Nevertheless, it is quite strange to find a treatment which relies on oral reading showing no effects on an oral reading assessment.

Very few other treatment reports have even approached the Ottoni (1974) or Ost, Gotestam, and Melin (1976) studies in terms of treatment description and assessment methodology—which gives a reasonable guide to the quality of those therapy studies. There have been some interesting variations on shadowing treatment, however, which, in turn, provide useful pointers on how this technique could be used more profitably in stuttering therapy.

Kondas and Pukacova (1977) gave a very abbreviated account of a shadowing treatment with 50 stutterers (10-15 years). They had subjects shadow the repeated oral readings of a 200-word passage, which was combined with verbal reinforcement for fluency. No data was reported, but they claim their findings "indicated that the decrease of disfluency moments remained stable and significant" at a two-month follow-up evaluation. They also mentioned that the procedure was not beneficial for severe cases.

Another useful example of shadowing treatment was outlined by Peins, Lee, and McGough (1970). They constructed a tape recorded program of masking and shadowing treatments. The procedure was used with a 13-year-old male stutterer who had received Van Riperian therapy some time before the introduction of this technique. The 40-minute recording was constructed with periods of masking, shadowing exercises, and instructions to speak spontaneously without assistance. The subject recorded his speech on a parallel track and then listened to the results afterwards. The procedure was used at home and then checked every 2 weeks by the clinician. This continued for 2 months before another recording was prepared. Over the 5 months of treatment, three tapes were constructed. The treatment results were based upon stuttering ratings and oral readings made immediately before and after treatment, and then 5 months later. They show that he was a "moderate stutterer" immediately before treatment, and "mild" immediately after treatment; 5 months later, he was rated a "very mild stutterer." The oral reading data showed a related trend: a passage was reread five times at each assessment and the first readings on each of the three assessment occasions show the mean words stuttered were approximately 44, 18, and 7 respectively. Although this treatment appeared beneficial, the clinicians report that it suffered from the subject's flagging enthusiasm.

Peins, McGough, and Lee (1972) provided what they described as an evaluation of their therapy procedure in a study which compared Van Riper's therapy and no treatment. Thirty-six stutterers were divided equally among the treatment conditions and compared over 6 months of therapy time. The difficulty in evaluating this study is that the shadowing treatment methodology was changed quite markedly. The subjects in the tape recorder therapy group received a 30-minute recording which involved shadowing exercises accompanied by instructions on how "to speak more slowly and smoothly in a manner of speaking termed legato style" (1972, p. 365). Since this appears to describe a speech pattern resembling "prolonged speech," their study will be considered in Chapter 10. Suffice to say, ratings of subject performance, made before, during, and after treatment revealed no differences between the two treatment procedures.

Shelton (1975) also used tape-recorded shadowing exercises to treat a 21-year-old male stutterer. The recording was a 200-word passage which contained subject-identified "difficult" words. The subject was instructed to shadow the passage once daily for 2 weeks, then another passage was introduced. This self-directed treatment continued for 6 weeks, with the subject scoring his total stutterings per day for a week before treatment, immediately after treatment, and 1 month later. He judged that he had 7 to 10 stutterings per day before treatment, and 2 to 0 per day a month later. No independent assessment of these data was reported.

Conclusions from Therapy Studies

In an earlier review of the use of shadowing and chorus reading in stuttering treatment, this writer and Andrews reached the conclusion that:

> the reported studies tend to imply that shadowing needs to be combined with other procedures when used in therapy. But these studies are characterized by methodological inadequacies and omissions which make it difficult to reach any firm conclusions on the efficacy of shadowing in stuttering therapy (Ingham & Andrews, 1973, p. 416).

The findings from the present review reveal nothing to suggest that this conclusion should be changed. This is most disappointing because the procedure lends itself to a variety of clinical situations—especially with children. For, in spite of the inadequacies of these reports, the findings, with respect to children, are uniformly positive. It is to be hoped that clinicians will regard this technique more seriously in future and convey their findings in the professional literature.

References

Adamczyk, B., Kuniszyk-Jozkowiak, W., and Sakowska, E. Correction effect in chorus speaking by stuttering people. In *XVIth International Congress on Logopedics and Phoniatrics, Interlaken, 1974,* Basal: Karger, 1976.

Adams, M.R., & Ramig, P. Vocal characteristics of normal speakers and stutterers during choral reading. *Journal of Speech and Hearing Research,* 1980, *23,* 457-469.

Andrews, G., Howie, P.M., Dozsa, M., & Guitar, B.E. Stuttering: Speech pattern characteristics under fluency-inducing conditions. *Journal of Speech and Hearing Research,* 1982, *25,* 208-216.

Barber, V. Studies in the psychology of stuttering: XV. Chorus reading as a distraction in stuttering. *Journal of Speech Disorders,* 1939, *4,* 371-383.

Bloodstein, O. Conditions under which stuttering is reduced or absent: A review of literature. *Journal of Speech and Hearing Disorders,* 1949, *14,* 295-302.

Bloodstein, O. A rating scale of conditions under which stuttering is reduced or absent. *Journal of Speech and Hearing Disorders,* 1950, *15,* 29-36.

Bluemel, C.S. *Stammering and allied disorders.* New York: Macmillan, 1935.

Cherry, E.C. Some experiments on the recognition of speech, with one and with two ears. *Journal of the Acoustical Society of America,* 1953, *25,* 975-979.

Cherry, C., & Sayers, B. McA. Experiments upon the total inhibition of stammering by external control, and some clinical results. *Journal of Psychosomatic Research,* 1956, *1,* 233-246.

Cooper, E.B. Intervention procedures for the young stutterer. In H.H. Gregory (Ed.), *Controversies about stuttering therapy,* Baltimore: University Park Press, 1979.

Eisenson, J., & Wells, C. A study of the influence of communicative responsibility in a choral speech situation for stutterers. *Journal of Speech Disorders,* 1942, 7, 259-262.

Fletcher, J.M. *The Problem of stuttering.* New York: Longmans, 1928.

Frank, A., & Bloodstein,O. Frequency of stuttering following repeated unison readings. *Journal of Speech and Hearing Research,* 1971, *14,* 519-524.

Ingham, R.J., & Andrews, G. Behavior therapy and stuttering: A review. *Journal of Speech and Hearing Disorders,* 1973, *38,* 405-441.

Ingham, R.J., & Carroll, P.J. Listener judgement of differences in stutterers' nonstuttered speech during chorus- and nonchorus-reading conditions. *Journal of Speech and Hearing Research,* 1977, *22,* 787-793.

Johnson, R.J. & Packman, A. A further evaluation of the speech of stutterers during chorus- and nonchorus-rading conditions. *Journal of Speech and Hearing Research*, 1979, *22*, 787-793.

Johnson, W., & Rosen, L. Studies in the psychology of stuttering: VII Effect of certain changes in speech pattern upon frequency of stuttering. *Journal of Speech Disorders.*, 1937, *2*, 105-109.

Jones, H.G. Behavior therapy and stuttering: The need for a multifarious approach to a multiplex problem. In B.B. Gray & G. England (Eds.), *Stuttering and the conditioning therapies*. Monterey, Calif.: Monterey Institute of Speech and Hearing, 1969.

Jones, H.G. Stuttering. In C.G. Costello (Ed.), *Symptoms of Psychopathology. A handbok*. New York: Wiley, 1970.

Kelham, R., & McHale, A. The application of learning theory to the treatment of stuttering. *British Jouranl of Disorders of Communication*, 1966, *1*, 114-118.

Kingdon-Ward, W. *Stammering*. London: Hamish Hamilton, 1941.

Klingbeil, G.M. The historical background of the modern speech clinic. *Journal of Speech Disorders*, 1939, *4*, 115-132.

Kondas, O. The treatment of stammering in children by the shadowing method. *Behaviour Research and Therapy*, 1967, *5*, 325-329.

Kondas, O., & Pukacova, M. Speech shadowing under the adaptation effect condition in the treatment of stammering. *Behavior Therapy*, 1977, *8*, 274-275.

Lee, B.A. Artificial stutter. *Journal of Speech and Hearing Disorders*, 1951, *16*, 53-55.

Maclaren, J. The treatment of stuttering by the Chery-Sayers method: Clinical impressions. In H.J. Eysenck (Ed.), *Behaviour therapy and the neuroses*. Oxford: Permagon Press, 1960.

Marland, P.M. Shadowing: A contribution to the treatment of stammering. *Folia Phoniatrica*, 1957, *9*, 242-245.

May, A.E. & Hackwood, A. Some effect of masking and eliminating low frequency feedback on the speech of stammerers. *Behaviour Research and Therapy*, 1968, *6*, 219-223.

Ost, L.G., Gotestam, K.G., & Melin, L. A controlled study of two behavioral methods in the treatment of stuttering. *Behavior Therapy*, 1976, *7*, 587-592.

Ottoni, T.M. Uso de la tecnica delineamento del habla para cambiar la conducta verbal. *Revista Interamericana de Psicologia*, 1974, *8*, 197-203.

Pattie, F.A., & Knight, B.B. Why does the speech of stutterers improve in chorus reading? *Journal of Abnormal and Social Psychology*, 1944, *35*, 362-367.

Peins, M., Lee, B.J. & McGough, W.E. A tape recorded therapy method for stutterers: A case study. *Journal of Speech and Hearing Disorders*, 1970, *35*, 188-193.

Peins, M., McGough, W.E., & Lee, B.S. Evaluation of a tape-recorded method of stuttering therapy: Improvement in a speaking tast. *Journal of Speech and Hearing Reseach*, 1972, *15*, 364-371.

Sergeant, R.L. Concurrent repetition of a flow of words. *Journal of Speech and Hearing Research*, 1961, *4*, 373-380.

Sheehan, J.G. Conflict theory and avoidance-reduction therapy. In J. Eisenson (Ed.), *Stuttering: A second symposium*. New York: Harper & Row, 1975.

Shelton, J.L. The elimination of persistent stuttering by the use of homework assignements involving speech shadowing: A case report. *Behavior Therapy*, 1975, *6*, 392-393.

Van Riper, C. Binaural speech therapy. *Journal of Speech and Hearing Disorders*, 1959, *24*, 62-63.

Van Riper, C. *Speech correction: Principles and methods*. Englewood Cliffs, N.J.: Prentice-Hall, 1963.

Walton, D. Learning theory, personality, drug-action, and the treatment of stammering. *Bulletin of the British Psychological Society*, 1958, *36* 37-38.

Walton, D., & Black, D.A. The application of learning theory to the treatment of stammering. *Journal of Psychosomatic Research*, 1958, *3*, 170-179.

Walton, D., & Mather, M.C. The relevance of generalization techniques to the treatment of stammering and phobic symptoms. *Behaviour Research and Therapy*, 1963, *1*, 121-125.

Wingate, M.E. Sound and pattern in 'artificial' fluency. *Journal of Speech and Hearing Research*, 1969, *12*, 677-686.

Wingate, M.E. Change of speech performance in choral speaking. Unpublished research, 1973.

Wingate, M.E. *Stuttering: Theory and treatment*. New York: Irvington, 1976.

9

Operant Methodology And Stuttering

Introduction

One of the main claims argued in previous chapters is that the past two decades have witnessed the diminishing influence of the nonbehavioral preparadigm and the increasing influence of the behavioral preparadigm on therapy practices. The epistomological foundations of these competing approaches to therapy practice can be largely traced to two figures: Sigmund Freud and B.F. Skinner. It is tempting to refer to them as influential theoreticians, but in the case of Skinner, his influence stems from an approach to the analysis of behavior which has disavowed theory.

It is almost indisputable that Freud's Psychodynamic Theory created a conceptual approach to treatment which dominated a diversity of therapy practices throughout the first half of this century. Its influence extended well beyond the relatively formalized strictures of psychoanalysis and can be recognized in many of the nonbehavioral stuttering treatments during that period. By way of comparison, it is probably not too premature to claim that Skinner's approach to the science of behavior will emerge as the most prominent influence on therapy practices during the last half of this century. Skinner's analysis of behaviors that are conceptualized to produce environmental consequences shifted the basic emphasis of treatment towards control over the relationship between behavioral responses and environmental stimuli or events.

Skinner's early influence on psychology stemmed from his endeavors to distinguish between the learning, or conditioning, models of Pavlov and Thorndike. Pavlov had identified the conditions that produce a relationship between a new stimulus, a conditioned stimulus, and a response. Thorndike's contribution was to describe the relationship between a given stimulus and a new response, as is expressed in his Law of Effect. Skinner (1937) suggested that these learning models could be viewed as involving two different types or classes of responses and two different types of conditioning. The response classes could be divided into those that were respondent and those that were operant. Respondents were those behaviors that are elicited; for example, the movement rections to painful stimuli or the salivatory actions in the presence of appetitive stimuli.

Operants were classes of responses that are not elicited, but are emitted spontaneously in the absence of stimuli. The classes of reponses were also related to two types of conditioning. Type S conditioning involved the stimulus conditioning of respondent behaviors. In this form of conditioning, the reinforcer is correlated with the stimulus. Type R conditioning involved stimulus conditioning of operant behavior, in which the reinforcer is correlated with the response. In short, Skinner's conceptualization led to the former (Type S) being referred to as respondent conditioning and the latter (Type R) operant conditioning.

There were, however, some areas of overlap between both types of conditioning. A pseudotype of conditioning may appear when operant behavior is induced in the presence of a particular stimulus. This behavior is referred to as a "discriminated operant." The usual circumstances are that the stimulus serves as a cue for reinforcing consequences that are likely to follow, and which increase the probability of a response. In this case, the operant response is stimulus correlated. Similarly, behaviors that may begin as respondents may also become operants. For example, a child's cry may shift from being a respondent behavior to one which generates consequences.

Skinner's analysis of operant conditioning shifted the emphasis and conceptual foundations of learning research. There was a move away from speculation about the physiological processes involved in conditioning (such as those advanced by Pavlov) and a move toward identifying lawful relationships between behavior and the environment. It also led to a research methodology that involved intensive study of individual subjects and frequency-of-response measurement which, in turn, has profoundly influenced the methods of investigating human behavior.

Operant-Conditioning Principles

The basic principles of operant conditioning and variables that contribute to operant performance were largely extracted from Skinner's research on animal behavior (Skinner, 1956). They are also principles and variables that have formed the framework for behavior modification techniques, and are used extensively in behavior therapy practices with human problem behaviors. These basic principles are as follows:

Reinforcement.

Any increase in the frequency of occurrence of a response that is immediately followed by certain consequences is referred to as reinforcement. The consequential event in this case is referred to as a reinforcer. Such reinforcers may be both positive and negative. A positive reinforcer is an event presented after a response which increases its frequency. A negative reinforcer is an event which, when removed after a response, also increases the frequency of that response. Like all the principles that follow, the events are defined solely by the effects they produce on behavior, and can only be identified by investigating the relationship between behavior and environmental events. Thus positive reinforcement describes an increase in the frequency of a response which is followed by a positive reinforcer, and negative reinforcement describes an increse in the frequency of a response which is followed by a negative reinforcer.

Punishment.

This term is still occasionally misunderstood in this context because common usage connotes the employment of aversive or painful stimuli. In the context of operant conditioning principles, however, it has a somewhat broader meaning; it describes the presentation or removal of an event contingent on a response which decreases the frequency of that response. Like reinforcement, there are positive and negative events that will decrease the frequency of the response they follow—except that their effects are reversed. The presentation of an event contingent on a response, which also decreases the frequency of that response, defines the event as a punisher. The event may be aversive in that it produces unconditioned respondent behaviors. Such events could be shock or loud noise. But it may also be nonaversive, or not produce unconditioned resondent behavior. The withdrawal of an event contingent on a response may also decrease the frequency of a response. This usually designates the event as a positive stimulus condition. The principle is referred to as "time-out from reinforcement" if the positive event is withdrawn for a specific period of time.

Extinction.

This refers to the cessation of delivery of a reinforcer after a response. The effect of this operation is to decrease the frequency of a response, or produce effects which resemble punishment. But it differs from punishment in that the event no longer follows the response.

Stimulus Control.

A response may have punishing or reinforcing consequences in the presence of other stimuli or antecedent events. Thus, a response may produce a positive or negative event in the presence of one stimulus or situation, but not in the presence of other situations. In these circumstances, the response may come under the control of different stimuli or situations. Thus, the stimuli previously associated with reinforcement or punishment will increase the probability that the organism has made a *discrimination* and the response is under *stimulus control.* Stimuli which achieve the same effects as the reinforcer or punisher are termed S^0 or discriminative stimuli. These stimuli may be positive or negative events. Custom has determined that an S^0 is referred to as an S+ stimulus or positive stimulus, while an SΔ or S- stimulus produces a reverse or negative stimulus effect. The stimulus conditions alter the frequency of the response according to the different contingencies with which these stimuli are associated.

Schedules of Reinforcement.

These are the rule systems that are used for delivering reinforcing or discriminative stimuli. There is no reason why these rules might not also apply to punishing stimuli, but they are usually related to procedures that sustain a response at a higher frequency than that which preceded the introduction of the contingency schedule. The most commonly studied schedules are those involving the delivery of events contingent upon the number of responses and the time interval between responses. These schedules are also based on fixed or variable numbers of responses, or time intervals, before the consequence is delivered. Other schedules may be time-dependent, rather than response-dependent. Extremely complex schedules, which combine both response and time patterns for the delivery of consequences, have been used mainly in animal research, in order to sustain a variety of responses. Increasingly, they are being investigated for their relevance to the maintenance of behavior change in humans.

Secondary Principles.

In addition to the primary principles, there are some important derived principles. These include conditioned reinforcement, shaping, chaining, generalizaton, and the Premack Principle.

Conditioned reinforcement may occur when previously nonreinforcing (or even nonpunishing) stimuli are paired with reinforcing stimuli. Low frequency or nonoccurring responses may also be shaped to a target response. In a related way, a sequence of responses may be systematically linked by a schedule of reinforcement. This may ultimately produce a chain of responses, or what might be termed, a new operant response class. The generalization of conditioned responses or response frequency refers to the maintenance of the response in the absence of scheduled contingent stimuli. The procedures used to produce generalization in human behavior have become more complex in recent years (Stokes & Baer, 1977), and will be considered in more detail in a later chapter. For the purpose of this summary, it is worth noting that two broad principles have been used in generalization; training a response that will come under the control of naturally occurring contingencies, and the systematic fading of the rate of delivery of contingent stimuli. The Premack Principle refers to the discovery by David Premack (1959) that the probability of occurrence of a low frequency response may be increased by arranging a high frequency response to be contingent on the low frequency response. The circumstances under which the Premack Principle may operate, particularly with humans, have become a source of debate (Knapp, 1976). In some respects, this debate testifies to the complex relationships that have been discovered in relating antecedent and consequent events to behavior change.

The starting point for many of the complexities of operant conditioning begins with the problem of defining operant behavior. In considering this issue, Schick (1971) concluded that the term "operant" refers to a class of behaviors related to a consequential event(s). This reponse class must contain members that possess the property upon which reinforcement may be contingent. But, as Schick noted, the difficulty with this approach towards finding a definition is that operant behaviors are also measured in the absence of consequential events; for example, during extinction or before contingencies are introduced. Also, the vulnerability of operant behavior—and the principles of operant analysis—to circular definition has never been entirely removed. The paradox of describing events in terms of their effects is usually resolved by referring to the replicability of the operations that produce changes in response frequency. In other word, in the final analysis, operant behavior is a classifiable set of empirical operations that relate a response and a contingent event, and increase the probability of occurrence of the response.

There are numerous other complex functional arrangements of behavior and consequential events which show that the previously mentioned principles are far from simple. The history of the organism, in terms of deprivation and previous training, may produce quite unpredictable effects. For instance, aversive stimuli, such as shock, may actually serve to reinforce behavior under some conditions. The magnitude, intensity, and duration of the consequential event may also determine whether it acts as a positive reinforcer or a punishing event. Similarly, there are characteristics of the response which suggest that some are more readily modifiable than others (Dunham, 1977). Also, the rate of responding may have a substantial bearing on the effects of contingent stimulation.

Recently, far more complex aspects of operant conditioning have been revealed through investigations with different animals. The work of Breland and Breland (1961; 1966) showed that, after the successful conditioning of certain response patterns, other seemingly species-specific responses may emerge to compete and interfere with the procurement of reinforcers. This has led to a belief that the relationship between operant behaviors and reinforcing events is far from arbitrary. Teitelbaum (1977), for instance, concluded that there are compelling suggestions "that learned associations between stimuli and physiological states undergo transformations and become less arbitrary as they are tied to sensory and motor systems which develop earlier in ontogeny or recover differentially after brain damage" (p. 24). In other words, the less related the response is to integrated patterns which govern simpler components of human behavior—such as reflexes or instinctive fixed actions—then the more responsive it is to consequential events. This evidence may also have important implications for the investigation of stuttering within an operant conditioning model.

The Experimental Analysis of Behavior

While the development of the principles of operant conditioning introduced an entirely new area of human learning investigation, it was accompanied by an experimental methodology which transcends those principles and has opened a multitude of new avenues for investigating and modifying human behavior. Skinner's methodology became known as the "experimental analysis of behavior" (Skinner, 1956), and stemmed from a rejection of theory-based research and the search for variables that will control the variability of behavior. Skinner regarded theory as a construct to offset inadequate data, or indicative of imperfect control over experimental subject matter:

> When we have achieved a practical control over the organism, theories of behavior lose their point. In representing and managing relevant variables, a conceptual model is useless; we come to grips with behavior itself. When behavior shows order and consistency, we are much less likely to be

> concerned with physiological or mentalistic causes. A datum emerges which takes the place of our theoretical fantasy. In the experimental analysis of behavior we address ourselves to a subject matter which is not only manifestly the behavior of an individual and hence accessible without the usual statistical aids but also "objective" and "actual" without recourse to deductive theorizing (p. 231).

The experimental analysis of behavior involves the systematic manipulation of stimulus and response conditions in order to identify unambiguous functional relationships between behavior and environmental events. The procedures used to establish this relationship require the identification of a response class, the use of frequency or response rate as the experimental datum, and the investigation of the individual organism. It is a methodology which has applicability for procedures involving other than operant-conditioning principles and has contributed much to the widespread use of single-subject experimental designs as a methodology for demonstrating an association between treatment and behavior change (Hersen & Barlow, 1976). The almost standard features of single-subject experimentation are that the subject is run until a steady response-rate pattern is identified, and then a treatment variable is introduced, in order to relate its introduction to any change, or otherwise, in response rate. If the rate decelerates, or accelerates, then the variable is removed, to assess whether the pretreatment rate is retrieved. This usually amounts to a comparison between the response rate in the treatment and nontreatment conditions. The treatment variable may then be reintroduced to determine the replicability of the treatment effect, or used with a negative value to observe whether the response rate shows reversed trend. By this means, a functional relationship between the dependent and independent variables may be systematically established (Sidman, 1960). There now exist numerous variations on this time-series design. But the essence of this form of experimentation is that the subject forms his own control and the generality, or specificity, of the treatment effect, with respect to other subjects, is determined by replication.

Yates (1970; 1975) has pointed out that single-subject research methods were used in cliinical psychology long before Skinner's experimental analysis of behavior began to influence the investigation of human problem behaviors. But there was a dramatic increase in the use of these methods during the 1960s, following repeated demonstrations that the principles of operant conditioning could serve to modify, with therapeutic purpose, a wide variety of problem behaviors (Kazdin, 1978). What emerged was "applied behavior analysis" (Baer, Wolf, & Risley, 1968), in which socially important behaviors were investigated to identify the controlling variables. But of most interest to clinicians was the conceptualization of problem behaviors as response classes, and awareness that the dimensions of a problem and its relationship to therapy objectives could be expressed in terms of the frequency of a response class. When this concept was blended with research designs that could discern the efficacy of a treatment, a fruitful fusion transpired between research practices and clinical practices which has virtually structured behavior therapy practice.

The growth and diversity in applications of the principles of operant conditioning to the treatment of problem behaviors in children and adults has been so great since the middle of the 1960s that the literature almost defies adequate review (Thoresen & Coates, 1978). Procedures derived from these principles have been used in the analysis and treatment of virtually every problem behavior dealt with by clinical psychologists and psychiatrists. It has also had considerable impact on the practices of many other professionals, particularly those concerned with health, education, sport, law enforcement, and, of course, the speech and hearing sciences.

Along with the increased use of operant conditioning principles, there have also been diverse and complex developments in the systems that employ these principles. These developments have taken the methodology for arranging contingencies to alter behavior well beyond those commonly employed in animal research. The developments may be broadly classified into those that employ external controls over the management of contingencies and those that use self-management of consequential events. Perhaps the most extreme development in the area of external contingency management has been the use of conditioned reinforcers in the context of a token economy (Kazdin & Bootzin, 1972). This has not only extended the possibilities of contingency management, but has led to the identification of a relationship between the laws governing token economies and economic theory (Winkler, 1971). The investigation of self-managed contingency arrangements has also widened the avenues of therapy practice. Virtually all of the principles of operant conditioning, including developments such as token reinforcement, have been used in a self-management context. Moreover, through the investigation of covert operants (coverants), modeling, and self-evaluation methods, other more complex systems of behavior management have emerged in the field of behavior therapy (Thoresen & Mahoney, 1974).

The apparent external and internal validity of these principles in the analysis and modification of behavior has not occurred without challenge. The most telling challenge to the wider advocacy of operant analysis of behavior stemmed from Skinner's attempts to investigate language behavior. Chomsky's (1959) now-famous critical review of Skinner's *Verbal Behavior* (1957), particularly with respect to Skinner's conceptualization of the development of grammatical structure, signaled the revival of cognitive model explanations for behavior change. The most visible extension of this alternative conceptualization has been cognitive therapy (Mahoney, 1974). It is interesting to observe, though, that some of these therapy practices bear a strong resemblance to the self-management techniques. But the most substantive challenges have related to the ethics of certain therapy practices (Yates, 1975), its lack of explanatory value for some problem behaviors (Eysenck, 1979), and, more significantly, the efficacy of the procedures in achieving long-term changes in behavior—especially changes that are greater than those achieved by nonbehaviorally based procedures (Kazdin & Wilson, 1978). This last-mentioned challenge has been partly met by experimental investigations of a growing "technology of generalization" (Stokes & Baer, 1977). Nevertheless, it remains the Achilles heel of many endeavors to translate the principles of operant conditioning into effective therapies for problem behaviors.

Response-Contingent Stimulation Experimentation with Stuttering

Investigations using the principles of operant conditioning, or operant methodology, with stuttering behavior had both relatively informal and formal beginnings. Before the appearance of experimental studies couched in the format of experimental analysis of behavior, there were some that did measure the effects of arranging consequential events on stuttering, but for other reasons. At least three that were reported in the speech pathology literature contain information which is pertinent to the response-contingent stimulation (RCS) research and findings obtained by later researchers.

The first of the "informal studies" was reported by Fahmy (1950), and was conducted to determine the therapeutic results of negative practice (Dunlap, 1932). The eight adult stutterers in this study were described as mainly "tonoclonic" or "tonic" stutterers, and were treated for short intervals by a procedure which required stuttering be imitated at least three times immediately after it occurred during oral reading or talking on a topic. If the same error occurred when the subject next attempted that word, then his negative practice was repeated. An oral reading task, scheduled over at least eight weeks, revealed that four "tono-clonic" subjects improved, and four described as mainly "pure tonus" tended to regress. Although the data from this study did not relate directly to the procedure, they did suggest that its effects may differ widely within any group of stutterers.

Sheehan's (1951) investigation of the effects of "nonreinforcement" of stuttering also required subjects to immediately repeat the stuttered word. He had 20 adult stutterers (18-25 years) orally reread a passage, during which they had to repeat a stuttered word until it was said fluently. The frequency of stuttering throughout these readings was compared with a controlled repeated reading of another passage. Since this data produced an "adaptation effect," the conclusions had to be drawn from comparisons between stuttering frequencies on each reading occasion. These show the experimental condition was associated with less stuttering than the control, although inspection reveals these differences were significant on only two of the six reading occasions.

Wingate (1959) compared two contingency schedules within an oral-reading task with 18 stutterers (15-39 years). In one condition, the subject was interrupted each time he began to stutter and was not permitted to continue until the word was said fluently. In the other experimental condition, the subject was "told to speak as fluently as possible," but was "reminded" by a counter which registered each stuttering. Both experimental conditions were compared with a repeated reading control condition. The group data show that both experimental conditions produced indistinguishably low levels of stuttering that were significantly lower than those found in the control condition. Unhappily, the findings from this study are difficult to interpret. This is mainly because in the second experimental condition it was not possible to identify effects attributable to the instructions or the counter, and because the experimental readings always followed the control reading. The data are also revealing, however, because of obvious individual differences; when the graphed data for all 18 subjects are inspected (see 1959, p. 330), at least seven subjects failed to display evident differences among stuttering frequencies from any of the reading conditions.

Although these "informal RCS studies" did not involve the systematic investigation of individual subjects, they did provide a data pattern which foreshadows the findings in many of the formal studies. They suggested that the effect of arranging a consequential event (albeit the subject's verbal response) or perhaps inducing attention to stuttering may cause it to be reduced. They also indicated that these procedures may be associated with marked individual differences.

The Initial Studies

The first formal investigation of the effects of RCS on stuttering behavior within an experimental analysis of behavior design was reported by Flanagan, Goldiamond, and Azrin, in 1958. Following an investigation by Azrin (1958), which demonstrated the punishing effects of response-contingent loud noise on behavior, a related method was applied during the oral reading of three male stutterers (15, 22, and 37 years). This study's methodology incorporates most of the essential ingredients for investigating response-contingent control of behavior. Each subject was run individually through two sequences of experimental conditions, commonly referred to as an ABA single-subject design. In the A, or base rate condition, the subject orally read (a continuous passage) until "a curve of stuttering frequency considered smooth was obtained." These data were collected "on-line," and analyzed from their cumulative frequency trends. The minimum speaking time for a subject in any base rate condition was a little over 20 minutes. Then, in one experimental run, the subject orally read for 30 minutes in a B (treatment) condition, with a one-second burst of 6000Hz 105dB white noise delivered immediately after each stuttering. In the next 30 minutes of oral reading, the A (extinction) condition, was reintroduced (that is, noise was removed). In a second ABA experimental run, the same conditions applied, except that in the B condition the white noise condition was arranged to shutoff for five seconds immediately after a stuttering. For all subjects, the trend of stuttering frequency during the first experimental run declined during the B, or aversive stimulation condition, compared with the first A condition. Stuttering showed an immediate increase in frequency during the extinction phase. In the second experiment, the B, or escape, condition was reported to increase stuttering frequency. When the data trends for at least two subjects are inspected (Flanagan et al., 1958, p. 174), the effect is quite ambiguous, however. To some extent, this ambiguity may be attributed to the cumulative data display which was commonly used in this type of research. It is a procedure which does not always lend itself to clear definition of differences between the frequencies of behavior in A and B conditions. (For this reason it has been largely replaced by graphs which permit easier data retrieval and frequency comparisons.) Nevertheless, Flanagan and colleagues' (1958) data for the avoidance experiment do show that at least one subject's stuttering decreased to about zero during the B conditions, and his oral reading rate (expressed in pages read per minute) indicated that the treatment effect was not confounded by a reduced speaking rate.

A year later, Flanagan, Goldiamond, and Azrin (1959) reported a similar study with four normally fluent speakers, except that electric shock was used during B condition and only the escape condition (10 shocks per second, shut off for 10 seconds contingent on stuttering) was investigated. "Stuttering" by these subjects was defined as "any hesitation, stoppage, repetition or prolongation in the rhythmic form of vocal behavior" (1959, p. 980). The results showed that stuttering increased during the B condition for two subjects, although for one subject it decreased very slowly during the extinction condition. The third subject failed to respond initially, but when the B condition was modified so that shock was occasionally presented when a light was extinguished for 10 seconds contingent on stuttering, his response pattern was also consistent with a treatment effect. The fourth subject failed to respond to the procedure. Both of the Flanagan et al. studies signalled the possibility that stuttering behavior might be profitably regarded as operant behavior. For some researchers this was evident because it could be shown to decrease when a stimulus condition was made contingent on its appearance and then increase when it served to shutoff a punishing stimulus. To some extent this view point was aided by Felty's (1959) unpublished successful replication of the Flanagan et al. (1958) experiment (see Bijou & Baer, 1966, p. 749-51). This included "children as young as 12 years" who stuttered. But it received the most positive expression in Goldiamond's (1965) account of experimental manipulation of stuttering by contingent delayed auditory feedback.

Goldiamond's research program began in the late 1950s and was largely organized around single-subject experimental designs that involved the systematic investigation of the effects of escape and avoidance conditions with DAF. In the initial study (Goldiamond, 1962), four adult stutterers orally read until a stable frequency of stuttering, as measured by both the experimenter and subject, was identified. Thereafter, the contingencies were attached to the subject's definition of stuttering (Goldiamond, 1965, p. 116). During the aversive condition, the data trend led to the conclusion that DAF functioned as a punishing stimulus, just as noise or shock had in the Flanagan et al. studies. When the escape conditions were introduced in later sessions (DAF was shut off for 10 seconds contingent on stuttering), some subjects reduced (rather than increased) their stutterings. This led Goldiamond to conclude that the escape conditions permitted the introduction of a new speech pattern which he elected to term "prolonged speech."

In subsequent studies on this DAF escape schedule, Goldiamond (1965) also investigated the prolonged speech pattern within an operant methodology framework. The results of these investigations will be reviewed in the next chapter. Suffice to say, at this point, that the findings from these initial studies were not expected within this response-contingent experimental strategy. Nevertheless, it was a finding which, as we shall see, led directly to one of the most influential therapy procedures found in stuttering and served to renew interest in the role of phonatory activity in stuttering. It also sparked interest in the possible role played by other forms of vocal behavior during response-contingent treatment procedures.

Before leaving Goldiamond's early work on RCS, it is worth mentioning that the procedure used in his studies is actually the first recorded use of a self-managed response-contingent schedule with stutterers. The literature on RCS research with stuttering appears to have inadequately recognized that Goldiamond's procedure involved subject-controlled, rather than experimenter-controlled, delivery of contingent events. Moreover, in establishing the base rate for subjects, the self-definition procedure also provided an opportunity to examine the effect of this self-recording process on stuttering. Interestingly, these data did show the procedure produced a transient reduction in one subject's stuttering, a finding which has special relevance to later RCS studies.

During the early 1960s, another research program for investigating RCS procedures with stutterers (and normally fluent speakers) was initiated at the University of Minnesota under the direction of Martin and Siegel. This has been far and away the most consistently productive program of research into the principles of experimental analysis of behavior with stuttering. The initial investigations were designed to explore the effects of various stimuli made contingent on stuttering. But these investigations had other purposes. For example, they were designed to investigate the effect of procedures generally thought to have negative effects on stuttering (Johnson, 1967; Van Riper, 1937). There was also particular interest in the effects of RCS on specific stuttering behaviors during spontaneous speech (rather than oral reading) and whether neutral stimuli gain punishing properties after being paired with response-contingent stimuli.

Martin and Siegel (1966a) first investigated the effects of response-contingent shock on stuttering behavior with three adult stutterers. In one subject "nose wrinkling" and "uh-uh-uh" were monitored. Initially, shock was made contingent on "nose wrinkling," and decreased from around 24-25 times per two minutes down to near zero. Subsequently, the electrodes alone were found to decrease stuttering, but the "uh-uh-uh" response remained unaffected until shock was also made contingent on this behavior. Then, it, too, was dramatically reduced to almost zero. In a latter session, electrode attachment was found to produce essentially the same effect as response-contingent shock. In another subject, tongue protrusion and /s/ prolongation responses were target behaviors. After response-contingent shock was demonstrated to reduce the subject's tongue-protrusion response to near zero, a nylon wrist strap was paired with the shock condition. And in later sessions, the wrist strap alone was shown to reduce this response. The /s/ prolongation was demonstrated to be unaffected by these treatment procedures until it, too, was treated by shock. Finally, a third subject's "moments of stuttering" were found to reduce from around five or six per two minutes to near zero when shock was made contingent on this response. In later sessions, a blue light, previously paired with the shock condition, was found to behave as a discriminative stimulus. It is noteworthy, however, that when the blue light condition was run for one final session, stuttering eventually returned to base rate levels. The word-output rate for two of the subjects remained generally unchanged, and increased during the treatment condition for the other subject. The findings of this study clearly replicated part of those obtained by Flanagan et all. (1958), and showed that certain stuttering behaviors could be manipulated independently and brought under stimulus control.

In another early study from Minnesota, Martin and Siegel (1966b) investigated the effect of arranging verbal consequences on stuttering and intervals of fluency during oral reading. Two stutterers (19 and 21 years) were run individually in conditions where "not good" was presented contingent on stuttering and "good" contingent on 30 seconds of fluency. For both subjects, moments of stuttering were reduced to near zero during the treatment conditions, but returned close to base-rate frequency in the nontreatment conditions. In a subsequent session, a wrist strap was attached during the treatment condition and then, in a later session, tested for its discriminative stimulus properties. For both subjects, the strap alone was shown to produce substantial treatment effects, even when the subjects orally read to other listeners or over a telephone. It was stated that the subject's oral-reading rates did not change in any systematic way throughout the experiment.

One recurring criticism of the Martin and Siegel (1966b) study is that the treatments were confounded by the experimenter's instructions preceding all treatment conditions: "Now I want you to read very carefully. Don't worry about keeping the sentence going, just say each word fluently." To some extent this effect was controlled by showing, in one session, that when instructions were presented alone (that is, as a treatment), there was a transient and less substantial reduction than was found with all other treatment conditions. But there were other problems. One quite significant design flaw was their failure to demonstrate that the wrist strap was indeed "neutral" before it was paired with treatment conditions. The experimenters also failed to identify the separate or conjoint effects of the two response-contingent stimuli. Nevertheless, the study did suggest that response-contingent verbal stimuli, rather than ostensibly noxious stimuli, such as loud noise or shock, might also behave as punishing stimuli.

The punishing effects of a verbal stimulus were demonstrated more clearly in a study by Quist and Martin (1967). Three adult subjects spoke spontaneously in sessions where the verbal stimulus "wrong" was delivered contingent on either a moment of stuttering or specific stuttering behaviors. An interesting feature of this study is that it incorporated criteria for base-rate and treatment measurement which predetermined aspects of the experimental procedure. For example, subjects were run in repeated experimental sessions in which extinction conditions were introduced to the session only if the subject's base-rate stuttering frequency decreased by more than 50% during treatment conditions. Across repeated sessions, the subject's frequency of moments of stuttering, and another's prolonged nasal "n-n-n," were reduced by 30-40% in treatment conditions. In the other subject, the stuttering response was an "inappropriate 'uh' " which almost ceased during treatment conditions (compared to between 10 and 11 every two minutes during base rate). The word-output rate for two of these subjects appeared to either increase or decrease very slowly during treatment conditions.

In 1968, Martin reviewed the preceding research and provided some interesting additional data. These data indicate that while the treatment procedures almost always produced quite substantial reductions in stuttering (at least for some subjects), such effects were not always reliable over time. For example, one subject (Martin, 1968, p. 337-39) was run in conditions where the verbal stimulus "good" was made contingent on 15 seconds of stutter-free spontaneous speech. In an initial experimental session, the contingency produced a 20% decrease in stuttering, but in subsequent sessions the treatment effect diminished completely. Then the treatment condition was changed to "wrong" contingent on a moment of stuttering, and the subject almost ceased stuttering during that and a following session. Once again, the treatment condition was associated with increased word output. The point of interest in this finding is that it not only alludes to variability among subjects, but also highlights a procedure that has been overlooked in many RCS studies—the investigative process necessary to identify a functional relationship between a contingency and stuttering. At the same time, Martin's report testifies to the strict empiricism which has characterized this research, and the guarded conclusions drawn from its contentious findings.

One other early RCS investigation failed to produce findings as decisive as those reported above. Daly and Cooper (1967) arranged for 18 stutterers (18-32 years) to orally read passages five consecutive times under three different conditions: shock contingent on stuttering, shock delivered "as soon as the investigator perceived the initiation of a moment of stuttering" (1967, p. 50), and when the subject was wired to receive shock but it was not delivered. The group data show percentages of stuttering were reduced from one reading to the next in all conditions, but there was no significant difference between the mean scores in each condition—even though there appeared to be less stuttering in the experimental conditions than in the control condition. The findings from this study are difficult to evaluate fully because of some methodological difficulties. One is the absence of data indicating that shock was presented differently in the two experimental conditions, but the main difficulty is caused by the experimental design. In this regard, Martin and Ingham (1973) noted:

> The experimental procedure employed by Daly and Cooper poses a problem that has plagued research in stuttering for years. When subjects read a given passage five times in control and five times in experimental conditions, it generally happens that stuttering frequency decreases with each reading even if no treatment is introduced. Treatment effects can be "teased out" of such a design only by observing variations in adaptation corresponding to introduction and cessation of treatments. However, the data from such a design always are confounded by the so-called "adaptation effect" and by the possible interaction of this effect with the treatment effect (p. 95-96).

The general findings from these early RCS studies were mainly positive and decisive. They showed that when various stimuli, previously thought to aggravate stuttering, were arranged as contingencies, they could substantially reduce or eliminate stuttering during oral reading or spontaneous speech.

Challenges to the Initial Studies

The challenge that these early studies offered prevailing theoretical and clinical approaches to stuttering during the early 1960s was quite profound. Some of the flavor of this challenge can be easily gleaned from the writings of Van Riper (1971; 1973) and Sheehan (1970). The most contentious element in these studies was that, to some, they suggested that stuttering could be treated by punishing with noxious stimuli, such as shock or loud noise. This provoked objections from both an ethical and conceptual viewpoint. The former objections were put forcibly by a number of clinicians and theorists and are well summarized by the above-mentioned writers. They certainly raised some concerns that had to be dealt with before these procedures could find their way to therapy settings.

The conceptual objections related to existing research findings. The notion that stuttering could improve during punishment had been regarded generally as contraindicated by findings from research by Van Riper (1937) and Frick (1951). It will be recalled from Chapter 6 that Van Riper (1937) had observed a deleterious effect when shock was threatened for stuttering during adaptation conditions. The group's data had shown increased stuttering when shock was threatened (to occur at the end of a passage) for stuttering during the course of that reading. Even more stuttering was reported when the threat was for the same number of shocks as stutterings. Nevertheless, the procedure in this study was not essentially response-contingent, since the stimulus was not arranged to immediately follow the response. Furthermore, at least one other related study[1] found that threatened shock produced variable effects. Toomey and Sidman (1970), as previously mentioned, found that when shock was not only threatened but actually delivered after oral reading, two subjects decreased their stutterings, another increased stutterings, and the fourth subject's stuttering remained unchanged. By contrast, Frick's (1951) unpublished doctoral dissertation described a study in which shock had been made contingent on stuttering during oral reading, but did not alter its frequency. Though, as Siegel (1970) observed, one reason for this "may have been because the stutterers were required to read single words and, as might be expected, there were very few instances of stuttering in the first place" (p. 680). But these were relatively minor challenges to the generality of the results of the early RCS studies.

At least four studies appeared during the late 1960s and early 1970s that posed more substantial questions about the generality of the effects of RCS procedures and the relevance of their findings to operant conditioning. The first appears to have been quite overlooked among reviews of response-contingent studies. This

[1] Bloodstein (1981, p. 272) has referred to others.

was a study by Murray (1969) on the effects of masking on stuttering. In two (of four) conditions, 30 stutterers (14-59) orally read a 300-word passage, while one second of white noise (loud enough in a continuous-noise condition to prevent the subject hearing his own voice) was delievered by the subject or the experimenter "after he [the subject] commenced a moment, and during that moment, of stuttering" (p.110). The mean number of moments of stuttering during these conditions was reported not significantly less than that observed during a control reading. However, the mean scores in these two experimental conditions were still numerically lower than in the control condition. (This was also true with respect to the measured length of moments of stuttering.)

The findings of the Flanagan, Goldiamond, and Azrin (1958) study were also subjected to two other challenges. The first came in the form of a comment on the study's methodology by Brutten and Shoemaker (1967). In the course of reviewing studies using RCS with stuttering, they made the following comment on the Flanagan et al. study: "we have chosen not to discuss these findings because of methodological difficulties that were brought to our attention and because Biggs and Sheehan. . .were unable to substantiate these findings in an attempted replication of this study." (p. 26). The source or form of those "methodological difficulties" has never been revealed to evaluate their challenge, but the Biggs and Sheehan study is available for consideration.

Biggs and Sheehan (1969) assessed the effects of a partial replication of the Flanagan et al. (1958) study by comparing three different methods of delivering a 4000Hz tone at 108dB.[2] They had six stutterers (18-20 years) orally reread three different passages throughout three conditions: base line, conditioning, and extinction. The reading interval averaged about 15 minutes during base line and was always 20 minutes in the conditioning and extinction conditions. Each subject completed, in random order, three different experimental runs. The conditioning period was either a one-second tone contingent on stuttering, cessation of continuous tone contingent on stuttering, or random delivery of tone (duration and frequency were not described). The data was subjected to an analysis of variance and presented along with mean-stuttering frequency scores for each subject in each condition. The group data show that stuttering decreased in all these conditions, and there were no significant differences between conditions. The authors concluded that because the data trend in all conditions was similar, the most expedient explanation for the findings was that the tone functioned as a distraction rather than as a response-contingent punishing stimulus.

The Biggs and Sheehan study stood as a serious challenge to the Flanagan et al. study (indeed to the findings of all the early response-contingent studies) and posed questions about the methodology employed in this type of research. But the findings were also flawed by a methodological error in their design. When the individual data are considered, there are 18 experimental runs (six subjects x three experimental runs). In 14 of the 18, the mean-stuttering frequency de-

[2] The 4000 Hz signal was preferred to the 6000 Hz signal, which was used by Flanagan et al. (1958) in order to avoid potential hearing damage.

creased from the base line to conditioning and, then again, from conditioning to extinction intervals. It is a data trend consistent with an effect that might have been obtained had the subjects simply orally reread for the same length of time with no tone present.[3]

The third study of interest was reported by Hegde (1971) in the Indian speech pathology literature. This described the results from five adult stutterers (18-23 years) who orally read during the presence and absence of shock contingent on stuttering. The summarized data from both conditions revealed that without shock 1532 words were stuttered, but during response-contingent shock 1992 words were stuttered, and the pattern was consistent across all five subjects. These data also appear to question the generality of findings such as those reported by Martin and Siegel (1966a). But, on closer examination, there are also important methodological weaknesses in Hegde's study. To begin with, the data were collected only by the experimenter, without audio-recording assistance, and in less than desirable circumstances. For example, the experimenter alone had to count the stutterings and deliver the response-contingent shock (during treatment sessions). Furthermore, the reliability of these data were not estimated, and no record was provided on the number of words actually read. This means it is quite possible that had percentage-of-words-stuttered scores been estimated, they may have yielded a different data trend.

Finally, a study by Cooper, Cady, and Robbins (1970) emerged as yet another interesting challenge to the generality and meaning of the results obtained by some of the Minnesota studies. They had 14 stutterers (15-23 years) and 14 nonstutterers (18-45 years) orally read a passage across three counterbalanced 21-minute experimental sequences. Each sequence involved an ABA experiment in which the two seven-minute A conditions were stimulus-free and the seven-minute B condition involved delivery of the verbal stimulus "wrong," "right," or "tree" contingent on each disfluency. The stuttering group's data showed that all three B conditions produced a significant reduction in disfluencies, when compared with the A conditions. But there was no significant difference between the A conditions or between the B conditions. (The nonstuttering group's data failed to indicate a significant treatment effect; there were no significant differences between the A and B conditions).

To a certain extent, the Cooper et al. (1970) findings simply indicated that the presumed affective content of the verbal-contingent stimulus may not be a significant factor in the changes in stuttering rate reported in RCS studies. And from one viewpoint, their data merely replicated a trend suggested by studies that had arranged a stimulus event to be contingent on stuttering. On the other hand, they also appeared to challenge a traditional learning-theory explanation, such as might be derived from the Law of Effect, wherein a positive stimulus event would be expected to increase certain types of behavior. But the individual

[3]The effects obtained in this study may also be closely related to those produced under masking conditions. As noted in Chapter 7, the effect of variable masking on stuttering has yet to be clearly identified. Consequently, it is entirely possible that variable masking may actually produce effects on stuttering that are similar to those found in continuous and random noise conditions.

subject data, presented by Cooper, et al., also showed considerable variability. For instance, if their stuttering subjects' disfluency counts are considered with respect to the reported "treatment effect" (that is, a decrease in stuttering from the first A condition to the B condition, and an increase from the B condition to the final A condition), then only five of the 14 produced the group's data pattern across the three experimental runs.

The "early challenge" certainly raised some questions about the generality and the conclusions that could be drawn from the initial RCS studies. Perhaps the most interesting of these related to methodology. For instance, they highlighted a need for control procedures that could provide a clearer definition of any functional relationship between a stimulus condition and stuttering. But the differences between these "challenge" studies and the initial RCS studies were largely methodological. Whereas the latter were characterized by experimental analysis of behavior methodology, or the systematic investigation of individual subject data, the "challenge" studies, for the most part, used average scores from across groups and across conditions. It was a difference that quickly evaporated in later investigations.

The suggested distinction between the early and later RCS studies is, of course, quite artificial, and is made only to provide some sense of the historical developments in this research. That is difficult to retain when considering the diverse investigations that began during the next decade. They are more easily reviewed by organizing them according to their principal stimulus procedures. We shall then return to "history" to review issues that have arisen from these studies in more recent evaluations of RCS research.

Punishment of Stuttering

Investigations on the effects of non-noxious stimuli in response-contingent research were continued at the University of Minnesota, where the first studies were conducted on the effects of time-out from speaking or stuttering. Time-out from positive reinforcement already had a well-founded history as a procedure which produces punishing effects on animal and human behavior, although its aversive properties were less clear (Leitenberg, 1965). But, as a consequential event on stuttering, it appeared to carry the most neutral properties of all response-contingent stimuli.

The first of the time-out studies was reported by Haroldson, Martin, and Starr (1968). They arranged for four adult stutterers to speak spontaneously throughout a single-subject ABAB experimental procedure involving 15 one-hour sessions (each separated by at least one day). During the B conditions, the subject was treated by response-contingent time-out (he was instructed to stop speaking immediately when a red light was illuminated, and to remain silent until it was extinguished 10 seconds later) which was not present during A conditions. However, unlike previous Minnesota studies, the A and B intervals were predetermined. The first A condition involved two sessions, followed by four sessions in which B conditions were presented for the first 40 minutes and then by 20 minutes of A conditions. Thereafter the subjects received four B sessions and two A sessions. The mean percentage of words stuttered in these conditions showed that most B conditions contained less stuttering than their preceding A condition. A "step-wise reduction" in stuttering was also evident over the three A phases. These trends were common to the four subjects, and thereby revealed less evidence of extinction than was found in studies which used either verbal stimuli or shock as a contingency. It was also reported (Haroldson et al., 1968, p. 565) that, before and after the experiment, three subjects had not changed stuttering when the 10-second light alone (that is, no time-out) was contingent on stuttering, although no data accompanied this additional information.

A subsequent study by Martin and Haroldson (1969) revealed that the suggested "carryover effects" of time-out on stuttering were not particularly durable. They compared the performance of two groups of 10 stutterers (18 years and older) across eight 50-minute once weekly treatment sessions. The subjects in one group were treated individually by Haroldson, Martin, and Starr's (1968) procedure, while the other group's members received equivalent periods of "Information-Attitude" therapy (the clinician discussed certain aspects of stuttering, including the role of anticipation and avoidance). In addition, each subject was assessed one week before and after the eight-week treatment period. The mean percentage of words stuttered for both groups over the course of treatment was strikingly different. The "information-attitude" group showed no evidence of any systematic change either during treatment or between the pre- and posttreatment sessions. By contrast, the "conditioning," or time-out group, decreased from around 18% to about 5% of words stuttered between the first and eighth treatment sessions. But they also showed no appreciable difference between their pre- and posttreatment assessment session scores. In other words, any treatment effect extinguished almost entirely a week after treatment ceased. One further finding was that the average words spoken during the time-out group's treatment sessions tended to increase, though it failed to reach the level recorded during session one. However, the complicating effects of the time-out interval, when assessing word output in this type of study, are obvious, and (as will be discussed) have become a point of concern in determining the efficacy of this procedure.

A single-subject study by Martin and Berndt (1970) provided further information on the potential clinical benefits of time-out. They reported an ABA-designed study with a 12-year-old boy who orally read for 15 40-minute sessions (the interval between these sessions was not reported). After four base rate sessions, response-contingent time-out was introduced during the next seven sessions and removed for the final four sessions. The mean stutterings (per two minutes) declined from around 25-32, during base rate, to zero by the last time-out session, and only increased slightly over subsequent extinction sessions. By the end of the treatment sessions, the words read per two minutes was virtually the same as base rate, and remained so during extinction sessions.

The preceding studies had strongly suggested that time-out from speaking was an aversive event. Some support for this was provided in Martin and Gaviser's (1971) study on three adult normal speakers. Each was required to talk spontaneously and press buttons which could activate a white light for seven seconds. The subjects were also instructed that whenever a red light appeared they were to cease talking until it extinguished after seven seconds. During these red-light conditions, the rate of button pressing decreased to almost zero for all subjects and then returned to near base rate during the extinction, or white light, conditions.

The aversive effects of time-out were also suggested in a study by Martin and Haroldson (1971) which included two pairs of adult stutterers. In base rate sessions, the subjects first conversed with each other, and were then given a hand switch with instructions to register each stuttering by their partner. In the first treatment session, each hand switch depresson activated 10 seconds of time-out for the partner. In a subsequent treatment phase, the experimenter also delivered time-out. Following extinction sessions, partner-controlled delivery of time-out was then re-introduced. The percentage of words stuttered by all four subjects shows that the initial partner-controlled procedure did not alter the base rate frequency of stuttering. It was also noted, however, that the subject's partners delivered time-out after no more than 2% of stutterings. By contrast, when the experimenter also delivered time-out, the stuttering rates for all subjects moved from between 2 and 20% to virtually zero, and thereafter showed a trend in extinction and treatment sessions consistent with a treatment effect. (The improvement during the final treatment sessions may be related as much to re-introduction of the time-out paraphenalia as to the procedure.) In general terms, therefore, the Martin and Gaviser (1971) and Martin and Haroldson (1971) studies gave some substance to the claim that time-out was an avoidable aversive stimulus.

A study by Adams and Popelka (1971) on the effects of time-out during oral reading also addressed the question of the aversive properties of time-out. They arranged for eight stutterers (18-27 years) to orally reread, five times, two different (but matched) 300-word passages under two conditions. In one, a 10-second 1000Hz tone was used to "time-out" specific types of dysfluencies (sic); "repetition or prolongation of a sound or syllable" (p. 336). In the other condition (preceding or following time-out readings by two to four days), the subject orally read without time-out. Comparisons between each reading, across occasions, showed all time-out readings contained 50% less stuttering than was found in control readings. Nevertheless, as mentioned in connection with the Daly and Cooper (1967) study, it is not clear how these procedures interacted with the adaptation effect. Two other features of this study relate to interesting issues in time-out research. The first concerns the extent of "contingency" in the delivery of time-out. Adams and Popelka reported that between 47% and 100% of stutterings were immediately followed by time-out, though the reliability of these estimates was not provided.[4] This implies that for some subjects the contingency arrangement was not necessarily responsible for the treatment effect. The second issue to emerge from Adams and Popelka's survey of their subjects' reactions to

[4] This is also true with respect to the reliability of the data measures. The peculiar reason for this was stated as follows: "the internal and external reliability of the senior experimenter's judgments of stuttering had been demonstrated to be better than +.85 on three separate occasions during the past year" (Adams & Popelka, 1971, p. 336).

time-out was that six of the eight said "time-out periods afforded them a chance to relax," another said it served as a cue to "strive for a higher level of fluency," but only one said it indicated failure or disapproval.

Some further doubts about the aversive properties of time-out also appeared to be demonstrated in a study by James (1976). He assessed the effect of 1, 5, 10, and 30 seconds of time-out with four experimental groups and a control group, with nine stutterers (15-65 years) in each group. Each subject spoke spontaneously for 10 minutes in a base rate condition and then 20 minutes in either a response-contingent time-out or control condition. (Only the final 10 minutes of this interval were used to compare base rate and treatment/control intervals.[5]) Comparisons between the percentage-of-syllables-stuttered and syllables-spoken-per-minute scores of the experimental groups revealed a significant reduction in stuttering, but no change in speech rate during treatment conditions. There was no significant difference between the treatment groups on both speech measures, and the control group showed no change in these measures over the experimental period. In other words, the magnitude of the time-out interval appeared unrelated to its treatment effect. It was also noteworthy that the reliability with which time-out was administered contingently (no more than one second after a stuttering) produced percentage scores resembling those obtained by Adams and Popelka (1971). In general terms, James's data suggested that time-out may not be an aversive stimulus for stuttering—at least, not in the way that different time-out intervals have been shown to have correlated effects on other response rates (Ferster & Appel, 1961; Zimmerman & Ferster, 1963).

The search for variables that may help explain the time-out effect also led to a consideration of the interaction between the stutterer's expectancy for improved fluency and the introduction of time-out conditions. It is an effect long recognized in other areas of behavioral research (Rosenthal, 1966) as contributing much to treatment variance. One test of this effect is to examine the effect of manipulating treatment instructions. To this end, James and Ingham (1974) conducted a time-out study with 14 male stutterers (15-29 years), using a fixed-duration ABAB experimental design in which the response-contingent time-out conditions were introduced by two different sets of instructions. For half the subjects, the first B condition was preceded by ingestion of a "tranquilizer" (placebo) which, it was stated, would interact with the pauses following each stuttering "to produce immediate reductions in stuttered speech." Before the second B condition, the "tranquilizer" was not taken, and subjects were told that therefore "the severity of your stutter will most likely stay at its usual level" (p. 89). The other group received the instructions in reverse order. The combined data showed that the time-out procedure was completely unaffected by the instructions; both treatment procedures yielded at least 68% reductions in mean-percentage-of-syllables-stuttered scores (relative to nontreatment), with no significant difference between the A conditions or between the B conditions. There was also no

[5]One interesting feature of this study was that the time-out intervals were compensated by adding comparable talking time during the treatment interval.

significant variation in speech rate across the four conditions. Another interesting finding was the failure to replicate Adams and Popelka's (1971) results on subject reactions to time-out: only two of the 14 reported that it helped them to relax, whereas the others were evenly distributed between unpleasant reactions and "time to think."

One recurring characteristic in the time-out studies has been that the treatment effects appeared to be somewhat more substantial and general than those obtained with response-contingent verbal stimuli. This suggestion appeared to receive some support in yet another (group) study by Martin and Haroldson (1979). This previously mentioned study (see Chapter 7) compared a number of treatments, including response-contingent time-out (five seconds) and the verbal stimulus "wrong." The data were derived from comparisons between 20 minutes of spontaneous speech in base rate, and a following 30-minute treatment condition. Twenty adult stutterers were run through these and other treatment conditions, but not before they completed a 20-minute pre-experimental condition (10 minutes of spontaneous speech followed by another 10 minutes of speaking, introduced with instructions "to try very hard not to stutter"). This pre-experimental condition also yielded data germane to the role of instructions on stuttering. And, unlike some suggestions regarding earlier response-contingent studies, there was no significant difference between the percentage of words stuttered in the two 10-minute conditions. With respect to the two response-contingent treatment conditions, there were some interesting similarities and differences. Both treatments produced significant reductions in mean percentage of words stuttered and duration of moments of stuttering. Furthermore, the changes in stuttering in these conditions were also significantly correlated (0.66). However, the "wrong" condition was not associated with changed-word output, while the "time-out" condition did decrease that output (a difference which will be discussed later). In addition, all subjects decreased stuttering during the time-out condition, but this was true for only 60% of subjects during the "wrong" conditions.

Another study by James (1981c) compared the effects of time-out and noise during either contingent or noncontingent stimulus conditions. Thirty-six subjects (16-57 years) were assigned to one of four groups: 10 seconds time-out from speaking contingent on stuttering (CTO), noncontingent 10 seconds time-out from speaking (NTO), 10 seconds tone signal contingent on stuttering, but without cessation of speaking (CTONE), and 10 seconds tone signal not contingent on stuttering, and also without cessation of speaking (NTONE). Percentage of syllables stuttered (%SS) and syllables spoken per minute (SPM), during spontaneous speech, were recorded during a 10-minute base rate and the following 20-minute experimental session (this was extended to a maximum of 40 minutes in CTO and NTO sessions to compensate for time lost to time-out). The data show that only the CTO condition produced a significant reduction in mean %SS scores (46% reduction), and this was accompanied by a significant increase in SPM scores (common to all four conditions). The surprising feature of these data was that the CTONE group did not also significantly reduce stutterings in the experimental conditions. This may be due to an important procedural problem, however; there was no control for the possibility that stutterings might have occurred during the "tone on" interval, thereby precluding delivery of a contingent stimulus. In short, CTONE may have been an intermittent RCS procedure, and certainly not a suitable comparative for CTO and CTONE conditions. A partial post hoc control for this procedural problem was evidence that the percentage of stutterings followed (within one second) by a stimulus was virtually the same in the CTO and CTONE conditions.

The findings from the time-out studies have yielded the most consistently positive data of all the response-contingent procedures (including those yet to be reviewed). The effects produced are remarkable for their consistency across subjects and their age groupings. To some extent, the consistency of the effect has been more adequately demonstrated than have the parameters of its effect, especially with respect to individual subjects. Ironically, the generality of the effect appears to have sustained group or parametric research on this procedure, rather than an experimental analysis of behavior approach. There are also many elements in the effect that need identification in order to establish its clinical utility. Perhaps the most notable is the limited research demonstrating that the contingency arrangement is critical to the time-out effect. The subjective, or qualitative, aversive properties of time-out also remain unclear, though one clue to this issue exists by comparing the findings across the reviewed studies. This reveals some interesting differences between studies that used spontaneous speech and those that used oral reading. For instance, the subjective reports of adverse reactions to time-out occur more often in the spontaneous speech studies. Another aspect of this difference relates to the "instruction to be fluent" effect. It will be recalled that this effect was evident during the oral-reading studies of Martin and Siegel (1966b) and Wingate (1959), but not during the spontaneous speech study of Martin and Haroldson (1979). Martin and Siegel's (1966b) relatively systematic investigation of the association between treatment and instructions suggests, however, that these differences are not too significant. There is, generally, sufficient evidence that instructional control over stuttering is either a weak source of control or, at best, interactive.

Reinforcement of Fluency

The converse of stuttering is, of course, stutter-free speech, so any increase in its frequency would logically result in less frequent stuttering. Thus, by using intervals of stutter-free speech as a response class, some researchers have investigated whether consequential events may reinforce fluency. The extent to which this has been demonstrated by their investigations will be reviewed here.

The first experimental attempt to reinforce stutter-free speech was reported by Martin and Siegel (1966b), but, unfortunately, it did not permit the effects of the reinforcer to be isolated. There was also a brief report by Martin (1968) on the transient effects of "good" contingent on 15 seconds of fluent spontaneous speech. In addition, some early therapy reports by Rickard and Mundy (1965) and Leach (1969) endeavored to reinforce fluency. The earliest RCS experimental study of fluency, which reported positive results, was conducted by Shaw and Shrum (1972).

Shaw and Shrum reported the effects of offering presumed conditioned reinforcement contingent on either fluent intervals or stutterings with three children (9-10 years). Each child spoke spontaneously in four daily 20-minute sessions. After an initial base rate session, the subsequent sessions included (in order) contingencies for fluent intervals, for stutterings and, again, for fluent intervals. The contingency was a mark which contributed to the purchase of a previously selected toy or candy. The total number of fluent intervals in each session (10-second intervals for two children, five seconds for the other) for each child was shown to follow a trend consistent with the contingency acting as a reinforcer. However, this was not as evident with respect to the frequency counts of stuttering: only one child's stuttering clearly increased above base rate when contingencies were offered for stutterings. But the main difficulty in interpreting these data is that all treatment sessions were confounded by instructions to the child on how to speak in each session. The child was told "to talk without stuttering," or with stuttering, but the instructions' effects were not separately identified. In addition, no speech-rate data are reported. These are relatively crucial data for a study in which reduced rate could have increased the number of fluency intervals.[6] The investigators do state, though, that the subjects "appeared to talk more during the conditioning [treatment] sessions" (Shaw & Shrum, 1972, p. 85).

Some of the same concerns apply to a study by Manning, Trutna, and Shaw (1976) with three children (6-9 years). Their design resembled that used by Shaw and Shrum. They combined verbal and tangible contingencies, along with instructions for the children to use either "hard" or "easy" speech during spontaneous speaking.[7] Each subject was run in a 15-minute base rate session, followed by three experimental sessions divided into three 10-minute intervals. In the first experimental session, marks were awarded contingent on individually determined intervals of "easy" speech (2.5 secs. intervals for two subjects and 1.5 secs. for the other). Only marks were given initially, then they accompanied individually selected verbal rewards, and, finally, the marks could earn previously chosen toys, etc. In the second experimental session, the same sequence of contingency arrangements was used with "hard" speech and specifically for stutterings. In the final session, the marks were again contingent on fluent intervals, but the order of contingency conditions was reversed (that is, "marks only" were given in the final interval). In general, the variations of stutterings and fluent intervals appeared to indicate that the verbal and tangible consequences acted as reinforcers (although the "marks only" condition may have

[6] When a time interval of stutter-free speech is used as a response class, the possibility exists that during treatment the subject may offer one or many words during such intervals.

[7] These terms were used by the child's clinician to describe either disfluent or fluent speech during the therapy they were receiving at the time of this study. In other words, the therapy procedures may have interacted with the contingency schedule, even though the experiment was supposed to "tease-out" this effect.

been an equally potent reinforcer for fluent intervals in at least one subject). But this conclusion is difficult to defend. The main difficulty is that the data presentation format does not make it possible to isolate any treatment procedure's effect within a condition. Since only one average score was presented to describe response rate for a treatment, it is impossible to learn whether the data trends changed in concert with treatment conditions. Some speech-rate data are presented for one subject indicating improved fluency was not accompanied by a slowed speech rate, but these data are conspicuously absent for the other subjects. Some "carryover" data are also presented from a 15-minute clinic session two months later, but, since the subjects were receiving therapy during this time, that data is of little interest.

Finally, there is a study by Hegde and Brutten (1977) which used money as a contingency for periods of fluent oral reading by three adult stutterers. All subjects were run through a fixed-duration ABA experimental design involving six 45-minute sessions: two base rate, two "experimental," and two extinction sessions. During all sessions, five-minute frequency counts of fluent periods and disfluencies were collected. In the "experimental" sessions, the subject observed a counter which contingently recorded the fluent units (these were 10-, or 12-sec units) during reading; it thereby provided a cumulative record of earnings. The frequency of fluent periods and disfluencies per session suggest the contingency increased fluent intervals and concomitantly decreased disfluencies. But when the five-minute interval data are carefully inspected, the treatment effect is far from clear. All subjects showed a confusing trend in either their fluent interval or disfluency data across some boundaries between the experimental conditions. In fact, the study illustrates the hazards of not seeking stability in data trends before the experimental condition is either introduced or removed.[8]

Unfortunately, the "reinforcement of fluency" studies have failed to yield "good data" (Sidman, 1960) which indicate that time intervals of stutter-free speech may be a manipulable response class. There is certainly evidence of change in the frequency of this response class in at least two studies (Manning, Trutna, & Shaw, 1976; Shaw & Shrum, 1972), but both rely on data which may have been confounded by substantial instruction effects. Quite obviously, clarifying studies are needed. What does seem rather surprising is that the response class chosen in these studies should be so vulnerable to alterations in speech rate; time periods of fluency, for instance, could support a wide range of stutter-free utterances. On the face of it, there would appear to be much less threat to internal experimental validity if numbers of stutter-free words or syllables were used as a response.

Some of the problems mentioned above were addressed in two other studies which endeavored to disentangle the effects of consequences for nonstuttered

[8] Also, the reliability measures obtained by Hegde and Brutten were surprisingly low. The interobserver reliability correlation coefficients ranged between only 0.69 and 0.81. In the absence of other information on the relationship between these second scores and the original scores (e.g., data trends of both sets of scores), it is quite possible that these correlations might have hidden a further source of ambiguity in the data trends.

speech and for stuttering. The first, by Moore and Ritterman (1973), arranged for 12 stutterers (16-26 years) to read orally in experimental conditions involving response-contingent shock, either following or during stuttering, plus (in one condition) 10 cents contingent on uttering three fluent words. These stimuli were also paired with either a red light for shock or a green light for fluency. Each experimental run involved base rate readings followed by the contingency schedule and, finally, an assessment of the stimulus control properties of the lights alone. The group's data show that each condition produced a mean frequency of stuttering progressively lower across each condition in each of the experimental runs. However, when the data were subjected to an analysis of variance, no significant difference was found within or between any of the experimental or stimulus control conditions, although both contained significantly less stutterings than the base rate conditions. In other words, there was no evidence that the shock-plus-monetary contingency was more effective in reducing stuttering (at least over the prescribed period) than the shock-only contingency. There was also no evidence of a return to base rate in the stimulus control condition, although the experimental design did not permit identification of the effects of using the light-alone stimulus conditions. One interesting finding was that only one subject's data failed to emulate the group's data trend.

The second study was reported by Mowrer (1978) and involved a relatively unusual stimulus delivery condition: verbal contingencies were delivered by an audience listening to a stutterer. Six stutterers (12-38 years) spoke spontaneously before 14 listeners whose reactions were programmed to vary across conditions. The conditions were, in order, (1) audience attentive only; (2) audience said "good" after three fluent words and "stop" after a stuttering; (3) return to condition (1); (4) audience said "stop" after a stuttering; (5) audience said "good after three fluent words; (6) same as condition (2); (7) same as condition (1); (8) subject says "good" after three fluent words and "stop" after a stuttering. Only total-words-stuttered-per-minute and disfluencies-per-minute data for each condition are provided, and they were subjected to an analysis of variance procedure. This showed that all the "treatments" reduced disfluencies, when compared with nontreatment conditions, but there was no significant difference between the treatment procedures. The speech-rate data were reported to be not significantly different between the treatment and nontreatment conditions (although the reported F score is identical to $p=.05$). At first glance, these data appear to suggest that contingencies were equally effective in reducing disfluencies, but the individual data provide a more complex picture. Only two of the six subjects showed a pattern of scores across the experiment which correlated with the conclusions drawn from the group data. And, in the absence of trend data within each of the conditions, absolutely no conclusions can be drawn from the findings of the other four subjects.

It should be clear, at this point, that most of the studies reported since the initial response-contingent studies were published have favored group rather than single-subject designs. In some cases this has yielded information regarding generality of treatment effects, but it has done little to demonstrate whether the stuttering or intervals of fluency in individual subjects definitely respond to reinforcement or punishment procedures. In fact, in the case of studies that have used combined contingencies, the procedure's efficacy is clouded by the inherent weakness of group data. For instance, at present, there are no data which show that any individual's speech behavior has been definitely improved by combining contingencies for stutter-free speech with contingencies for stuttering, or vice versa.

Studies Using Different Response Classes

The previously reviewed studies did introduce one important variation to the response classes used in response-contingent studies; that is, periods, or numbers, of stutter-free utterances. But more radical variations have also been used. These include changes in percentages of stuttering, expectancy to stutter, and language behavior. The findings from this group of studies have much relevance to clinical applications of operant conditioning principles.

A series of group studies by Ingham and Andrews (1973a) were concerned with assessing the clinical effectiveness of a token economy in the treatment of stuttering. In the course of these studies, three groups of stutterers (18-56 years) were run through a series of "rating sessions," in which tokens were delivered immediately after the session contingent on a relative decrease in percentage of syllables stuttered (%SS), or they were withdrawn contingent on an increase in %SS scores. The subjects were hospital patients, and the tokens were used as the means of purchasing all food, drink and luxuries in that setting. In one group (n=12), a comparison was made between noncontingent token consequences (A) and contingent token consequences (B). The A conditions were maintained for eight rating sessions, followed by six B, four A, and three B condition sessions. The group's trend of %SS scores were consistently lower in B, when compared with A conditions. In another study, the same experimental session design was used with eight stutterers, except that the A condition was the contingent-token system used in the first experiment. In B conditions, tokens earned for decreased %SS scores were doubled. Once again, the group data demonstrated that the B condition produced a greater rate of decrease in %SS scores. In the third study, the same design was used with 12 stutterers who spoke initially in the same token-system conditions, except that tokens could be earned but not lost. In the B condition, the token reinforcing and punishing consequences were restored. The findings from this third study were not conclusive: there is some slight suggestion that the B condition showed a treatment effect, but the data trends across conditions are too similar to justify this finding. One general finding across all three experiments was that the syllable-per-minute rate in each of the treatment conditions tended to rise as stuttering decreased. Subsequently, Ingham (1975) analyzed the individual-subject data for each of these studies and reported that four of the 20 stutterers involved in the first two experiments failed to demonstrate changes in stuttering that were consistent with those found in the group data. Nevertheless, the overall findings from this study strongly supported the suggestion that the response class, percentage of syllables stuttered, could be modified, at least within token-economy conditions. (This study, and the related therapy procedure, will be discussed further in Chapter 10). At the same time, it is interesting that this study also failed to demonstrate a benefit from combining essentially punishing and reinforcing consequences.

Another program of research applying operant methodology to stuttering was begun in the mid-1960s by George Shames. His earlier investigations were mainly concerned with determining the effects of manipulating the thematic content of the stutterers' speech behavior. In the main, they investigated the results of arranging clinician-delivered positive verbal responses contingent on statements judged to be clinically desirable, and negative verbal responses contingent on statements judged incompatible with recovery from stuttering.

Some of the clinical findings from Shames's work will be discussed later, but an experimental study by Rhodes, Shames, and Egolf (1971) is described here because of its relevance to RCS procedures. This study used two groups of four adult stutterers, and was designed to measure the effects of "awareness" in verbal conditioning.[9] Each group of subjects was run through 22 40-minute therapy sessions, beginning with one "base rate session" and ending with one "extinction session." One group was told the clinician would paraphrase certain target phrases immediately after they were spoken and then either verbally approve or disapprove of their content. Approval followed "statements deemed desirable" (TR+) and disapproval followed statements "incompatible with recovery" (TR-). The other group was not informed about the contingency schedule. The trend of TR+ and TR- responses for the informed group appeared to either increase or decrease, as hypothesized, throughout the 20 therapy sessions, but this trend was less evident in the "uninformed" group (although the TR- responses decreased during therapy and returned to pretreatment levels in the "extinction session"). By contrast, stuttering showed no clear change in the "informed" group but decreased approximately 50% in the "uninformed group. It is not at all clear what conclusion can be drawn from this study with respect to stuttering. It may simply imply a relationship between language content and stuttering for some subjects—a connection which was considered in later therapy studies (Shames, Egolf, & Rhodes, 1969). At best, the Rhodes et al. study shows that language content may be manipulated by the affective content of contingent verbal stimuli.[10]

One of the most-quoted Johnsonian concepts of stuttering is that the problem is essentially those behaviors that occur to avoid expected stuttering (Johnson, Brown, Curtis, & Keaster, 1948). Thus, if the expectancy to stutter were reduced, then it should follow that stuttering would also be reduced. From this viewpoint, it made sense to assess the effects of RCS on expectancy to stutter, as much as

[9] This study primarily addressed itself to an issue which was relatively controversial in RCS research during the early 1960s; the significance of knowledge about the response/contingency arrangement to operant conditioning. The issue has receded in importance and relevance in the course of later RCS research.

[10] Rhodes et al. (1971) claimed it justified using client-centered therapy with stutterers.

stuttering behavior per se. At least three studies have reported investigating the effects of applying consequences to the expectancy to stutter. Curlee and Perkins (1968) initiated these investigations by measuring the effect of shock on signaled expectancies to stutter. Twelve stutterers (17-36 years) were assigned to three groups: a control, experimental, and yoked group. During a base-rate condition, the experimental group responded to 40 stimulus words with a 5-6 word sentence containing the word. Before saying the sentence, the subject signaled, via a red light, if he expected to stutter. In the treatment condition, the subject illuminated the light if he expected stuttering in the sentence, but received shock on a variable-ratio. However, unless a variably activated green light appeared after the red light signal, the subject did not then speak the sentence. During extinction, the base-rate conditions were repeated. The yoked-control group received shock on a predetermined schedule, and the time-control group completed equivalent sentences with unchanged conditions. Expectancy counts and stuttering-frequency data, collected in the base-rate and treatment conditions for all groups, showed that only the experimental group decreased the expectancies and frequency of stutterings. Their expectancy counts declined by 95%, although stutterings reduced by only 51%. This pointed to some association between the two behaviors but, possibly, less than Johnsonian theory might have suggested.[11]

Daly and Frick (1970) refined Curlee and Perkins's procedure. They had three groups of 12 stutterers (17-42) exposed to ABA conditions while orally reading single words in each condition. During the B condition, one group received shock contingent on every signaled expectancy to stutter, another received shock contingent on stuttering, and the third received shock contingent on both signaled expectancy to stutter and stuttering. The main difficulty in comparing the data from these groups is that, before treatment, the first experimental group had about 50% more expectancy counts than the other groups. Nevertheless, all subjects reduced their expectancy and stuttering counts by virtually identical amounts, with the shock-contingent-on-stuttering and combined-contingency groups showing, apparently, more substantial reductions during the treatment conditions. But group comparisons of subject performance under different conditions make it difficult, if not impossible, to clearly identify the differences between these two contingency schedules on either stuttering or stuttering expectations.

A single-subject experimental design by Harris, Martin, and Haroldson (1971) managed to get somewhat closer to discerning evidence of expectancy control over stuttering. Three adult subjects spoke spontaneously throughout conditions in which stuttering changes determined the scheduling of response-contingent events. After a base-rate was established, the subject signaled whenever he expected to stutter. If this contingency did not reduce stuttering (by 40%), then in subsequent sessions the subject activated 10 seconds time-out from speaking.

[11] These data may also be interpreted as demonstrating stimulus control of "expectancy button pushing" in the extinction condition. There is also at least one other explanation for their findings. When subjects in the experimental group signaled an expectancy to stutter, they were not always allowed to speak the sentence. So, in one sense, they were also exposed to a time-out condition.

Extinction sessions followed either contingency schedule if the criterion reductions in stuttering occurred. The results across subjects were about as variable as is possible. One subject decreased expectancy counts during time-out, but this had no effect on percentage of words stuttered. Another's expectancy counts dramatically reduced his stuttering. However, the third subject's stuttering was reduced during the time-out condition, while his expectancy counts decreased fairly systematically across the two contingency conditions. These data tend to confirm that stuttering expectations may be a manipulable response class, but they also show the variable effect that this may have on stuttering.

Self-Control Studies

It has already been observed that some of the early response-contingent studies were concerned with subject-identified rather than experimenter-identified responses. In fact, as was noted, Goldiamond's (1965) research program was built mainly around subject-identified stutterings, so that the findings from this research should be interpreted as demonstrating the effects of either self-monitoring or self-punishment on stuttering. The data, from at least one stutterer investigated by Goldiamond, demonstrated that when the subject was instructed to signal stutterings they reduced by about 37%, but the reduction was only transient—other subjects showed no such effect.

Attempts to define the characteristics of self-managed behavior have produced some of the most contentious issues in the field of behavior therapy. One of the principal issues boils down to isolating the contribution of external control on self-control in procedures which purport to use only subject-managed contingencies (Jones, Nelson, & Kazdin, 1977; Nelson & Hayes, 1981). Another concerns the relationship between observed measures and the subject's measures. In the case of self-monitoring research, for example, there may be wide differences in monitoring accuracy. This is exceptionally problematic where instructions emphasize recording accuracy, yet the subject is supposed to be free to respond to the instruction to self-monitor. The effect of monitoring accuracy on performance is unclear at present. But, it is clear that considerable differences exist between the self-monitoring methodologies that are employed in many studies. This makes it difficult to decide which variable might have reasonable claim to treatment effects. Some of those difficulties will become apparent in the course of this overview of the use of self-monitoring within stuttering.

Perhaps the most provocative study using self-monitoring of stuttering was LaCroix's (1973) therapy study with an adolescent and adult stutterer. In the case of one stutterer, a 30-minute conversation with the clinician formed a base-rate session, and was followed by 19 sessions in which he was instructed to count each "disfluency" on a hand-held digital counter. This permitted the subject access to his accumulated disfluencies at the end of each session. Separately recorded disfluency counts showed they dropped from around 8% per session to about 1% for the final 10 sessions. The second subject had three base-rate sessions, and then he counted his disfluencies during the next 11 sessions. His disfluencies went from around 9-11% to below 2% for most of the final treatment sessions. LaCroix also noted a wide disparity between the apparent accuracy of self-monitoring by both subjects: agreement between subject and clinician counts was 96.5% and 63.2%.

A veritable cornucopia of experimental and clinical possibilities seemed to be revealed by LaCroix's findings—particularly if they could be replicated, and yet, surprisingly, they have not been. Remarkably few studies (at least at this time) have looked at this area. One relevant investigation was reported by Hanson (1978). The object of this study was to identify the effects of highlighting self-recorded moments of stuttering. Two adult female stutterers spoke spontaneously in conditions in which, initially, they pressed a hand switch for each stuttering; then, in later conditions, this switch activated a light. In the first condition, pressing the hand switch alone appeared to substantially reduce stuttering in one subject (about 92%), but less so in the other (about 17%). There was some evidence of carry-over effects in the first subject, but the contingent light condition showed about the same level of stuttering as the hand switch pressing. In the second subject, the light contingency had no effect on stuttering. The difficulty with Hanson's findings is that the first subject actually counted very few of her stutterings (less than 14% of the experimenter's counts), while the second subject's counts generally agreed with the experimenter's.

Hanson's data not only pointed to the variability of effects in self-monitoring, or self-delivered contingencies, but also raised the possibility that, for some subjects, simply performing some activity while speaking may produce reductions. This could be true, but it is somewhat unlikely in view of the earlier-reviewed studies of Fransella (1967) and Brady (1969). Another alternative is that simply counting speech behaviors may be responsible for some portion of the effect. To control for this possibility, Ingham, Adams, and Reynolds (1978) arranged for three stutterers (16-23 years) to speak spontaneously in conditions in which they counted the verbal response "the," or their stuttering. Once again the results were variable, but informative. One subject failed to respond to the procedure, another decreased stuttering almost completely (from 6% of syllables during base rate) only when counting stutterings, and a third actually increased stutterings whenever he counted either "the" or stutterings. Rather intriguingly, the subject who benefited most from this procedure also showed least agreement with the experimenter's stuttering counts, and also counted only 66% of the experimenter's counts.

The possibility has now emerged that there may even be a negative correlation between subject-experimenter agreement and the effects of self-monitoring. This was evident in a study by James (1981a) involving 33 subjects (16-58 years). Each was required to speak spontaneously in base rate and self-monitoring conditions (pressing a handswitch immediately a stuttering occurred). When the subject's percent syllables stuttered data were partitioned, according to the "accuracy" with which subject and experimenter counts agreed, it was found that only the "low accuracy" group (mean 26% agreement; n=11) significantly reduced their stutterings during the self-monitoring conditions (approximately 41%). Another notable finding was that seven subjects actually increased stuttering during self-monitoring conditions, which means that for these subjects the procedure was self-reinforcing.

Before considering these puzzling findings, it is worth noting that this sequence of studies provides a useful illustration of an advantageous interaction between single-subject and group-research methods. For example, the peculiar responses to self-monitoring may not be as idiosyncratic as was suggested by the single-subject findings. James (1981a) suggests that one explanation for these strange findings is that they relate to the severity rather than frequency of stuttering. That is possible, but it is noteworthy that studies reporting the reactivity to self-monitoring of other behaviors have also reported low agreement between subject and experimenter response counts (Kazdin, 1974). Nelson and Hayes (1981) reviewed studies which suggest that some minimal level of accuracy may still be necessary to self-monitoring effects, though it can be surprisingly low. A study by Hayes and Cavior (1977) compared the responses of face touching, value judgments, and nonfluences during conversations by six normally fluent speakers. They found that correlations between subject and experimenter on nonfluencies was 0.00, yet this was the most reactive to self-monitoring of the three responses.

At least two other studies have ostensibly used punishing and reinforcing self-administered consequences on stuttering. To some extent, both have attempted to compare the effects of self-administered and experimenter-administered consequences. The first, by Cross and Cooper (1976), compared self-administered and experimenter-administered monetary rewards for judged improved fluency during oral readings. By comparison with control readings, the two experimental conditions produced significantly less (but not distinguishably different) stuttering counts. All but one of their 17 subjects reduced stuttering in the self-administered contingency condition, relative to the control conditions. Mowrer (1978) also used self-delivered verbal stimuli contingent on stutterings and stutter-free utterances in one of a number of treatments using an audience. The data show that all six subjects had fewer disfluencies, relative to a preceding base-rate condition. Unfortunately, neither study provided data concerning the comparative accuracy of self-ratings and experimenter ratings of performance. Both studies, however, were characterized by procedures that make it difficult to ignore the role of external controls on behavior. In Cross and Cooper's study, it would seem likely that subjects were aware the experimenter would know if they made inaccurate judgments, especially since "judged improvement required [that they] take from the investigator a token redeemable for $0.25" (Cross & Cooper, 1976, p. 242). The possibilities of the subject freely delivering contingencies also appear to have been constrained in Mowrer's study. His subjects had to say "stop" contingent on stuttering and "good" following three fluent utterances, in front of 14 observers. While these conditions may not entirely "explain" the findings, they do indicate sources of external control that limit their relevance to investigations of self-control.

A final study relevant to self-management research was reported by Martin and Haroldson (1977). They arranged for 20 adult stutterers to observe three different 10-minute video tapes between three pairs of spontaneous speaking conditions. One video was of a normal speaker, the other a severe stutterer, and the third showed a severe stutterer responding favorably to a time-out procedure. The post-video speaking behavior of subjects was unchanged following the first two viewings, but after watching the time-out condition tape there was a significant reduction in stuttering (about 27%). In fact, 18 of the 20 subjects reduced their percentage of words stuttered. Of course, it is possible that these data might relate to viewing changes in stuttering, rather than watching time-out effects. They also suggest that self-awareness of the possibility of reducing stuttering might be encouraged by a variety of external conditions. Self-delivery of consequences may only be a method of self-evaluating the ability to control the frequency of a behavior.

The present data on the effects of self-monitoring, or self-delivered consequences, for stuttering (or nonstuttering) present some fascinating research questions—as well as interesting clinical possibilities. Much of the data may simply derive from procedures that trigger the subject's use of different means of reducing stuttering. Indeed, there is actually insufficient evidence to prove that response-contingent self-delivered stimulation is responsible for altering stuttering.

Almost all the relevant studies have shown that the measurable accuracy with which self-stimulation is performed may be quite unrelated to its effects. This presents a number of interesting research issues. It may be that contingency, as such, is quite unimportant to the changes produced by these procedures. There may also be some unrecognized potency in intermittent, rather than continuous, stimulation with stuttering. There is also evidence that the contingency procedure (however it is used) sometimes punishes, reinforces, or only briefly alters stuttering.

In summary, there is still remarkably little information on the critical parameters relating to self-management effects. Perhaps the only clues are (1) the stimulus event may not be important, (2) it should be directed in some way towards stuttering (at least when it acts as a punisher), and (3) it may be connected in some way to the subject's awareness of his/her stuttering performance. Otherwise, the procedure simply offers experimental clinical promise.

The Later Challenge

The preceding review of some of the main areas of research stemming from early investigations of the use of operant methodology with stuttering largely testifies to the utility and generality of response-contingencies in modifying stuttering. That should not be interpreted to mean that either the utility or generality of these findings has gone unchallenged. Far from it. Generally, most of the initial challenges have been met, principally by replication, but there are some puzzling experimental findings, contentious methodological issues, and theoretical considerations that fuel the debate about these findings. Many of these issues are interrelated, but for purposes of presentation they will be described under separate headings.

The Experimental Challenge

Perhaps the most puzzling response-contingent research findings are those that seem contrary to what might be expected from the valence of the contingency. For instance, as was previously noted, Cooper, Cady, and Robbins (1970) found that when "right" or "tree" was made contingent on stuttering they reduced stuttering in the same manner as contingent "wrong." The effect was replicated (even more distinctively) by Daly and Kimbarow (1978), but with a slightly younger age group of stutterers. Quite a number of issues were raised by these findings. One was that if a "reinforcing" stimulus could punish stuttering, then it should not be regarded as operant behavior. It will be seen immediately that the effects, not the presumed properties of a stimulus, serve to describe a stimulus as a punisher—however incongruous the consequence and punishment relationship may appear. But while these data suggested that the affective content of a verbal response-contingent stimulus may not be important, an operant behavior should not be expected to generate manifestly aversive stimuli such as shock, or loss of common reinforcers such as money. Yet, some data implied that this could be so.

The possibility that stuttering could be reinforced was first suggested by Flanagan et al. (1958; 1959), but their data, with respect to the stutterers, were somewhat ambiguous. Their findings were based on cumulative record displays which failed to show distinct differences between the escape and base rate/extinction data trends. Some relevant data were also collected in the course of a study by Halvorson (1971). Three stutterers were run individually through conditions in which they were instructed to earn as many points on a counter as possible. In punishment (response cost) conditions, each stuttering subtracted a point. In "pairing" conditions, each stuttering also subtracted a point, except if the next word was spoken fluently, and then 10 points were added. As Martin and Ingham (1973) observed, it is conceivable that the subject would perceive this as earning points for stuttering. Unfortunately, however, the resulting data trends do not permit easy resolution of the findings. For all subjects, the punishment condition produced less stuttering than a preceding nontreatment condition. But the pairing condition did not consistently increase stuttering for any subject—certainly not in excess of the nontreatment conditions.[12]

More evidence of stuttering reinforcement occurred in previously mentioned studies by Shaw and Shrum (1972) and Manning, Trutna, and Shaw (1976). In both studies, children received marks (permitting purchase of a toy or candy) for disfluencies or stutterings in one experimental condition. Also, most children showed a higher frequency of stuttering in this condition than in the base-rate or reinforcement-for-fluent-intervals conditions. The difficulty in deciding whether this effect was due solely to the response-contingent arrangement in these studies is that this was integrated with quite obvious instruction effects.

Contrasting findings emerged in later studies. They appeared to demonstrate

[12] Halvorson hypothesized that stuttering frequency would increase during the pairing condition because punishment (point loss) would become a discriminative stimulus for positive reinforcement of the next fluent word.

that presumably reinforcing stimuli may punish stuttering. The first suggestions of this effect were reported in studies by Lanyon and Barocas (1973; 1975). (The data and procedure of the 1973 study are virtually identical to those reported in 1975, so only the later study will be discussed here.) Two experiments were reported, the first with four stutterers (8-65 years) and the second with six stutterers (17-34 years). In the first, each subject orally read 1000-word blocks in which each nonfluency (stuttering) contingently recorded a gain or loss of five cents. A "gain" or "loss" condition session was interspersed with readings free of contingencies. Also, comparisons were made with conditions in which the subject's counter operated randomly, even though he was told he would still receive the contingency. The resulting data show that both the "gain" or "loss" conditions decreased nonfluencies, relative to nontreatment conditions, and the differences between these conditions were not consistent across individuals. In the second experiment, they compared the effects of "gain" or "loss" (also with "no treatment" conditions) of money contingent on a stutter-free line of reading. Here the results are not quite as conclusive. In the gain condition, five (of six) subjects increased their number of fluent lines (relative to nontreatment conditions), but in the loss condition only three increased their production of fluent lines.

A study by Patty and Quarrington (1974) reported somewhat related findings. They compared three groups of seven stutterers (17-30 years) on three different experimental runs. Subjects spoke spontaneously throughout base-line (5 minutes), experimental (10 minutes), and extinction (5 minutes) conditions in which a red light flashed contingent on stuttering during experimental conditions for two groups. Only one group was told that each light flash would earn 5¢. The third group was simply told they would be paid 5¢ for each stuttering. The stuttering response class in this study contained only certain disfluencies, those described as Factor I and II behaviors by Brutten and Shoemaker (1967). The data trends of repetitions of single sounds and syllables, prolongations, and "visual struggle behavior" showed that only visual struggle behavior was altered by RCS conditions. This response decreased within the groups receiving rewards, but increased for the group receiving the response-contingent light flash. In other words, with this limited response class, the data trend was contrary to that expected by the different consequential events.

To some extent, Patty and Quarrington's findings are also consistent with those obtained in studies by Starkweather and Lucker (1978) and Corcoran (1980). In the Starkweather and Lucker study, four children (10-12 years) were assessed during 15-minute sessions in which the middle five minutes of some sessions permitted subjects to earn tokens for stutterings. The tokens were exchangeable for treats, and were given contingent on Factor I stutterings, but with the rather vague instructions, "You may be given a token while you speak." The summarized data are really quite inconclusive. Two subjects showed control-condition data trends that were the same as those found in the experimental-condition data. One other subject decreased stuttering and another increased stuttering (with what were described as "faked" stutterings). In Corcoran's (1980) study, eight stutterers (20-36 years) were paid to speak spontaneously during conditions in which a light flashed contingent on stuttering, and in another where each contingent light flash also earned 5¢ The percentage of words stuttered in these conditions was compared with that in the preliminary nontreatment condition, and showed no evidence of significant changes in stuttering.

Finally, Cross and Cooper's (1976) data are also relevant to the effects of reinforcement on stuttering. Their subjects (n=17; 18-66 years) either self-reinforced or were experimenter-reinforced for judged improvements in fluency during a preceding one-minute of oral reading. Their data showed decreased stuttering during these conditions. However, Cross and Cooper also reported more stutterings in the one-minute intervals that preceded reinforced one-minute intervals.

The findings from the "reinforcement of stuttering" studies present a fairly confusing picture. There is certainly ample evidence that some findings are contrary to those expected if stuttering is regarded as operant behavior. But there are other ways of explaining these confusing data. To begin with, in none of these studies did the subject actually fail to receive payment for speaking during the experimental conditions; thus, regardless of performance, they were "rewarded." Consequently, the "punishing" effects of highlighted stuttering may have been greater than the reinforcement of "more money." Also, in Cross and Cooper's (1976) study the subjects' response pattern appears to be eminently sensible—increased stuttering in one interval may have made it easier to earn in the next, particularly when increased stuttering was not penalized. A final consideration is the value of the presumed reinforcer. It may be hazardous to predict the reinforcing properties of the stimulus before an event, but this writer would be prepared to wager that markedly different data trends might have appeared in many of these studies if the contingency had been, say, $10 per stuttering, instead of 10¢.

Anticipating the effects of presumably potent stimuli can be extremely questionable. Consider the findings of a study by Martin, St. Louis, Haroldson, and Hasbrouck (1975). They used subjectively rated painful shock, as either a discrete or continuous stimulus, in single-subject experiments with five adult stutterers. During spontaneous speaking, shock was either contingent on stuttering, continuous but shut-off for five seconds contingent on stuttering, or the subject could choose either of these conditions.[13] None of the findings were consistent with the notion that stuttering is operant behavior. They even failed to replicate findings from previous response-contingent shock experiments: only two subjects decreased their frequency (and percentage) of words stuttered during this condition. And only three subjects appeared to increase stutterings during the continuous shock condition. The choice conditions were seemingly unrelated to performance. The conclusions reached by Martin et al. nicely summarized their findings:

> Results of the present experiment yield only very equivocal support to the

[13] A feature of this study is the duration of treatment conditions, a minimum of six 50-minute sessions in each condition.

> notion that stuttering is an operant response class. The results do accord with those of other recent single-subject experiments with stutterers; namely, when stuttering subjects are run under similar experimental procedures for long periods of time, there emerge as many distinct patterns of behavior as there are subjects (p. 489)

The Martin et al. (1975) data are a timely reminder of the dangers involved in presuming responsiveness to aversive contingent stimuli, plus the value in investigating subjects for extended periods. The temporal factors in RCS investigations have only been alluded to in this chapter. They may be particularly relevant, since there is every reason to expect that the punishing or reinforcing properties of stimuli may vary as much across time as they do across individuals. In other words, the conclusions drawn from such specific procedures may be as time-related as they are individually-related.

The Methodological Challenge

The preceding section has already touched on some methodological issues which limit the conclusions of many RCS studies. These mainly relate to the camouflaging effects that group experimental designs have on individual data, and differences that may be due to different treatment durations. There are also methodological considerations that relate to the properties of the stimulus event. For example, a particular stimulus procedure may not be indicative of an individual stutterer's responsiveness to an RCS procedure. This is illustrated in studies by Reed and Lingwall (1976), Martin and Haroldson (1979), and Costello and Hurst (1981), where individuals were found to respond quite differently to various response-contingent stimuli. However, the principal "methodological challenge" is that RCS studies often fail to control for factors which might better explain their results.

Alternative explanations for the results of RCS studies have been based on, at least, three general concerns about their methodologies: experimental design issues, instructional effects, and speech behavior changes. Each of these will be briefly reviewed.

Some claims have been made that single-subject experimental designs contain numerous possibilities for drawing false conclusions from data trends (Adams, 1970; Starkweather, 1971; Watts, 1973). Perhaps the main criticism is that comparisons between base rate and treatment data may be confounded by stuttering variability, sequence effects, and contrast effects. Clearly, the ABA design's strength depends on data trends during the B condition being visibly distinct from those in A conditions. Conversely, it is weakened if systematic trends occur in data preceding changes in experimental conditions, and evidence of that trend in succeeding conditions. At least two examples of this can be found in the previously reviewed studies. The first occurs in a report by Halvorson wherein the base-rate stuttering frequencies of Subject B (Halvorson, 1971, p. 360) systematically declined from base rate into the punishment condition. The second is a study by Hegde and Brutten (1977), in which the graphed data of all three subjects "blended" across some conditions.

In some cases, ironically, summarized data have disguised a quite powerful treatment effect. A notable example emerged from an exchange between Adams (1970) and Martin, Haroldson, and Starr (1971). Adams suggested that variability in the base-rate data reported by Haroldson, Martin, and Starr (1968) overlapped that found in the time-out conditions. Only when Martin et al. (1971) presented the data for shorter intervals (at least for one subject) were the treatment effects shown to be unambiguous.

Another concern is that the B interval in ABA designs may simply reflect time effects (Starkweather, 1971). This could transpire if a decrease in stuttering, due only to time, happened to coincide with the introduction of treatment. For the most part, this concern and that related to base-rate variability, can be answered by the use of lengthy and stable base-rate data, plus replication. In view of many studies that have adequately controlled these variables, it is reasonable to dismiss these explanations for the effects attained in most RCS studies.

A more serious challenge is raised by absence of control for effects due to the contrast between the base-rate and treatment conditions in many RCS studies. Simply introducing a new condition, such as shock or time-out from speaking, may be sufficient to reduce (or increase) stuttering. Perhaps the only counters to this criticism are the surprisingly few studies that have compared response-contingent and noncontingent stimulation conditions. Martin and Haroldson (see Martin & Ingham, 1973) reported an unpublished study in which two adult stutterers spoke spontaneously while time-out was delivered either randomly or response-contingently. They reported that both subjects decreased their percentage of words stuttered in the response-contingent condition, but not in the random condition. Similarly, Ingham and Andrews (1973a) compared noncontingent and response-contingent token reinforcement for reduced stuttering across twelve subjects, and reported that group treatment effects occurred only during the response-contingent conditions. James (1981c) also reported that a group of stutterers who received contingent time-out significantly reduced their stuttering, while another group who experienced noncontingent time-out failed to show this effect. A related finding, with respect to self-recording of stuttering, was reported for an individual stutterer in a study by Ingham, Adams, and Reynolds (1978). Perhaps less convincing control conditions have been used in studies that compare escape and avoidance aversive stimulation conditions (Flanagan, Goldiamond, & Azrin, 1958; Martin, St. Louis, Haroldson, & Hasbrouck, 1975). Some of their data show that the stimulus condition alone was not responsible for treatment effects. The confusing findings reported in the self-managed RCS studies have increased the cogency of this criticism.

The contribution that overtly (and covertly) conveyed instructions may play in RCS effects gain greatest impetus from the responsiveness that stuttering appears to have shown to instructions "to speak more fluently." This is partly demonstrated in findings reported by Wingate (1959), and has been claimed, particularly by Wingate (1970; 1980), to be a plausible source of treatment effects in many RCS studies. It has already been suggested that this variable may contribute to some RCS treatment effects, but it is difficult to believe that this accounts for all such effects. The point is illustrated by taking up Wingate's (1980) claim with respect to Martin and Siegel's (1966b) study. It will be recalled that Martin and Siegel introduced their treatment conditions with the instructions, "Now I want you to read very carefully. Don't worry about keeping the sentence going, just say each word fluently" (p. 469). This preceded the contingent stimulus conditions or noncontingent conditions, such as when just these instructions were given, or when a wrist strap (previously paired with contingent conditions) was attached. Wingate claims, "These subjects performed as well in the noncontingent as in the contingent conditions" (1980, p. 218). This simply is not true; the data trends from both conditions were quite dissimilar. Subject N's data show that his stuttering stabilized at less than five per minute in the contingent condition, but in the noncontingent conditions was mainly between 10 and 20 per minute. More importantly, the instruction-alone condition produced a sharp decline in stuttering for four minutes, but then it consistently increased over the rest of the session. This trend never appeared in the other experimental conditions. Other studies have also assessed the contribution of instruction effects. Martin and Haroldson (1979) compared the effects of instructions "to try very hard not to stutter" on stuttering during spontaneous speech, and found it produced no significant changes relative to noninstructed conditions. By contrast, response-contingent "wrong," or time-out, produced significant reductions in the group's (n=20) stuttering frequency scores. James and Ingham (1974) assessed the effects of instructions which suggested that one response-contingent time-out condition would reduce stuttering, while the other would not. They also found no evidence that these instructions altered their subjects' responsiveness to time-out. However, other studies have used potentially confounding instructions without isolating their role in treatment effects. Perhaps the most obvious examples are contained in studies by Shaw and Shrum (1972), and Manning, Trutna, and Shaw (1976).

Another explanation is that the entire RCS procedure may simply amount to subjects receiving knowledge of results. This explanation also derives from a criticism offered by Wingate (1970), and reiterated (Wingate, 1976) as a "cognitively-based" explanation for RCS data. Quite obviously, procedures that involve signaling events, particularly when accompanied by a counter, may have to sustain a knowledge-of-results explanation for all RCS treatment effects when stimuli, that are just as likely to provide knowledge of results, also produce different treatment effects. For example, Reed and Lingwall (1976), Martin and Haroldson (1979), and Costello and Hurst (1981) all described subjects who failed to respond to one response-contingent stimulus but did respond to another. There are also group data reported by Ingham and Andrews (1973a) which show that the rate of reductions in stuttering could be increased or decreased according to whether the response-contingent token stimuli were increased or decreased in value. This is not to deny that knowledge-of-results or cognition could be a substantial and even necessary condition for RCS effects, but they are probably less than sufficient explanations for the present findings.

One other way in which stuttering might be reduced during response-contingent stimulation is for the subject to use an unusual speech pattern. The possible ways in which this might occur have been described generally in Chapter 2, and may amount to the most "challenging" alternative explanation. The challenge can be considered from two viewpoints. First, it can be stated as a description of speech behaviors that could always be present whenever stuttering is reduced or eliminated. In other words, the challenge can only be met by demonstrating that one of these behaviors coincided with the RCS conditions, or that their presence was controlled. Second, evidence can be cited to show that some of the more obvious speech pattern changes were present and may have confounded treatment effects. Quite clearly, it is virtually impossible to answer the first challenge —at least with present methods of measuring speech behavior. It might be possible to demonstrate that RCS treatment effects exceed those obtained by the subject adopting different speech patterns, but this would not show that they were actually implicated. The only alternative is to seek evidence of the presence of some measurable or identifiable speech pattern in these studies.

Another explanation for RCS treatment effects is that subjects may reduce their speech rate during these procedures. It is well known (even self-evident) that stuttering will decrease if word output is reduced (Adams, Lewis, & Besozzi, 1973; Ingham, Martin & Kuhl, 1974; Johnson & Rosen, 1937). It is also a ruse which subjects could have used in some studies to either reduce shock or acquire reinforcers. Moreoever, some studies do report subjects who altered their rate of speaking coincident with treatment conditions (Martin, St. Louis, Haroldson, & Hasbrouck, 1975). On the other hand, there is ample evidence that when stuttering is reduced, in most RCS studies, it is accompanied by unaltered or increased speech rate. Consequently, the explanatory value of speech-rate change is likely to be slight. This is underscored by the distinct possibility that simply reducing speech rate may not always reduce stuttering. Ingham, Martin, and Kuhl (1974) reported that 50% reductions in base speaking rate reduced stuttering in some, but not all of their stutterers. In addition, reduced word output during a treatment may not mean that the speaker uniformly reduces speaking rate; subjects could introduce more frequent pauses, while their periods of connected speech remain at the basal speaking rate.

The problem of speech-rate comes down to the different ways in which rate can be quantified (see Chapter 2). This is well illustrated in a recent exchange of letters in the *Journal of Speech and Hearing Research* concerning Martin and Haroldson's (1979) study. Adams (1980) drew attention to the fact that the word-output data during Martin and Haroldson's treatment conditions showed either no significant change, or in the case of time-out, a reduction relative to the base-rate condition. Adams argued that the reduced moments of stuttering during the treatment conditions should have produced increased speaking rates, and since this "trade off" did not occur, the treatment effects may have been due to reduced speaking rate. To clarify the issue, Adams suggested a formula to recalculate Martin and Haroldson's data. Martin and Haroldson's (1980) response included Adams's suggested recalculations of their data. These showed that when time "lost" to stuttering was removed there was no significant change from base rate to treatment in any treatment condition. But, more importantly, Martin and Haroldson highlighted other sources of invalidity in attributing changes in word-per-minute data to reduced speed of utterance. Much of the variability, as they pointed out, can be attributed equally to "thinking of topics and formulating expressions" during spontaneous speaking.

Other types of alterations in speech behavior have only been vaguely identified within some RCS studies. It will be recalled, for instance, that Toomey and Sidman (1970) described how their subjects radically altered their manner of speaking during noncontingent shock conditions. Such reports have not usually accompanied RCS studies, which could imply that such obvious changes may not typify the effects of RCS conditions. But there are exceptions. For example, Goldiamond (1965) described a prolonged speech pattern which appeared during the course of a DAF-escape condition. This is a well-known modifier of stuttering. Also, Manning, Trutna, and Shaw (1976) instructed their children to speak in a "hard" or "easy" speech pattern during the course of response-contingent schedules. These are the most explicit indications that altered speech patterns may occur in RCS conditions. But the extent to which such changes may have occurred during RCS treatments, and were critical to their effects, remains unknown. This is a much-needed area of investigation that might yield functional dimensions relevant to the experimental analysis of stuttering.

In short, most challenges to RCS research findings, which are based on methodological grounds, have been adequately answered. Undoubtedly, these studies are not flawless, but thus far the findings have been remarkably durable as a result of the best possible test—replication. There may be additional "necessary conditions" for RCS effects, but these have yet to be clearly identified. There is still a paucity of studies which actually exploit the principles of experimental analysis of behavior. Such studies would seem to have better chances of identifying the interrelationship between temporal factors, stimulus conditions, and accompanying variables. The extent to which there is clinical "payoff" for this type of research will be considered later in this chapter.

The Conceptual Challenge

Throughout the period of RCS research there has been a consistent challenge to the "meaning" of these findings with respect to explanatory models of stuttering. The challenge has been mainly mounted by those who argue that these experimental studies are addressed to the notion that stuttering is, or is not, operant behavior. There has also been a recurring challenge to those findings from the perspective of Brutten and Shoemaker's (1967) Two-Factor Theory of stuttering.

The history of RCS research on stuttering is characterized, in one sense, by an unfortunate confusion between its relevance to the concept of stuttering as operant behavior and its contribution to the experimental analysis of behavior. This confusion was probably fostered, unwittingly, by two publications: Shames and Sherrick (1963) and Goldiamond (1965). Shames and Sherrick published their review at a time when operant methodology was first applied to stuttering. They argued that stuttering might be considered an operant behavior which "is maintained by positive and negative reinforcements on complex, multiple schedules" (1963, p. 17). Goldiamond, too, outlined a "consideration of stuttering and fluency as behaviors maintained by differential reinforcement in complex, but systematic relation to the environment" (1965, p. 109). It is not hard, therefore, to see how this led to the belief that the RCS studies were essentially concerned with the "operant model of stuttering" (Bloodstein, 1975; 1979), or even to an "operant or one factor" learning theory of stuttering (Patty & Quarrington, 1974, pp. 72-73). Of course, the RCS studies never had a necessary connection with operant conditioning, or to the concept of stuttering as an operant. This point has been made by those concerned with investigating these procedures (Ingham, 1975, p. 336; Martin & Ingham, 1973, p. 126), plus reviewers of these procedures (Wingate, 1980). The criterion used to decide "whether or not a behavior is operant is mainly that its properties may be modified by the effects that result from its appearance" (Shames & Sherrick, 1963, p. 4). But this is a property shared by many behaviors that would hardly be considered operants. Heart-beat rate, for example, has often been shown to be manipulable by arranging consequential events on certain frequency levels (Yates, 1980). Yet it would be almost ludicrous to describe it as a behavior maintained by environmental consequences. The plain fact is that the RCS studies have done nothing more than demonstrate that some individuals' stutterings may be either decreased (or sometimes increased) when stimuli closely follow the occurrence of this behavior. The resulting data say absolutely nothing about whether that behavior is developed or sustained by environmental stimuli. In fact, under some circumstances, it is evident that stuttering has not behaved as "an operant" (for example, Martin, St. Louis, Haroldson, & Hasbrouck, 1975). The confusion between the conclusions that can be drawn from RCS research, with respect to stuttering, and the concept of stuttering as operant behavior, is not difficult to understand. The wonder is that those conducting this research have not been more forthright in emphasizing this distinction. Whatever meaning is able to be drawn from this research about stuttering largely depends on research creativity. It will be argued later in this chapter that the principal relevance that this has to stuttering, at present, is in the clinical context.

Perhaps the most sustained challenge to the RCS research findings has been from those who advocate a Two-Factor Theory of stuttering (Brutten & Shoemaker, 1967). It will be recalled that the essence of this theory is that stuttering is, by definition, a negative emotional event which, in its behavioral manifestations, is composed of involuntary and voluntary behaviors. The former are, as Webster and Brutten (1974) state, "involuntary repetitions and prolongations of sounds or syllables that are the disruptive result of. . .emotional arousal. It is this fluency failure, and this failure of fluency *only*, that we refer to as stuttering" (p. 202).

In effect, the presence of any "contingent negative stimulation" would be expected to increase the rate of this Factor I behavior. By contrast, Factor II behaviors are voluntary avoidance responses, such as "interjections, whole-word and phrase repetitions, circumlocutions, changes in speaking rate and intensity, eye blinks, lip purses, head shakes, foot taps, and arm swings" (Webster & Brutten, 1974, p. 202). Since they are voluntary they can also be modified by instructions, or they tend to increase with rewards and to decrease with punishment (see Brutten, 1975). It is important to recognize that these behaviors are only defined by paper and pencil tests, physiological measures and behavioral reactions which substantiate that "speech associated emotional arousal is related to these episodes of fluency failure" (Webster & Brutten, 1974, p. 200). Consequently, it is quite possible that the so-called stuttering behavior referred to throughout the present review of RCS research may not always be stuttering, according to the strictly defined criteria used by Two Factor theorists. Of course, it is equally incumbent on those who issue challenges from the perspective of Two Factor Theory to demonstrate that the behaviors referred to in RCS studies were stutterings or voluntary accessory behaviors, as defined by that theory. At the very outset, therefore, it will be evident that a satisfactory answer to this challenge is unlikely, since few studies have carefully defined stuttering in accordance with Two Factor Theory.

Generally, most of the early evidence used to support the claim that stutterings would increase during contingent-aversive or "negative" stimulation was derived from unpublished studies which, in almost every instance, have not ultimately appeared in the professional literature (see, for example, papers listed by Brutten & Shoemaker, 1967; 1971). One unpublished study (Martin, Brookshire, & Siegel, 1964) from those produced in the course of the University of Minnesota research program has been referred to with striking regularity by Brutten and Shoemaker, Webster, Starkweather, and other advocates of Two Factor Theory, as evidence that certain behaviors within a "moment of stuttering" (such as prolongations) increase during response-contingent shock conditions. However, in recent years, the challenge has drawn from a more accessible literature.

A study by Janssen and Brutten (1973) is one endeavor to measure the effects of response-contingent shock on different types of Factor I and II behaviors. Four adult stutterers (29-39 years) were treated in a single-subject experimental design in which shock was contingent on all prolongations (for some reason, this behavior was not identified before the experiment as Factor I stuttering). The results

> indicated no systematic effect of punishment on prolongations. For two subjects shock did not significantly affect oral prolongations. Two subjects showed a significant increase, but whether or not this change was occasioned by the introduction of the electric shock could not be clearly demonstrated (p. 74).

One questionable feature of this study was the wide range in the correlations between observer and experimenter scores. These range from .53 to .93 "depending on the behaviors measured." Unfortunately they were not listed. With such low reliability measures on some behaviors, it is quite possible that the marginal trend differences in the graphed cumulative data could have disguised directionally different trends.

Other studies have yielded more decisive data with respect to the independent responsiveness of different types of stuttering behaviors and the effects of RCS procedures. Oelschlaeger and Brutten (1976) measured the effects of instructions to reduce either Factor I or II behaviors in the spontaneous speech of four stutterers. Two subjects were instructed to try "to speak without repeating sounds or syllables'' (repetitions) and the other two were instructed to ''try not to interject sounds'' (interjections). Those behaviors were counted throughout an ABA design in which the instructions to change speech behavior formed the B segment. Interpreting this study's data is not easy, since only total responses in each experimental segment were reported (and there is reliance on statistical, rather than graphic, comparisons between the segment data). The experimenters reported the instructions had no effect on repetitions by the first two subjects, although the noninstructed behavior, interjections, did decrease. With the other subjects, the instruction to cease interjections reduced that behavior, although it continued to decrease during the last A segment for one subject, but not the other. Also, their repetition responses were unaffected by changes in the experimental conditions. In another study, Oelschlaeger and Brutten (1975) assessed the impact of response-contingent ''positive stimulation'' (money) on part-word repetitions by four subjects ''diagnosed as stutterers.'' These subjects orally read throughout an ABA experimental design in which 10¢ was earned for each part-word repetition within the B period. (The data in this study were also collapsed and analyzed statistically.) The results indicated that the RCS procedure did not significantly alter the response.[14] These findings are also closely related to those reported by Patty and Quarrington (1974) who, as mentioned earlier, investigated the effects of earning 5¢ for each Factor I or II stuttering. The data for their group of stutterers (n=7) showed that Factor I repetitions and prolongations were unaffected by this procedure, but the Factor II ''struggle behaviors'' actually decreased during the RCS procedure.

The response class mentioned in the previous studies appears to react in a manner anticipated by Two Factor Theory, although it is interesting that not one study indicated that the responses were ''diagnosed'' as Factor I or II behaviors. The only study which appears to have taken this precaution was conducted by Brutten (1980). He assessed effects of RCS using a presumed negative verbal stimulus, ''wrong'', on Factor I prolongations during a subject's oral reading. Repeated ABA experimental conditions were used, with either nontreatment, noncontingent stimulation, or response-contingent stimulation introduced to the B condition on different experimental runs. The data showed that, in all but one experimental run, the B condition contained more prolongations than either A conditions (the exception was the first of three runs in which no treatment was used during the B interval). The repeated experimental runs appeared to show no difference between the effects of all three experimental conditions, but a statistical analysis of the subject's data (at best a questionable procedure) revealed that only the response-contingent ''wrong'' condition significantly increased sound prolongations. Brutten then concluded that response-contingent ''wrong'' increased the frequency of the sound prolongations. There are, however, a number of ways in which these data can be considered. One is to notice that all experimental conditions increased the frequency of sound prolongations (albeit

[14] As previously mentioned, the effect of more available reinforcers (for example, more money) may provide a more exacting assessment of the effects of this type of contingency on such behaviors.

not necessarily via a Wilcoxon's t-test). Indeed, the percentage of differences between the A condition frequencies (average scores) and the B condition (in each ABA sequence) shows that the two nontreatment runs, plus the noncontingent and contingent stimulation runs, all produced greater than 33⅓% increases in prolongations—in fact, the nontreatment condition "produced" a 65.6% increase in prolongations! It therefore seems wiser to adopt a more conservative conclusion—that the subject displayed no distinguishable treatment effect.

The foregoing studies revealed some reasonably consistent data with respect to the effects of RCS on Factor I- and II-type behaviors. They yielded no evidence that either RCS procedures or instructions consistently increase or decrease Factor I behaviors. But, they did show that Factor II behaviors decrease under both conditions. By contrast, other RCS studies suggested that both types of behavior decreased when, presumably, aversive stimuli were contingent on moments of stuttering. Reed and Lingwall (1976; 1980) described two RCS studies (see Chapter 6) on a total of 20 adult stutterers. In these studies either response-contingent noise (one second 95dB SPL white noise), "wrong," or laughter (one second of recorded female laughter) produced significant reductions in stuttering. In all ABA conditions subjects spoke spontaneously while the following six "stuttering-behavior types" were recorded; part-word repetitions, word repetitions, phrase repetitions, prolongations, hesitations, and interjections. The mean frequency of moments of stuttering decreased by more than 50% during B conditions (relative to the combined A conditions), yet the proportions of stuttering-behavior types remained unchanged across experimental conditions. In other words, Factor I and II behaviors showed the same pattern of decrease during the B conditions.

Another relevant study was reported by Costello and Hurst (1981). They used a repeated ABAB single-subject design with three stutterers (40, 19, and 18 years) to identify the effects of different RCS procedures on certain types of stuttering. During either spontaneous speech or oral reading, contingencies were paired with one disfluency category while at leat one other was monitored. In one subject "jaw tremors" were treated by time-out (5-10 seconds) while repetitions ("of phonemes, syllables, and monosyllabic words") were monitored. This showed that time-out conditions reduced both behaviors. In a final session, time-out was contingent on repetitions which then decreased, but the jaw tremors were unaffected. In another subject, part-word and monosyllabic word repetitions were treated by time-out (10 seconds), while "hard contacts" ("silent prolongations") and "inhalation interjections" were monitored for most sessions. The data show that repetitions were consistently reduced during the treatment conditions and, for most sessions, the other two behaviors followed suit. During the last steps, treatment was shifted from repetitions to all disfluencies, and in both cases these behaviors almost ceased. The third subject first received time-out contingent on audible prolongation while repetitions ("of phonemes, syllables, and monosyllabic words") and "hard contacts" were monitored. The source of treatment effects for this subject are not as obvious. This is because the time-out duration varied and, in a later session, response-contingent noise was paired with a pep talk "to encourage [the subject's] harder work at fluency" (1981, p. 253). At this point a rather nondistinctive data trend showed correlated reductions in all three disfluency responses over this and later treatment sessions. Costello and Hurst claim their data show that the treatments produced "direct behavioral covariation," or evidence that contingencies may alter the frequency of a response class.

On the face of it, Reed and Lingwall, and Costello and Hurst have reported data that contradict the findings of Oelschlaeger, Brutten, Patty, and Quarrington. There are some differences between the studies that could explain this contradiction, however. In the first place, Reed and Lingwall and Costello and Hurst's data relate to behaviors that were not "diagnosed" as Factor I or II. Though it seems unlikely that all their subjects had stutterings which were not of the type referred to by Two Factor theorists—especially since the same criteria were not used in studies reporting findings consistent with Two Factory Theory. Secondly, the data reported by Reed and Lingwall were grouped and do not necessarily reflect individual trends. Yet, if Factor I and II behaviors are expected to have common responses to contingent stimuli (albeit in different directions), then group data might be expected to express those patterns. The only other option is that differences between findings from these studies simply reflect individual reactions to RCS procedures.

In general, at least as much evidence has been gathered to reject the challenge from Two Factor Theory as has been gathered to support that challenge. On balance, it would seem fair to conclude that very little data support Brutten's (1980) contention with respect to Factor I type stutterings that "the use of punishment is unwarranted with this form of fluency failure even if the stimulus employed is not strongly aversive... Though punishment has been found to suppress Factor II responses like arm swings, nose wrinkles, and tongue thrusts it can augment the occurrence of Factor I prolongations" (p. 83). From the vantage point of the present review of RCS research, the weight of evidence suggests that this warning is neither warranted nor supportable.

Conclusions from Experimental Studies

This has been a rather lengthy review and it is not intended to augment it with a drawn-out account of the findings. It does, however, beg some comment on the current status of RCS research on stuttering. At one point in this review mention was made of RCS research on heart rate. There may be profit in relating the direction of that work to stuttering research. Yates (1980) recently summarized the history and direction of that research, and showed that the initial demonstrations of the modifiability of heart rate led to exacting investigations of the methodology, the role of feedback, and the variables necessary to these effects. In addition, efforts were then made to identify the contribution of self-managed variables. The resemblance between the apparent operant nature of the heart rate response and the factors found to be critical to producing similar effects is difficult to recognize, but it has not impugned the validity of the initial findings. In the case of stuttering research, it would seem justifiable to conclude that this behavior can be decreased by the arrangement of certain types of response-contingent stimuli during the speech of many stutterers of most age groups. There is also some evidence that nonstuttered intervals of speech can be reinforced so that stuttering is concomitantly decreased. The interaction between the duration of treatment by this procedure and specific contingencies is unclear at present. Nevertheless, most of the more striking effects relate to intervals of talking that extend over many hours. The current direction of research into the RCS effect on stuttering now appears to be moving down the same paths followed by heart rate research.

The investigation of self-managed RCS procedures has led to an exceedingly interesting, if not bewildering, development in this research area. It is not at all clear why the effects of contingencies appear to be quite substantial when they are delivered in seemingly random or intermittent fashion. But, then, there has also been no serious research on the effects of intermittent RCS on stuttering. It may be that subjects are more capable than their experimenters of leading this research towards the critical parameters of RCS effects.

There appear to be numerous avenues to choose from in trying to chase down the variables relevant to the effects of RCS procedures. There may be gains in following the path concerned with the role of other aspects of speech behavior, or even physiological factors, that relate to the effect. The path concerned with the role of feedback and its relationship to certain types of contingencies may also yield benefit. Undoubtedly, the avenue opened by self-control over contingencies must also be attractive. Whatever the case, the notion that the effect of these procedures is reducible to knowledge-of-results or increased-attention-to-fluency reflects a measure of ignorance about the intriguing effects reported thus far in this field.

Perhaps the only disappointing trend in the latest RCS research is the limited use made of the principles of experimental analysis of behavior. There is a crying need for research that systematically investigates the variables possibly critical to contingency effects in individual subjects. Here, surely, is an area needing creativity and imagination, in contrast to the sterile image this field of research often projects.

In the final analysis, the use of response-contingent methodology should find its most fruitful expression in therapy practice. The following section will consider whether that is so.

Therapy Procedures Using Response-Contingent Methodology

Introduction

At the start of this chapter it was argued that Skinner's influence on therapy for many problems could be the most dominant of all influences over the last half of this century. That may turn out to be a difficult claim to support, since many procedures emerging from fundamentally different backgrounds share a lot in common with contingency-management techniques. For instance, the graduated steps in systematic desensitization hierarchies certainly resemble operant-response classes, since success or failure on a hierarchy step invokes a contingent event: introducing a new step, repeating a step, or returning to a previous step. Even more pertinent is biofeedback practice with its fairly obvious use of feedback as a "consequential event." Indeed, efforts to determine a distinction between operant-conditioning principles and biofeedback methodology have become a point of controversy (Hatch & Gatchel, 1981; Yates, 1980). Perhaps the only distinctive feature of operant methodology is its use of a response-contingent schedule which alters the frequency or topography of a target behavior. This means that the absence of a therapy design which makes it possible to discern the impact of such a schedule should exclude it from consideration. It is recognized that this would not distinguish between operant and biofeedback methodologies, but, for purposes of description, biofeedback will be regarded as a special form of this procedure.

The pervasive influence of operant methodology also makes it increasingly difficult to clearly identify its boundaries within the stuttering therapies. In many cases, for example, operant methodology has an adjunct rather than principal role in treatment. This has been evident in some of the syllable-timed speech (see Chapter 5) or desensitization (Chapter 6) treatments which have been amalgamated with response-contingent schedules. Consequently, in order to organize the boundaries of an account of operant methodology and stuttering, a review of therapies that use this methodology mainly in a supplementary capacity will be deferred. Thus, treatments involving modification of the subject's speech pattern by delayed auditory feedback, prolonged speech, or other related methods will be reviewed in Chapter 10. Also the growing generalization of maintenance "technology," which uses response-contingent schedules, will be considered separately. Less defensible will be the inclusion of response-contingent treatments which use Van Riper's (1963) techniques, modify verbal content, alter cognitive factors, or manipulate other types of behavior. They are included because their application has been relatively limited and involves no more than a few studies.

Reinforcement Procedures

The first type of applications of RCS procedures in stuttering therapy were somewhat surprising. Almost all the initial experimental investigations of RCS on stuttering used punishment principles, yet virtually all the early therapeutic studies used reinforcement principles. Perhaps the only exception was the "informal" response-contingent study by Fahmy (1950) mentioned earlier in this chapter.

The first planned use of operant conditioning principles in a therapy context appears to have been a study by Rickard and Mundy (1965). They treated a 9-year-old boy whose speech was "characterized by repetitions and blockages." The treatment incorporated "successive approximation" steps designed to reduce "repetition errors" on phrases, sentences, paragraphs, conversation, and generalization tasks. In the "phrases" step, the subject was reinforced (verbally, and then with ice cream) for reading pronoun and verb combinations with fewer than base-rate repetitions. When (presumably) 100 percent success was achieved with two-word phrases, the subject earned points (leading to the purchase of a yo-yo) for zero repetitions on six-word sentences. The same procedure was then followed with paragraphs and oral reading of short stories. The criterion used to judge success on these tasks is not mentioned. The first three steps were completed in daily sessions over 12 days, followed by 23 sessions of conversational practice. In this last step, secondary reinforcers were earned for either talking with reduced errors or for error-free five-minute intervals of spontaneous speech. This step was also blended with a generalization phase involving the child's parents. Ultimately, the parents reinforced error-free conversation outside the clinic during a vacation and at home. Over this eight-month period they also recorded the subject's performance. A follow-up interview was conducted six months later. Oral reading assessments were made before, during, and after treatment, as well as during the follow-up session. Within-treatment session data generally showed that when each treatment step was introduced repetition errors declined, as counted by the clinician or assessed by the subject's parents. The oral-reading data also show that repetition errors went from around 128 (per 173 words) to zero over the course of treatment, but increased to 16 on follow-up. The parents also reported that, by follow-up, "much of his stuttering behavior had been reinstated in the home and school environment" (1965, p. 273).

Rickard and Mundy's study illustrates a number of points about the clinical use of operant-conditioning principles which appear in many later studies and are pertinent in gauging their value. It describes a procedure which is designed to instate clinic-based fluency by successive steps, then transfer these gains to nonclinic conditions with "hoped-for" generalization over time. It also sought to determine therapy effects by the use of within- and beyond-treatment measures. The internal and external validity of their study was enhanced by this measurement methodology, but it was compromised by a dubious measure of stuttering: "stuttering behavior was defined by repetition errors per task unit ('g-g-g-going' as one-word task unit would yield a score of three repetition errors) blocking, flushing, and other concomitants of stuttering were not recorded" (1965, p. 270). Consequently, while repetition errors may have been reduced, other aspects of stuttering, such as blocks, were not included. This might be one explanation for the child's relapse on follow-up.

Leach (1969, actually reported in 1966) described an experimental treatment in which stutter-free intervals of speech were reinforced. A 12-year-old boy received 42 twice-weekly sessions (30-minutes) in which he orally read or spoke spontaneously, and earned two cents for each minute of talking. After four of these sessions, the second half of each session enabled the subject to earn an additional one cent for each 15 seconds of fluency. The subject was simply told "it was a period in which he could earn additional money" (1969, p. 122). Only first-half session data were reported. They showed his disfluencies went from roughly eight to less than one per minute by the end of treatment. Unfortunately, neither reliability nor speech rate data were recorded, and two months after treatment ceased there was "a partial return of the disfluent behavior" which required further therapy.

Another essentially within-clinic experimental treatment was reported by Russell, Clark, & Van Sommers (1968). They treated three stutterers (48, 40, and 15 years) individually in one-hour sessions (usually once a week), using oral reading of slide-projected stimulus words or phrases. In the treatment procedure "some correct [fluent] responses were rewarded not only by the exposure of a new stimulus but also by the sounding of a buzzer and a flashing green light in the corner of the screen. At the same time a counter mounted on the screen counted backwards to zero" (p. 448). This intermittent and, presumably, reinforcing procedure was investigated in experiments on one subject, and was shown to decrease his "errors" from around 35 to 8 percent. The two other subjects treated by this method decreased their speech errors from 8-10 percent down to 2 percent. Only unsolicited and dataless reports supported a claim that two subjects had shown improved speech beyond the clinic. Yet, again, no reliability or speech-rate data are reported. There is also a probability that reinforcement was accompanied by a punishment procedure, since each stuttering caused the slide to be "exposed for five seconds before a new slide was presented."

Bar (1971; 1973) reported using verbal and sometimes tangible reinforcement for fluent intervals spoken by two 13-year-old stutterers. Graphic illustration techniques were used to identify children who were aware of their speech problem. In Bar's 1971 report, 44 of 48 children "became fluent," and in the 1973 report, 67 of 83 children were stated to be fluent at the end of the therapy. Absolutely no data were provided in support of these extravagant claims.

The previously reviewed experimental studies by Shaw and Shrum (1972) and Manning, Trutna, and Shaw (1976), which evaluated the effects of reinforcing intervals of fluency, also provided some follow-up information. In the former study, with three children (9-10 years), spontaneous carry-over of reduced stuttering was claimed for two subjects (two months posttreatment for one subject, no time interval reported for the other) via informal contacts at varying intervals after the experiment. The problem with this claim is that the children were also receiving another therapy; however, carry-over efects were claimed because these therapy sessions preceded the experiment and had not yielded improved fluency. Each child's clinician also reported improved fluency in the three subjects over a two-to-four-month period, but supportive data were not provided. Manning, Trutna, and Shaw (1976) also treated three chidren (6-9 years) and reported what they termed carry-over data from a 15-minute session two months after the experiment. But these data are also extremely difficult to interpret. To begin with, the children may have continued with another therapy during the carry-over interval (nothing is stated to suggest otherwise): also, their data are only reported in terms of fluent time intervals and stutterings per five minutes. Such data do not clearly indicate whether there was an actual improvement in the percentage of words stuttered. The problem is pointedly illustrated by the only subject's (SK) data to include word-per-minute scores. By using these scores to calculate the actual percentage of words stuttered, SK averaged 10.2

percent-words-stuttered at base rate, 11.5 percent at the end of the experimental treatment, and 6.9 percent at carry-over. The other two subjects showed relatively reduced stutterings per-five-minutes and increased fluent intervals over the same occasions, but in the absence of speech-rate data this has little clinical significance: one subject still had 50 stutterings per five minutes and the other 12 per five minutes during carry-over sessions.

The only other relevant therapy study (to date) was reported by Peters (1977). This described the treatment of two mild stutterers (8 years) in short sessions (3 to 12 minutes), once or twice weekly, using a mixture of monologue and conversational speech. Following base-rate sessons, 30 seconds of fluent speech was rewarded with a chip convertable to various other reinforcers (both used their reinforcers to bring a friend to the treatment session). When base-rate disfluencies were reduced by 90 percent for two consecutive sessions, the treatment was removed, and only reintroduced if disfluencies per 30 seconds increased during subsequent extinction sessions. For one subject, whole-word repetitions decreased from 2.64 to below 0.26 and remained near that level over six extinction sessions. A month later, an 11-minute session of oral reading, conversation, and monologue produced 0.27 repetitions per 30 seconds. The second child averaged 1.58 interjections during base rate, which decreased to less than 0.15 over 13 consecutive treatment sessions. They remained at that level over three extinction sessions. This subject produced no interjections during a 30-minute follow-up session. The report benefited from reliability data and extemporaneous reports by significant others, but it was weakened by the total absence of word output data (although Peters reported "it did not appear that fluency increased because the subject spoke less").

The findings from all reinforcement of fluency studies are uniformly positive (at least in the direction of their findings), but they contain no information which would inspire reasonable confidence in the clinical value of their results. In fact, the threats to the validity of the results by the absence of nonclinic data, limited follow-up (with evidence of relapse even in some clinic conditions), and infrequent reliability measures are so substantial that only minimal confidence can be placed in the direction of their findings.

Punishment Procedures

The findings from clinical studies that have used response-contingent stimulation for stuttering present a rather more encouraging therapy picture. In one sense, this mirrors the previously reviewed differences between the experimental studies which have used reinforcement or punishment principles. It will be recalled that punishment was more frequently reported to reduce stuttering than was the case with reinforcement. The clinical applications of punishment have involved the different types of stimuli that have been used over the course of experimental studies on punishment.

In spite of the ethical concerns about the clinical use of response-contingent shock, it does not seem to have been used very often in a stuttering therapy setting. Nevertheless, the clinical setting in which it was used first may justify some ethical concerns. That was for a study by Crowder and Harbin (1971), who reported treating a 21-year-old mild stutterer with response-contingent shock in the psychiatric clinic of a prison. During 29 treatment sessions (unspecified duration), the first third of each session was "untreated," but, in the last part of each session, the subject received "shock once for every five stutters." The subject orally read or conversed while his stutterings (repetitions of single and multisyllable words) were monitored. Only data from untreated parts of the session were reported, and they show a decline from about 40 to less than five per session. it was also noted that only 15 shocks were delivered over the course of treatment. An informal one-month follow-up was used to claim "stability of improvement," but confidence in that result is lessened by a 0.66 correlation between original and repeat scores from 48 percent of the treatment sessions.

Shock was also used in a stuttering therapy procedure reported by Beattie (1973) for a 20-year-old female. The subject's speech problem was divided into eight stuttering categories and shock was delivered contingent on some categories using a 1:3 schedule during oral reading. Oral-reading data from before and after the shock sessions showed that target behaviors and some untreated behaviors were reduced over treatment. Some stuttering still remained after nine months of irregular 30-40 minute sessions, and so systematic desensitization techniques were introduced to her treatment. Some generalization of the gains achieved during oral reading to beyond-clinic settings was claimed, but no supportive data were provided. The complete absence of relevant within-treatment data, conversational speech assessment, reliability, and word output data make it impossible to place too much importance on these findings.

The possibility that response-contingent time-out from speaking may have therapy benefits gained impetus from some early experimental time-out studies which showed carry-over or resistance to extinction (Haroldson, Martin, and Starr, 1968; Martin & Berndt, 1970). The Martin and Berndt (1970) study, in particular, had obvious clinical implications, since it showed that a child's stuttering (at least during oral reading) could be reduced to virtually zero during time-out conditions and remain near that level during extinction sessions.[15]

One of the first attempts to use time-out in a therapy context was by Egolf, Shames, and Seltzer (1971). They used an interesting variation on the conventional experimental application of time-out with 10 stutterers (22-52 years) during five 90-minute group therapy sessions which were organized to form an ADADA experimental design. During the A sessions the change in speakers followed customary conversational rules. But, in B sessions, subjects spoke only until a stuttering occurred, then another speaker immediately "took over" the speaking time in the group. The mean number of words spoken before a first stuttering in each B session was about 740 percent greater than in A sessions, with about the same word-per-minute rates in A and B sessions. Eight of the 10 subjects' scores followed a pattern in which B session scores always exceeded A session scores.

[15] It should be recognized that it is difficult to define an extinction condition within a punishment schedule which actually eliminates a response. For in such circumstances the punishment condition is, ostensibly, removed.

This was principally an experimental study with little therapeutic purpose, but it did suggest the method's viability in controlling stuttering under these conditions.

Perhaps the most clinically (if not conceptually) important of all response-contingent treatment studies was reported by Martin, Kuhl, and Haroldson (1972). Known as the "Puppet Study," it was carried out individually with two young boys (ages 3.5 and 4.5 years). Each child was run in weekly 20-minute sessions. During base-rate sessions the child conversed with a puppet, known as "Suzybelle," located on an illuminated stage. During treatment sessions the stage was darkened and Suzybelle ceased talking for 10 seconds contingent on a stuttering. With the younger child, who often displayed 15-second moments of stuttering, the time-out condition was initially contingent on two-second intervals of stuttering for almost 13 sessions. During a further 15 sessions it was contingent on an entire stuttering moment. The base-rate conditions were then restored for 10 additional sessions. The number of stutterings and words spoken during these sessions revealed that the child produced around 6% words stuttered during base-rate sessions, but his stuttering declined to near zero by the latter part of treatment, and remained at that level during the extinction sessions. By contrast, the child's word output showed a concomitant increase over the course of treatment. These data trends and levels were also reflected in monthly 20-minute conversations with the experimenter in another room. They were also evidently sustained outside the clinic, as revealed by covert home recordings; only six stutterings in 2,146 words were produced during conversations with family members. A follow-up session in the clinic 11 months later showed 0.82 percent words stuttered. Virtually identical results were produced by the older child, but over fewer sessions. During base-rate sessions this child averaged round 2.5 percent words stuttered, but this percentage declined to zero shortly after the introduction of 10 treatment sessions and remained at that level over 12 extinction sessions. Concurrent nontreatment sessions, involving conversations between mother and child, produced an identical data trend. Zero stutterings were also recorded on covert recordings made in the child's home (not clear when). Finally, 13 months later in another city, the child produced 0.55 percent-words-stuttered while speaking to a clinician.

The Martin et al. (1972) study is not entirely free of problems. For example, it is feasible that the treatment conditions might not have been solely responsible for the treatment effects. The principal claim for the treatment's responsibility is the immediacy of its effect on stuttering and replication of this effect across two subjects. There is also an unfortunate absence of beyond-clinic data collected before or during treatment. Nevertheless, the findings clearly show that a clinically significant change in stuttering was durable across pertinent speaking situations and over a substantial interval. They also show the beneficial effects of a procedure which clearly drew attention to stuttering (during treatment one child remarked "Hey, Suzybelle, how come you turn out when I'm stuttering, how come" 1972, p. 751).

The "Puppet Study" findings were replicated, in principle, by Reed and Godden (1977). They described another response-contingent treatment for two preschool stutterers (a 5-year-old boy and nearly 4-year-old girl) in which the puppet condition was replaced by clinician-directed conversation. The children were treated individually in twice-weekly 20-minute sessions using the contingent verbal stimulus "slow down." During base-rate sessions the oldest child averaged around 8% words stuttered and then demonstrated responsiveness to the contingency during a following within-session ABA experiment. Over 15 subsequent treatment sessions his stuttering reduced to 1%, along with a 13.27% decrease in word rate. Home recordings, concurrent with treatment, showed a variable beyond-clinic data trend, with stutterings reduced to 3% by treatment end. A follow-up session (11 minutes) eight months later showed 1% words stuttered. The younger child stuttered on a mean of 18% during base-rate sessions, which then decreased to 1% after 10 treatment sessions; her word output actually increased by 8.7% by the end of treatment. The concurrent home recordings for this subject revealed a data trend paralleling clinic scores. An eight-month follow-up session produced 0.6% words stuttered.

Reed and Godden's findings, and those reported by Martin et al. (1972), demonstrated a range of clinical possibilities in RCS procedures that have immense potential for clinicians. At the same time, these findings also confronted the long-nourished belief that any stuttering therapy for children which directs their attention to their speech behavior is especially inadvisable—even dangerous (Bloodstein, 1969; Johnson, 1967; Luper & Mulder, 1964). In fact, in a very important respect, these were pivotal studies since their procedures and findings presented a direct challenge to the nonbehavioral preparadigm.

The only other clinician-managed time-out therapy report (to date) is Costello's (1975) account of the treatment of three mild stutterers (16, 18, and 20 years). These subjects were treated individually in 40- or 50-minute sessions held twice weekly. Each session actually contained an ABA experimental condition which permitted carry-over effects to be distinguished from treatment effects.[16] "Time-out" was not the only treatment procedure in this study, however, so that the results should also be related to other treatment methods. Subject One began therapy with around 15 disfluencies per minute at 178 words per minute (wpm) while speaking spontaneously. During six sessions, the time-out condition (the clinician said "stop" and looked away for 10 seconds contingent on stuttering) showed consistent within-session treatment effects. By session seven the subject's disfluency rate stabilized around 1.2 per minute (196 wpm), and in nontreatment conditions at around 3 or 4 per minute (200 wpm). After instructions "to remain fluent," the subject's disfluencies stabilized at around 0.5 per minute across A and B conditions. One reasonable interpretation of this subject's data over the subsequent sessions was that the instructions actually sustained his improved performance. Subject Two used oral reading and monologues during a treatment which combined positive reinforcement (praise plus points for tangible reinforcers contingent on one minute of fluent speech) and time-out. Initially, this subject's stutterings went from 3 to 7.7 per minute (100-120 wpm) during A

[16] This is an interesting application of this design since it permits some indication as to when nontreatment and treatment condition effects may blend.

conditions, but reduced to around 2 per minute during treatment conditions. When the time-out and reinforcement schedules were investigated separately, the data generally indicated that reinforcement was redundant. Nevertheless, the schedule was continued and was later augmented by the formerly mentioned "fluency instructions." Once again, the instructions appear to have been responsible for maintaining 0.5 disfluencies per minute with no evident change in speech rate. Subject Three averaged 6.2 disfluencies per minute (125 wpm) prior to treatment, which reduced to about 0.5 per minute (156 wpm) before the "fluency instructions" were introduced. Self-managed counting and time-out were finally alternated with clinician-administered counting or time-out for stuttering. The data show that self-counting produced a comparative reduction in stuttering relative to clinician counts, but this pattern changed during the time-out conditions. These data are difficult to interpret, however, because they also followed the introduction of "fluency instructions."

Carry-over and follow-up data in Costello's study were gathered informally. They indicated that 27 months after treatment "no stuttering was noted" from Subject One, while Subject Two continued to receive treatment, and Subject Three still had difficulties in some situations. In general, these findings show that a combination of treatment procedures, which included time-out, produced improved performance in all subjects during clinic conditions. This improvement may have been sustained in only one subject. But in the absence of independent evaluation of the effects of the "fluency instructions," it is quite possible that this procedure alone might have produced the same, or superior, gains to those reported from time-out, however unlikely that may seem from previous research.

There have been other therapy reports which described the use of punishment schedules. Perhaps the best known are part of a clinical research program directed by Bruce Ryan. These treatment studies will be discussed later since they are more easily understood within the context of various other programs that Ryan has directed. Occasionally, RCS punishment procedures have also been embedded within other therapy procedures. For example, Rustin (1978) described a therapy program which used a variety of techniques, including time-out, for subjects who failed to respond totally to relaxation or slow speech. Intriguingly, this data-less report recommended that if "the general level of anxiety is high 'time-out' is not indicated, as it will increse anxiety which would cause deterioration in the speech" (1978, p. 89). No basis for this recommendation was provided. In another example, Poppen, Nunn, and Hook (1977) described a method for identifying an appropriate treatment via a behavioral approach. A 23-year-old stutterer[17] received a variety of treatment techniques, including a very simple application of time-out: "each time a disfluency occurred, the therapist raised his finger, stopping the client, who paused and then continued speaking" (p. 37). Over 10 30-minute time-out sessions the subject apparently reduced stuttering, but the effect deteriorated towards the end of these sessions. Unfortunately, no supportive data were provided for this interpretation.

[17] This subject was included in Jones and Azrin's (1969) experiment on metronomic stimulation.

The therapeutic effects of RCS procedures, particularly for children, have been among the most promising in the stuttering therapy literature. But they appear to have had a relatively limited impact on therapy practice, especially in view of the positive and clinically significant findings by Martin et al. (1972) and Reed and Godden (1977). It is remarkable that such simple and efficient therapy procedures appear to have received such a relatively lukewarm reception from the clinical community—at least in terms of subsequent publications. It may still be too early to recognize their impact, but there is a disconcerting suggestion in this quietness that more-than-positive data might be necessary to alter clinical practice.

Combination Reinforcement and Punishment Procedures

On the face of it there is much to be gained by joining reinforcement and punishment schedules in therapy. But impressions do not always accord with reality: one of the surprising findings from the experimental RCS studies was that combining these contingency schedules has not yielded additive gains. Nevertheless, there appear to be numerous ways in which these schedules could be combined for therapeutic benefit, some of which merit consideration. For example, the gains achieved by a punishment schedule may be supplemented by a subsequent reinforcement schedule in order to sustain such gains. In the following review it will be observed that this organization of RCS schedules is often used. But it is not always clear when either the reinforcement or punishment schedule was effective, or which was responsible for therapy benefits.

The last point is partly illustrated in one of the first stuttering treatment reports which used behavioral procedures, that by Browning (1967). In this unusual study, a 9-year-old schizophrenic stutterer (who also displayed psychomotor seizures) was treated in a hospital setting, first by reciprocal inhibition, and then by reinforcement of successive approximations to spontaneous fluent speech. This was followed by social reinforcement of fluent responses by the hospital staff. The punishment procedure is not described as such by Browning, but during the social reinforcement phase it was reported that the staff had to ensure that the subject repeated a statement correctly whenever he made an error (stuttering). The subject's percentage of words "stuttered or blocked" was obtained from daily samples of conversational speech and oral reading (amounts unspecified). They show that reduced stuttering occurred in conversational speech whenever the staff issued social reinforcers contingent on fluency (and punishment for stuttering). Parallel effects were observed in the subject's oral reading. By the end of this treatment (140 days), the subject's stuttering had declined from around 22% to 2 or 3% words stuttered. The difficulties with this study are that the data was not supported by reliability estimates, specifications of the amount of speech measured, or posttreatment data.

In 1969, Griffin and Van Kirk also reported a relatively unusual therapy using reinforcement and punishment schedules. In this report (eventually published by Ryan, 1974), a lecturer, who was a stutterer, was treated during teaching by organizing some students in his class to cough contingent on stuttering, and smile, or be attentive, "during periods of fluency." The subject had relapsed after earlier treatment, and displayed about 2.5 stuttered words per minute (sw/m) during lectures (instructions "to be fluent" showed he could produce 0.07 sw/m). During the treatment his stutterings reduced to 0.4 sw/m and remained below this level in three subsequent classes. Thereafter, the students were scheduled to converse with the subject in different locations. It was claimed (without data) that his low level of stuttering was sustained for two terms. Unfortunately, no reliability data were collected to bolster this finding.

A report by McDermott (1971) illustrated a sequential application of punishment and reinforcement in a therapy study on a 9-year-old stutterer. During 24-minute sessions, conducted once or twice weekly, his stuttering was treated first by 10 seconds time-out for speaking, and then with the addition of points for two minutes of stutter-free speech. Finally, listeners were added to the sessions and the subject recorded any stutterings on a hand-held counter. The data show that during base rate the subject averaged around 40% words stuttered and this declined to less than 1% over the course of therapy (this was an estimate, since words were not counted during treatment). A follow-up session 15 weeks after therapy showed about 3% words stuttered. The boy's mother also reported some variability in stuttering. Once again, however, no reliability measures were provided in support of these data.

The treatment studies conducted or directed by Bruce Ryan, and more recently Ryan and Barbara Van Kirk, form one of the most extensive and productive applications of RCS principles to stuttering therapy. This work began in the mid-1960s with the use of performance-criteria schedules designed to integrate a nonbehavioral treatment, primarily Van Riper's (1963) methods, and reinforcement/punishment schedules. In recent years these schedules have been combined with methods developed by Rickard and Mundy (1965), Haroldson, Martin and Starr (1968), and Goldiamond (1965). In turn, this has resulted in studies (Ryan, 1974) which have been designed to compare the efficacy of these methods. Most of Ryan's work will be reviewed here. The exception will be those studies that have used either DAF or prolonged speech techniques based upon Goldiamond's work.

The first published description of Ryan's treatment procedures (Ryan, 1970) outlined a therapy schedule which has remained relatively unchanged over subsequent publications. The subject passes through establishment, transfer, and maintenance phases by achieving (usually) less than 0.5 sw/m over a hierarchy of speaking tasks within each phase. A 14-year-old stutterer's therapy illustrated the procedure. During establishment the subject received a programmatic version of Van Riper's (1963) methods for reducing stutterings. This involved training the subject to identify, cancel and then prolong anticipated stutterings during increasing amounts of oral reading, monologue, and conversational speech. Then the subject had to sustain criterion performance over a transfer phase. This phase was composed of different physical settings, audiences, and telephone tasks with and without the clinician. In the maintenance phase, the subject's contact with the clinician was systematically decreased via telephone, written reports, and tape recordings. This maintenance phase is also checked across different settings while the subject's use of self-controlling activities is presumed to fade. The subject began treatment with a base rate of between four and 24 sw/m during oral reading and monologue. He completed part of the maintenance phase (for a second time) and had maintained less than 0.5 sw/m for six months.

In 1971, Ryan reported the treatment of five children (6-9 years), including three who were treated mainly by praise or points (exchangeable for game-playing time or toys) contingent on fluent utterances. (The other two were treated with DAF or prolonged speech.) These children were also contingently punished for stutterings by either repeating a stuttered word, counting stutterings with a hand-counter, or loss of points. Maintenance programs using the same reinforcement or punishment schedules were conducted in the home or school. It was reported that sw/m scores in clinic conditions decreased to less than 0.5 (from between 7.3 and 15.0 before treatment), which was generally maintained for between 8 and 18 months after treatment., The difficulties with these findings are that no beyond-clinic data were collected, and the reliability of the treatment measures was not determined. Another important problem is the absence of word output or speech rate data, which leads to the possibility that the stuttered words-per-minute scores were simply varied by rate of speaking (see Ingham & Andrews, 1973b).

The most detailed evaluation of Ryan's therapy programs appears in his book written in 1974. This provides extensive data from four different establishment-phase treatment procedures: "traditional" (the programmed version of Van Riper's methods), "punishment" (response-contingent verbal stimulation), "GILCU" (a gradual-increase-in-length-and-complexity-utterance procedure derived from Rickard and Mundy, 1965), and DAF. An important feature of this report was that the treatment data were supplemented by scores from a "Criterion Test" (five minutes of oral reading, monologue, and conversation) given at intervals across the therapy phases, plus measures of words spoken per minute. It is almost impossible to do justice to the vast amount of data reported in this publication. Some notion of the clinical value of the procedures, however, can be gauged by confining this review to the two procedures which have most relevance to RCS therapy practice: "punishment" and "GILCU".[18]

Only two subjects (DC, 15 years; DH_3, 20 years) were treated by the punishment schedule during the establishment phase. No specific information was provided on session length (probably 10-40 minutes, one to five times a week), or responsiveness to the schedule. It was indicated that DC was treated by response-contingent "no," and DH_3 experienced tape-recorded replay of his stuttering as a contingency. This occurred during oral reading, monologue, and conversational speech. Both subjects stuttered in excess of 8.6 occasions per minute before establishment and 0.7 per minute (or less) after this phase on a monologue- and conversation-based Criterion Test. Only subject DC proceeded through the transfer tasks, and, during the phase, averaged 0.2 sw/m. DC actually received only part of the transfer phase and no maintenance phase, and when

[18]To some extent the omission of the "traditional" group from this review is also justified because no information was provided on the reliability with which response classes, such as "cancellation" or "pullouts," were recorded by clinicians.

followed up three months later recorded 1.3 sw/m (presumably on the Criterion Test). Also, no nonclinic data were provided. Since much incidental feedback of performance, positive social reinforcement, and even instructions to be fluent were reported to have been included with the punishment procedure (1974, p. 125), it is difficult to identify the main treatment agent within the therapy for these subjects.

Ryan's (1974) GILCU program, involving 54 steps, "starts with reading a single word and works up to five minutes of fluent conversation." Also included were various "branch programs" to deal with constant failure at any step. Nine subjects (7-35 years), six of whom were 7 to 9 years old, were treated by this program in the establishment phase. On the Criterion Test, these children produced 0.6 to 15.0 sw/m scores before "establishment," and less than 0.5 sw/m scores after this treatment phase. The three older subjects had higher pretreatment and slightly higher posttreatment scores (1.5-0.0 sw/m) than their younger counterparts. Only one subject completed the transfer and maintenance procedures, and follow-up data were reported for only five subjects (all children). All were reported speaking with less than 0.5 sw/m 8 to 21 months after their treatment ceased. Subject BH, who completed all treatment phases, was assessed as stutter-free 21 months after treatment. He was, incidentally, one of the three children mentioned in Ryan's earlier (1971) treatment report. In the present report, his treatment was described in some detail which revealed that a parent-managed program, involving points contingent on fluency, was also instituted during the maintenance phase (1974, p. 128). Furthermore, the follow-up data were derived from a 3.5-minute telephone conversation, rather than the Criterion Test. This suggests that the rather formalized treatment format was supplemented by treatment and measurement methods which make it difficult to confidently judge the therapeutic strength of the procedures. In fact, most criticisms leveled at Ryan's 1971 report also apply in this case: no beyond-clinic treatment measures (other than the telephone conversations), or speech-rate scores supported the findings.

From a clinical perspective, the most interesting data on Ryan's treatment procedures have appeared in some recent general accounts of his work. For example, in 1979 Ryan reported comparisons between sw/m scores of subjects on the Criterion Test (five minutes of oral reading, monologue, and conversation), the Fluency Interview (14 or 20 speaking tasks, which include speaking with others and telephone conversations), and a Natural Speech Sample (from recordings made in home and school settings). These data were described by Ryan to "reveal similarity among the three measures" (1979, p. 156). In fact, as can be seen from the reproduction of this table (Table 9.1), "similarity" may be in the eye of the beholder. For this beholder, it indicates that during the course of treatment the Natural Speech Sample means were either 280% or 100% greater than the Criterion Test means! It is intriguing to imagine the differences that may have also existed within the scores of individual subjects across these measures.

Other pertinent information on Ryan's treatment program has appeared in a more recent report (Ryàn, 1981). This included follow-up data on 10 children (9-16

Table 9-1
Assessment-procedure data from across treatment conditions reported by Ryan (1979, p. 156).

	PRE-ESTABLISHMENT SW/M Mean (n=40)	POST ESTABLISHMENT SW/M Mean (n=39)	POST TRANSFER SW/M Mean (n=27)
Criterion Test	7.2	1.0	0.8
Fluency Interview	7.4	3.7	1.0
Natural Speech Sample	7.5	3.8	1.6

years) who were treated by either the GILCU (n=9) or punishment (n=1) procedures during the establishment phase. At the end of the maintenance phase, five children were stutter-free (only one had scores above 0.8 sw/m) and seven had increased their speech rate from that recorded before treatment. However, at follow-up (7-20 months later), none of the children were stutter-free, although five had scores of less than 0.5 sw/m. These data are certainly encouraging, especially since they were derived from programs conducted by a variety of clinicians. This fact alone highlights the durability of this treatment procedure. But the extent to which these data can be claimed to represent the child's customary speaking behavior is debatable.

In fairness, only part of the therapy programs that Ryan has reported have been reviewed in this chapter (the DAF therapy will be considered in Chapter 10). Nevertheless, they provide an impressive picture of considerable therapeutic benefit, particularly in the case of children. There is some unfortunate laxity in the measurement methodology and the specificity of treatment procedures, but the reviewed studies provide a fairly consistent record of benefits from well conceived procedures that have obvious utility in many settings.

Other examples of the GILCU treatment procedure have been provided by Mowrer (1975), Johnson, Coleman, and Rasmussen (1978), and Costello (1980). Mowrer also provided a relatively detailed description of an establishment, transfer, and maintenance treatment schedule which incorporated graduated steps through different speaking tasks and situations. This was followed by decreasingly frequent clinic visits and telephone conversations. Fifteen stutterers (8-43 years) were treated by this schedule for four to six hours daily (presumably in the establishment phase), and were assessed before and after treatment on Ryan's (1974) Fluency Interview Test. But only five subjects (10-31 years) were reported to have completed the transfer or maintenance phases. Their data show that pretreatment and post-treatment mean sw/m scores were, respectively, 8.1 and 0.36. But these data were also unaccompanied by either speech rate or reliability measures. The same is true of Johnson, Coleman, and Rasmussen's (1978) report on the treatment of a 6-year-old male stutterer. The child required 21 hours of therapy time (three one-hour sessions per week) in order to progress from isolated vowels and consonants through to eight-word utterances, with additional word games to assist generalization. The stuttering interview (Ryan, 1974) data show stutterings reduced from 17.4 to 4.4 sw/m over the treatment period, and by a month later to 3.7 sw/m. The proportion of stuttered prolongations, part-word repetitions, and whole-word repetitions changed over the course of these assessments. But no beyond-clinic data were reported. Costello's (1980) report described the treatment of an 11-year-old mild stutterer by a series of steps leading from two-syllable words through to five-minute monologues. No transfer or maintenance procedure was described, although the subject's speech behavior in the home was reported to have been concurrently monitored during the establishment phase. Each stuttering was consequated by "no" or "stop," and target behaviors were rewarded by tokens exchangable for "free time" in the session. Pre- and posttreatment data plus treatment time information were provided; the former shows that the subject's monologue and conversational speech performance went from between 12.0 and 20.0 percent syllables stuttered down to between 0.7 and 1.2 percent syllables stuttered. There was also a concomitant increase in syllables-per-minute scores and improvements in ratings of tension and prosody in the subject's speech. Clinician agreement scores of 87% on stuttered and nonstuttered utterances were judged to be evidence of measurement reliability. The clinical value of these data are weakened by the absence of nonclinic or follow-up measures of performance, however.

The four GILCU treatment reports provide some interesting issues with respect to the internal validity of their procedures. For instance, none of them provided clear evidence that the introduction of any treatment step altered a preceding rate of performance on the target behavior for a particular step. The only way that this could be adequately recognized would be by comparisons with ongoing independent measures of the targets (for example, multisyllables, phrases, etc) during the course of the GILCU procedures. There is also a possibility that a modicum of stuttering may have been constantly reinforced throughout each of the GILCU steps. For example, the criterion of success at any step in Ryan's, Mowrer's and Johnson and colleagues' procedure was, respectively, less than 0.5 sw/m, 95, and 90 percent success; in effect, their subjects could "succeed," yet continue to stutter. This may partially explain why the outcome findings from these treatments rarely included subjects who were stutter-free. In fact pre- and posttreatment data from Mowrer's study equate almost perfectly with his "success" criterion: the mean pretreatment scores for the five subjects, who completed either the transfer or maintenance phases, was 8.1 sw/m, and after treatment it reduced to 0.36 sw/m; this is equivalent to a 95.5 percent decrease. On the other hand, Costello's subject was required to achieve 100% success in order to pass a step, yet still achieved only about 95% fewer stutterings. Nevertheless, it is an aspect of this procedure which merits investigation. A final issue relates to the method used to construct steps within GILCU programs. No clear rationale has been enunciated for defining the number of steps or the number of "successes" required on a step. The general rationale appears to be that gradual increments in task difficulty is an efficient method of learning. In fact, it is quite possible that this may be an inefficient method of changing behavior: concurrent and independent measures of performance might show that some steps could be bypassed without threatening this treatment design or its efficacy.

The importance of a concurrent and beyond-clinic data base is evident in a combined reinforcement and punishment experimental treatment reported by Ingham and Packman (1977). A 42-year-old female stutterer was treated in daily 40-minute clinic sessions, while her beyond-clinic speech behavior was recorded throughout every second day over most of the treatment period. During the first treatment phase, a response-contingent bone-conducted tone produced marginal changes in percentage of syllables stuttered (%SS) scores during spontaneous speech. But the addition of a time-out contingency reduced her stutterings to near zero. The subsequent replication of these experimental phases showed that the time-out control of stuttering faded over time. An assessment of speech-rate control then showed her stutterings could be substantially reduced whenever she spoke at between 150 and 170 syllables per minute (target rate), but this effect was not sustained until the response-contingent bone-conducted signal was added. The subject was then weaned from daily clinic-sessions contingent on maintaining zero stuttering and the target rate. Over this final 95-day phase, the clinic measures revealed she stuttered on two syllables out of 104,698! By contrast she had produced 4.0 %SS during base-rate clinic sessions. But the overall within-clinic data bore almost no resemblance to her beyond-clinic data. Throughout treatment the subject carried a recorder which was designed to record all her speech (from the beginning to the end of the day) every second day. These recordings showed that her %SS score tended to decrease in some settings, but there was considerable variability, and in no situation, other than the clinic, was she stutter-free.[19] Six months after treatment the subject returned to the clinic and was again recorded as stutter-free and within the target speech rate range. However, her beyond-clinic data were quite different. This is essentially an experimental therapy study, but it does illustrate the lack of correspondence between within-clinic and beyond-clinic data, as well as the potential irrelevance of within-clinic "maintenance" data.

There have been other examples of combined punishment and reinforcement schedules in treatments that have used procedures such as "prolonged speech," or in the context of maintenance schedules. These will be considered in other chapters. But some applications of these schedules have occurred within treatment packages designed to deal with different aspects of stuttering. One "package approach" to behavior therapy has been advocated by Lazarus (1976). This is based upon his "multi-modal behavior model," and was used by Beaty (1980) to treat a 15-year-old stutterer. Part of Beaty's package included a "response cost system with rewards for fluent speech." In many ways this study is almost a travesty of the concept of behavior therapy: no details were provided

[19] The method by which such data are subdivided into situational categories has never been addressed in this form of research. Ingham (1981) described how it was possible to categorize such nonclinic data in terms of time dimensions as well as situation dimensions in order to assess generalization. In other words, data categorization procedures may obscure important sources of variance if the method by which data are classified is not recognized.

on the treatment procedures and no objective data were provided to support the claim (from subject-recorded data) of stutter-free speech two months after treatment.

In summary, the combined reinforcement and punishment procedures have provided much promise, but yielded remarkably little clinically useful substance. Without doubt, the GILCU procedure is one of the more interesting approaches to stuttering therapy. It is almost overloaded with face validity as a therapy approach for children and, to a lesser extent, adults. But the therapy evaluation procedures have limited, even scant, external validity. In almost every report of its application, the findings are weakened by the absence of reasonably satisfactory beyond-clinic data. Children may have responded quite well to this procedure, but there is a dire need to demonstrate this responsiveness in clinically meaningful conditions. The importance of this is underscored by the type of data collected by Ingham and Packman (1977).

The Treatment of Nonstuttering Behaviors

Treatments using reinforcement of fluent, or stutter-free speech, showed that modifying nonstuttering behavior may sometimes decrease stuttering. This somewhat indirect approach to treating this disability is not new and has been applied using many types of behavior. In fact, the manipulation of certain speech and nonspeech behaviors (other than stutterings) have been an integral feature of many behavioral and nonbehavioral therapies. In this section the treatments that blend indirect therapy procedures and RCS schedules will be reviewed.

In the preceding section it was noted that Ryan (1970; 1974) had described programming some of Van Riper's (1963) stuttering treatment techniques ("cancellations," "pullouts," and "prolongations") within punishment and reinforcement schedules. Much of this type of therapy appears to have been instigated by George Shames. In his 1969 paper (actually presented in 1966), Shames suggested that the thematic content of clinician-client exchanges might be profitably viewed as a pattern of behaviors that could be systematized and modified by verbal reinforcement procedures. The clinical rationale, which formed the basis of these exchanges, was used to determine which client responses would be strengthened or weakened by these procedures. Some data from interviews with a 20-year-old mild stutterer showed that his frequency of independent decision-making statements (those that defined or described clinical goals) were increased from 60% to 89%. Before- and after-treatment data also showed differences in the number of repetitions during a 60-minute session. An 18-year-old mild stutterer was also treated by a verbal reinforcement schedule which was appended to Van Riper's procedures. The therapy process required him to succeed on 80% or more of the occasions within each step of an eight-step program. The program involved procedures such as identifying stutterings and prolonging the first sound of a word on which he thought he would stutter. Only five treatment steps were described and the data show that the subject's stutterings declined from 2.5 per minute to about one every 25 minutes. From one perspective this program actually involved a "disfluency trade-off": the subject's apparent blocks were replaced by prolongations—albeit of a voluntary type. Unfortunately, neither reliability nor nonclinic data were included with the data for either subject.

The clinical efficacy of manipulating the thematic content and certain types of speech behavior was investigated in a number of reports by Shames and colleagues. The first of these was by Shames, Egolf, and Rhodes (1969). This described two programs: "the stuttering behavior program" and the "thematic content modification program" (TCMP). The first was usually applied to stutterers "who exhibit overt struggle behavior to the extent that communication is seriously impaired." A 30-year-old housewife, who began therapy with 14% words stuttered, was treated in an abridged version of the schedule described by Shames (1969). Her within-clinic data show her stutterings decreased to 2% over six sessions, but again no reliability or beyond-clinic measures were provided. Three other subjects were treated by different versions of TCMP. A 25-year-old was treated by a "TCMP1" schedule—which involves favorable clinician responses to TR+ statements and unfavorable clinician responses to TR− statements. Her data are extremely difficult to interpret: TR+ statements increased inconsistently and TR− statements decreased, but stutterings increased and then decreased back to initial-session level over the 14 sessions. The absence of a stable base rate really precludes any meaningful interpretation of these data. A 41-year-old mild stutterer was treated by "TCMP2." This required the clinician to verbally reinforce only TR+ responses. But over 12 sessions the TR+ responses actually tended to decrease, rather than increase, and eventually reached the level found in the first session! Also, this subject's percentage of words stuttered at the final session was only marginally less than what it was in the first session. The final subject (a 37-year-old female) received a "TCMP3" schedule (which resembles TCMP1, except that the clinician omits noncontingent responses) and did show relative increases in TR+ and decreases in TR− statements over 14 sessions. In addition, her stutterings declined from 8 to 3% of words spoken over the same period. However, all of these data were unaccompanied by reliability or beyond-clinic measures. More importantly, they also provided little or no evidence that the reinforcement/punishment schedule was responsible for any change in thematic content or stutterings. In fact, only one subject's data showed changes that are consistent with a treatment effect, though not necessarily proof of that effect.

The methodological problems in the preceding study appear to have continued in a report by Egolf, Shames, and Blind (1971). The same treatment principles were adapted to the therapy for a 47-year-old female stutterer. Over the initial treatment sessions, the subject's eye contact problems were treated by instructions to "look at me" each time she looked away from the clinician while conversing. In the next treatment stage, the subject was treated by a TCMP3 schedule outlined by Shames, Egolf, and Rhodes (1969). And in a final stage, she was verbally reinforced for following behavioral rules (talking whenever she wished, being unconcerned about her stuttering, comparing her behavior with what others do in similar situations) outside of the clinic. The subject's stuttering frequency declined across all treatment stages, as well as in follow-up sessions 6 and 12 months later, until no stuttering was recorded during that final session. But it is unclear why this occurred. Martin and Ingham's (1973) description of this study highlights its problems:

> The Egolf, Shames and Blind study is noteworthy in that the authors reported carefully collected data on the reliability of the various response classes. On the other hand, this study suffers serious methodological shortcomings. It is entirely possible that the reduction in stuttering frequency is independent of any of the three treatments. This is particularly problematic because the stuttering frequency reduced across sessions irrespective of treatment (p. 118).

The previously described study by Rhodes, Shames, and Egolf (1971) formed another unit in the package of therapy studies that Shames and colleagues reported during this period. This involved the application of TCMP1 in the course of group therapy sessions for two groups (n=4) of adult stutterers. One group was informed about the schedule, while the other group was kept "uninformed." The target thematic content behaviors appeared to change appropriately in the "informed" group, but only in the "uninformed" group was stuttering decreased (approximately 50%).

Shames and Egolf's (1976) book on the management of stuttering using operant conditioning principles also included some findings (p. 115) from the use of TCMP procedures. In a way, these findings illustrate the clinical potency of this procedure. Thirteen adult stutterers were treated by one of the three TCMP procedures, and, though only limited data are provided, they are quite suggestive. Three subjects were treated for between 6 and 18 sessions (time unspecified) by TCMP1. During base-line they exhibited 4 to 14% words stuttered and in the final session 2 to 3%; but only two subjects changed their TR+ and TR− responses in the hypothesized directions. Three other subjects were treated by TCMP2 over 7 to 14 sessions. Only one of these subjects increased TR+ responses and decreased stuttering by the final session. The seven other subjects on TCMP3 (4 to 18 sessions) showed an even more inconsistent pattern: only one subject showed hypothesized changes in TR+ and TR− responses, as well as a decrease in stuttering. In summary, only four of the 13 subjects altered their thematic content and reduced stuttering in accordance with the purpose of this therapy.

To some extent the last-mentioned findings add to a recurring implication in the data from TCMP studies; that is, the procedure has inconsistent effects and rarely shows a consistent relationship with stuttering. At best, it appears to be a not very powerful procedure for altering either thematic content or stuttering. One plausible indication of the clinical merit of both of these procedures is expressed by the direction of Shames's later clinical research. This shows much more interest in the use of procedures derived from DAF effects on stuttering and self-management procedures (Shames, 1975; Shames and Florance, 1980).

The child stutterer's pattern of interaction with his parents has been an area of speculation and theory in the stuttering literature over many years. One therapeutic approach to this aspect of the disorder is to implement techniques that directly alter these patterns of interaction. Two experimental therapy reports have described such an approach, one without and one with the use of formalized response-contingent schedules.

Egolf, Shames, Johnson and Kasprisin-Burrelli (1972) used a method designed to alter the pattern of parent-child interactions during therapy for nine children (5-13 years) who stuttered. Before treatment, each child-parent pattern of interaction was described in terms of broad categories (for example, "mother did not react differentially to fluent and stuttered speech", p. 224) and the clinician was instructed to interact "in a manner different from that of the parent" (p. 226). However, in Stage One of the two-stage therapy process (involving an unspecified number of 40-minute sessions), the children's recorded efforts at achieving fluency were replayed in each session so that they could evaluate their performances. After achieving less than 1% stuttering in a session, the child moved to Stage Two, wherein the parent also interacted with the child during treatment sessions. The researchers hypothesized that parent-child interaction patterns were "maintaining factors of stuttering" and that their results "support the hypothesized relationship" (p. 222). But their data did not invite such convincing conclusions. Some reductions in mean-stuttering frequencies were reported from comparisons before and after treatment (40.2% reduction in a controlled waiting-room situation and 85.3% reduction in the treatment situation). However, four of the nine subjects showed higher stuttering frequencies on the final "controlled waiting room" or "treatment session" when compared with their average first half of Stage One scores. In fact, on inspection, neither the procedure nor the reported data support the researchers' conclusions. The procedures were clearly confounded by the speech-performance-evaluation technique, which had ample claim as a cause for any alterations in stuttering. More importantly, no data were provided to show that the interaction patterns were actually changed, or that the introduction of this procedure coincided with changes in stuttering.

The second study of interest was reported by Wahler, Sperling, Thomas, Teeter, and Luper (1970). Theirs was also concerned with interaction patterns, but in the form of problem behaviors that were treated by contingency schedules. The study by Wahler et al. was founded upon research by Lovaas (1961), Sherman (1964), and Wahler and Pollio (1968), which had shown some functional relationships between verbal and nonverbal behavior. It involved the treatment of a 4- and a 9-year-old stutterer, both of whom displayed what the parents labeled as problem behaviors. The 4-year-old displayed "oppostional behavior" to parent requests, and the 9-year-old exhibited "activity shifts" (failure to sustain interactions on one object, person, or topic). The 4-year-old was run in an ABAB schedule of playroom sessions (duration unspecified) managed by the child's mother. The child's oppositional behavior and stutterings were monitored in weekly A sessions. In B sessions, five minutes of time-out (removal from the clinic room) was contingent on instances of oppositional behavior. This technique was also combined with verbal reinforcement for cooperative behavior. The results show that oppositional behavior and stutterings (per 10-second intervals) were concomitantly reduced. The same procedure was then continued in the home. Following 5 base-rate sessions, 4 treatment sessions produced almost complete elimination of both behaviors, and that gain was sustained in 11 follow-up sessions over a six-month period. The 9-year-old was first treated at home by parents who were instructed "to respond differentially to his fluent and stuttered speech." This showed some reduction in clinic sessions, but not at home. Then followed an ABAB sequence of therapy sessions in which activity shifts and stutterings (per 10-second units) were recorded. In the B sessions, the clinician and the parents contingently ignored the subject until he returned to the discontinued activity. The data trends over these sessions clearly indicated that activity shifts and stutterings were reduced by about 90% during the B conditions. In subsequent home sessions, the procedure was repeated and stuttering was virtually eliminated; it remained that way throughout a six-month follow-up interval (though activity-shift data were not recorded). The data were supplemented by satisfactory indicators of scorer reliability, plus measures showing the independence of the problem behaviors and stuttering during treatment and nontreatment sessions. There is also clear evidence that the subject's verbal output tended to increase whenever stuttering decreased.

In summary, the therapy studies that have used RCS procedures with nonstuttering behaviors are probably best described as uneven in both quality and outcome. Most have emerged from efforts by Shames and his colleagues to demonstrate the manipulability of behaviors used by Van Riper to control stuttering, and verbal behaviors claimed to improve or retard therapy progress. In general, these studies have failed to yield any conclusive data. There is certainly little evidence to suggest that the thematic content of stutterers' speech is functionally related to stuttering. At the very least, these concepts need further investigation in more controlled contexts before their therapeutic utility can be deduced. By contrast, the findings by the Wahler et al. study are among the most provocative in the stuttering literature. Their findings—admittedly from only two children—show strong evidence of the therapeutic potential in treating certain nonstuttering behaviors. However, a decade has passed since that study was conducted. It is therefore surprising that other clinicians have not reported even a partial replication of the procedure, let alone the findings.

Self-Managed Response-Contingent Procedures

The advantages of self-managed treatments over clinician-managed treatments for stuttering are virtually self-evident. The very ubiquitous nature of speech behavior means that any procedure that relies on other-person management is likely to be weakened by its failure to control all speech during treatment. Self-managed procedures also have obvious economic advantages with respect to clinician time. When these advantages are coupled with promising findings from experimental studies, it is remarkable that they have found so little application in therapy.

One of the earliest endeavors to employ subject-management of RCS procedures in stuttering therapy was a "shaping group" program described by Leith and Uhlemann (1972) and Leith (1979). Strictly speaking, this was a group-managed rather than subject-managed treatment, since the group directed the therapy process. In this treatment, the group members were instructed first in the principles of operant conditioning and then trained (presumably by the model of a group leader) to respond accordingly to each member's self-identified positive and negative behaviors. Applications of these programs have included the use of token and verbal reinforcement techniques (Leith, 1979). The only data-based report of this therapy procedure is by Leith and Uhlemann (1972), which describes the treatment of four stutterers and six nonstutterers (presumably adults). The group met for two 20-hour "marathon" sessions and, in the case of the stutterers, weekly two-hour sessions in the five-week interval between the marathon sessions. The only objective speech behavior measures were derived from pre- and posttreatment oral readings of "The Rainbow Passage" (Fairbanks, 1940) before a class of students: two subjects decreased their disfluencies (20% and 37% reductions) but two actually increased their disfluencies. This finding does little to recommend the treatment, especially since the pre- and posttherapy differences may not have exceeded within-subject variability preceding treatment (such data were not provided).

Another relatively unusual application of self-management methods is a "cognitive conditioning therapy" program reported by Berecz (1973; 1976). In this procedure the subject self-delivers shock while imagining situations or cues "which trigger stuttering," then the subject is instructed to "relax, and think about talking fluently." A male adult stutterer was reported to have received this therapy for four sessions, but he then requested termination of therapy. He was persuaded to continue with a treatment in which the clinician delivered the shock during descriptions of relevant situations. The only semblance of data within this report is the subject's judgment (six weeks after a break from therapy) that "his stuttering was down to 35 or 40 percent of the original level" (1973, p. 265). In a subsequent report, Berecz (1976) described treating a 29-year-old female stutterer solely by the self-administered shock procedure over 70 25-minute sessions (the frequency of these sessions was not specified). Once again, only self-report data were used to support the claim that she had reduced her stuttering by 75% over the course of treatment. In evaluating these data, it is noteworthy that Leith and Uhlemann (1972) reported that all subjects overestimated their rate of improvement when compared with objective data.

In the experimental section of this chapter, a description was given of La Croix's (1973) study on the effects of self-counting stuttering by two subjects. As mentioned, this study reported the most promising data yet recorded on self-management with stuttering. Only disfluency counts were recorded, but these were reduced from 8 to 1% in one subject and from 9-11% to around 2% for the other over the course of sessions involving 30-minute conversations. The posttreatment performance was not recorded, but informal reports indicated one subject maintained improved fluency while the other had little carry-over.

In another previously reviewed study, Costello (1975) reported the self-administered use of time-out, or counting stutterings, by one subject during the last phases of a response-contingent treatment. But a more extensive and conclusive assessment of such a procedure was described by James (1981b). This study, which reported a self-managed time-out treatment of an 18-year-old male stutterer, is, in many respects, one of the best designed in the treatment literature.

The merit in James's study is that it integrated experimental and clinical procedures in a therapy format that permitted within- and beyond-clinic treatment effects to be reasonably well established. The subject's speech was repeatedly recorded in five situations: alone and in conversation within the clinic, outside the clinic on the telephone, at home, and during shopping assignments. These assessments produced measures of percentage of syllables stuttered, percentage of interjections, and syllables per minute. In the first experimental treatment, a multiple base-line design was used to isolate the effects of introducing, first, clinician-administered time-out (at least two seconds), followed by self-initiated time-out during monologue and conversational speech. (Immediately afterwards, the subject made four- to five-minute recordings in the home and during phone conversations; also, less frequently, speech behavior while shopping.) The data show that the percentage of disfluencies (stutterings plus interjections) decreased from a base rate of around 8-12% in the clinic to approximately 2% in both time-out conditions. (This was demonstrated independently during monologue and conversational speech.) In the beyond-clinic setting, there were reduced disfluencies when the subject covertly "timed-out" stutterings. In the final extinction sessions, the percentages of disfluency returned to near base rate levels. During the first experiment, it was observed that the subject initiated time-out contingent on only 45.5% of his disfluencies. Thus a response-cost procedure (loss of 5¢ contingent on failure to initiate time-out) was combined with time-out procedure, and its effects were measured over a multiple base line ABB'A experimental design in which the final condition was follow-up data collected six and 12 months after treatment sessions. This second experiment's data showed that fewer than 1% of disfluencies remained over almost all assessment sessions, and the percentage of self-initiated time-out increased to 62.8%. The follow-up data show that these low levels were generally sustained. The only exception was percentage of interjections; they returned to near base-rate levels during some beyond-clinic assessments. It is difficult to judge the clinical significance of this rise in interjections, but it may suggest that this remained a continuing problem. In addition to the data summarized above, measures of reliability and speech-rate data indicate these findings were not vulnerable to error from either source (the subject's treatment and follow-up speech-rate scores were consistently above base-rate scores).

The limited number of self-managed RCS therapy studies is likely to be a temporary phenomenon. This will be evident in the next chapter, which will review the growing number of studies that have combined this procedure with treatments using variations of the prolonged speech pattern (Goldiamond, 1965). In the midst of presently reported self-managed RCS therapy studies, there exist some guides on how this procedure may be applied with profit. Perhaps the most useful guide is the method and procedures used by La Croix (1973) and James (1981b). The James study also provides a useful indication of the quality of treatment research that is needed to discern the clinical value of this therapy approach. Indeed, when this study is considered in relation to many RCS therapy studies it provides one measure of the difference between poor and well designed therapy research.

Conclusions on RCS Therapy Studies

Over the past decade there have been a number of reviews on the contribution that response-contingent methodology has made to stuttering therapy. Some of the early reviews of these therapy approaches were far from complimentary, and drew attention to the wide disparity between the sophisticated methodology used in the experimental investigations of RCS and the inadequacies of most clinical applications of these procedures (Bloodstein, 1975; Ingham & Andrews, 1973b). Others saw the whole enterprise as almost destined to failure (Murphy, 1970; Sheehan, 1970; Van Riper, 1970). One of the more frequently quoted descriptions of the earlier clinical studies is by Martin and Ingham (1973):

> The extent to which laboratory data can be used to develop reliable therapeutic procedures for stutterers is. . .encouraging, but considerable work remains to be done. The reports of response-contingent stuttering therapy programs or techniques. . .are far from satisfactory. There is evidence that the procedures may affect changes within some therapy programs, but the data are difficult to evaluate. Most reports are premature and do not include carefully obtained carry-over or follow up data. Most reports contain no information at all about the reliability of the observers. Many reports do not employ a carefully specified and unambiguous stuttering response class. Many reports do not make it clear that the treatment variable under study is in fact responsible for the change in stuttering. Most reports contain no data about the extent to which speech parameters other than fluency are modified. Hopefully, future clinical studies will take account of these shortcomings, even though it may be expensive. In the interim, there is little reliable evidence to support the use of response-contingent treatment procedures in stuttering therapy. (p. 126-127.)

The obvious question to ask now is, "Has the situation changed since the time of that review?"

The past decade has certainly delivered a mixed bag of treatments from which to determine support for the use of RCS procedures in stuttering therapy. In the final analysis, the real test is whether the decade has yielded studies which, first of all, can be reasonably described as producing findings that have adequate internal and external validity, and second, which show that improved fluency is durable across time and situations. The fact that the former feature may obtain is no guarantee that the latter has occurred. But, when even the most liberal criteria are used to judge these studies from both vantage points, the list that emerges is remarkably small. In fact, such studies can be easily listed.

Among the reinforcement-procedure studies, Peters's (1977) has some reasonable internal validity, but it provides unsatisfactory evidence of durability of effects. By contrast, Martin, Kuhl, and Haroldson's (1972) and Reed and Godden's

(1977) studies with children show durable gains from response-contingent punishment schedules, and in treatment designs that have reasonable internal and external validity. The Ingham and Packman (1977) study shows that stutter-free speech may be sustained in clinic conditions by combined punishment and reinforcement procedures, but these effects do not necessarily generalize beyond that setting. Finally, James's (1981b) study provides a convincing demonstration that useful treatment gains might be achieved within a self-managed time-out schedule. In this case, the strength of the evaluation procedure was also demonstrated by its capacity to detect situation-related variability. The GILCU studies by Ryan (1974) have also produced rather suggestive evidence of the durability of the procedure's effect on children, although the internal validity of the treatment evaluation method is somewhat suspect. In other words, only six studies have produced some within- and beyond-clinic data that might counter part of the criticism offered by Martin and Ingham (1973).

Few as these studies might be, they have provided some important findings with respect to therapy practices, particularly for children. The Martin et al. (1972), Reed and Godden (1977), and Ryan (1974) studies have directly challenged some long-held notions on stuttering treatment for young children. There now exists some fairly persuasive evidence that RCS procedures may assist in removing or markedly reducing stuttering in some children. They also provide some good reasons for reducing one of the clinician's "fears of stuttering" (Wingate, 1971); that is, concern about drawing attention to the disorder. These are findings which directly contradict the traditional, and even recent, arguments (Zwitman, 1978) that the child's stuttering should not be managed by either highlighting it or by advice to "slow down." But it is not at all clear that these data-based findings will be sufficient to relieve the concerns of some clinicians. Then again, it is not at all clear how these concerns may be assuaged.

It should be apparent by now that clinicians and clinical researchers who employ and investigate RCS procedures in stuttering therapy are exceptionally critical of both the methodology and findings of such studies. But there is a level of criticism that serves no useful purpose. For example, a recurring theme in criticism of RCS techniques by Van Riper (1970; 1973) and Sheehan (1970; 1979), plus others, is that most of these procedures "are mechanical methods routinely administered to the person without regard to his lifestyle or individual motivations" (Sheehan, 1979, p. 206). Such an interpretation of these treatments is probably warranted in some instances. But good therapy and poor therapy is practiced within any clinical orientation. The routine use of such procedures represents the antithesis of the way these approaches should be employed by clinicians. And, certainly, no therapeutic approach has a mortgage on compassion and clinical sensitivity; it should go without saying that they are likely to be necessary features of any effective therapy, including those described in this chapter.

References

Adams,M.R. Some comments on "Time-out as punishment for stuttering." *Journal of Speech and Hearing Research*, 1970, *13*, 218-220.

Adams, M.R. Some comments on "Effects of five experimental treatments on stuttering." *Journal of Speech and Hearing Research*, 1980, *23*, 210-213.

Adams, M.R., Lewis, J.I., & Besozzi, T.E. The effect of reduced reading rate on stuttering frequency. *Journal of Speech and Hearing Research*, 1973, *16*, 671-675.

Adams, M.R., & Popelka, G. The influence of "time-out" on stutterers and their dysfluency. *Behavior Therapy*, 1971, *2*, 334-339.

Azrin, N.H. Some effects of noise on human behavior. *Journal of the Experimental Analysis of Behavior*, 1958, *1*, 183-200.

Baer, D.M., Wolf, M.M., & Risley, T.R. Some current dimensions of applied behavior analysis. *Journal of Applied Behavior Analysis*, 1968, *1*, 91-97.

Bar, A. The shaping of fluency not the modification of stuttering. *Journal of Communication Disorders*, 1971, *4*, 1-8.

Bar, A. Increasing fluency in young stutterers vs decreasing stuttering: a clinical approach. *Journal of Communication Disorders*, 1973, *6*, 247-258.

Beattie, M.S. A behaviour therapy programme for stuttering. *British Journal of Disorders of Communication*, 1973, *8*, 120-130.

Beaty, D.T. A multimodal approach to elimination of stuttering. *Perceptual and Motor Skills*, 1980, *50*, 51-55.

Berecz, J.M. The treatment of stuttering through precision punishment and cognitive arousal. *Journal of Speech and Hearing Disorders*, 1973, *38*, 256-267.

Berecz, J.M. Cognitive conditioning therapy in the treatment of stuttering. *Journal of Communication Disorders*, 1976, *9*, 301-315.

Biggs, B., & Sheehan, J.G. Punishment or distraction? Operant stuttering revisited. *Journal of Abnormal Psychology*, 1969, *74*, 256-262.

Bijou, S.W., & Baer, D.M. Operant methods in child behavior and development. In W.K. Honig (Ed.), *Operant behavior: Areas of research and application*. New York: Appleton-Century-Crofts, 1966.

Bloodstein, O. *A handbook on stuttering*. Chicago: The National Easter Seal Society, 1969.

Bloodstein, O. *A handbook on stuttering*. (2nd ed.) Chicago: The National Easter Seal Society, 1975.

Bloodstein, O. The operant model of stuttering. *Journal of Speech and Hearing Research*, 1979, *22*, 665-666.

Bloodstein, O. *A handbook on stuttering*. (3rd ed.) Chicago: The National Easter Seal Society, 1981.

Brady, J.P. Studies on the metronome effect on stuttering. *Behaviour Research and Therapy*, 1969, *7*, 197-205.

Breland, K., & Breland, M. The misbehavior of organisms. *American Psychologist*, 1961, *16*, 681-684.

Breland, K., & Breland, M. *Animal behavior*. New York: MacMillan, 1966.

Brookshire, R.H. The use of consequences in speech pathology: Incentive and feedback functions. *Journal of Communication Disorders*, 1973, *6*, 88-92.

Browning, R.M. Behaviour therapy for stuttering in a schizophrenic child. *Behaviour Research and Therapy*, 1967, *5*, 27-35.

Brutten, G.J. Stuttering: Topography, assessment and behavior-change strategies. In J. Eisenson (Ed.), *Stuttering: A second symposium*. New York: Harper & Row, 1975.

Brutten, G.J. The effect of punishment on a Factor 1 stuttering behavior. *Journal of Fluency Disorders*, 1980, *5*, 77-85.

Brutten, G.J., & Shoemaker, D.J. *The modification of stuttering*. Englewood Cliffs, N.J.: Prentice-Hall, 1967.

Brutten, G.J., & Shoemaker, D.J. A two-factor learning theory of stuttering. In L.E. Travis (Ed.), *Handbook of speech pathology and audiology*. New York: Appleton-Century-Crofts, 1971.

Chomsky, N. Reviews: *Verbal Behavior* by B.F. Skinner, *Language*, 1959, *35*, 26-58.

Cooper, E.B., Cady, B.B. & Robbins, C.J. The effect of the verbal stimulus words, "wrong," "right" and "tree" on the disfluency rates of stutterers and nonstutterers. *Journal of Speech and Hearing Research*, 1970, *13*, 239-244.

Corcoran, J.A. Effects of neutral and positive stimuli on stuttering: "Calling attention to stuttering" revisited. *Journal of Fluency Disorders*, 1980, *5*, 99-114.

Costello, J.M. The establishment of fluency with time-out procedures: Three case studies. *Journal of Speech and Hearing Disorders*, 1975, *40*, 216-231.

Costello, J.M. Operant conditioning and the treatment of stuttering. In W.H. Perkins (Ed.), *Seminars in speech, language and hearing: Strategies in stuttering therapy* (Vol. 1). New York: Brian C. Decker, 1980.

Costello, J.M., & Hurst, M.R. An analysis of the relationship among stuttering behaviors. *Journal of Speech and Hearing Research*, 1981, *24*, 247-256.

Cross, D.E., & Cooper, E.B. Self- versus investigator-administered presumed fluency reinforcing stimuli. *Journal of Speech and Hearing Research*, 1976, *19*, 241-246.

Crowder, J.E. & Harbin, R. The effect of punishment on stuttering: A case study. *Psychotherapy: Theory, Research and Practice*, 1971, *8*, 179-180.

Curlee, R.F., & Perkins, W.H. The effect of punishment of expectancy to stutter on the frequencies of subsequent expectancies and stuttering. *Journal of Speech and Hearing Research*, 1968, *11*, 787-795.

Daly, D.A., & Cooper, E.B. Rate of stuttering adaptation under two electroshock conditions. *Behaviour Research and Therapy*, 1967, *5*, 49-54.

Daly, D.A., & Frick, J.V. The effects of punishing stuttering expectations and stuttering utterances: A comparative study. *Behavior Therapy*, 1970, *1*, 228-239.

Daly, D.A., & Kimbarow, M.L. Stuttering as operant behavior: Effects of the verbal stimuli *wrong*, *right*, and *tree* on the disfluency rates of school-age stutterers and nonstutterers. *Journal of Speech and Hearing Research*, 1978, *21*, 589-597.

Dunham, P. The nature of reinforcing stimuli. In W.K. Honig & J.E.R. Staddon (Eds.), *Handbook of operant behavior*. Englewood Cliffs, N.J.: Prentice-Hall, 1977.

Dunlap, K. *Habits: Their making and unmaking*. New York: Liveright, 1932.

Egolf, D.B., Shames, G.H., & Blind, J.J. The combined use of operant procedures and theoretical concepts in the treatment of an adult female stutterer. *Journal of Speech and Hearing Disorders*, 1971, *36*, 414-421.

Egolf, D.B., Shames, G.H., Johnson, P.R., & Kasprisin-Burrelli, A. The use of parent-child interaction patterns in therapy for young stutterers. *Journal of Speech and Hearing Disorders*, 1972, *37*, 222-232.

Egolf, D.B., Shames, G.H., & Seltzer, H.N. The effects of time-out on the fluency of stutterers in group therapy. *Journal of Communication Disorders*, 1971, 4, 111-118.

Eysenck, H.J. The conditioning model of neurosis. *The Behavioral and Brain Sciences*,

1979, *2*, 155-199.

Fahmy, M. The theory of habit control and negative practice as a curative method in the treatment of stammering. *Speech*, 1950, *14*, 24-30.

Fairbanks, G. *Voice and articulation drillbook*. New York: Harper, 1940.

Felty, J. The operant nature of stuttering behavior by adolescent boys. Unpublished Master's thesis, University of Washington, 1959.

Ferster, C.B., & Appel, J.B. Punishment of SΔ responding in matching to sample by time-out from positive reinforcement. *Journal of the Experimental Analysis of Behavior*, 1961, *4*, 45-56.

Flanagan, B., Goldiamond, I., & Azrin, N. Operant stuttering: The control of stuttering behavior through response-contingent consequences. *Journal of the Experimental Analysis of Behavior*, 1958, *1*, 173-177.

Flanagan, B., Goldiamond, I., & Azrin, N. Instatement of stuttering in normally fluent individuals through operant procedures. *Science*, 1959, *130*, 979-981.

Fransella, F. Rhythm as a distractor in the modification of stuttering. *Behaviour Research and Therapy*, 1967, *5*, 253-255.

Frick, J.A. An exploratory study of the effect of punishment (electric shock) upon stuttering. Unpublished doctoral dissertation, State University of Iowa, 1951.

Goldiamond, I. The maintenance of ongoing fluent behavior and stuttering. *Journal of Mathetics*, 1962, *1*, 57-95.

Goldiamond, I. Stuttering and fluency as manipulatable response classes. In L. Krasner & L.P. Ullmann (Eds.), *Research in behavior modification*. New York: Rinehart & Winston, 1965.

Griffin, K., and Van Kirk, B. Modification of stuttering behavior in a natural environment. In B.P. Ryan (Ed.), *Programmed therapy for stuttering in children and adults*. Springfield, Ill.: Charles C. Thomas, 1974.

Halvorson, J. The effects on stuttering frequency of pairing punishment (response cost) with reinforcement. *Journal of Speech and Hearing Research*, 1971, *14*, 356-364.

Hanson, B.R. The effects of contingent light-flash on stuttering and attention to stuttering. *Journal of Communication Disorders*, 1978, *11*, 451-458.

Haroldson, S.K., Martin, R.R., & Starr, C.D. Time-out as a punishment for stuttering. *Journal of Speech and Hearing Research*, 1968, *11*, 560-566.

Harris, C.M., Martin, R.R., & Haroldson, S.K. Punishment of expectancy responses by stutterers. *Journal of Speech and Hearing Research*, 1971, *14*, 710-717.

Hatch, J.P., & Gatchel, R.J. The role of biofeedback in the operant modification of human heart rate. *Biofeedback and Self-Regulation*, 1981, *6*, 139-167.

Hayes, S.C., & Cavior, N. Multiple tracking and the reactivity of self-monitoring: 1. Negative behaviors. *Behavior Therapy*, 1977, *8*, 819-831.

Hegde, M.N. The effect of shock on stuttering. *Journal of the All India Institute of Speech and Hearing*, 1971, *2*, 104-110.

Hegde, M.N., & Brutten, G.J. Reinforcing fluency in stutterers: An experimental study. *Journal of Fluency Disorders*, 1977, *2*, 315-328.

Hersen, M., & Barlow, D.H. *Single case experimental designs: Strategies for studying behavior change*. New York: Pergamon, 1976.

Ingham, R.J. Operant methodology in stuttering therapy. In J. Eisenson (Ed.), *Stuttering: A second symposium*. New York: Harper & Row, 1975.

Ingham, R.J. Evaluation and maintenance in stuttering treatment: A search for ecstasy with nothing but agony. In E. Boberg (Ed.), *Maintenance of fluency*. New York: Elsevier North-Holland, 1981.

Ingham, R.J., Adams, S., & Reynolds, G. The effects on stuttering of self-recording the frequency of stuttering or the word "the." *Journal of Speech and Hearing Research*, 1978, *21*, 459-469.

Ingham, R.J., & Andrews, G. An analysis of a token economy in stuttering therapy. *Journal of Applied Behavior Analysis*, 1973, *6*, 219-229. (a)

Ingham, R.J., & Andrews, G. Behavior therapy and stuttering: A review. *Journal of Speech and Hearing Disorders*, 1973, *38*, 405-411. (b)

Ingham, R.J., Martin, R.R., & Kuhl, P. Modification and control of rate of speaking by stutterers. *Journal of Speech and Hearing Research*, 1974, *17*, 489-496.

Ingham, R.J., & Packman, A. Treatment and generalization effects in an experimental treatment for a stutterer using contingency management and speech rate control. *Journal of Speech and Hearing Disorders*, 1977, *42*, 394-407.

James, J.E. The influence of duration on the effects of time-out from speaking. *Journal of Speech and Hearing Research*, 1976, *19*, 206-215.

James, J.E. Self-monitoring of stuttering: Reactivity and accuracy. *Behaviour Research and Therapy*, 1981, *19*, 291-296. (a)

James, J.E. Behavioral self-control of stuttering using time-out from speaking. *Journal of Applied Behavior Analysis*, 1981, *14*, 25-37. (b)

James, J.E. Punishment of stuttering: Contingency and stimulus parameters. *Journal of Communication Disorders*, 1981, *14*, 375-386. (c)

James, J.E., & Ingham, R.J. The influence of stutterer's expectancies of improvement upon response to time-out. *Journal of Speech and Hearing Research*, 1974, *17*, 86-93.

Janssen, P., & Brutten, G.J. The differential effects of punishment of oral prolongations. In Y. Lebrun & R. Hoops (Eds.), *Neurolinguistic approaches to stuttering*. The Hague: Mouton, 1973.

Johnson, G.F., Coleman, K., & Rasmussen, K. Multidays: Multidimensional approach for the young stutterer. *Language, Speech and Hearing Services in Schools*, 1978, *9*, 129-132.

Johnson, W. An open letter to the mother of a stuttering child. In W. Johnson & D. Moeller (Eds.), *Speech handicapped school children* (3rd ed.). New York: Harper and Row, 1967.

Johnson, W., Brown, S., Curtis, J., & Keaster, J. *Speech handicapped children*. New York: Harper & Row, 1948.

Johnson, W., & Rosen, L. Studies in the psychology of stuttering: VII. Effect of certain changes in speech pattern upon frequency of stuttering. *Journal of Speech Disorders*, 1937, *2*, 105-109.

Jones, R.J., & Azrin, N.H. Behavioral engineering: Stuttering as a function of stimulus duration during speech synchronization. *Journal of Applied Behavior Analysis*, 1969, *2*, 223-229.

Jones, R.T., Nelson, R.E., & Kazdin, A.E. The role of external variables in self-reinforcement: A review. *Behavior Modification*, 1977, *1*, 147-178.

Kazdin, A.E. Self-monitoring and behavior change. In M.J. Mahoney & C.E. Thoresen (Eds.), *Self-control: Power to the person*. Monterey, Calif.: Brooks/Cole, 1974.

Kazdin, A.E. *History of behavior modification: Experimental foundations of contemporary research*. Baltimore: University Park Press, 1978.

Kazdin, A.E., & Bootzin, R.B. The token economy: An evaluation review. *Journal of Applied Behavior Analysis*, 1972, *5*, 343-372.

Kazdin, A.E., & Wilson, G.T. *Evaluation of behavior therapy*. Cambridge, Mass: Ballinger, 1978.

Knapp, T.J. The Premack principle in human experimental and applied settings. *Behaviour Research and Therapy*, 1976, *14*, 133-147.

LaCroix, Z.E. Management of disfluent speech through self-recording procedures. *Journal of Speech and Hearing Disorders*, 1973, *38*, 272-274.

Lanyon, R.I., & Barocas, V.S. Effects of contingent stimuli on stuttering. *Proceedings 81st Annual Convention American Psychological Association,* 1973, 539-540.

Lanyon, R.I., & Barocas, V.S. Effects of contingent events on stuttering and fluency. *Journal of Consulting and Clinical Psychology,* 1975, *43,* 786-793.

Lazarus, A.A. *Multimodal behavior therapy.* New York: Springer, 1976.

Leach, E. Stuttering: Clinical applications of response-contingent procedures. In B. Gray & G. England (Eds.), *Stuttering and the conditioning therapies.* Monterey, Calif.: Monterey Institute for Speech and Hearing, 1969.

Leitenberg, H. Is time-out from positive reinforcement an aversive event? *Psychological Bulletin,* 1965, *64,* 428-441.

Leith, W.R. The shaping group: Habituating new behaviors in the stutterer. In N. Lass (Ed.), *Speech and language: Advances in basic research and practice* (Vol. 2). New York: Academic Press, 1979.

Leith, W.R., & Uhlemann, M.R. The shaping group approach to stuttering: A pilot study. *Journal of Comparative Group Studies,* 1972, *3,* 175-199.

Lovaas, O.I. Interaction between verbal and non-verbal behavior. *Child Development,* 1961, *32,* 329-336.

Luper, H., & Mulder, R. *Stuttering therapy for children.* Englewood Cliffs, N.J.: Prentice-Hall, 1964.

Mahoney, M.J. *Cognition and behavior modification.* Cambridge, Mass.: Ballinger, 1974.

Manning, W.H., Trutna, P.A., & Shaw, C.K. Verbal versus tangible reward for children who stutter. *Journal of Speech and Hearing Disorders,* 1976, *41,* 52-62.

Martin, R.R. The experimental manipulation of stuttering behaviors. In H.N. Sloane, Jr., & B.D. Macaulay (Eds.), *Operant procedures in remedial speech and language training.* Boston: Houghton-Mifflin, 1968.

Martin, R.R., & Berndt, L.A. The effects of time-out on stuttering in a 12 year old boy. *Exceptional Children,* 1970, *36,* 303-304.

Martin, R.R., Brookshire, R., & Siegel, G.M. The effects of resonse contingent punishment on various behaviors emitted during a "moment of stuttering." Unpublished manuscript, University of Minnesota, 1964.

Martin, R.R., & Gaviser, J. Time-out as a punishment for button pushing. *Journal of Speech and Hearing Research,* 1971, *14,* 144-148.

Martin, R.R., & Haroldson, S.K. The effects of two treatment procedures on stuttering. *Journal of Communication Disorders,* 1969, *2,* 115-125.

Martin, R.R., & Haroldson, S.K. Time-out as a punishment for stuttering during conversation. *Journal of Communication Disorders,* 1971, *4,* 15-19.

Martin, R.R., & Haroldson, S.K. Effect of vicarious punishment on stuttering frequency. *Journal of Speech and Hearing Research,* 1977, *20,* 21-26.

Martin, R.R., & Haroldson, S.K. Effects of five experimental treatments on stuttering. *Journal of Speech and Hearing Research,* 1979, *22,* 132-146.

Martin, R.R., & Haroldson, S.K. Some comments on "Effects of five experimental treatments on stuttering": A reply. *Journal of Speech and Hearing Research,* 1980, *23,* 214-216.

Martin, R.R., Haroldson, S.K., & Starr, C.D. Time-out as punishment for stuttering: A reply to Martin Adams. *Journal of Speech and Hearing Research,* 1971, *14,* 220-222.

Martin, R.R., & Ingham, R.J. Stuttering. In B. Lahey (Ed.), *The modification of language behavior.* Springfield, Ill.: Charles C. Thomas, 1973.

Martin, R.R., Kuhl, P., & Haroldson, S.K. An experimental treatment with two preschool stuttering children. *Journal of Speech and Hearing Research,* 1972, *15,* 743-752.

Martin, R.R., & Siegel, G.M. The effects of response contingent shock on stuttering.

Journal of Speech and Hearing Research, 1966, *9*, 340-352. (a)

Martin, R.R., & Siegel, G.M. The effects of simultaneously punishing stuttering and rewarding fluency. *Journal of Speech and Hearing Research*, 1966, *9*, 466-475. (b)

Martin, R.R., St. Louis, K., Haroldson, S.K., & Hasbrouck, J. Punishment and negative reinforcement of stuttering using electric shock. *Journal of Speech and Hearing Research*, 1975, *18*, 478-490.

McDermott, L.D. Clinical management of stuttering behavior: A case study. *Feedback*, 1971, *1*, 6-7.

Moore, Jr., W.H., & Ritterman, S.I. The effects of response contingent reinforcement and response contingent punishment upon the frequency of stuttered verbal behavior. *Behaviour Research and Therapy*. 1973, *11*, 43-48.

Mowrer, D. An instructional program to increase fluent speech of stutterers. *Journal of Fluency Disorders*, 1975, *1*, 25-35.

Mowrer, D.E. Effect of audience reaction upon fluency rates of six stutterers. *Journal of Fluency Disorders*, 1978, *3*, 193-203.

Murphy, A.T. Stuttering, behavior modification and the person. In Speech Foundation of America, Publication No. 7; *Conditioning in stuttering therapy*. Memphis: Speech Foundation of America, 1970.

Murray, F.P. An investigation of variably induced white noise upon moments of stuttering. *Journal of Communication Disorders*, 1969, *2*, 109-114.

Nelson, R.O., & Hayes, S.C. Theoretical explanations for reactivity in self-monitoring. *Behavior Modification*, 1981, *5*, 3-14.

Oelschlaeger, M.L., & Brutten, G.J. Response-contingent positive stimulation of the part-word repetitions displayed by four stutterers. *Journal of Fluency Disorders*, 1975, *2*, 10-17.

Oelschlaeger, M.L., & Brutten, G.J. The effect of instructional stimulation on the frequency of repetitions, interjections, and words spoken during the spontaneous speech of four stutterers. *Behavior Therapy*, 1976, *7*, 37-46.

Patty, J., & Quarrington, B. The effects of reward on types of stuttering. *Journal of Communication Disorders*, 1974, *7*, 65-77.

Peters, A.D. The effect of positive reinforcement on fluency: Two case studies. *Language, Speech and Hearing Services in Schools*, 1977, *8*, 15-22.

Poppen, R., Nunn, R.G., & Hook, S. Effects of several therapies on stuttering in a single case. *Journal of Fluency Disorders*, 1977, *2*, 35-44.

Premack, D. Toward empirical behavior laws: 1. Positive reinforcement. *Psychological Review*, 1959. *66*, 219-233.

Quist, R.W., & Martin, R.R. The effect of response contingent verbal punishment. *Journal of Speech and Hearing Research*, 1967, *10*, 795-800.

Reed, C.G., & Godden, A.L. An experimental treatment using verbal punishment with two preschool stutterers. *Journal of Fluency Disorders*, 1977, *2*, 225-233.

Reed, C.G., & Lingwall, J.B. Some relationships between punishment, stuttering, and galvanic skin resonses. *Journal of Speech and Hearing Research*, 1976, *19*, 197-205.

Reed, C.G., & Lingwall, J.B. Conditioned stimulus effects on stuttering and GSRs. *Journal of Speech and Hearing Research*, 1980, *23*, 336-343.

Rhodes, R., Shames, G., & Egolf, D. "Awareness" in verbal conditioning of language themes during therapy with stutterers. *Journal of Communication Disorders*, 1971, *4*, 30-39.

Rickard, H.C., & Mundy, M.B. Direct manipulation of stuttering behavior. An experimental-clinical approach. In L.P. Ullman & L. Krasner (Eds.), *Case studies in behavior modification*. New York: Holt, Rinehart & Winston, 1965.

Rosenthal, R. *Experimental effects in behavioral research*. New York: Appleton-Century-

Crofts, 1966.
Russell, J.C., Clark, A.W., & Van Sommers, P. Treatment of stammering by reinforcement of fluent speech. *Behaviour Research and Therapy*, 1968, *6*, 447-453.
Rustin, L. An intensive group programme for adolescent stammerers. *British Journal of Disorders of Communication*, 1978, *13*, 85-92.
Ryan, B. An illustration of operant conditioning therapy for stuttering. In Speech Foundation of America, Publication No. 7, *Conditioning in stuttering therapy*. Memphis: Speech Foundation of America, 1970.
Ryan, B.P. Operant procedures applied to stuttering therapy for children. *Journal of Speech and Hearing Disorders*, 1971, *36*, 264-280.
Ryan, B.P. *Programmed therapy for stuttering in children and adults*. Springfield, Ill.: Charles C. Thomas, 1974.
Ryan, B.P. Stuttering therapy in a framework of operant conditioning and programmed learning. In H.H. Gregory (Ed.), *Controversies about stuttering therapy*. Baltimore: University Park Press, 1979.
Ryan, B.P. Maintenance programs in progress—II. In E. Boberg (Ed.), *Maintenance of fluency*. New York: Elsevier North-Holland, 1981.
Schick, K. Operants. *Journal of the Experimental Analysis of Behavior*, 1971, *15*, 413-423.
Shames, G.H. Verbal reinforcement during therapy interviews with stutterers. In B.B. Gray & G. England (Eds.), *Stuttering and the conditioning therapies*. Monterey, Calif.: Monterey Institute of Speech and Hearing, 1969.
Shames, G.H. Operant conditioning and stuttering. In J. Eisenson (Ed.), *Stuttering: A second symposium*. New York: Harper & Row, 1975.
Shames, G.H., & Egolf, D.B. *Operant conditioning and the management of stuttering*. Englewood Cliffs, N.J.: Prentice-Hall, 1976.
Shames, G.H., Egolf, D.B., & Rhodes, R.C. Experimental programs in stuttering therapy. *Journal of Speech and Hearing Disorders*, 1969, *34*, 30-47.
Shames, G.H., & Florance, C.L. *Stutter-free speech: A goal for therapy*. Columbus, O.: Charles E. Merrill, 1980.
Shames, G., & Sherrick, C.E. A discussion of nonfluency and stuttering as operant behavior. *Journal of Speech and Hearing Disorders*, 1963, *28*, 3-18.
Shaw, C.K., & Shrum, W.F. The effects of response-contingent reward on the connected speech of children who stutter. *Journal of Speech and Hearing Disorders*, 1972, *37*, 75-88.
Sheehan, J.G. The modification of stuttering through non-reinforcement. *Journal of Abnormal Psychology*, 1951, *46*, 51-63.
Sheehan, J.G. Reflections on the behavioral modification of stuttering. In Speech Foundation of America, Publication No. 7, *Conditioning in stuttering therapy*. Memphis: Speech Foundation of America, 1970.
Sheehan, J.G. Current issues on stuttering and recovery. In H.H. Gregory (Ed.), *Controversies about stuttering therapy*. Baltimore: University Park Press, 1979.
Sherman, J.A. Modification of non-verbal behavior through reinforcement of related verbal behavior. *Child Development*, 1964, *35*, 717-723.
Sidman, M. *Tactics of scientific research: Evaluating experimental data in psychology*. New York: Basic Books, 1960.
Siegel, G.M. Punishment, stuttering and disfluency. *Journal of Speech and Hearing Research*, 1970, *13*, 677-714.
Skinner, B.F. Two types of conditioned reflex: A reply to Konorski and Miller. *Journal of General Psychology*, 1937, *16*, 272-279.
Skinner, B.F. A case history in scientific method. *American Psychologist*, 1956, *11*, 221-233.
Skinner, B.F. *Verbal behavior*. New York: Appleton-Century-Crofts, 1957.

Starkweather, C.W. The case against base rate comparisons in stuttering experimentation. *Journal of Communication Disorders,* 1971, *4,* 247-258.

Starkweather, C.W., & Lucker, J. Tokens for stuttering. *Journal of Fluency Disorders,* 1978, *3,* 167-180.

Stokes, T.F., & Baer, D.M. An implicit technology of generalization. *Journal of Applied Behavior Analysis,* 1977, *10,* 349-367.

Teitelbaum, P. Levels of integration of the operant. In W.K. Honig & J.E.R. Staddon (Eds.), *Handbook of operant behavior.* Englewood Cliffs, N.J.: Prentice-Hall, 1977.

Thoresen, C.E., & Coates, T.J. What does it mean to be a behavior therapist? *The Counseling Psychologist,* 1978, *7,* 3-21.

Thoresen, C.E., & Mahoney, M.J. *Behavioral self-control.* New York: Holt, Rinehart & Winston, 1974.

Toomey, G.L., & Sidman, M. An experimental analogue of the anxiety-stuttering relationship. *Journal of Speech and Hearing Research,* 1970, *13,* 122-129.

Van Riper, C. The effect of penalty upon frequency of stuttering spasms. *Journal of Genetic Psychology,* 1937, *50,* 193-195.

Van Riper, C. *Speech correction: Principles and methods.* (4th Ed.). Englewood Cliffs, N.J.: Prentice-Hall, 1963.

Van Riper, C. Behavior modification: An overview. In Speech Foundation of America, Publication No. 7, *Conditioning in stuttering therapy.* Memphis: Speech Foundation of America, 1970.

Van Riper, C. *The nature of stuttering.* Englewood Cliffs, N.J.: Prentice-Hall, 1971.

Van Riper, C. *The treatment of stuttering.* Englewood Cliffs, N.J.: Prentice-Hall, 1973.

Wahler, R.G., & Pollio, H.R. Behavior and insight: A case study in behavior therapy. *Journal of Experimental Research in Personality,* 1968, *3,* 45-56.

Wahler, R.G., Sperling, K.A., Thomas, M.R., Teeter, N.C., & Luper, H.L. The modification of childhood stuttering: Some response-response relationships. *Journal of Experimental Child Psychology,* 1970, *9,* 411-428.

Watts, F. Mechanisms of fluency control in stutterers. *British Journal of Disorders of Communication.* 1973, *8,* 131-138.

Webster, L.M., & Brutten, G.J. The modification of stuttering and associated behaviors. In S. Dickson (Ed.), *Communication disorders.* Glenview, Ill.: Scott Foresman, 1974.

Wingate, M.E. Calling attention to stuttering. *Journal of Speech and Hearing Research,* 1959, *2,* 326-335.

Wingate, M.E. Stuttering, 1970: Where do we stand? *Journal of Speech and Hearing Research,* 1970, *13,* 5-8.

Wingate, M.E. The fear of stuttering. *Asha,* 1971, *13,* 3-5.

Wingate, M.E. *Stuttering: Theory and treatment.* New York: Irvington, 1976.

Wingate, M.E. On the Hegde-Daly and Kimbarow exchange. *Journal of Speech and Hearing Research,* 1980, *23,* 217-219.

Winkler, R.C. The relevance of economic theory and technology to token reinforcement systems. *Behaviour Research and Therapy,* 1971, *9,* 81-88.

Yates, A.J. *Behavior therapy.* New York: Wiley, 1970.

Yates, A.J. *Theory and practice in behavior therapy.* New York: Wiley, 1975.

Yates, A.J. *Biofeedback and the modification of behavior.* New York: Plenum, 1980.

Zimmerman, J., & Ferster, C.B. Intermittent punishment of SΔ responding in matching to sample. *Journal of the Experimental Analysis of Behavior.* 1963, 6, 349-356.

Zwitman, D.H. *The disfluent child.* Baltimore: University Park Press, 1978.

10

Prolonged Speech, Its Variants, and Stuttering

Introduction

One of the interesting problems faced in preparing this chapter was the choice of an appropriate title. "Prolonged speech" is only one of many that could have been used. The problem was to find a title that represented both the procedures and the various "speaking techniques" that came to prominence during the 1960s largely as a result of delayed auditory feedback (DAF) research. The title also had to reflect procedures and techniques that now have virtually no connection with DAF. "DAF-induced Fluency," "Breathstream Management," "Rate Control," or "Vocal Tract Dynamics," were other titles that could have been chosen since they describe prominent characteristics of the research and clinical procedures whose lineage can be traced to the earlier DAF investigations. Indeed, serious consideration was also given to "The Return of the Heavy Breathing Therapies," since the clinical procedures that will be reviewed have a striking resemblance to the breath-control techniques used in past decades—even past centuries. Part of this uncertainty also reflects one of the more troublesome features of this topic area: how to consider allegedly behavioral techniques that have not been operationalized. Masking, response-contingent procedures, and rhythmic stimulation, for instance, are usually connected with reproducible operations. But prolonged speech, and its multitudinous variants, are simply labels given to a speech pattern(s) that may emergy from many relatively ill-defined operations. It might be expected, therefore, that this would raise some serious concerns about the relevance of these methods to behavior therapy. But this has certainly not deterred the application of these speech patterns within a behavior therapy context. In fact, their use has grown enormously over the past decade and they have instigated some of the most interesting experimental and clinical research on stuttering.

The purpose of this chapter is to review the research that has led to the development and application of prolonged speech in clinical settings. This is a rather formidable task since it is now a remarkably diverse literature. Its formative stages occur in the field of audiology, but its development is associated with operant-conditioning research and, more recently, investigations on speech physiology. Nevertheless, what follows is an attempt to trace the history of this research in order to identify its origins, directions, and influences. In general, this involves a review of the emergence of DAF, and its role in stuttering research, followed by an account of "modified vocalization" and "vocal tract dynamics" research that has relevance to procedures that modify stuttering. From this vantage point, it is anticipated that the strengths and weaknesses of the clinical practices that have emerged from this diverse field will be more easily recognized.

DAF Research

The Initial Studies

Previous chapters have provided many instances of the role played by auditory factors in the theory and treatment of stuttering. The continuing interest in audition stems from the relatively consistent ameliorative effect that altered audition produces on stuttering and, to a lesser extent, the relationship between this effect and altered prosody. Therefore, it should not be surprising that modifying the speaker's perception of his voice signal by delaying its feedback might also have implications for stuttering.

The disturbances to speaking caused by breaking the phase relationship between oral-sensory activities and audition is a reasonably familiar phenomenon and prompted some of the initial investigations of DAF. In 1950, Black reported that oral reading in rooms of different shape, size, and reverberation quality changed the rate and intensity of the voice signal. He concluded that the speakers were apparently monitoring their altered sidetone (air-conducted signal) and adjusted their speech to this feedback as a way of "maintaining a 'normal' experience at the ear" (Black 1950, p.176). By coincidence, in the same year, Lee (1950a) first described the disruptive effects of speaking during delayed-auditory-feedback conditions produced by a tape recorder. Shortly afterwards, Lee (1950b) also provided supportive data from oral reading and recitation tasks by five normal speakers while each experienced 40, 140, and 280 msec DAF. The time that subjects took to read a passage or recite syllables was generally slower with each increase in the delay interval. Lee also observed that the effect depended on the feedback signal being loud enough to mask any bone-conducted voice signal feedback.

Lee's initial findings, and his description of the effect of DAF, were both provocative and influential. To begin with, he drew attention to "stuttering errors" that occurred when the speaker attempted to use his normal speech rate during DAF. Subsequently, Lee (1951) described these errors as "artificial stutter," even though, as Wingate (1970) has pointed out, the accounts of this "stuttering" ("The word, *aluminum,* becomes *aluminum-num, lum-lum* becomes *lum-lum-lum*") did not resemble chronic stuttering. Such stuttering is typified by repetitions on initial rather than final syllables (Wingate, 1964). However, three conclusions in Lee's report were remarkably portentive. The first was his suggestion that the speed-governing effects of DAF would likely "provide the more useful information," The second was the variability in his data: two of the five subjects failed to speak more slowly as the delay interval increased. And, finally, there was the connection that Lee (1950a; 1951) made between the DAF effect and cybernetics.

One of the important explanatory influences on early DAF research, especially with respect to stuttering, was Norbert Wiener's (1948) book *Cybernetics: Or Control and Communication in the Animal and the Machine*. Many of Wiener's ideas molded the conceptual basis of much behavioral research at that time. Cybernetic theory drew parallels between the critical role of feedback in artificial control systems and the biochemical and cognitive systems operating in humans. The pervasive influence of cybernetics has diminished somewhat in recent years, but its impact is still evident in the continuing interest in feedback concepts to explain findings in speech production investigations.

Perhaps the earliest speech production model to exhibit the influence of cybernetics, was Fairbanks's (1954) model of the speech mechanism as a "servosystem," with a closed-cycle operation. In an open-cycle system, the operations that produce outputs, such as speech, are controlled by events independent of that output. However, the closed cycle servosystem almost exclusively utilizes feedback from output signals to manage control—principally via comparisons between input and output signals. The model predicted that speech output was constantly responsive to a controller unit which synthesizes signals via acoustic, tactile, and proprioceptive pathways. Thus, the validity of the model can only be inferred by assessing the effect on speech output of interruptions to these feedback pathways. Fairbanks predicted that the "model can be caused to repeat, prolong and hesitate by several different manipulations, one of which is feedback delay" (1954, p.138).Thus any perceptual dysfunction associated with the voice signal (such as occurs during DAF) should also produce aberrant speech behavior. Quite naturally, this led some to speculate about the model's relevance to an explanation of stuttering.

The initial clinical and research applications of DAF were concerned with assessing hearing loss and, arguably, this continues to be its most practical area of application. Azzi and Invernizzi (1951) were the first to report the suitability of this procedure for detecting psychogenic deafness. Shortly afterwards, Tiffany and Hanley (1952) investigated the effects of feedback intensity in connection with malingering and/or psychogenic deafness. They found that during 140 msec DAF conditions, oral reading was progressively retarded as the feedback signal was increased from 35 to 75dBs above threshold. In subsequent reports, Hanley and Tiffany (1954a; 1954b) showed that even at 20dB above threshold, at least 70% of speech samples made under these conditions could be detected by listeners (principally from speech rate) as originating from DAF conditions. They also noted that "whistling was even more markedly disturbed" under DAF (though without supportive data). One of their most interesting findings (Tiffany & Hanley, 1956) was that repeated exposure to DAF (180 msec; 80dB SL) reduced its disruptive effects on fluency. But there were also marked individual departures from this trend, and reduced disfluencies during DAF are often reported to have occurred at some cost to speech quality.

Tiffany and Hanley's research typified the direction of much of the early work on DAF with normal speakers. Since that time, a massive amount of DAF research has identified virtually all of the parameters of its effects on normally fluent speakers. Nevertheless, the durability of the early findings is quite impressive; very few surprises have emerged in subsequent research. What follows is an attempt to organize the findings of that research. This attempt will review the research in terms of an experimental design; that is, the principal independent variable manipulations will be followed by an overview of the major dependent variable findings.

DAF and Normally Fluent Speakers: Independent Variables

Delay Times

Lee (1950b) assessed the effects of 40, 140, and 280msec DAF, and showed that three out of five subjects produced correlated increases in oral reading time across the delays, with a peak effect at 140 msec for the other two subjects. Black (1951) found a peak effect on oral-reading rate at 180 msec when 22 subjects were assessed on delays ranging from 0 to 300 msecs. Vocal intensity increased by slightly over 5dBs at 90 msec delay, but did not alter significantly over longer delays. Rather similar findings were found in Atkinson's (1954) investigation on the effects of 30 to 270 msec delays, but articulation intelligibility was reported to show maximum deterioration at around 100 msec. Fairbanks (1955) assessed 0, 100, 200, 400, and 800 msec delays with 16 subjects, and found that maximum articulation errors and oral-reading-rate retardation occurred at 200 msec.

Some effects of accelerated air-conducted feedback have also been investigated. Stromsta's (1959; 1962) studies show that the minimum feedback interval for air-conducted sidetone was about .001 secs. Thus Peters's (1956) use of .0003, .001, and .00015 secs "delayed" sidetone during oral reading measured the effects of accelerated and normal feedback rates. This showed that reading rate may increase during accelerated feedback conditions. Essentially similar findings were reported by Davidson (1959) with .0005, .001, and .0015 sec delays, plus an additional finding of correlated effects on the extent and rate of inflection.

Intensity of Sidetone Signal

As previously mentioned, Tiffany and Hanley's research found oral-reading rate to be systematically reduced with increments in SRT levels during 140 msec DAF. Using controlled reading rate, Butler and Galloway (1957) assessed 85 to 340 msec delays at 20 to 80dB SL and found the peak number of errors occurred at 170 msec and 80dB SL. Chase and Guilfoyle (1962) manipulated concurrent presentation of simultaneous and delayed feedback (300 msec) so that the former signal varied in intensity relative to the latter. The median correct words during oral reading approached the level attained during no-delay conditions, but when the simultaneous signal was faded to one-third intensity, correct-word rate and oral-reading rate were markedly affected. Taken together, these findings support Lee's contentions on the contribution of signal intensity to the DAF effect.

Task Variables

There has been little variety among the speech activities measured during DAF. These activities have been mainly confined to oral-reading tasks, although interesting effects have been reported occasionally with other activities such as whistling (Hanley & Tiffany, 1954b). Schwartz (1961; 1967) compared oral and whispered reading under 0-300 msec and found a slightly shorter peak slow-rate in the case of whispering. MacKay (1969) compared the effects of nasal distortion (holding the nose), nasal articulation (nasal accent), and normal speaking during controlled oral-reading rates with 175 and 200 msec DAF, and found, essentially, that nasal articulation was less disrupted by DAF. In other words, this finding suggested that prosody rather than articulation is more vulnerable to DAF effects. Another somewhat related finding was reported by Bradshaw, Nettleton, and Geffen (1972); they were primarily interested in laterality effects of DAF and reported that tapping and whistling tasks were more disrupted by left than right ear feedback. One intriguing finding was that as a rhythmic pattern was introduced to a speaking task, the slowing effects of DAF were substantially reduced. In general, both MacKay's and Bradshaw and associates' findings suggested that DAF's effects were likely to be dampened when speakers altered their customary manner of speaking.

The usefulness of DAF to medico-legal audiometry has continued over the years, but mainly in conjunction with nonverbal tasks such as key tapping. The reliability with which rhythmic key tapping is disrupted during DAF has been reported by Ruhm and Cooper (1964) and Cooper, Strokinger, and Billings (1976).

Duration of DAF Exposure

The extent of changes in speech that relate to DAF exposure time has been studied, but with the use of surprisingly brief speech samples. Aktinson (1953) compared 15 and 60 five-word phrases uttered under 0 to 300 msec DAF and reported relatively insignificant vocal intensity and reading-time effects. Unfortunately, the study failed to measure errors or disfluencies. The importance of this oversight is shown by Tiffany and Hanley's (1956) finding that when subjects reread a passage a week later under 180 msec DAF their nonfluencies declined significantly. In a comparison between 8 and 53 secs (at least) of oral reading during a 140 msec delay, Hanley, Tiffany, and Brungard (1958) reported that judges found fewer samples from the longer period were affected by DAF. Gibbons, Winchester, and Krebs (1958) and Winchester, Gibbons, and Krebs (1959) provided studies which make it possible to gain some idea of the effects of relatively longer periods of DAF exposure. The former study showed that oral readings of 10 200-word passages, without DAF, resulted in virtually unchanged oral-reading rate. In the Winchester et al. study, the same task was performed under 160 msec DAF and produced an initial reduction in reading time, followed by increasingly faster readings—but still short of the rate produced without DAF.

Much longer periods of DAF exposure have been investigated, but with relatively abbreviated data. Krombholz and Rubeling (1974) arranged for a subject to speak 12 hours a day under either 100, 200, or 300 msec DAF on each of 3 days. It was reported that "articulatory accuracy" improved during the course of each day, but there was only slight variation in speech rate. This finding is consistent with more detailed findings from Goldiamond, Atkinson, and Bilger (1962) on the effects of daily 90-minute oral-reading sessions by two subjects under either 200, 300, or 400 msec DAF. They reported (without data) no functional association between these delay times and oral-reading rates. But their most interesting finding was that when subjects were instructed to either listen or ignore their voice signal during DAF ("at an intensity level judged sufficient to overcome bone conduction"), their oral-reading rates varied accordingly; ignoring their voice signal resulted in oral-reading rates that clearly exceeded those found when subjects were instructed to listen to their oral reading. Consequently, part of the variability associated with prolonged (or even brief) exposure to DAF may depend on whether the subject chooses to attend to the feedback signal, undoubtedly a bothersome variable in any attempt to predict DAF's effect.

Utterance Rate

At least two studies have shown there is likely to be an association between nonfluency and utterance rate during DAF. Kodman (1961) had subjects (n=20) orally read at 132, 96, 72, and 60 wpm during 200 msec DAF, and showed that the mean number of reading errors declined substantially from 132 to 72 wpm. In fact, zero errors were produced at 72 wpm. But at 60 wpm, the subject's speech was described as "closer to singing" than speaking. Robinson (1972) used four subjects to assess the effect of varying oral-reading rate across delays ranging from 90 to 360 msecs. He concluded that the delay leading to maximum disruption was a function of speech rate.

Sidetone-Signal Effects

Investigations on the characteristics and source of the feedback signal have yielded some of the most interesting findings in DAF research. One of the least investigated (and most fascinating) occurs in an anecdotal account by Cherry and Sayers (1956) on the effect of delayed bone-conducted feedback. They claimed its effect was "considerably more severe than that of a correspondingly loud sound impressed through telephones by air conduction" (p.238). However, most researchers have been concerned with modifications to the air-conducted signal.

Spuehler (1962) measured the results of 0 to 3000 interruptions per second during delays ranging from 0 to 350 msec. He found that phonation time increased as the interruption rate was increased to 300 per second, while word rate was maximally retarded at the 3000 per second level. Fillenbaum (1965) varied the delay level (100 to 280 msec) irregularly during oral reading, and found that reading rate was virtually the same as was obtained during a 200 msec delay.

Some particularly interesting findings in relation to stuttering have emerged from studies by Courtney Stromsta. Stromsta's initial research (1959) was prompted by some earlier reports on the effects of out-of-phase air-conducted sidetone. In the first investigation, subjects (n=8) sustained a 350Hz vowel /u/ while experiencing 62.5% nonlinear delivery of their sidetone. Comparisons between this distorted sidetone condition and a nondistorted sidetone condition showed that the former produced nearly seven times more phonation blockage. The subjects' (n=32; 11-50 years) reports on the procedure's effects showed that they also experienced shortness of breath, tension at the larynx, and some uncontrollable rapid lip tremors. A summarized account of a similar study by Homann (1964) with 20 subjects produced almost identical findings, plus evidence of shifts in fundamental frequency immediately before and after phonation blockages. Apart from the resemblance between these behaviors and stuttering, however, it is not clear what implications these findings hold for any particular model of stuttering.

Stromsta's research on sidetone also extended to measurement of the temporal delays in the speaker's internal-sidetone pathways (Stromsta, 1962). This showed that signal transmission rates, via bone and tissue conduction, vary greatly in relation to each other, and also with respect to sidetone air conduction. This is quite evident at certain frequency levels, so that a speaker probably always experiences a natural disparity in voice feedback intervals. In other words, a speaker is always obliged to accommodate to delayed feedback, albeit with delays ranging from less than 0.5 to about 9 msec—well below the disruptive delay levels used in DAF research.

Subject Susceptibility

An enormous amount of research effort has been expended on attempts to relate subject characteristics to DAF efforts. Since this effort has produced little return, only an abbreviated account of some typical studies will be considered. Beaumont and Foss (1957) reported finding some evidence of an association between high performance on tests of preservation ability and responsiveness to DAF. A rather more direct attack on the role of "responsiveness" occurred in a study by Burke (1975a). He identified subjects who showed relatively high rates of disfluency and slow oral reading rates under 180 msec DAF, plus others who showed low disfluency rates and fast reading rates under the same conditions. These "high" and "low" susceptibility subjects were found not to differ in their reactions to masking or whispering. Also, a subgroup from each set of subjects showed no differences in their reactions to local oral anaesthesia. The principal consequence of this finding was that it failed to verify a notion advanced by Yates (1963; 1965); that is, speakers who are highly susceptible to DAF depend on auditory feedback, while the less susceptible depend mainly on oral sensory feedback.

An example of a search for more fundamental sources of DAF susceptibility is a study by Timmons and Rankin (1970). They compared identical and fraternal twins for their oral-reading time during 200 msec DAF, and found the rates of the identical pairs correlated 0.85, while the fraternal pairs rates correlated − 0.64. Unfortunately, their study failed to control for sex differences between the two groups, a factor which might have contributed much to this finding.

Sex Differences

There is some evidence that males and females tend to differ in their responsiveness to DAF, although the reason is unclear. Spuehler (1962) and Mahaffey and Stromsta (1965), for example, found that peak effects in college-age males and females were significantly different. But in Spuehler's study, females reacted maximally at a shorter delay than males, while in Mahaffey and Stromsta's study the reverse was true. At least part of the reason may be due to the different sidetone characteristics used in these studies. Bachrach (1964) also reported (anecdotally) differentiating effects on the sexes of 200 to 800 msec delays. However, Timmons (1971) found no differences in the oral-reading rates of both sexes at 100 to 500 msec delays, although the female subjects showed more evidence of adaptation to DAF.

There appears to be little substantial evidence of a sex factor influencing DAF susceptibility in children. Timmons and Boudreau (1976) compared 5- to 13-year-old males and females on their oral-reading time and disfluencies during 113 to 520 msec delays. Their reading rates differed at some age and delay levels, but they showed no differences with respect to disfluencies.

Age Factors

Once again, an extensive amount of research has addressed itself to the age factor. For the most part, it has been concerned with the contribution of auditory feedback to speech development. These considerations originated with a series of studies at John Hopkins University Hospital. Studies by Chase, Sutton, First, and Zubin (1961), Cullen, Fargo, Chase, and Baker (1968) and Yeni-Komshian, Chase, and Mobley (1968), generally demonstrated the modifying effects of 200 mesc DAF on phonation time (even in the form of crying) in infants as young as 24 hours and children up to age 9.

Older age factors have been identified in studies by Smith and Tierney (1971) and MacKay (1968). Smith and Tierney measured the number of oral-reading errors produced by age groups, 10-18, 23-38, and 42-68 (n=6 in each group) during 200 msec delay conditions. This showed the age 23-38 group had significantly fewer errors than the other groups. MacKay used variable delays to identify peak oral-reading and articulatory errors produced by subjects within age groups 4-6, 7-9, and 20-26 years. The peak, or critical delay, effects occurred at 200 msec for the 20-26 age group, 375 msec for the 7- to 9-year-olds and 524 msec (750 msec for articulatory errors) in the youngest group. A partial replication of this study by Siegel, Fehst, Garber, and Pick (1980), using 5- and 8-year-old children, plus adults, also found the younger children were most affected by the longer delays. But they also found no evidence of a critical delay level in any of the age levels. In passing, it is important to note that neither the MacKay nor the Smith and Tierney study were supported by measurement reliability data. Nevertheless, there is some consistency in the finding that young subjects are more responsive than adult subjects to substantially longer delay levels.

Linguistic Factors

Only relatively general linguistic factors, such as verbal ability and the speakers' language, have shown some evidence of effects in DAF investigations.

Arens and Popplestone (1959) compared the oral-reading rates (using an unspecified delay condition) produced by speakers divided into high and low "verbal facility" (based on verbal IQ scores), and reported (without data) that the less facile group was more affected by DAF. That finding is consistent with Tiffany and Hanley's (1956) report that subjects judged as effective speakers by an audience "learned to resist delay distortion."

DAF may also have different effects with different languages. Hanley (1968) compared the effects of 400 msec DAF on females whose first language was either American English, Spanish, Japanese, or Tagalog (a language spoken in the Philippine Islands). He found the Japanese speakers to be much less affected in terms of their oral-reading rate and phonation/time ratio. MacKay (1970) compared speakers who spoke German and English (with either as their first language) during 0-300 msec DAF. The peak effect (independent of speech rate) was more pronounced in the second than the first language, but it was most pronounced when these speakers used an unfamiliar language (Congolese).

Siegel (1981) reviewed the research in this area and argued that age and linguistic contributions to DAF's effects can be understood more easily by reference to articulatory and prosodic variables. He points out that the main disruptive effects of DAF during childhood are probably associated with articulation, but with development, auditory feedback becomes a less important source of control. This conclusion is supported by some evidence showing that DAF is more disruptive with a less customary (second) language, and that it affects nasal distortion more than nasal articulation in adults (MacKay, 1970).

DAF Experiments with Normally Fluent Speakers: Dependent Variables

Nonfluencies

For many years, the type of nonfluencies that occur during DAF was one of the more contentious issues in stuttering research. Lee's (1950b; 1951) initial description of this speech as "artificial stuttering" led naturally to speculation about its relevance to "true" stuttering. Lee's description of the nonfluencies that occurred during DAF certainly resembled some typical stuttering nonfluencies;

when speaking, the subject "halts or repeats syllables and continuant sounds." But data from other studies showed the resemblance was far from complete. Fairbanks and Guttman (1958), for example, observed that "substitutions" and "omissions" were most prominent under DAF and were followed by "additions" (70% of the "additions" were classed "repetitions"). Substitutions and omissions are not usually regarded as stutterings. On the other hand, Chase (1958) found that normal speakers were highly susceptible to increases in repetitions during DAF.

One notable attempt to determine whether DAF nonfluencies resemble stutterings was Neelley's (1961) investigation of stutterers' and nonstutterers' speech in the presence and absence of 140 msec DAF. He found that listeners generally failed to judge nonstutterers' speech during DAF as identical to stutterers' speech (without DAF). Yates (1963) disputed the relevance of this finding to a perceptual defect theory of stuttering. He argued that use of a fixed delay level and the relative novelty of the nonstutterers' experience with DAF makes it useless to compare the speech from both groups: Yates argued that if stutterers constantly experience something akin to DAF, then their speech would differ from someone who only experiences that phenomenon for a short period. But, as Wingate (1976) has retorted, it was also the speech of nonstutterers during DAF which gave rise to the notion that it resembled chronic stuttering. Therefore, its dissimilarity can be reasonably argued as grounds for rejecting some or all of that claim. In passing, it is interesting to note that the nonstutterers in Neelley's study also had a higher proportion of additions, substitutions, and omissions than nonstutterers during DAF.

Part of the controversy over the type of nonfluencies nonstutterers produce during DAF stems from the imprecision of nonfluency categories. The point is illustrated by Neelley's study in which some of the nonfluencies of "relatively fluent stutterers" were said to be similar to those produced by stutterers during DAF. But, unfortunately, Neelley's listeners were never asked whether they would also describe these (or any others) as "stutterings." Venkatigiri (1980) claimed that when nonstutterers orally read under 200 msec DAF, their disfluencies resembled those that Wingate (1964) cites as forming the "kernel" of stuttering. Not only did disrhythmic phonation and part-word repetitions constitute the majority of disfluencies (70.9%), but Venkatigiri also found that part-word repetitions occurred mainly on the initial syllable. This finding challenged Wingate's (1976) claim that DAF-induced part-word repetitions invariably involve the final syllable. It is unfortunate that Venkatigiri failed to provide evidence of actual equivalence between the nonstutterers' and stutterers' repetitions.

Intelligibility Effects

Another method of describing DAF-affected speech has been in terms of its intelligiblity. Atkinson (1954), for example, found that the judged intelligibility of speech produced during 30-270 msec delays showed most obvious deterioration when the sidetone signal level was increased. This is an interesting finding when related to the claimed similarities between the effect of DAF and masking. In this regard, Draegert (1951) observed that during masking conditions, intelligibility ratings of speech also deteriorated. Those subjects with "superior" intelligibility under masking produced speech samples distinguished by longer syllable durations and greater intensity. Rate change was not shown to discriminate "inferior" and "superior" intelligibility ratings. A related finding emerges from Tiffany and Hanley's (1956) listener assessment of speech effectiveness during 180 msec DAF conditions. Their listeners rated "highly effective" speakers in nondelay conditions as much less effective in DAF conditions. Indeed, they were judged even less effective in DAF than those rated "less effective" without DAF. The level of intelligibility of speech produced during DAF conditions may therefore be an additional feature of the nonfluent speech produced during DAF. In short, DAF may not only produce nonfluent speech, but may also "scramble" the speaker's message.

Rate Effects

Numerous DAF studies have realized Lee's (1951) forecast that the speed-governing effects of DAF "probably will provide the more useful information"; though it now appears that speed reduction is not an invariant effect of DAF. Many early DAF studies chose oral-reading rate as a measure of its effects (Black,1951; Mahaffey and Stromsta, 1965; Spilka, 1954). Spilka's findings on the effects of short periods of oral reading under 94 to 375 msec delays are particularly informative—that the rate effect is associated with greater phonation time and increased vocal intensity. In this respect, therefore, it shares something in common with the effects produced by auditory masking.

The pattern of speech parameters that change during reduced speech rate under DAF may be related to some typical variations that transpire in speech production. Fonagy and Fonagy (1966), for example, showed that when speakers read loudly their vowel durations increase, but the duration of their voiceless sounds remain unchanged. Syllable duration change has also been reported during reduced oral-reading rate. Healey and Adams (1981a) showed that syllable *and* pause duration tend to increase when speakers (children and adults) are instructed to halve their oral-reading rate. DAF is often claimed to interrupt speaking, but an increase in pause time is not one of its typical effects. Therefore, it is unlikely that DAF's effects are the same as those caused by slow speaking, though they may resemble effects found during increased vocal intensity.

The consistency of DAF's rate reduction effect is uncertain. Brokaw, Singh, and Black (1966), for example, found the duration of oral readings increased by a ratio of 1.3:1, regardless of delays in the range 90-270 msec, although each delay increment was accompanied by increased intersubject variability. More significantly, Goldiamond, Atkinson, and Bilger (1962) found that rate varied during DAF according to whether or not speakers attended to their voice signals. Consequently, the speed-governing effect of DAF cannot be confidently regarded as a straightforward invariant effect.

Intensity Effects

Vocal intensity increases during DAF have been reported almost as consistently as nonfluency or rate reduction. The findings by Black (1951) and Spilka (1954) suggested that vocal intensity increases when relatively short delay levels are used, but does not increase during longer delay levels. However, the main effect of DAF on vocal intensity is probably directly related to sidetone level. Zalosh and Salzman (1965), for instance, found that an increase in sidetone level at different delay levels produced an associated increase in vocal intensity.

The positive effect of DAF sidetone manipulations on vocal intensity suggests that a portion of DAF's effect may be due to masking effects. Siegel and Pick (1974) observed that a speaker's usual response to an increase in nondelayed sidetone is to reduce vocal intensity, whereas, during masking conditions, vocal intensity is increased (the Lombard Effect). In other words, changes in vocal intensity during DAF probably resemble those produced by loud noise rather than the speaker's "stepped-up" voice signal.

Phonation Time

It is generally agreed that DAF may extend the duration of phonated sounds. And, as will be seen, it is an effect that has wide-ranging theoretical and clinical implications for stuttering.

Throughout this review it has been noted that increased syllable duration, vowel duration, and phonation time occurs during DAF with almost all age groups. Consequently, it would labor the point to review the relevant studies. Like the reduced rate effect, it obviously occurs frequently, but it is not an invariant effect. One interesting demonstration of this occurs in a study by Goldiamond, Atkinson, and Bilger (1962). They investigated their subjects' speech patterns using daily 90-minute oral readings under various delays and reported variable effects. One of the most prominent was "stretching out each word," but it was not the only one; "Others solved the problem of delayed feedback without slowing down. Some lowered their voices; others 'spat out' the words or read without normal inflection" (p.437). Quite obviously, therefore, increased phonation time was only one speech pattern that emerged in these conditions.

Conclusions from DAF Experiments with Normally Fluent Speakers

DAF research has revealed that the procedure produces remarkably diverse effects. Generally, they emerge as consequences of disruptions to the normal speech pattern during certain delay levels, signal intensity levels, and speaking rates. The effects also partially depend on the age and sex of the subjects. These consequences appear to vary with the time of DAF exposure, but over short periods they usually take the form of increased nonfluency, decreased intelligibility, reduced speech rate, increased vocal intensity, and increased phonation time. All of these response patterns may also be modified, or completely removed, however, according to the level of attention that the subject chooses to offer the delayed voice signal.

The variability of the DAF response, both within and between subjects, suggests that DAF has relatively unreliable effects, particularly over lengthy periods. That finding alone should have given pause to considerations on the relevance of DAF's effects to some models of speech behavior. But even if its effects were consistent, it is not at all clear what meaning they might have for a servosystem model of speech production. For instance, Lane and Tranel (1971) have noted that rhythmic tapping is disrupted whenever an associated light-signal is delayed, but that does not prove that visual feedback has a role in tapping. Indeed, it is more easily understood to be an unusual environmental condition that *may* disrupt that tapping. DAF's relevance to any explanation of the speech-production process is probably equally tenuous. Of more interest, though, are the strategies that speakers adopt to control the DAF effect. These have proven to be of far greater significance to clinicians concerned with medico-legal audiometry and, as will be seen, stuttering.

DAF Investigations with Stutterers

The Initial Studies

The almost predictable ameliorative effect of any novel stimulus on stuttering made it likely that DAF would have similar effects. That expectation should have been bolstered by evidence from normal speakers that DAF's effects included reduced speech rate, increased vocal intensity, and increased phonation time. Likewise, from the perspective of perceptual defect theories that had claimed stuttering resulted from aberrant auditory feedback (for example, Webster & Lubker, 1968; Yates, 1963; 1970), DAF's "corrective" effects were also predictable. Although, as will be seen, even the necessity of DAF to theoretical exlanations of its beneficial effects has turned out to be debatable. Indeed, DAF treatment research provides an excellent example of how history may repeat itself.

The initial DAF studies with stutterers provided only vague indications of its beneficial effects. The first indication occurred almost incidentally in a study by Naylor (1953) which was concerned with measures of stuttering severity. In one condition, stutterers (n=24) orally read an "adaptation passage" six times, the first five being under 180 msec DAF. A negative correlation emerged from comparisons between listener severity ratings (and, to a lesser extent, the subjects' severity ratings) of the subjects' speech during DAF and normal auditory feedback (NAF). Evidently, the more severe stutterers reduced the severity of their stutterings during DAF, while the less severe subjects reacted like nonstutterers. Naylor's study was followed by Nessel's (1958) assessment of speech rate and "errors" by stutterers (n=32) and nonstutterers (n=18) during oral reading of a 135-word passage in NAF and 130 msec DAF conditions.

Generally, the stutterers' speech rate did not differ under either condition, but they had fewer errors (including stutterings) under DAF. Three years later, Chase and colleagues reviewed their extensive work with DAF and indicated that they had "observed marked improvement of speech under delayed auditory feedback for 10 or 30 stutterers tested" (Chase, Sutton, & Rapin, 1961, p.216).

Soderberg was probably the first to recognize that any gains stutterers might receive from DAF could be related to different delay levels. He investigated this connection in his PhD thesis, which was subsequently published in summarized form (Soderberg, 1960). This described assessment of oral reading, spontaneous speech, and vowel production by 30 stutterers during DAF which *averaged* 140 msec delay: in pre-experimental trials, the "precise [delay] time was individually predetermined as a time that seemed to reduce the severity of the subject's stuttering" (p.253). When the group was divided into "most" and "least severe," it was found that the most-severe group tended to reduce frequency and duration of blocks during DAF, while the least-severe group showed more reduction in speech rate. Both groups increased their vocal pitch, which was also the only change that was retained when DAF conditions ceased.

The differential effects of DAF delay levels was also investigated by Lotzman (1961). Fifty stutterers and 43 nonstutterers made different oral readings (verse and prose) during six delay conditions (50, 100, 150, 200, 250, and 300 msecs). The entire assessment involved about 35 minutes of oral reading. The stutterers, in particular, showed individualized maximum and minimum beneficial effects at different delay levels, although most speech reductions (with minimal rate reductions) occurred at 50 and 100 msec delays. At longer delays, the effects resembled those found in the nonstutterers. The size of these effects is illustrated by data from 15 stutterers who showed approximately 88% reduction in speech errors at their most "beneficial-delay," but with quite variable effects on speech rate (one subject's reading time increased by 462% while another's decreased by 51%). An interesting observation by Lotzman was that some of the stutterers and nonstutterers' errors could be attributed to "pseudostuttering."

An attempt to assess the resemblance between nonfluency and true stuttering during DAF was made by Neelley (1961). He compared stutterers (n=23; 17-36 years) and nonstutterers (n=23; 19-32 years) during repeated oral readings under NAF and 140 msec DAF. In addition to measuring the frequency of nonfluencies and correct word rate, listeners (n=20) rated speech samples on a nine-point "speech disturbance" scale and attempted to distinguish samples from stutterers and nonstutterers made under the different reading conditions. Intriguingly, Neelley found no significant differences between the nonfluent response frequencies in both groups under DAF, except that the stutterers had fewer "additions" (mainly repetitions). Furthermore, listeners were unable to detect differences in the speech-disturbance ratings of both groups during DAF. But the study's most frequently cited finding was that listeners were generally able to identify the stutterers' NAF samples from the nonstutterers' DAF samples. This led Neelley to claim that nonstutterers' DAF-induced "stutterings" are not of the same type as chronic stutterings. The controversy over this finding was discussed earlier (see page 282, paragraph 1). One important and overlooked aspect of the controversy is that Neelley's data were also derived from "adaptation effect" conditions. This means that the speech quality of both groups should be considered as influenced by both DAF *and* repeated oral-reading conditions.

The Goldiamond Studies

The preceding studies exposed subjects to relatively brief periods of DAF. Yet, even during these short intervals, it was evident that DAF's beneficial effects would be quite variable. The importance of this variability became much clearer when stutterers were exposed to much longer intervals of DAF. This was particularly evident in a monumental series of studies by Israel Goldiamond. In many respects, Goldiamond's studies (Goldiamond, 1962; 1965; 1967; Goldiamond, Atkinson, & Bilger, 1962) cut a virtual swath across the whole field of DAF research. In retrospect, it becomes clear that these studies caused one of the most dramatic and productive shifts in the history of stuttering research. Ironically, the contribution of this research to stuttering appears to be quite unrelated to the reasons that Goldiamond advanced to explain his findings. The point should become clearer later in this chapter.

The variable effects on stutterers of long periods of DAF were not unexpected. The previously reviewed research has produced many indications that speech rate and disfluencies change over time during DAF (Tiffany & Hanley, 1956; Winchester, Gibbons, & Krebs, 1959). However, it was Goldiamond, Atkinson, and Bilger's (1962) study that drew attention to the remarkably different patterns that could be expected both within and between normal speakers; a finding which was also evident in later studies that Goldiamond conducted with stutterers.

Goldiamond's (1962, 1965) DAF investigations with stutterers contained three unusual features. First, they used DAF as either a 10-second consequence for stuttering, or it was eliminated for 10 seconds contingent on stuttering. Second, DAF was used over relatively long periods of oral reading; usually 90 minutes per day. And, finally, Goldiamond used 250 msec delay *plus* "masking noise in the [experimental] booth as well as through the headphones to mask bone conduction" (1965, p.121). No further details on this masking were provided in Goldiamond's reports, nor were efforts made to isolate masking's contribution to the studies' findings.

Goldiamond's (1962) initial findings were obtained with two (presumably adult male) stutterers who, incidentally, also gave a vivid demonstration of variability during DAF. The first subject (S) had two different responses to the elimination conditioning: a high rate of reading and stuttering, or a low rate of reading and stuttering. The latter pattern also involved prolonged vocalization and was described as "prolonged speech." It was this pattern that was eventually maintained when DAF was removed, and was later shaped towards normal speech rate using systematically increased reading speed. These procedures appear to have produced a 90% reduction in S's stuttering and a threefold increase in speech rate. In the other subject (K), the same procedure was reported to reduce stuttering by about 90%, while virtually retaining the subject's pretreatment speech rate. The carry-over effects were demonstrated 6 weeks later when K displayed the same behavior pattern in the absence of DAF conditions.

Goldiamond's (1965) procedure for instating and shaping prolonged speech was eventually developed into a relatively standardized method for treating stuttering. In summary, it involved (1) establishing prolonged speech with 250 msec DAF contingent-elimination conditions during oral reading sessions, (2) systematically fading DAF conditions by reducing the delay level in 50 msec steps while stuttering was maintained at a relatively low rate, (3) shaping the new speech pattern into more normal-sounding speech by increasing oral-reading rate and retaining a low frequency of stuttering, and (4) introducing self-control procedures to assist use of the new speech pattern beyond the clinic. The results of this methodology will be considered later. At this juncture, the principal interest is in the procedure that Goldiamond instituted to ensure that the prolonged speech pattern could be reproduced.

There is ample evidence in Goldiamond's 1965 report that prolonged speech was neither a reliable nor replicable derivative of oral reading during 250 msec DAF. This problem might have been due to the 10-second elimination condition, though later applications of this technique, using continuous DAF, have also required additional strategies to ensure the consistent appearance of prolonged speech. In Goldiamond's report, such strategies were needed to ensure that only one of "four possible novel patterns" emerged during DAF: "prolongation, voice lowering, proprioceptive increase, tuning out" (p.139). In fact, just running the subject until prolongation occurred was contraindicated; Goldiamond argued that this might cause the other competing patterns to be maintained. For this reason, verbal instructions, reading-rate control, and/or reinforcement were recommended to ensure the appearance of prolongation. This leads to an interesting problem which, in many ways, has been the procedure's Achilles heel with respect to stuttering treatment. The problem is the use of clinician judgments to identify and virtually cajole the appearance of prolonged speech during DAF. Admittedly, the descriptions of prolonged speech included "prolonged vocalization" at a low reading and stuttering rate, but this also describes a huge variety of speech patterns. This may seem a moot point in a context where judgments are needed even to identify stuttering. But, unlike stuttering judgments, the reliability with which experimenters or clinicians identified the distinguishing features of prolonged speech was never established—an oversight that continues to plague all clinical uses of prolonged speech.

The impact that Goldiamond's research had on DAF research was not immediate. It arrived via a rather circuitous route that began when other clinicians employed his treatment method and generally replicated many of its effects. Some began to draw attention to factors in the speech pattern that could be even more responsible than DAF for procuring stutter-free speech. That was accentuated by growing awareness that DAF was not even essential to the treatment: the relevant speech pattern could be produced simply by instruction (Goldiamond, 1967). In the midst of this, it also became obvious that Goldiamond's research had touched on a number of important issues concerning DAF's effect on stuttering. It had certainly highlighted the significance of speech rate, the controlling effects of attention to the feedback signal, and the unreliability of effects derived from either short- or long-term DAF conditions. But, more importantly, the findings also highlighted the possibility that the speech pattern, as such, was far more responsible for DAF's control over stuttering than delayed feedback of the voice signal. In fact, Goldiamond's standardized method for instating prolonged speech probably turns out to be a successful method for controlling the unpredictable nature of DAF's effects.

The greatest legacy from Goldiamond's research may well be the inadvertent attention it gave to the role of vocalization in modifying stuttering. For, shortly afterwards, the pervasive role that vocalization occupied in procedures or conditions that modify stuttering was brought to the fore in two influential theoretical papers by Wingate (1969b; 1970). Both papers drew attention to the regularity with which altered vocalization accompanied many conditions that reduce stuttering (for example, rhythm, masking, chorus reading, singing, and DAF). But they placed equal emphasis on the temporary or "artificial fluency" that accompanied use of these procedures. Indeed, Wingate's thesis implied that DAF-induced fluency was as much related to normal fluency as "artificial" stuttering was to chronic stuttering: both simply relied on procedures that could temporally disrupt the subject's customary manner of speaking. The sudden interest that this provoked in vocalization, or more specifically, phonation, was virtually matched by the sudden loss of interest in DAF research on stuttering. To some extent, this decline in DAF research was aided, at that time, by growing disenchantment with the explanatory strength of auditory feedback models of stuttering.

The "Post-Goldiamond" Studies

Research on DAF and stuttering did not end after the mid-1960s. Quite a number of investigations were conducted on the effects of manipulating the frequency and intensity of the feedback signals, comparing DAF and masking, assessing age effects, and closer examination of the types of disfluencies produced by DAF. But almost all of these studies used relatively brief periods of DAF, and appear to have had little impact on either the theory or treatment of stuttering. For the sake of completeness—and to support that claim—the relevant research is reviewed below.

Feedback-Signal Manipulations

Manipulations of frequency and intensity of the feedback signal have revealed some variable effects of DAF on stuttering. Ham and Steer (1967) assessed 100 to 800 msec DAF with college-age stutterers (n=10) during oral reading. They found the most desired effect on "blocks" and speech rate occurred when the feedback signal was conditioned by an 800Hz HP filter at 60 or 75dB (above individualized SRT scores). But they failed to find a "peak effect" at any delay level. Gibney (1973) assessed the interaction between 100, 200, and 400 msec delay levels and 65,

75, and 85dB SPL during oral reading. In contrast to Ham and Steer, Gibney showed that disfluencies were minimized and reading rate maximized during 100 msec delay at 65dB SPL. Langova, Moravek, Novak, and Petrik (1970) reported using 500-1100Hz pass filtering of 145 (or 415)[1] msec DAF with 71 stutterers. But no data were provided to support their claim that relative increases in speech rate were associated with the filtered DAF condition.

DAF and Masking Comparisons

The contribution that masking makes to DAF's effect on stuttering has not been seriously investigated, yet there is reason to suspect that it might be influential. For instance, when prolonged speech accompanies 250 msec DAF then a relatively continuous audible signal is generated that must share something in common with masking. Goldiamond (1965) made this more manifest by actually organizing for masking to accompany DAF in his treatment studies. On the other hand, it is likely that some masking studies may have induced DAF effects. For instance, the silent-masking conditions in the Sutton and Chase (1961) experiment produced a "delayed masking" condition that may have resembled DAF effects: each pause after an utterance was filled with a signal condition as is true of DAF. But comparisons between DAF and masking would be more significant if it were found that they produced similar effects.

At least five studies have included comparisons between DAF and masking with stutterers. Lotzman (1961) had subjects (n=62) orally read under conditions in which all speech signal frequencies below 500 Hz were masked by a signal 10dBs above vocal intensity. A comparison was made between the effects of this condition and the delay level for each subject (n=48) that produced maximum reductions in stuttering and minimum reductions in speech rate. The findings show the masking conditions produced an average of 236% more "speech errors," although three subjects did have more "speech errors" during DAF. But the comparison is complicated because 42 of the 48 subjects also spoke more slowly in the DAF conditions. Another difficulty is that the DAF condition was individualized, while the masking condition's signal intensity was fixed. Hutchinson and Norris (1977) compared 300 msec DAF, 80dB SPL masking, and 60 bpm metronome conditions; they showed no significant reductions in stuttering during conversational speech (3 minutes) with DAF and masking. But, in an oral reading task (250 syllables), there were similar reductions in stuttering during DAF and masking. Lechner (1979) assessed NAF, 140 msec DAF, and 90dB SPL masking during oral reading by 15 stutterers and 15 nonstutterers. Lechner's most relevant finding, regarding the stutterers, was that both masking and DAF increased fundamental frequency, with DAF producing more impact on the frequency of inflections. In addition, DAF reduced utterance rate but, surprisingly, no condition altered percentage of vocalization time. Stephen and Haggard's (1980) study used 100 msec DAF in which the feedback signal was also low-frequency

[1]This confusion exists because of typographical errors in the article.

masking or an amplitude envelope derived from the speech signal. They also used continuous or amplitude-modulated masking conditions to yield various analyses of the effects of DAF and masking on their stutterers' (n=11) oral reading. In summary, their findings showed DAF and contingent masking conditions were equally effective in improving reading rates and reducing reading errors. Finally, Martin and Haroldson (1979) compared 250 msec DAF and 100dB SPL white noise (5 minutes "on" followed by 5 minutes "off") over 30 minutes of spontaneous speech by 20 stutterers (19-46 years). Generally the effects were quite similar: 85% of the subjects reduced stuttering during DAF, while 80% reduced stuttering during masking. The mean reductions in stuttering were very similar, although the mean duration of stuttering during DAF was significantly shorter. However, this comparison is based on continuous DAF conditions and intermittent masking conditions. Andrews, Howie, Dozsa, and Guitar (1982) assessed mean phonation duration, pause proportions, articulation rate, fluent speech rate, mean sentence length, and percentage of syllables stuttered by three adult stutterers during DAF (250 msec) and wide-band 80-dB binaural masking (plus other conditions). The mean percentage of stuttering during 10 minutes of spontaneous speech decreased, relative to base rates, by a mean of 98% during DAF, but only 52% during masking. Predictably, the DAF conditions increased mean phonation duration, while this increase was not evident during masking. But this finding is confounded by differences in speech rates and stutterings in both conditions.

Some tentative conclusions can be drawn from these studies. For example, DAF's effects on stuttering are probably quite similar to those produced during masking, except when an "optimum masking level" is used, although this finding is weakened by the absence of a study using an individually "optimum masking level." Actually, the similarities between the findings are rather surprising, since relatively short periods of DAF and fixed-delay levels (in all but one study) might be expected to yield dissimilar, rather than similar, findings. The fact that they did not suggests that the two conditions might have much in common. In other words, there is a good likelihood that DAF effects may be partially influenced by auditory masking.

Age Variables

Because age variables produced quite prominent differences in DAF effects with normal speakers, some interest in their implications for stuttering continued. Burke (1975b) investigated the effects of 0-300 msec DAF on stutterers in the 7-12 (n=10) and 13-18 (n=10) age range during 1-minute periods of oral reading and spontaneous speech (interestingly, 11 subjects failed to stutter during the 0 msec DAF condition). Comparisons between "high" and "low disfluent" subgroups at both age levels showed maximum effects occurred within the "high disfluent" subgroups. Like Lotzman's (1961) finding, these were also found mainly during 50 and 100 msec delays. Negative effects tended to appear at the longer delay levels. Timmons and Boudreau (1978a; 1978b) assessed the effects of 113-520 msec DAF on 5- to 13-year-old subjects. Their data, from brief oral readings, show that the 5-8 (n=10) and the 9-13 (n=15) age groups significantly reduced disfluencies at all delay levels, with the younger group benefiting more from the longer delay (520 msecs). The significance of these findings is not at all obvious, because it is uncertain whether the effects were independent of other alterations to fluency. This last point becomes relevant when related to studies that have used more refined measures of speech behavior during DAF.

Disfluency Changes by Stutterers during DAF

The effects of brief periods of DAF on stutterers' disfluency categories is rather ambiguous. It will be recalled from Neelley's (1961) findings that the disfluency categories showed differential changes during DAF. This finding received further support in two other studies. Hayden, Scott, and Addicott (1977) measured various disfluency categories in the oral readings (196 words) of 10 stutterers (14-21 years) under NAF and 200 msec DAF, and found that the total number of disfluencies actually increased during DAF. The changes within specific disfluency categories turned out to be quite different. As expected, prolongations increased, but blocking decreased. Meanwhile, the frequency of repetitions (of most types) remained unchanged: only medial syllable repetitions significantly increased during DAF. By contrast, Hutchinson and Norris (1977) found no increase in total disfluencies during either oral reading or conversational speech by 12 stutterers during 300 msec DAF. The "dysfluency" categories used by Hutchinson and Norris (1977) do not readily equate with those used by Hayden et al. (1977), but they do share a common "repetition" category. This category shows evidence of reduction in DAF conditions within the Hutchinson and Norris data, but not in the Hayden et al. data. At least part of the differences between the findings from both studies could be due to their different delay levels. Unfortunately, none of these findings shed any light on individual behavior changes that may appear over longer DAF intervals, using different delays and/or oral reading rates. Although Hayden et al. did observe that very wide-ranging changes occurred within each disfluency category.

Extended DAF Conditions and Stuttering

Two studies have produced more findings concerning the effects of lengthy exposure to DAF. Webster, Schumacher, and Lubker (1970) used 0-500 msec DAF during oral reading by six stutterers (14-28 years). Over a 5-day interval, each subject read for 5 minutes during 0, 100, 200, 300, 400, and 500 msec DAF (each delay level was tested on each day). In general, measures of oral-reading time and number of blocks showed that most benefits appeared at 100 and 200 msec. These gains were associated with markedly different speaking rates, however, the two subjects showing greatest reductions in blocks produced the fastest and slowest reading rates. Treon and Tamayo (1974) treated two stutterers (19 years) with 28 1-hour sessions of 200-300 msec DAF (with and without GSR biofeedback conditions) and showed that fewer blocks were associated with the DAF conditions. Unfortunately, no reliability or speech-rate data accompanied these findings. Nevertheless, both Webster et al. and Treon and Tamayo did find that blocking behaviors were reduced during extended DAF.

DAF and Stuttering Theories

Auditory feedback provided the conceptual base for a number of stuttering theories that emerged during the 1960s. In fact, most of these theories virtually rested on the findings from DAF research. The zeal with which some theorists seized on the DAF effect to explain stuttering is quite amazing in retrospect. Perhaps an extreme example is an explanatory model offered by Wolf and Wolf (1959). They argued that stuttering may be a byproduct of a "deadtime lag" that occurs intermittently in the neural speech centers, thereby producing delayed comparisons between speech production and error detection. Their suggested treatment was surgery designed to provide compensatory networks: "The compensatory networks will consist of nerve-like tissue which will be collected in a bank and connected to the proper part of the brain to reduce or even correct these anomalies" (p.53). Many feedback theories of stuttering appear to have been influenced by Cherry and Sayer's (1956) speculation that stuttering "is mediated by the subject's perceptions of his low-frequency-voice sounds" (p.243). Only a brief account of these theories will be provided in order to illustrate their common elements and their attempts to account for various types of stuttering.

Mysak (1960) argued that both open- and closed-cycle servosystems are required to sustain "verbal automaticity." He claimed this automaticity is due to "disturbances in reflexive and automatic mechanisms in various parts of the total linguistic circuitry" (p.195). The sources of disturbance, he conjectured, were "aberrations in bone conduction, the organ of Corti as well as the auditory pathways, [that] may produce conditions that simulate experimental delay times and which may result in similar [to DAF's effect on normals] fluency anomalies" (p.190).

Yates (1963) claimed the DAF findings provided grounds for concluding "that a major breakthrough has been made in the understanding of stammering." He argued that the empirical results indicate "that the locus of the basic defect is in the bone conduction channel which is 'out-of-phase' with the other feedback channels" (Yates, 1969, p.161-2). Yates also theorized, though, that stuttering was an end-product of a variety of learned factors which may modify the predictable disruptions from this defect. Gruber (1965) produced a perceptual defect theory which shifted the focus to the airborne feedback channel. He theorized that a stutterer is "arrested at the auditory level of speech monitoring and has failed to make the transition to the tactual and proprioceptive avenues" (p.379). To resolve this difficulty, Gruber recommended therapy procedures which, somehow, intensify speech monitoring via the tactual and proprioceptive channels in order to counteract a "malfunctioning auditory monitoring system" (Gruber, 1970).

Two theories implicated middle-ear dysfunction as a source of feedback disruption. Butler and Stanley (1966) postulated that the source of instability in the stutterer's auditory feedback system is a flawed "sidetone suppression loop." This was a theorized byproduct of the stutterer's "overdeveloped" response to social pressure, and it manifested itself in the middle-ear tympanic muscle's failure to adjust to variations in auditory gain; this prevented normal neural feedback and produced stuttering. A rather related theory was proposed by Webster and Lubker (1968). They argued that auditory feedback blocks the "output signals" for speech control, mainly because of an aberrant interaction between air-conducted and bone-conducted components of the feedback system. The operative interfering agent was the middle-ear reflex which, presumably, malfunctioned because of momentary phase or frequency-induced distortions to the feedback signal. Webster and Lubker argued that DAF's beneficial effect on stuttering occurs because "the delay interval serves to hold back the return of the interfering air-conducted auditory signal until the speech act which originated the signal is well underway or completed" (1968, p.760).

Two theories have been proposed to integrate anxiety factors and auditory feedback factors. One was suggested by Martin (1970). He argued that speech anxiety leads to unusual signal detection operations that become excessively conservative in stutterers. This delays the operation of a comparator which distinguishes between noise and speech signals. The result is similar to DAF'S effect, except that it produces an even more conservative detection criterion in order to avoid more unintelligible speech. It is not at all clear how this self-perpetuating system could end. Timmons and Boudreau (1972) also claimed that anxiety may cause muscle tightening which (among other effects) slightly alters the oral cavity's contour. The result is a change in auditory feedback which, in turn, disrupts the ongoing speech output.

The only feedback theory which locates the source of auditory disruption at a more peripheral level is one suggested by Sklar (1969). In this model, stuttering was regarded as a manifestation of an oscillating closed loop feedback system. The object of Sklar's model was to provide a logical basis for removing stuttering by using engineering principles for dampening oscillation. This involved reducing signal feedback which arrived from any sense modalities involved in speaking (Sklar recommended masking, hearing reduction, or tranquilizers).

This survey of the perceptual-defect theories may have blurred some of their distinguishing features, but they all share a common assumption: the stutterer lives with a malfunctioning auditory feedback system which produces continuous or intermittent DAF conditions. Most also claim that for the chronic stutterer, in particular, this asynchronous feedback is made synchronous during DAF conditions, thereby accounting for its fluency-inducing effects. The model was simple and obviously engaging as is demonstrated by the number of theories it produced. The only problem was that it bypassed the subtleties and complexities of the relationship between DAF and stuttering.

Criticisms of Auditory-Interference Models of Stuttering

One fairly fundamental criticism of an auditory defect model of stuttering is that it rests on a shaky model of speech production. Garber and Siegel (1981), for instance, criticized Fairbanks's (1954) model because it assumes that speakers have the capacity to constantly regulate or correct errors in phonemes or syllables. But their claim that this is impossible may be a little premature. Netsell (1981) recently concluded that the current evidence on reaction time rates within the speech motor system make it possible that such regulation could occur: "Whether the [speech motor control] system is under 'open or closed loop control' or both, or whether it is 'preprogrammed' and playing out a 'motor tape' while oblivious to its 'senses' remain matters of essential conjecture." (p.6.)

Nevertheless, it is unclear how evidence on the effects of delaying the auditory feedback process necessarily implicates auditory regulation. As mentioned earlier, Lane and Tranel (1971) illustrated this point by reference to the Chase et al. (1961) experiment in which rhythmic key tapping was disrupted by a delayed, but correlated, light flash. As they pointed out, it does not follow, therefore, that tapping is regulated by visual feedback. Another criticism was offered by Smith (1966), who argued that DAF effects are so variable that it is difficult to believe that there exists a direct relationship between auditory feedback and speech production. He also noted that since the sources of "feedback" in the speech system are so multitudinous it would be naive to ascribe any primacy to auditory feedback.

Any attempt to cement a relationship between stuttering and DAF must deal with some important features of stuttering, as well as DAF's impact on stuttering. To begin with, many theories are based on the resemblance between oscillation in a servosystem and stuttering. While there may be some similarity between repetitions during DAF and stuttering (Venkatigiri, 1980), not all stutterings are repetitions. More importantly, a substantial number of stutterings occur on the initial sound of an utterance, that is, before any disruptive feedback could occur. In fact, many severe stutterers are often unable to utter a sound for quite lengthy periods; at such times the auditory feedback channels would seemingly fail to convey any signals, let alone disruptive feedback.

Another problem is that the effect of continuous DAF (presumably a necessary condition within some feedback theories) is far from predictable. Among normal speakers some evidence shows that a substantial amount of adaptation can be expected from continuous DAF. And although no carefully documented account exists on the effect of weeks or months of speaking under these conditions, there is some evidence that constant DAF would produce a considerable amount of compensatory behavior. In fact, as Goldiamond, Atkinson, and Bilger (1962) found, some speakers have no difficulty at all in ignoring DAF. Moreover, most theorists have drawn on the brief effects of continuous DAF to support their claims, when there is more likelihood that studies which have used lengthy and intermittent DAF conditions would be much more relevant to their theories. Unfortunately, to date, no such study has been reported.

Another difficulty for auditory interference theories has been the failure to replicate some important experimental findings on which these theories are based. For example, it will be recalled that Cherry and Sayer's findings were regarded as cornerstones for Yates's (1963; 1969; 1970) theory. However, not only have these findings not been replicated (Conture, 1974; May & Hackwood, 1968), but also the parallel notion—that speakers who are susceptible to DAF effects would improve during reduced bone-conducted feedback—has not been supported (Burke, 1975a).

Perhaps the most important criticism levelled against the auditory intereference theories is their reliance on the "beneficial" effects of DAF with stutterers. As mentioned earlier, these effects were also far from predictable. Certainly some stutterers—usually severe stutterers—reduce stuttering during DAF, but this almost always emerges in conjunction with abnormal speech quality. Indeed, in short-term studies this speech quality might be aptly described as disfluent speech (Hayden, Scott & Addicott, 1977) since it is largely composed of prolongations. Moreover, many descriptions of DAF's effects on stutterers (for example, Goldiamond, Atkinson, & Bilger, 1962; Langova, Moravek, Novak, & Petrik, 1970; Soderberg, 1968) emphasized the appearance of an unusual speech pattern as much as they emphasized reduced stuttering. What emerged, therefore, was not so much a finding supportive of auditory interference theories, but an abundance of possible explanations for DAF's modifying effects on stuttering. It should also be added that no auditory interference theory explained DAF's negative effects on less severe stutterers. They also failed to account for such odd findings as DAF's differential effects on conversational speech and oral reading (Burke, 1975b).

In many respects, the "artificial" fluency (Wingate, 1969b; 1970a) that DAF appeared to generate for stutterers can be "explained" by most auditory interference theories. The prolonged speech pattern can be conceived of as establishing an overlapping signal which removes a disruptive delay or aberrant mixture of feedback speech signals. Alternatively, since DAF's "fluency" is usually—though not always (Webster, Schumacher, & Lubker, 1970)—produced at a slow speech rate, this may be the principal agent modifying stuttering. Of course, reduced rate may also be a means of reducing feedback.[2] But, more importantly, the altered manner of speaking during DAF incorporates some factors that might be as responsible for reducing stuttering as aberrant feedback regulation, factors that Wingate has jointly labelled "modified vocalization."

The Revival of Auditory-Interference Postulates

Before examining the research sparked by the "modified vocalization hypothesis," some mention should be made of investigations into characteristics of the auditory system of stutterers. Much of this research was reviewed in Chapter 7, and was also considered recently by Garber and Siegel (1981). But there are some important studies in this area which have produced findings that have revived interest in auditory interference theories.

The rate of the stapedial reflex in stutterers has been central to some theories

[2] Recall, even with normal speakers, Kodman (1961) found that reduced rate removed the disruptive effects of DAF.

(for example, Butler & Stanley, 1966; Webster & Lubker, 1968). The evidence that it may function abnormally in stutterers, or has a role in stuttering, is certainly suggestive. The first investigation of the reflex in stutterers, by Shearer and Simmons (1965), was inconclusive; they found no differences in the reflex-action time preceding phonation by stutterers and nonstutterers. However, Horovitz, Johnson, Pearlman, Schaffer, and Hedin (1978) observed that when stutterers and nonstutterers visualized anxiety-evoking scenes, only their stutterers produced significantly altered mean stapedial reflexes. Perhaps a related finding is Panconcelli-Calzia's (1955) report that only 25% of stutterers showed the Lombard Sign, compared with 70% of voice-disorder patients and 80% of normal speakers. Other evidence of unusual audition occurs in Delaney's (1979) investigation of middle-ear muscle function in stutterers and normals (4-14 years), some of whom had a history of middle ear problems: the stutterers without a problem history and nonstutterers with a problem history showed greater, and more variable, contractions than stutterers with a problem history and nonstutterers without a problem history.

Perhaps the most pertinent evidence regarding a hypothesized disparity in stutterers' air- and bone-conduction system was provided by Stromsta (1972). He compared the point at which stutterers (n=25) cancelled the auditory sensation of bone-conducted sinusoidal signals at frequencies ranging from 150Hz to 2400Hz. Phase differences were found at 150, 300, and 1200Hz, and were interpreted to mean that stutterers experience generally slower transmission times than nonstutterers at those frequencies. From earlier research, Stromsta (1959) concluded that stutterers may be more vulnerable to phonation blockage as a result of these slower transmission times.

Another interesting finding, relative to feedback concepts, is Martin, Lawrence, Haroldson, and Gunderson's (1981) investigation of oral stereognosis in stutterers and nonstutterers. Contrary to earlier findings of Jensen, Sheehan, Williams, and LaPointe (1975), they found that stutterers (n=20) were generally poorer than nonstutterers (n=20) in recognizing various shapes placed inside their mouths. The stutterers' apparent inability to accurately perceive proprioceptive information was also found to be reliable over time.

These are some of the more intriguing findings that have served to revive interest in auditory interference theories. They provide some support for the possibility that stutterers may, after all, be handicapped by unusual, if not abnormal, feedback systems.

Speech-Pattern-Change Factors and Stuttering Modification

The main contribution to stuttering from the years of delayed-auditory-feedback research now appears to be that it forced researchers and clinicians to attend (yet again) to variables that change in the stutterer's speech pattern whenever stuttering is reduced. It led, particularly, to an interest in the prominent feature in the "fluency" produced by DAF or other "fluency-inducing" conditions. The investigations stemming from this interest implicated almost all aspects of the speech production process that had any relevance to fluency or stuttering. The initial and, in many respects, continuing impetus behind many of these investigations were some relatively vague postulates that Wingate (1969b; 1970) advanced, and which have come to be known, jointly, as the "modified vocalization hypothesis." In many ways, this hypothesis is responsible for stimulating revived interest in the contribution that certain respiratory, phonatory, and articulatory factors might make to cardinal changes in a fluency-inducing speech pattern. In turn, this has led to a surge of investigations on physiologic, aerodynamic, and perceptual variables that might distinguish between the speech pattern of stutterers and nonstutterers. The development and current state of this area of research will be examined in the following sections.

Wingate's Modified Vocalization Hypothesis

Just as auditory feedback concepts dominated much stuttering research during the 1960s, so Wingate's "modified vocalization hypothesis" appears to have influenced the bulk of stuttering research in the 1970s. Its influence is all the more remarkable because, as we shall see, the exact terms of the hypothesis were never clearly enunciated. The terms simply emerged from some speculations that Wingate (1969b; 1970) offered regarding factors that seem to be common (and necessary) to conditions reliably reported to reduce or remove stuttering. He argued that rhythmic speech, singing, choral reading, shadowing, masking, and delayed auditory feedback all have one common feature—they alter the sound and pattern of speech. More specifically: "In almost all circumstances where stuttering is substantially reduced, certain changes in vocal expression seem to be significantly involved if not, in fact, responsible for the improved fluency" (Wingate, 1970, p.871). This observation was not original. Johnson and Rosen (1937) and Bloodstein (1950), for example, had also drawn attention to the involvement of speech-pattern change in many of these conditions. But none had attached significance to one aspect of this pattern change—emphasized vocalization. And, for many reasons, their observations failed to provoke the extraordinary interest that Wingate's speculations achieved.

The main reason for the impact of the modified vocalization hypothesis may well be that it simply appeared at the right time. Its appearance coincided with the growing popularity of therapy programs based on Goldiamond's methodology (for example, Curlee & Perkins, 1969; Ryan, 1971; Webster & Lubker, 1968) that were beginning to dispense with DAF as a means for procuring the prolonged speech pattern. In doing so, both the theoretical and clinical focus on factors that might be necessary to reduce stuttering shifted towards the vocal and motoric variables that obviously accompanied the prolonged speech pattern. This should have been a predictable area of investigation, given the abundant evidence that DAF's effects—even with normal speakers—involved modified and extended vocalization. But the appealing feature of Wingate's hypothesis was that it introduced a possibility that emphasized vocalization was not only crucial to DAF's fluency-inducing effects, but might always be present whenever stuttering decreases. The hypothesis then led many to conclude that this might mean that the processes involved in vocalization are especially significant to stuttering. And it was this prospect that effectively launched a wide-ranging search for stuttering-related variables that has ultimately implicated almost every part of the speech-production process.

Before considering the search for the "proof" of the modified vocalization hypothesis, it is important to recognize that it is linked to Wingate's claim that stuttering is a "phonetic transition defect" (Wingate, 1969a). This concept of stuttering emphasized that the disorder was literally the action involved "in getting 'off' or progressing 'beyond' the sound" (p.107). It suggested that stuttering is mainly discoordination of the phonatory and articulatory actions needed in the transitional process that forms much of a fluent utterance. One of the first investigations related to this concept was Wingate's (1966a) own, which was concerned with the relationship between the adaptation effect and altered prosody: the effect was found to occur when punctuation was unchanged across readings, but it was not evident when punctuation was altered for each reading. Wingate concluded, therefore, that the adaptation effect was produced by general familiarity with a situation, plus increased familiarity with the passage's prosody. Conversely, it was suggested that changes in suprasegmental features, such as juncture, intonation, and stress produced by altered punctuation, reduced familiarity with the passage's prosody and reactivated stuttering. This led Wingate to the "suspicion" that stuttering is largely caused by quick changes in phonation and articulation—a suspicion fostered by the likelihood that emphasized vocalization does not usually involve such quick changes.

In later writings, Wingate (1976; 1977) has argued that much of the alleged "grammatical factor" in stuttering—such as more frequent stuttering on initial consonants rather than vowels (Johnson & Brown, 1953)—is better explained by reference to linguistic stress. As a result of a analysis of earlier research on word position effects (Wingate, 1976), plus his own research (Wingate, 1979a), he argued that the level of emphasis that speakers place on sounds during speech directly contributes to stuttering. For instance, stuttering is often reported to be more frequent on initial words in a sentence, particularly if they are "content" words. However, by using sentences with changes in the typical ratio of "content" to "function" words in the first three words of a sentence, Wingate (1979a) demonstrated that total stutterings on those first three words was not dissimilar to its frequency later in a sentence. The linguistic stress that usually accompanies content words was assumed to be less evident on function words. As a result, the typical finding of more stuttering at the beginning of sentences was not reproduced.

Wingate's conceptualization of stuttering as defective management of shifts between phonation and articulation, or activated by unusual demands on the phonatory process, was inevitably implicated in the research that pursued the modified vocalization hypothesis. As will be seen, investigations on the pattern and management of phonation became almost synonymous with investigations on

Wingate's "hypothesis." This was the logical consequence of the relatively flimsy specifications on the form or extent of vocalization change that the hypothesis predicted in fluency-inducing conditions. Nevertheless, almost every dimension of speech behavior has been examined in endeavors to test the hypothesis. That research will be traced in the proceeding sections, and will be followed by a further appraisal of Wingate's speculations—both original and current—regarding fluency-inducing conditions and stuttering.

In previous sections, much credit for the direction of current stuttering research has been given to Israel Goldiamond—particularly his 1965 research program. To some extent, as was noted, much of that credit is accidentally deserved. At the very least, it should be shared with Marcel Wingate, whose contribution was far from accidental. Wingate's influence on stuttering research has come in two phases. The initial phase, as was mentioned earlier (see Chapter 4), prompted many to reconsider the tenability of the influential propositions derived from Johnson's Diagnosogenic Theory. In the same vein, incidentally, he has also been a trenchant critic of many propositions spawned within the behavioral preparadigm. But this second phase, which has involved many speculations about factors that might be crucial to stuttering modification, has had *the* most dramatic directional influence on stuttering research over the past decade.

Martin Adams's Contributions

One of the first research programs largely directed towards investigating aspects of the modified vocalization hypothesis was initiated by Martin Adams and colleagues at Purdue University. Adams is also a major contributor to the revived interest in physiologic and aerodynamic analyses of stuttering and fluency. Much of this work is based on the notion that "speech fluency depends, at least in part, upon the correct timing and prompt smooth initiation, and maintenance of air flow and glottal vibration. These effects result from the harmonious integration of subglottic pressure, glottal resistance and supraglottic pressure" (1974, p. 37). Consequently, muscle activities that cause "the disintegration of subglottic pressure, glottal resistance and supraglottic pressure [also] prevent the timing, starting and maintenance of air flow and concomitant vocalization. Therefore these muscle actions might well be the motor determinants of stuttering" (1974, p.38).

This concept of fluency and stuttering has partly served to relate the modified vocalization hypothesis to propositions that could be investigated with the advantages of previously unavailable technology. At the same time, it also activated interest in the contribution that phonatory activities make to stuttering. The whole process of producing adequate and accurate phonation obviously relies on a subtle combination of air flow, muscle actions (at all levels of the vocal tract), and articulatory gesture. It probably also relies on some aspects of audition. When all of these factors must be related to the individual's state of arousal, and the high degree of synergy which the system requires to ensure "fluency," it is obvious that any research on aberrant phonation is faced with some immense technical problems. But these problems have not been aided by the conceptual basis of the research methodology used in many investigations in this area. It is an issue which merits some comment.

The research area that emerged in association with Martin Adams's analyses of the physiologic and aerodynamic variables associated with the speech of stutterers has become known as "vocal tract dynamics." This general area of investigation has included perceptual, physiologic, and acoustic studies with particular emphasis on voice timing, laryngeal muscle activity, and air flow. Most of the research has been based on comparisons between stutterers and nonstutterers, fluent and stuttered utterances, and differences produced by conditions known to reduce stuttering. Naturally, the findings have led to conclusions based on these differences. However, this method of investigation, which typifies much stuttering research, has some obvious limitations; it might reveal important characteristics of stuttering, but it has limited possibilities for identifying causal factors. For instance, findings derived from comparisons between stutterers and nonstutterers, particularly adults, are inevitably confounded by the unpredictable effects that their widely different speaking histories may impose on orally related responses. Comparisons between fluent and stuttered utterances may be a very suitable means of identifying important differentiating factors. But, again, the causal nature of those factors only emerges when their independent and controlled manipulation concomitantly modifies stuttering. Unfortunately, until lately, this method of investigation has been virtually unused in this area of stuttering research.

Another research issue in this area concerns the use of the adaptation effect to test hypotheses. Stuttering researchers appear to have an unquenchable interest in this phenomenon, in spite of its questionable predictability (Bloodstein, 1981). Nevertheless, many investigators seem prepared to trade off this obvious disadvantage for the dubious experimental advantage of using identical oral readings—and this seems to be true of researchers working in this area. The issue has been made more complex because the adaptation effect has been freely used in order to investigate vocal tract dynamics, and has also been regarded as a phenomenon likely to be explained by vocal tract dynamics.

Laryngeal-Adjustment Investigations

As mentioned above, Wingate (1966a) found that manipulating prosodic structure during repeated oral readings served to impede the adaptation effect. This led him to conclude that stuttering is reduced whenever the speaker practices articulation-phonation coordination. Presumably, such practice is "disrupted when the prosodic pattern of each reading is altered" in various ways. On the face of it, the strength of this effect must be somewhat limited, since repeated oral readings may reduce stuttering but rarely remove the condition (Wingate, 1966b). Nevertheless, there exists some persuasive evidence in the following studies that oral-reading practice contributes more to the adaptation effect than does increased familiarity with reading material.

Besozzi and Adams (1969) arranged for stutterers (n=16) to orally read a passage, then silently reread it on three occasions, and finally read it orally once more. The median reduction in stuttering between the first and fifth reading was about 20%; the reduction was around 61% if all readings were read orally. In two subsequent studies, the articulation-phonation coordination factor was identified even more clearly. Brenner, Perkins, and Soderberg (1972) compared the effects of silent, lipped, whispered, and no-rehearsal of different sentences (three times), with loud rehearsals on stuttering frequency during a final reading aloud. The aloud readings by the stutterers (n=8) resulted in significantly fewer stutterings than all other reading conditions (which, incidentally, were not significantly different). However, any conclusions drawn from this study must be qualified by its relatively poor reliability data (66% agreement between three judges on stutterings), and absence of control over the duration of the task in each condition. These problems were partially controlled in a subsequent study by Bruce and Adams (1978), which essentially used Besozzi and Adams's (1969) design, except that readings two, three, and four were whispered, rather than read silently. By the end of the fifth reading, the experimental passage had produced a 39% reduction in stutterings, compared with 65% fewer stutterings during the control condition. The 98% between-judge scoring agreement was impressive, although the absence of information on reading rate is disappointing.

Various conclusions can be drawn from these adaptation studies. From the perspective of vocal tract dynamics, however, it has usually been concluded that the findings show stutterers have difficulty in coordinating the laryngeal adjustments needed to integrate respiration, phonation, and articulation, and that these coordinations are achieved more easily with practice. By inference, rapid laryngeal adjustments should make stutterers more vulnerable to discoordination and, presumably, stuttering. That inference has also gained some support from recent investigations on oral reading and voice-reaction time.

The recent burst of interest in voice-reaction time has virtually ignored some findings on this topic that emerged from much earlier research on the motor abilities of stutterers. Bloodstein (1981) recently reviewed this earlier research and concluded that, in general, it "does not give strong support to the assumption that they [stutterers] have more difficulty in the rapid or precise movement of the speech and related structures than is to be observed in any representative sample of the general population" (p.148). The more recent research in this area has benefited from the availability of more sophisticated technology. However, as will be seen, it is not at all clear that the findings from this research warrant a change in Bloodstein's conclusion.

If it is assumed that laryngeal adjustments are reduced when more voicing is employed, then it follows that less stuttering should occur when oral reading involves mainly voiced sounds. Acting on this assumption, Adams and Reis (1971; 1974) conducted two studies in which they had stutterers (14 subjects in each study) make five oral readings of one passage containing all-voiced sounds and of another which contained voiceless-voiced sound combinations. The results were derived from comparisons between rates of adaptation on both readings; they show the all-voiced passage generally produced a more rapid rate of reduction in median stuttering scores.

The Adams and Reis findings provoked a lot of interest; yet, by almost any yardstick, they were based on relatively weak experimental effects. For example, Young (1975) observed that the mean frequency of stuttering across both reading passages in both Adams and Reis studies was 11.8 and 11.5. In response to Young, Adams and Reis (1975) acknowledged that their data support only an "imperfect relationship between phonatory onset requirements in a passage and the frequency of stuttering, especially over the course of massed readings of that passage" (p.604). But the extreme fragility of this effect was well illustrated in a study by Adams, Riemenschneider, Metz, and Conture (1975). They compared three passages in which presumed requirements for rapid initiation of phonation and complete articulatory constriction during oral reading decreased across the passages; one contained all types of speech sounds, a second had mainly voiced sounds with some stops, while the third contained only voiced continuants. Once again, 14 stutterers were chosen as experimental subjects, but the data from only 7 were used because the others either stuttered insufficiently or, more surprisingly, only "adapted" on two passages. It, therefore, requires some courage to accept the researchers' conclusions that the passages containing a relative preponderance of voice showed more evidence of adaptation than the passage containing all types of sounds.

If the hypothesized relationship between laryngeal adjustment skill and stuttering frequency is theoretically and empirically imperfect, then it is difficult to understand how this could ever be a profitable line of investigation. That seems to be borne out in the studies that followed the Adams and Reis reports. Manning and Coufal (1976) investigated the relationship between different types of phonatory transistions and disfluencies by stutterers (n=11; 18-33 years) and nonstutterers (n=11; 19-31 years) during oral reading. Their data, shown in Table 10.1, reveal that the voiceless-voiced transitions were, indeed, associated with the

Table 10.1
Disfluencies occurring on phonatory transition categories from data provided by Manning & Coufal.*

	PERCENTAGE OF DISFLUENCIES	
***Phonation transition* categories**	*Stutterers*	*Nonstutterers*
Voiced—Voiced	7.7	0.49
Voiced—Voiceless	9.8	0.70
Voiceless—Voiced	11.4	0.75
Voiceless—Voiceless	11.1	1.48

* From Manning & Coufal, 1976, p.78.

highest percentage of stutterings. But they were closely followed by voiceless-voiceless transitions that do *not* involve phonatory activity. Some negative results were claimed by Hutchinson and Brown (1978) from a study which they incorrectly stated was "a replication of the Adams and Reis (1971, 1974) experiments" (Hutchinson and Brown, 1978, p.149). Their study involved only one oral reading of a passage containing voiced and voiceless phonemes, and another single oral reading of a passage which contained only voiced phonemes (both passages had roughly equal percentages of stops, affricatives, and continuants). The findings showed that the stutterers (n=20; 17-37 years) had, if anything, more stutterings on the all-voiced passage. In response, Reis and Adams (1978) simply reaffirmed their position that the "off-on" voicing effect only appears during repeated oral readings.

Two replications of the Adams and Reis experiment have been carried out with children. Each has served to delineate the "on-off" voicing effect's limited contribution to stuttering. McGee, Hutchinson, and Deputy (1981) used Adams and Reis's passages in a true replication of their procedure with 15 children (enrolled in third through seventh grades). McGee et al. found no difference in adaptation rates on both passages. Runyan and Bonifant (1981) provided partial support for that finding; they used the less relevant method of comparing only one reading of an all-voiced passage with one reading of a voiced-voiceless passage. Across 22 stutterers, aged 7 to 13 years, they found no significant differences between stuttering frequencies on both passages.

Taken together, the previous studies suggest that Adams and Reis's findings might be restricted to oral reading by adult stutterers, and then only during the course of repeated readings. In effect, the stutterers's ability to improve fluency through the coordination of respiration, phonation, and articulation with practice (if this is the factor involved) must be acquired with age.

Actually, the method of using different types of passages may have only partially tapped the fluency-enhancing effects of limited phonatory adjustments. The initial adaptation studies by Brenner et al. (1972), for example, appeared to produce much more definite evidence on the strength of phonation management practice on stuttering adaptation. This is also true in some more recent studies that have avoided the complicating features of the adaptation effect. Perkins, Rudas, Johnson, and Bell (1976) investigated the oral reading of different passages by 30 stutterers (14-67 years) when they either read aloud, whispered, or silently articulated (lipped) words. All subjects showed a similar pattern of progressively fewer disfluent syllables with progressively more syllables read per minute across these reading conditions.[3] The Perkins et al. (1976) results were virtually replicated in a similar study by Commodore and Cooper (1978). Their only variation was to have their stutterers (n=12; 16-33 years) read under conditions in which they knew they were going to be video recorded. This was

[3]It is interesting to note that in this study, and in the Bruce and Adams (1970) study, there was a surprisingly large amount of stuttering during whispering. For instance, Perkins et al. (1976) report 10.3% disfluent syllables during whispering and 24.6% during aloud reading. This seems to be an unexpectedly high level of stuttering (if the disfluencies were stutterings) under circumstances in which the laryngeal muscle adjustments during speech are virtually absent. That finding should also raise questions about the prominent role attributed to abductor-adductor laryngeal muscle action in stuttering.

supposed to form a "communicative stress" variable, but it failed to influence the results. Perkins, Bell, Johnson, and Stocks (1979) studied the effect on stuttering (presumably) of increasing the proportion of phonation (and thereby reducing the proportion of "off-on" voicing) during oral reading. The procedure required stutterers (n=19; 20-50 years) to orally read at their normal rate, then again at a controlled slow rate (30 words presented per minute), and finally with instructions to "prolong the phones in each syllable and stretch the word until it blended with the next word" (Perkins et al., 1979, p.749). Under the slow reading condition, the mean "percent syllables disfluent" declined by about 56%, but during the "prolong" condition their disfluencies declined by over 94%. Perkins et al, (1979) attributed the difference to reduced phone rate[4] in the latter condition.

In general, the findings from these studies highlight the effect of introducing substantial alterations to phonation time during oral reading. In other words, somewhere between the relatively insubstantial alterations in phonatory activity achieved within the Adams and Reis studies, and those procured by procedures used in Perkins's studies, there may yet exist a critical laryngeal adjustment factor that controls stuttering.

Voice-Reaction-Time Studies

For many years, voice reaction time has interested stuttering researchers, mainly because of reported differences in the speed with which stutterers and nonstutterers initiate and terminate phonation. A few earlier studies had pointed to the likely existence of such differences. West and Nusbaum (1929) reported that stutterers' jaw movements were slower than those of normal speakers, and Cross (1936) had reported that the diaphragm reaction times of stutterers were slower than those found among normal speakers. More significantly, Shaffer (1940) found that the time between the initiation of jaw movement and the initiation of phonation was greater among stutterers than among nonstutterers. Shaffer also found that stutterers had longer durations of phonation on voiced words and more interrupted phonation while saying words—findings which have special significance in the light of current research.

The revived interest in voice reaction time began with an unpublished report by Agnello and Wingate (1972) of differences between the voice onset time (VOT) of stutterers and nonstutterers. Subsequently, Agnello (1975) published an account of findings from his research program which included VOT and voice termination times (VTT) for 23 stutterers and 23 nonstutterers. The stutterers were found to be significantly slower than nonstutterers in initiating voice during the opening phase of a consonant release (VOT), or slower in approaching closure—or the VTT phase—on CV or VC sounds. This finding was effectively supported by Adams and Hayden (1976). They compared the speed with which stutterers (n=10; 18-20 years) and nonstutterers (n=10; 20-35 years) initiated (VIT) and

[4] "Phone rate" is syllables spoken divided by the total duration of phonation.

terminated (VTT) phonation in response to a series of 1000Hz tones lasting 1.5 to 4.5 seconds. The stutterers' VTT scores were found, generally, to be significantly slower. However, their VIT scores were actually significantly slower than the nonstutterers' VIT scores only on the final of three series of tones.

A veritable avalanche of studies followed the Adams and Hayden study. Starkweather, Hirschman, and Tannebaum's (1976) compared the VOT measures of 11 stutterers (19-42 years) and 11 matched nonstutterers when they rapidly uttered different syllables in response to a light signal. The VC or CV syllables contained controls for manner, place, and transition patterns. On most sounds, the stutterers were found to have significantly slower VOT scores, except with syllables initiated by voiceless consonants or terminated by voiced consonants. Hillman and Gilbert (1977) compared 10 stutterers and 10 normal speakers (ages unspecified) on VOT measures made from different intervocalic-voiceless-stop-consonant segments obtained during oral reading. Their principal finding was that the stutterers, generally, had significantly longer VOT values than the nonstutterers. Cross, Shadden, and Luper (1979) compared adult stutterers' (n=10; 17-37 years) and nonstutterers' (n=10; 17-38 years) VIT scores in response to five sets of 20 tones presented in either the left or right ear. The stutterers' VIT scores were consistently slower, and none of the differences were attributable to the ear presentation. Cross et al. (1979) also provided data relevant to the findings of Adams and Hayden and Starkweather et al. that stutterers tended to improve their scores over trials. Over a large number of trials, Cross et al. found their stutterers took longer to stabilize than the nonstutterers, but the stutterers still remained consistently slower in their optimum vocalization speed. One slightly discordant finding was reported by Metz, Conture, and Caruso (1979), who measured VOT, plus duration of frication and aspiration, in the fluent utterances of five stutterers (17-25 years) and five nonstutterers (19-23 years). They failed to find consistent differences between VOT scores and other sound durations from both groups, although this could be partly due to their small number of subjects.

The generally consistent differences between the speed with which stutterers and normal speakers initiate and terminate phonation raised the possibility that these differences may also extend to nonvocal activities. Once again, however, there existed a body of research from the past that suggested this was unlikely (Perkins, 1970). In any event, recent research has confirmed that suggestion. McFarlane and Prins (1978) measured the neural response time (lip closure and verbal response times following offset of either visual or audible signals) by adult stutterers (n=12; 21-38 years) and matched nonstutterers. They found that their stutterers did have significantly longer response times across all stimulus modes and response tasks, although the main differences related to the auditory mode for verbal responses, and only left ear signal presentations for lip closure. However, Prosek, Montgomery, Walden, and Schwartz (1979) found somewhat more distinctive differences between their stutterers (n=10; mean 25.6 years) and nonstutterers (n=10; mean 25.9 years) on manual and verbal response tasks. They recorded button press and verbal response times to either visual, audible, or word signals. In addition, voice activation and surface EMG laryngeal measures were made for the verbal response. Generally, they found that the subject groups were undifferentiated on their manual response or laryngeal region response times, but the stutterers' voice-activation times were significantly slower than their counterparts. This led Prosek et al. to conclude that for the stutterers "the initial gesture may occur with normal latency, but the release of the gesture or the onset of airflow may be abnormally long" (Prosek et al., 1979, p.277). In short, the stutterers were disadvantaged in the synergy needed for phonation. Reich, Till, and Goldsmith (1981) also measured laryngeal and manual reaction times in stutterers (n=13; 19-59 years) and nonstutterers (n=13; 19-59 years), and obtained fairly similar results. However, they identified rather more fine-grained distinctions. For example, the laryngeal-response-time measures (transduced signals from the laryngeal region) were obtained on two speech-related tasks (vowel or vowel-matched CVCs) and two allied nonspeech tasks (inspiratory or expiratory phonatory actions). They found that only on the speech-related tasks were the stutterers significantly slower than the nonstutterers. Another useful addition to this network of findings were data collected by Venkatagiri (1981) from comparisons between whispered and voiced /a/ response times to 1000Hz tones. In this case, the stutterers (n=10; 19-39 years) tended to be slower than the nonstutterers (n=10; 18-31 years) on the voiced task, but faster on the whispered task; although it is noteworthy that this was a directional difference which failed to reach statistical significance. Finally, there is a report by Mallard, Hicks, and Riggs (1982) of a comparison between stutterers (n=10; mean age 28 years) and nonstutterers (n=10; mean age 26 years) in their ability to control the intensity rise time of a phonated sound (/a/). It is of some significance to the later account of clinical applications of prolonged speech that Mallard et al. used a voice monitor devised by Webster (1977b). From comparisons between the number of attempts each subject required to achieve a criterion rise time, the percentage of correct productions, and the intensity level of each production, it was reported that there were no significant differences between the groups. In other words, on this task the stutterers were as able as the nonstutterers in making appropriate vocal and respiratory adjustments.

In general, therefore, the reaction-time studies have produced a remarkably uniform picture. The stuttering populations show a pattern of delayed-voice-reaction time that is seemingly specific to speech-related behavior. It even fails to occur with phonatory activity unless that activity relates to speech behavior and, apparently, only involves rapid onset. The picture has achieved even greater clarity, however, through the addition of voice-reaction-time studies with children. Cross and Luper (1979) used a procedure that was virtually identical to that used by Cross, Shadden, and Luper (1979), but with matched stuttering and nonstuttering children aged 5 (n=9.9), 9 (n=9.9), and 15 years (n=9.9). They found that the stutterers had significantly slower VIT scores at each age level (and also that an improvement trend in VIT scores over repeated trials was evident but not sustained). Cullinan and Springer (1980) conducted a rather more complex investigation on 5- to 11-year-old stutterers (n=20) and nonstutterers (n=20). The interesting aspect in their study was that 11 of the stuttering children were also found to have mild to moderate articulation, language, or learning disabilities. When the 9 "stuttering-only" children were compared with their nonstuttering counterparts, no significant differences appeared between the VIT and VTT scores of either group. But significant differences did emerge when the children with other problems were added. It was also observed that the overlap between scores of the "stuttering-only" and nonstuttering children was mainly confined to those who were 8 years old or younger. This finding was also nicely supported by Murphy and Baumgartner's (1981) investigation of VIT and VTT measures from stuttering (n=7) and nonstuttering (n=8) children aged 4 to 6 years. In this study, the stuttering children were described as "free of articulation, language and voice disorders," and they produced VIT and VTT scores that were indistinguishable from the nonstutterers' scores.

It would appear, therefore, that speech-related phonatory reaction time in stutterers is likely to be slower than for nonstutterers, simply because of their experience with speech difficulty. That is not to diminish its significance. But it is difficult to establish the nature of that difficulty from the present group of studies. For example, it is impossible to learn whether slower reaction time contributes to stuttering or is merely a byproduct of the disorder. Only direct manipulation of reaction times for either stutterers or normals would help resolve this issue. In any event, it seems likely that slow phonation onset would make the coordination of phonation and articulation relatively difficult, especially during rapid voiceless-voiced transitions.

There is a tenor of speculation within the area of "vocal tract dynamics" that the stutterer's poor ability to coordinate respiration, articulation, and phonation is not only evident in stuttering activity, but permeates all areas of speech behavior (Adams & Runyan, 1981). In other words, the stutterer's fluent speech is also characterized by unusual perceptual, aerodynamic, and physiological features. Adams and Runyan have argued that aberrant patterns of speech production may surround overt stuttering events, thereby causing "perceptible tenuous fluency" to occur during nonstuttered intervals. This would also imply that the stutterer's speech quality will differ in many ways from a nonstutterer's speech quality.

Adams and Runyan's (1981) proposition is rather awkward to test, since such tenuous fluency is claimed to be more evident in unspecified temporal areas adjacent to overt stutterings. It is also claimed to be a function of the level of severity of stuttering moments. Nevertheless, there is interesting evidence of differences between the stutter-free speech of stutterers and the fluent speech of nonstutterers that may have relevance to that proposition. That evidence comes from investigations of stutterers' "fluency" using perceptual, acoustic, and aerodynamic techniques. These investigations, and some physiological studies of the articulators that bear on Adams and Runyan's proposal, are considered in the following sections.

Perceptual-Evaluation Studies

Wendahl and Cole (1961) had listeners judge whether a pair of stutter-free speech samples (n=8) were from stutterers and/or nonstutterers: each sample in a pair had been obtained from oral readings by either a stutterer or a nonstutterer. Wendahl and Cole concluded that "stutterer" judgments were more often applied to the stutterer's sample than to the nonstutterer's sample. However, when this study was replicated by Young (1964), using a more appropriate data analysis procedure (binomial probability), the findings failed to support Wendahl and Cole's conclusion. In general, the listeners were unable to confidently differentiate between the stutter-free speech of a stutterer or nonstutterer. Few and Lingwall (1972) conducted a more detailed investigation of listener judgments on 10-second fluent speech samples from 14 adult stutters and 14 similar-aged nonstutterers. Not only were their listeners unable to distinguish between the stutterers' and nonstutterers' samples, but analyses of their articulation rates (phones per second) and cumulative pause time (via graphic displays) also failed to reveal significant differences between the samples from both groups. In general, therefore, the published studies on stutterers (who, presumably, have not received a speech-pattern-modification treatment[5]) have not shown that their fluent intervals of speech are perceptually distinctive.

Adams and Runyan (1981) have referred to either unpublished studies or studies involving stutterers who were "partially" or "successfully therapeutized" (Runyan & Adams, 1978; 1979) to support their claim that "stutterers' fluency is perceptibily different from that of normal speakers" (Adams & Runyan, 1981, p.202). Prosek and Runyan (1982) made a further investigation of some of Runyan and Adams's (1978; 1979) recordings of treated stutterers and nonstutterers. They found that speaking rate (the stutterers were slower), combined with either average number of pauses or average pause duration (the stutterers scored more), accounted for about 70% of the variance in listener responses. But, since all but one set of the "successfully therapeutized" stutterers in the Runyan and Adams study were treated by speech pattern procedures, it is quite possible that this was the main factor that influenced the perceptual judgments on the stutterers.

Acoustic-Evaluation Studies

More persuasive evidence of differences in stutterers' fluent speech has been derived from measures of the acoustic signal. Love and Jeffress (1971) showed that a trained clinician may fail to distinguish between stutter-free samples from stutterers and nonstutterers, whereas a signal-pause analysis of these samples showed notable differences: the stutterers' samples had significantly more 150-250 msec pauses. In fact, pause analysis alone accurately identified 74% of the samples as produced by a stutterer or nonstutterer. Di Simoni (1974) measured fluent vowel and consonant durations by stutterers and nonstutterers and showed that the stutterers had "greatly" longer vowels and consonants than the nonstutterers, and also showed much more variability during a repetition task. Such variability suggests that the stutterers' fluent utterances may also have relatively unstable timing characteristics.

[5] Few and Lingwall's (1972) subjects were the only ones described as "enrolled in a clinical program."

This last finding aligns with the results of a study by Cooper and Allen (1977). During repeated fluent utterances of sentences, paragraphs, and nursery rhymes, the interval between marker sounds was found to be much more variable for adult stutterers than it was for matched nonstutterers. This difference was also found on a finger-tapping task which, in turn, suggests that stutterers may have unstable general timing skills. In a way, this finding is also consistent with data obtained by Bills (1934) from measures of key pressing and vocal response rates by adult stutterers (n=28) and nonstutterers (n=33) during a color matching task. The stutterers' reaction times showed much greater variability with a decided "lack of rhythmicality in reacting" (Bills, 1934, p.578). Another indication of stutterers' odd timing skills is Ringel and Minifie's (1966) finding that their stutterers' ability to estimate the duration of a 10-second interval while speaking, reading (oral or silent), or listening was generally much poorer than that found among nonstutterers. The stutterers generally made longer duration judgments.

Returning to the characteristics of fluency, some investigations have suggested that only certain features of a stutterer's fluent speech are distinctive. For example, Schmitt and Cooper (1978) found no significant differences between the fundamental frequencies in the speech of male stutterers and nonstutterers who were matched for age, race, height, and weight. However, a careful analysis of the intervocalic interval (IVI) in the contextual fluent speech of stutterers and their controls, by Starkweather and Myers (1979), has revealed some interesting differences. Spectrographic analyses of one IVI showed that the stutterers were slower than the nonstutterers in producing transitional subsegments, but not in producing the steady state subsegment. These investigators concluded that this indicates that stutterers' movements of their tongue and larynx are likely to be slower than expected. Of course, this also implies that they will have relatively slow coordination of laryngeal and oral mechanisms in conjunction with respiration.

The evidence produced by the acoustic signal investigations is quite persuasive. It is apparent that brief pauses, unusual vowel and consonant durations, and timing variability are prominent features within nonstuttered speech intervals by stutterers. But these features have only been identified in the speech of adult stutterers; the speech of stuttering children has not been examined in the same fashion. Consequently, in the light of the voice-reaction-time research, it is quite possible that these features could turn out to be only relevant to adult stutterers.

Aerodynamic-Evaluation Studies

The recurring evidence that stutterers have unusual timing, initiations, and duations of phonatory behavior during speaking has revived interest in the way stutterers manage respiration. For, if the critical air pressure values at either a subglottic or supraglottic level are at variance with what is necessary to procure normal phonation, then a more fundamental discrepancy may exist between the fluent-sounding speech of stutterers and nonstutterers (Adams, 1974; 1975a).

Stutterers' breathing patterns have been a source of interest from many different perspectives. In fact, some early investigations take on added interest in the light of current research on vocal tract dynamics. For example, Van Riper (1936) measured the thoracic breathing of 37 stutterers (presumably children and adults) prior to a block or on a fluent utterance. He found that the inspiration-expiration duration ratio changed approaching a word utterance, and showed much greater variability when a block was expected. Two of Van Riper's comments on this study are particularly interesting. First, only six subjects showed stereotypic breathing abnormalities on all words, and secondly, two children in the study "showed no breathing abnormalities whatever. Their spasms were of the short clonic variety and they did not seem to react to their blocks with any noticeable forcing or grimaces" (Van Riper, 1936, p.71). In other words, while unusual breathing patterns might be expected from stutterers, they may be inconsistent byproducts of their disorder rather than necessary conditions for stuttering. Starbuck and Steer (1954) measured thoracic and abdominal breathing during adaptation conditions with stutterers and nonstutterers. Their findings failed to yield differences between the groups on either the depth or duration of thoracic or abdominal breathing, although the number of thoracic breathing cycles per period was significantly larger in the stutterers, and over repeated readings they reduced the number of cycles of abdominal or thoracic breathing. In short, the stutterers did show some differences from nonstutterers in their respiration patterns, although the implications of these differences are unclear.

As previously mentioned, much of the revived interest in respiration or aerodynamic factors is due to theory and research publications by Adams (1974; 1975a) and colleagues. Adams, Runyan, and Mallard (1975) measured peak air flow rates on initial and final consonants, air-flow duration and flow volume between peaks within CVC's (uttered aloud or whispered) by 6 adult normals and 6 adult stutterers (it is noteworthy that 5 subjects were in the midst of a therapy program). Their findings showed that the stutterers had longer durations and larger volumes of air flow during voiced and whispered utterances. Adams et al. (1975) argue that because the stutterers had higher air flow and longer durational features in their articulatory movements, this may have also contributed to the very low number of disfluencies (two) that subjects produced during this task. Another pertinent investigation was the previously described (Chapter 5) study by Hutchinson and Navarre (1977). It will be recalled that they compared peak intraoral air pressure, intraoral air pressure onset and offset duration, total intraoral air pressure duration, and peak air flow rate during oral reading by 5 adult stutterers and their age-matched controls. Comparisons were made between the subjects' range of scores on these measures on selected CVC's with and without a 60 bpm metronome condition. Inspection of their graphed data shows no clear evidence that the stutterers or nonstutterers had distinguishably different scores on any of these measures. However, as in the Adams et al. (1975) study, these comparisons may have been confounded by the subjects' extensive therapy history. For example, Hutchinson and Navarre's stutterers had received between 60 and 350 hours of unspecified therapy.

The evidence derived from aerodynamic analyses of the fluent speech of stutterers is obviously not sufficient to permit meaningful conclusions.

Furthermore, if the methodology used in these studies continues to rely upon comparisons between stutterers (some of whom may be exhibiting therapy effects) and nonstutterers, or between fluent and stuttered utterances, then it is difficult to see how this research will ever identify causal factors. It would be surprising, for instance, if unusual breathing patterns were not associated with any form of speaking that is typified by unusual phonatory activity (including stuttering). Perhaps a more interesting task will be identification of factors responsible for that unusual breathing. Then, presumably, these factors could be manipulated for the purpose of rectifying any abnormal respiratory activity, and relating such changes to stuttering.

The Rush to the Larynx

The principal bodily system involved in coordinating respiration and phonation is the larynx. And in recent years close examination of the function of this organ has become possible with advances in technology. These advances have also contributed much to the recent rush of investigations and speculations about the role of laryngeal factors in stuttering.

There have been numerous claims made for the contribution that abnormal laryngeal activity makes to stuttering; some, as Freeman (1975) has observed, are centuries old. In recent decades the most developed argument for this contribution was put by Kenyon (1943). He claimed that stuttering is *only* associated with actions of the larynx and is "a compulsory interpolation (for an act of speech sound production) of a normal but misplaced psychophysiological act, namely vocal cord adduction" (p.347). More recently, at least two theorists—Wyke and Schwartz—have accorded abnormal laryngeal activity a primary role in stuttering. Wyke (1970; 1971; 1974)[6] has suggested that neurological factors may explain these laryngeal actions. He postulated that this produces two types of stuttering:

> (1) "abnormally slow or inaccurate voluntary presetting of the laryngeal and respiratory musculature" or (2) "inefficient or disorganized reflex maintenance of this preset pattern of muscle tone, because of the abnormal operations of one or more of the laryngeal mucosal myotatic and articular reflex systems" (1970, p.13).

Perhaps the most controversial theoretical position is that taken by Schwartz (1974). He argues that the stuttering block is the result of a stress-activated rise in subglottic air pressure which produces a vigorous abductory response by the posterior cricoarytenoid muscle in the larynx. In response, the speaker's actions involve forceful adduction of the vocal folds or a tensing of the lips and tongue—actions which result in a blockage of phonation. Critics of Schwartz's theory (Adams, 1975c; Freeman, Ushijima, & Hirose, 1975; Zimmerman & Allen, 1975) have cast doubts on the adequacy of this model, including its limitations as an

[6] The content in each of these publications is surprisingly similar.

explanation of stutterings that do not involve an absence of phonation.

The claims made for the primacy of aberrant laryngeal muscle action in stuttering have activated some of the most interesting physiological studies on the disorder. Four different techniques have been used to investigate laryngeal activity among these studies; they involve either the glottograph, laryngograph, fiberscope, or the electromyograph (EMG).

Glottographic investigations of the larynx produce recordings of the size of the glottis via light refraction from the glottal opening. Using this method with 29 stutterers, Chevrie-Muller (1963) observed unexpected glottal openings, and an absence of voicing during glottal activity. These actions were ascribed to unusual laryngeal patterns. A somewhat vague account of glottograph analysis of stuttering was provided by Gautheron, Liorzou, Even, and Vallancien (1973). They reported that in four stutterers the initiation of voicing with a hard attack (glottis closed and probably under stress) was prominent on 60% of utterances, but this only occurred on 8.7% of utterances by nonstutterers. Unhappily, they provided no data to support an additional claim that visual display of this abnormal glottal action enabled their stutterers to correct this pattern. Such information might have provided useful evidence of a connection between this self-managed alteration in glottal activity and fluency.

The laryngograph procedure involves a radiographic examination of the larynx, with techniques that enable delineation of the laryngeal structures. Freeman (1975; 1979) has described a study by Fujita (1966) which used this method with one stutterer and showed "(1) irregular or inconsistent opening and closing of the pharyngolaryngeal cavity and (2) asymetric tight closure of the pharyngeal cavity" (Freeman, 1979, p.84). McCall (1975) also used this method to examine spastic dysphonia, and showed that this disorder may also be associated with atypical movement patterns in the larynx (during quiet respiration, as well as during speaking).

The advantages of fiberoptics have permitted some investigators to actually film the operation of a stutterer's glottis during speaking conditions. A description of a Japanese-produced film of a stutterer's glottal actions by Ushijima, Kamiyama, Hirose, and Niimi, in 1965, has been given in a number of places. Freeman (1975) describes the presentation as showing tight closure of the laryngeal aperture along with moments of stuttering, but also "irregular, intermittent and/or unpredictable opening and closing of the glottis" (p.236). However, the most extensive fiberoptic investigation of stuttering was reported by Conture, McCall, and Brewer (1977). They observed various laryngeal actions in 10 stutterers (17-47 years) during stuttering moments. Out of 159 identified stutterings, 101 could be related to three types of laryngeal muscle action; laryngeal abduction, adduction, or a combination of both. Ninety-four of the stutterings were related to either abduction or adduction. The relationship between these actions and different types of stutterings was also interesting: 60% of the part-word repetitions involved abduction, 72% of sound prolongations were related to adduction, and all broken words were typified by adduction. But the extent of invariance in the relationship between laryngeal behaviors and fluent or stuttered utterances was not established. The researchers claimed that part-word repetition stutterings were different from fluent productions of the same segment, but this was not true for sound prolongations, though no supportive data were provided to justify this claim. Healey and Turton (1979) also criticized this study for its failure to provide quantitative information on the duration of laryngeal actions, vis-á-vis stutterings and fluent productions.

Each of the preceding techniques provides graphic, though somewhat nonspecific, evidence that the laryngeal activities associated with stuttering are relatively unusual (which should not be surprising), and may also display abnormalcy during a stutterer's periods of fluent speech. A more quantified and detailed account of laryngeal muscle action has been sought via direct electromyographic recording from the principal muscles in the larynx. This approach has been used in a series of investigations by Freeman and Ushijima (1975, 1978; Freeman, 1975; 1979). A preliminary EMG investigation by Freeman and Ushijima (1975), mainly with one stutterer, provided some evidence that abductor-adductor muscle reciprocity is disrupted during stuttering. They also noted that one muscle in particular, the lateral cricoarytenoid, tends to become much less active during fluent utterances. A much more detailed EMG analysis of the laryngeal muscles and the upper airway articulators occurred in another study by Freeman and Ushijima (1978) with four adult male stutterers. Not all the target muscles were measured, and for only two subjects were the abductor and adductor muscles recorded. The speech of these subjects was recorded from oral readings made during chorus reading, rhythmic reading, white noise, DAF, and without accompanying stimulation. For two subjects, all the measured laryngeal muscles decreased their activity during the fluency-inducing conditions. But this failed to occur in another subject who also reduced stuttering during these conditions. However, decreased activity did occur when this subject orally read slowly. A fourth subject failed to stutter during oral reading, and so muscle activity comparisons were made between this subject's stuttered and nonstuttered utterances of two words: this revealed reduced peak activity in all measured muscles during fluent utterances.

The overall data from Freeman and Ushijima's subjects is certainly suggestive, but it contains numerous ambiguities—which is not at all surprising considering the fearsome technical difficulties involved in this type of research. Nevertheless, definite negative correlations between abductor and adductor laryngeal muscles were found during stutter-free speech. Also, positive correlations (indicating lack of reciprocity) occurred during many stuttered utterances. But these findings reflected trends rather than invariance. In other words, their data were not sufficiently unambiguous to support the claim that antagonistic laryngeal muscle activity is a necessary condition for stuttering. The strength of that claim might have been clearer had Freeman and Ushijima also assessed their subjects' speech in conditions that are known to induce co-contracting abductor-adductor muscle patterns.

The source of ambiguity in Freeman and Ushijima's findings becomes more obvious and meaningful from data reported by Shapiro (1980). He obtained EMG laryngeal muscle activity data from 4 adult stutterers and a nonstutterer. Only 1 stutterer had verified measures made on abductor and adductor laryngeal muscles, and these showed rather inconsistent antagonistic activity during stutterings ("long blocks"). The conclusions that Shapiro reached were particularly interesting in this respect:

> most often no consistency could be found in the muscular activity across stuttering blocks. That is, each subject often looked muscularly different even if dysfluencies on the same exact word were compared. Even when cocontraction of intrinsic laryngeal muscles was clearly evident on one block with a particular subject, the very next block might have revealed perfect reciprocity although abnormally high levels of activity. This variability of intrasubject stuttering behavior was not seen when the nonstutterer control subject faked these same blocks (pp.229-230).

It bears restating that the methodological difficulties associated with these procedures are formidable. In fact, each study provides ample testimony to the extraordinary problems involved in reliably locating and recording specific laryngeal muscles. For this reason, it would be surprising if these studies did yield clear-cut findings. However, Shapiro's findings suggest that it is unlikely that antagonistic laryngeal muscle activity is a necessary conditon for stuttering. If anything, the overall evidence suggests that only a high level of laryngeal muscle activity might be a necessary condition. Moreover, Freeman and Ushijima's (1978) findings from a subject who reduced stuttering, without heightened muscle activity, would raise problems even for that proposal.

If exaggerated laryngeal muscle activity does tend to accompany stuttering, then it may still have functional value. For, if such activity preceded audible moments of stuttering, then it might be useful for feedback manipulation (see Chapter 11). But the available evidence suggests that this activity—albeit inconsistent activity—is confined to the actual interval of stuttering. For instance, McLean and Cooper (1978) traced laryngeal muscle activity in stutterers (n=19) during a 10-second interval preceding an utterance. They found, essentially, no significant differences between the level of laryngeal muscle activity that preceded either a stuttered or a fluent utterance. This was also true regardless of whether the stutterings (or fluent utterances) were expected or unexpected events.

The notion that laryngeal activity has a necessary role in stuttering has recently come under challenge because there is a possibility that stuttering may persist even after the larynx has been removed! Indeed the very existence of a laryngectomized stutterer would present almost as much of a challenge to vocal tract explanations of stuttering as did Red Indian stutterers for Wendell Johnson's Diagnosogenic Theory of Stuttering.

The obvious way to determine the effect of a laryngectomy on stuttering would be to collect evidence showing that stuttering ceased after such an operation. Unfortunately, the evidence that has been collected for this purpose is often vague and supported by poor documentation. For example, Van Riper (1953) claims that Oswald reported on a 58-year-old stutterer who ceased to stutter after a laryngectomy. But when Irving and Webb (1961) made personal contact with Oswald, she disclaimed any knowledge of the case. Nevertheless, Irving and

Webb did describe a 58-year-old laryngectomized stutterer who "was able to develop an esophageal speech which was fluent and free from pathological stuttering. Three months later the stuttering had not returned"(p.1078). Irving and Webb also surveyed neurologists, otolaryngologists, psychologists, and speech pathologists for laryngectomized stutterers; that search yielded 6 cases, but only 4 had subsequently ceased to stutter. Beck (1956; see Doms & Lissens, 1973) also reported on two stutterers who became fluent when taught esophageal speech. Other relevant evidence appears in a report by Wingate (1981b) on a survey of laryngectomees; all but 1 of 10 "bona fide laryngectomees" stated that they ceased stuttering following their operation. Wingate dismissed the significance of the exceptional case by claiming this subject's stuttering descriptions were contradictory. Nevertheless, the subject stated that his postoperative stuttering "occurred only when in large groups or when nervous in which case words starting a sentence would 'come out dah' " (p.276)—hardly the speech of a fluent esophageal speaker.

Two other reports have provided some rather persuasive evidence that stuttering may persist after the larynx is removed. Doms and Lissen (1973) described a 67-year-old multilingual Dutch Dominican father whose postoperative stutterings during esophageal speech included blocks, repetitions, word omissions, and irregular pauses for air intake. The prior of his monastery confirmed that he had stuttered before his operation, and that he had received irregular stuttering therapy before the operation. The other report, by Tuck (1979), described the speech of a 56-year-old male who claimed to have begun stuttering at 13 years of age after seeing a film about a stutterer. The wife and client gave a description of his preoperative speech that was consistent with stuttering. Tuck describes the subject's postoperative speech as including part-word repetitions, sound repetitions at the beginning of a phrase or sentence, and evident blocks. This side of pre- and postperative recording of these subjects, or perhaps an independent judge's assessment of their stutterings, it is difficult to regard these reports as less valid than those that are used to describe "fluent" laryngectomized stutterers. On the other hand, Freeman and Rosenfield (1982) have recently noted that laryngectomized nonstutterers may exhibit a large number of dysfluencies when learning to use esophageal or pharyngeal speech. They provided a transcript of a recording from a formerly normal speaker learning to use a surgically constructed neoglottis. The transcript included numerous instances that could be judged as stutterings. Such judgments may well have occurred in many of the previously mentioned assessments of laryngectomized stutterers.

Actually, the necessity of the larynx to stuttering is also doubtful because of evidence that stuttering may occur during whispering. Presumably, in whispering the vocal folds are held in a slightly abducted position and vocal fold vibration ceases. As a result, the laryngeal muscle actions which are required to produce phonation, also cease and, in theory, this should prevent stuttering. At least 2 recent studies have found quite substantial amounts of stuttering during whispering (Bruce & Adams, 1978; Perkins, Rudas, Johnson & Bell, 1976). They certainly reported there was less stuttering during whispering, but the fact that some stuttering did remain implies that laryngeal activity may not be an entirely necessary accompaniment to stuttering. It is noteworthy, though, that neither study provided independent corroboration that the subjects' "whispering" was completely voiceless.

Articulatory Dynamics

The recent upsurge in physiological research has not been confined to investigations of the larynx. Some of this research has produced evidence which suggests that there may be some important differences between the articulatory dynamics of stutterers and nonstutterers.

Zimmerman (1980a) compared the temporal and spatial patterning of lip and jaw movements, as well as voicing during perceptually fluent utterances by normal adult speakers (4 males and 3 females) and 6 adult male stutterers. Not surprisingly (in view of recent voice-reaction-time research), Zimmerman found the stutterers had a longer latency for the onset of movements for the lip and jaw, as well as voice onset time. But the stutterers also displayed longer transition times, longer steady state positions, and longer intervals between movement onset and peak velocity for the lip and jaw. One fairly logical consequence of these differences was that the normals had the presumed advantage of comparatively higher temporal correlations between these movements. In another study, Zimmerman (1980b) used cinefluorographic analysis techniques to compare disfluent and fluent productions of a syllable by four male stutterers and one female nonstutterer. In general, Zimmerman found that the articulators of the stutterers had a much less synchronous relationship during fluent and disfluent productions than did those of the nonstutterer. As a result of these findings, Zimmerman (1980c) has argued that part of the stuttering problem may relate to abnormal movement ranges of the speech structures. When this occurs "the afferent nerve impulses generated alter the gains of associated brainstem reflexes. Altering of the reflex gains throws the articulatory system out of balance and a breakdown in behavior occurs, often manifested as oscillations or static positioning" (p.122).

The attraction in Zimmerman's proposal is that it not only fails to rely on laryngeal activity as a proximal cause of stutterings, but it also provides an explanation for aberrant muscle activity in that region. Both Adams (1974) and Zimmerman (1980c) observed that unusual articulatory activities would provide almost sufficient cause for any alterations in supraglottic air pressure which, in turn, could impinge on glottal action. This proposal also carries a certain amount of face validity in view of the many visible components of stuttering that seem unrelated to laryngeal behavior. Another interesting, and germane, finding appears in a relatively brief report of an investigation by Stromsta and Fibiger (1980). They measured obicularis oris muscle activity via EMG in adult stutterers (n=8) and nonstutterers (n=10). In short intervals preceding syllable repetitions characterized by interphonemic disruptions,[7] they observed EMG activity to be

[7] Stromsta and Fibiger argue that this is the core behavior of stuttering.

considerably less than it was for normally uttered syllables by either stutterers or normals. In effect, the stutterers showed articulatory activities that were incompatible with a successful or fluent utterance. In passing, it is interesting to observe the compatibility between the findings of Zimmerman and Stromsta and Fibiger with those reported in the much earlier and technically disadvantaged study of Shaffer (1940).

Conclusions from Physiological Studies

The findings that have emerged from recent physiological studies on stuttering have not been especially helpful in identifying factors that either reduce or increase stuttering. Nevertheless, they have opened up enormously interesting areas of research on different aspects of stuttering.

For the most part, the laryngeal activity studies appear to have drawn attention to another level for describing stuttering, rather than identifying causal components of the disorder. This does not diminish their significance. For there is a possibility that these studies could help resolve what is possibly *the* major problem for stuttering research—an acceptable definition of the disorder. The failure to find the unique behaviors that distinguish stutterings from other forms of disfluent speech has undoubtedly hindered the search for acceptable explanations and treatments of stuttering. If these studies identified a unique set of physiological processes that are *always and only* synonymous with the moment of stuttering, then, presumably, this would permit manipulation and explanation of these physiological processes. It would also bypass the present questionable dependency on clinician judgment in research and treatment.

The main weakness in the findings of present physiological studies is that they have yet to identify an invariant process that is directly related to stuttering. Freeman and Ushijima's (1975; 1978) findings appeared to have some promise. But the limitations of their findings were well demonstrated by Shapiro's (1980) study, which showed extremely variable patterns of laryngeal muscle activity within (rather than across) subjects. The continuing vulnerability of this methodology to technical problems also makes it unlikely that a reliable operation for identifying a distinctive physiological stuttering pattern is about to appear.

The findings of Zimmerman and colleagues, as well as Stromsta and Fibiger, have interesting implications at two levels. First, they suggest that EMG measures of the articulators might yield certain causal and, thereby, definitive stuttering movement patterns. The evidence from Zimmerman's (1980a; 1980b) studies for instance, has been interpreted (Zimmerman, 1980c) to mean that in some way the stutterer's speech-neuromotor system might be more susceptible to destabilization than is the case for normal speakers. Secondly, the EMG data of Stromsta and Fibiger (1980) imply that there might be a pattern of activity leading up to a stuttering which is available for some form of feedback manipulation.

Zimmerman's proposals certainly point to alternative lines of investigation that need exploring. But before these lines are pursued, some consideration should be given to the internal validity of the foundation studies. For instance,

Zimmerman's (1980a) studies comparing articulatory movements of stutterers and nonstutterers during fluent utterances involve sources of variance that are, to say the least, considerable. There simply is no possibility that the different oral behavior histories of these subjects could be presumed an irrelevant variable. This may even be magnified by the limited and varied samples of subjects used in both of Zimmerman's studies (1980a; 1980b): an all-male stuttering group compared with a male and female normal-speaking group, and four male stutterers compared with one female nonstutterer. There certainly needs to be some assurance that the articulatory movement patterns of females are indistinguishable from males. But the importance, or otherwise, of the difference in movement patterns of stutterers and nonstuterers would take on much more significance if manipulation of the temporal correlations between oral movements was shown to influence stuttering. None of the foregoing should be interpreted as reflecting on the potential contained in Zimmerman's findings, but, rather, as cautionary observations on their methodological underpinnings. One other concern relates to the general use of EMG in order to identify critical muscle groups. A recent report of the problems involved in verifying EMG signals from the orofacial and mandibulor region by O'Dwyer, Quinn, Guitar, Andrews, and Neilson (1981) suggests that the validity of these signals is very debatable, especially when they purport to measure specific muscle groups. Until some of these problems are resolved, it would appear unwise to place too much confidence in the long-term implications of the current crop of physiological studies.

Reappraisal of the Modified Vocalization Hypothesis

Current Status

Throughout the 1970s, there were numerous interesting attempts to test Wingate's (1969b; 1970) claim that modified vocalization is responsible for most conditions in which stuttering is reduced or absent. But according to Wingate's (1979b) own interpretations of his hypothesis, most investigations were ill founded. It will be recalled that most researchers endeavored to operationalize "altered vocalization" in terms of air-flow management, voice-reaction-time control, and, ultimately, laryngeal muscle activity. The main implication in this research was that phonation was synonymous with the term "vocalization." This was a reasonable interpretation, since Wingate (1969b) argued that in many fluency-inducing conditions the "stutterer is induced to emphasize phonation and continuity of phonation in the production of some kind of melody or prosody" (p.682). Nevertheless, Wingate (1979b) has recently disclaimed this interpretation by pointing out that his reference to vocalization was essentially related to prosody. In fact, it would appear that Wingate's modified vocalization hypothesis might have been more appropriately labelled a "modified prosody hypothesis." This also becomes clear when investigations on some of the fluency-inducing conditions referred to by Wingate (1969b; 1970) are considered.

At its inception Wingate's modified vocalization hypothesis was never characterized by specificity. The essence of the hypothesis was that "in almost all circumstances where stuttering is substantially reduced, certain changes in vocal expression seem to be significantly involved if not, in fact, responsible for the improved fluency" (1970, p.871). In that form, which Wingate has never really altered or developed, the hypothesis is almost untestable. The vague reference to "certain" alterations in vocal expression, and the qualified responsibility of changed vocal expression for any improved fluency makes it easy to understand why it has attracted different interpretations. It is also interesting to consider just how the hypothesis might be falsified: What quantifiable indices of vocal expression might show *insufficient* change during reduced stuttering in order to reject modified vocalization as "involved" or "responsible"? Alternatively, a reduction in severe stuttering might be expected to produce altered utterance rate; would that qualify as a significant change in vocal expression? The explanatory strength of the hypothesis would certainly be clearer if it were possible to determine whether there are vocal expression changes that actually do induce improved fluency, or merely appear in conjunction with conditions that reduce stuttering. Thus, inspite of the undeniable productivity of this hypothesis, most research on the hypothesis has been concerned with identifying *any* speech quality changes during "artificial fluency" that might qualify as consistent with the hypothesis. Very little effort has been directed towards testing whether such changes might be responsible for that "fluency."

Many of the "artificial fluency" conditions that Wingate (1969b; 1970; 1976) referred to have been reviewed in previous chapters, as has the research on the modified vocalization hypotheses. What follows, therefore, is a summarized account of that research.

A number of studies have shown that when masking conditions reduce stuttering, there are associated changes in other dimensions of speech (Chapter 7). Adams and Moore (1972) and Brayton and Conture (1978), for example, found that vocal intensity increased significantly as stuttering decreased. Brayton and Conture (1978) and Lechner (1979) also observed an increase in fundamental frequency, but no alteration in vowel duration. Andrews, Howie, Dozsa, and Guitar (1982) showed that one of their three adult stutterers increased phonation duration in 80dB masking. The evidence implicating vocal intensity as necessary for reduced stuttering during masking is weakened by data from Garber and Martin (1977). They showed that when vocal intensity was manipulated, it failed to produce changes in stuttering frequency similar to those produced by noise conditions. This still leaves open the possibility, though, that changes in fundamental frequency, possibly combined with changes in vocal intensity, were necessary and sufficient for the changes that occurred during masking.

If changes in fundamental frequency do modify stuttering, then this may be the variable responsible for reduced stuttering during singing. However, many other factors have also been investigated for their relevance to this phenomenon. Healey, Mallard, and Adams (1976) assessed the contribution that familiarity with lyrics and vocalization changes make to reductions in stuttering during singing. They measured utterance duration and frequency of stuttering by eight stutterers (18-30 years) while they orally read or sang familiar and unfamiliar lyrics. Quite predictably, they found that during singing utterance durations were significantly longer and stutterings were significantly reduced. But they also concluded that the familiarity factor might be as important as the vocalization factor in reducing stuttering.[8] Colcord and Adams (1979) measured frequency of disfluencies, voicing duration, peak and average SPL during singing and oral reading of identical lyrics ("Home on the Range") by stutterers (n=8; 18-31 years) and nonstutterers (n=8; 18-31 years). They found that the stutterers' disfluencies were significantly reduced and their voicing duration significantly increased, but there were no appreciable changes in SPL measures. By contrast, the nonstutterers did not significantly change their disfluencies during singing, but did increase their voicing duration and SPL scores. Two interesting features of this study were the quite obvious differences in voicing duration by the stutterers and nonstutterers during oral reading, and the absence of measures of fundamental frequency. The first feature suggests one other source for preceived differences between the "fluent" speech of stutterers and nonstutterers. The second feature, which was also absent from the Healey, Mallard, and Adams (1976) study, is puzzling because it would seem to be a necessary measure in order to validate differences between singing and oral reading. However, the possible contribution of changes in fundamental frequency were considered in a study by Ramig and Adams (1981); they compared children and adult stutterers and nonstutterers (nine in each of the four groups) when they were instructed to orally read normally and then with a high or low pitch. Measures of fundamental frequency indicated that the instructed changes in speech quality were actually achieved. Both groups of speakers reduced their frequency of disfluencies during the high and low pitch conditions, but both groups also decreased their speaking rates. During the high pitch conditions vocal SPL measures also increased significantly.[9] In short, this finding suggests that variations in fundamental frequency may modify stuttering, but the finding is complicated by uncontrolled effects produced by reduced rate and vocal SPL. Actually this type of comparative study illustrates some of the complexities involved in isolating factors that may be "responsible" for reduced stuttering. All three of the reviewed studies have adequately identified changes in speaking behavior that may accompany a particular method for inducing fluency, but none has demonstrated that these changes are either necessary or sufficient to reduce stuttering.

Different levels of measurement might be necessary to identify changes in vocal expression in fluency-inducing conditions. This is illustrated in studies by Healey and Adams (1981a; 1981b) on variables related to reduced speaking rate by stutterers and nonstutterers. In both studies, children and adults repeated

[8] An interesting sidelight to this study was evidence of quite substantial amounts of stuttering during singing of both the familiar and unfamiliar lyrics (range across subjects: 0-16 for familiar lyrics and 0-33 for unfamiliar lyrics). It is a finding which runs counter to the generally held belief that stutterers rarely stutter during singing (Wingate, 1969b, p. 680).

[9] There is an interesting similarity between this finding and Brayton and Conture's (1978) findings with respect to masking.

sentences at both a basal rate and at a rate that each subject judged to be 50% below basal rate. Only fluent utterances under both conditions were assessed for phonetic and pause durations. The initial data reveal that both pause and phonetic duration were usually extended when subjects were instructed to reduce their speech rate. But when the same subjects' utterances were spectrographically analyzed for consonant, vowel, pause, and utterance duration, no consistent between- and within-group differences were evident. The findings appear to show that reduced rate may not be associated with predictable or consistent changes in typical measures of vocal expression. However, this conclusion is qualified by three questionable features in these studies; absence of speech rate control, measures derived from adaptation conditions, and the restricted variety of measures chosen to test the experimental question. That qualification is supported by data reported from a study by Andrews, Howie, Dozsa, and Guitar (1982), which showed that a 50% reduction in spontaneous speech rate by three adult stutterers actually decreased phonation duration and increased pause intervals.

One other description that Wingate (1969b) provided for "modified vocalization" was that the "stutterer is induced, in one way or another, to do something with his voice that he does not ordinarily do" (pp.884-85). Although this appears to be an extremely vague concept, it does convey the relatively simple notion that what the stutterers change is their customary speech quality in some obvious manner during "artificial fluency." In other words, these differences should be just as evident to listener judgments as they are via specified measures of the speech signal. This proposition was tested in two studies directed by this writer. Ingham and Carroll (1977) and Ingham and Packman (1979) had listeners judge pairs of samples of speech made by stutterers during the course of experiments on chorus reading. Twelve stutterers were used in these studies, but the listeners confidently identified differences between stutter-free samples drawn from chorus- and nonchorus-reading conditions for only half of these subjects. To some extent these indecisive findings are consistent with data reported by Adams and Ramig (1980). They also compared samples of speech made in chorus- and nonchorus-reading conditions by stutterers and nonstutterers and found no significant differences in peak vocal SPL or continuity of phonation under both conditions. However the stutterers actually shortened their vowel durations during chorus reading—a finding which is at odds with Wingate's claim that such conditions should emphasize "continuity of vocalization." By contrast, Andrews, Howie, Dozsa, and Guitar (1982) reported that their adult subjects (n=3) increased phonation duration during chorus-reading conditions.

Sufficient evidence has been presented in Chapter 5, and at the beginning of this chapter, to show that rhythmic stimulation and DAF usually changes the subject's customary voice quality. But again, there is virtually no evidence which demonstrates the exact changes necessary to produce the ameliorative effects of both procedures. In the case of DAF, the preceding review suggests that its main effects are likely to be derived from extended phonation. But remarkably little interest has been shown in identifying the crucial parameters of extended phonation. This writer recently directed one study which found that a reduction in the frequency of relatively short intervals of phonation may reduce or eliminate stuttering without excessively distorting speech quality. Ingham, Montgomery, and Ulliana (1983) had two adult stutterers speak spontaneously under conditions in which the frequency of intervals of phonation shorter than a prescribed duration were signalled to the subject. By this means, phonation intervals shorter than 100 msecs could be reduced or increased by one subject, as could intervals shorter than 150 msecs by the other subject. When these intervals were decreased by less than 50% of their base-rate occurrence, stuttering was virtually eliminated. But, when the subjects increased these intervals by at least 50%, their stuttering increased above basal frequency levels. In the case of the first subject, samples of speech drawn from the reduced-phonation-intervals condition were judged by listeners to be normal-sounding and indistinguishable from stutter-free speech samples obtained from base-rate conditions. The second subject clearly adopted an unusual speech pattern, probably resembling "prolonged speech," during the experimental conditions. The findings from this study suggest that relatively small and not unusual sounding increases in the duration of phonation may be sufficient to reduce stuttering. Conversely, increasing the frequency of relatively short periods of phonation may produce an increase in stuttering frequency. This study also demonstrates some of the advantages in exploring the manipulation of certain speech dimensions in a single-subject rather than group study. It may well be the case that the changes in voice quality referred to by Wingate are individualized and, on examination, share little in common with conditions known to produce "artificial fluency."

Some evidence of the differences that might be expected in "changes in voice quality" under the different conditions occurs in a spectrographic study by Wingate (1981a). This study compared a phrase spoken by four stutterers and four nonstutterers under chorus reading, rhythmic stimulation, shadowing, singing, and a control condition. From inspection of their spectrograms it was claimed that reduced variation in the intonation pattern was the most common feature across all experimental conditions. Yet, surprisingly little attention was drawn to quite obvious variations in speech rate: the rhythmic condition for all subjects always produced slower speech samples, while the shadowing or chorus reading conditions were all associated with faster utterance rates than those found in the control condition.[10] Actually Wingate's study only showed the great variations in speech that might be expected under each of the experimental conditions. It certainly revealed differences, but, like many of the previously reviewed studies, it also did nothing to identify their relevance to reduced stuttering.

Conclusions

The conclusions that can be drawn from research prompted by the modified vocalization hypothesis are surprisingly insubstantial. That research has, thus

[10] Ironically, Wingate (1981a) disparaged use of perceptual judgments to identify these effects, yet he also acknowledged that some of the common effects, such as a monotone quality, are "clearly perceptible in listening to the actual samples": a perceptible state that would be just as easily recognized via appropriate methods of assessment.

far, provided very little guidance on variables that might be necessary, or sufficient, to modify stuttering. In fact, at best, it has only yielded some indication that extended phonation, and possibly shifts in fundamental frequency during speaking, are related to—or possibly responsible in some way, for—reduced stuttering.

Part of the reason for the relatively insubstantial conclusions from this field concerns methodology. Reference was made earlier to the limited explanatory strength of any conclusion drawn from comparisons between the performance of stutterers and nonstutterers. The same limitations apply to comparisons between speech performed in the presence and absence of certain fluency-inducing conditions. For the most part, such studies have yielded evidence of differences across almost as many dimensions as the experimenters have cared to measure. In other words, it is an approach to research which lacks a commitment to the principal of "strong inference" (Platt, 1964). There is an almost desperate need in this field for experiments that will systematically cancel alternative hypotheses in order to track down the sources of variance that contribute most to fluency-inducing conditions. It is also becoming clearer that there is more likelihood these sources of variance will be traced by careful single-subject experimentation, rather than relying on the imprecision of error variance within group studies.

Another rather neglected aspect of modified vocalization research is the durability of any identified critical variables. If a slight shift in fundamental frequency, or change in phonatory activity, is found to be a controlling agent, then what implication does this have at either a theoretical or therapeutic level? If these variables prove to be necessary to remove stutter-free speech, does it mean that such changes would be sufficient to sustain that condition? The answer to these questions will certainly require much more inventive research than that which has been used thus far to test the modified vocalization hypothesis and/or its ramifications.

Prolonged Speech and Its Variants in Stuttering Therapy

Introduction

If a stuttering therapies "hit parade" existed, then "prolonged speech and its variants" would currently top the chart. There are many reasons for its popularity, but among the more likely is that this category of therapies simply includes so many techniques or combinations of techniques known to modify stuttering. The diffuseness of this treatment category is also matched, unhappily, by the diffuse procedural descriptions that accompany these treatments. And since it is almost impossible to operationally define many of the procedures in these therapies, they actually have questionable relevance for behavior therapy. What began as therapy using DAF to produce a particular speech pattern has now become synonymous with almost any therapy that uses either emphasized vocalization, de-emphasized articulatory gestures, or even reduced speech rate. At a more general level, the derivatives of the "DAF therapies" are usually described as relying on breathstream management and speech-rate control. It is certainly not at all clear whether "prolonged speech" now means something that is different from numerous therapy labels that have appeared in recent years—for example, "breathstream management," "fluency shaping," "regulated breathing," "rate control," "smooth motion speech," or "legato speech." The vague descriptions that occasionally accompany these labels usually share so many features that, for review purposes, it is simpler to describe them as variants of prolonged speech. In fact, as will be seen, there is very little evidence that they differ from each other in any important way.

The extent to which the derivatives of DAF-based therapies have influenced stuttering therapy in recent years is evident in many treatment reviews. For example, a recent treatment overview by Conture (1982) argued that only certain common denominators occur in therapeutically-induced fluency: "The two variables that seem most consistently related to increments in stutterers' fluency are (1) minimized variability of speech production ... and (2) lengthening of intra- and inter-segmental durations and transitions. ..." (p.146).

Also, a recent search for commonalities among behavioral approaches to stuttering therapy by Guitar and Peters (1980) yielded "Fluency Shaping Therapy" as representative of that approach. They described this as a procedure "based on operant conditioning and programming principles" and typified by the methods used by "Perkins (1973), Ryan (1974) and Webster (1974)." As will be seen, the treatments described by these clinicians mainly involve variants of prolonged speech. The pervasive influence of this speech pattern on stuttering therapy is also demonstrated by Cooper's (1980) recent overview of current treatments: it was literally restricted to programs that employ variants of prolonged speech. Finally, there is the comparative, or meta-analysis, investigation by Andrews, Guitar, and Howie (1980) of different stuttering treatments (mainly with adults). These investigators reached the surprisingly confident conclusion "that treatments based on training the stutterer in prolonged and gentle onset techniques are superior to other types of treatments" (p.305). As will be seen, the grounds for this conclusion are questionable, but the claim probably reflects the stature of this procedure in the eyes of many clinicians.

The Ancestry of Prolonged Speech and Its Variants

One constant criticism of the treatment procedures that constitute the behavioral preparadigm is that they are neither original nor dependent on one of the keystones of behavior therapy, replicable operations. Such criticism is undeniably well placed with respect to some therapies that will be reported in this chapter. In many respects their methodology has provided proponents of alternative stuttering treatments, such as Sheehan (1970; 1980), Van Riper (1973; 1979), and Gregory (1977; 1979), with ample weaponry to criticize many of these allegedly innovative therapies. There is, for example, good evidence that the descriptions of some behavioral treatments are almost indistinguishable from those applied to therapies that have been advocated since the 18th century. There is also good cause for the complaint that many current versions of these treatments use methodologies that do not rely on operationalized concepts; and, in this way, they certainly cannot be distinguished from their earlier counterparts.

Therapy practices that use emphasized phonation and reduced speech rate, or exaggerated respiration and vocalization, have appeared in different guises throughout the history of stuttering treatment. Borman (1969) published a treatise from 1724 by one Cotton Mather, a colorful early American medical practitioner, which gave advice to stutterers to

> first use yourself to a very deliberate Way of Speaking, a Drawling that shall be little short of Singing. Even this Drawling will be better than Stammering ... [as a result] ... the Organs of your Speech will be so habituated into Right Speaking, that you will by Degrees, and sooner than you imagine, grow able to speak as fast again, as you did when the Law of Deliberation first of all began to govern you. Tho' my Advice is, beware of speaking too fast, as long as you live. (from Borman, 1969, p.460).

Nearly 150 years later, a self-treatment pamphlet (Anonymous, 1870) described the following methods as among the then "most approved and most successful" for treating stuttering: "speak slowly, with an affected ease, in a style approaching to chanting as distinguished from staccato; in other words, let the words flow out rather than attempt to jerk them out" (p.30).

Virtually the same principles were recommended earlier this century by Alexander Melville Bell (1904). He encouraged his patients to use breath regulation and practice in prolonging vowels and voiced consonants. The emphasis on phonatory over articulatory action during speaking is captured in his recommendation that "no mouth-action must be allowed to interfere with the flow of throat-sound" (p.23). Van Riper's (1973) excellent overview of therapies that flourished during the same era also highlights the prominence of these methods. It shows that exaggerated breathing, prolonged vowels, and slowed speaking were almost integral to numerous therapies prescribed by European authorities around the turn of this century. In the United States, at roughly the same time, Samuel Robbins, famous for his association with the Boston Stammerers' Institute, recommended the following treatment exercises:

1. The easy start of the first word to be spoken on each breath
2. Keeping calm, relaxed, and unhurried in everything they do
3. Slow breathing
4. The relaxation pause on empty lungs
5. Never holding the breath between breathing and speaking
6. Joining all words smoothly and easily together
7. Getting the attention more on vowels and less on consonants

(from Cooper, 1979, p.76).

It will be seen that many of these features now form the centerpieces of most of the behavior therapies that employ prolonged speech or its variants. In fact, the descriptions provided for prolonged speech, breathstream management, gentle contacts, and the like often carry no more precision than the descriptions offered by these early clinicians.

The resemblance between the past and present-day therapies becomes even clearer by studying the procedural descriptions of many therapies used during the late 1930s and 1940s. One program that shares much in common with many current treatments was outlined by Bender and Kleinfeld (1938). They described a "rate-control technique" as part of a treatment schedule involving prolongation, concentration on phonation, softening of consonants, and "smooth slow motion speech." This last-mentioned speech pattern required the stutterer to "prolong the vowel sound in each syllable, whether the syllable contains one consonant or several consonants" (p.122). Thereafter, the procedure incorporated relaxation techniques and transfer recommendations. At about the same time that Bender and Kleinfeld were promoting their methods in the eastern United States, on the West Coast Mabel Gifford (1939; 1940) was advocating a very similar approach to stuttering treatment. She developed a relatively programmed method of therapy which involved relaxation practice, learning the "sigh principle" ("breathy outpouring of the voice on the sigh stream") and speaking in short phrases. This was followed by development of the "fluency pattern," which involved active but silent recollection of these principles while speaking (Gifford, 1939, pp.32-33).

Many of the techniques described by Bender and Kleinfeld and Gifford were used in a remarkable treatment program reported by Hahn (1941). The similarities between Hahn's program, which was conducted at the University of Southern California, and the features of programs promoted during the 1970s is almost uncanny. It included relaxation, practicing the "fluency pattern" along the lines described by Gifford, as well as relatively systematic within- and beyond-clinic transfer procedures. Some results of this program were described earlier, but in view of its relationship to some recent treatments, it is also interesting to read Hahn's description of the "new speech pattern" which was the focal point of his program:

> In speaking, [the stutterer] should have a feeling of pouring out the tone on the outgoing breath and he should emphasize the length of vowel sounds. He should speak in short phrases, pausing between phrases to replenish his breath and to re-establish the feeling of physical and emotional relaxation. The broken speech rhythm is then supplanted by an easy, rhythmical, controlled speech pattern. To the observer the stutterer's speech is characterized by a soft, breathy-tone quality, prolonged vowel sounds, short phrases, frequent pauses, and natural inflections. The rhythm is definite and rather slow. The bodily tensions and strains so prevalent among those who stutter are replaced by increased ease and calm.
>
> ...Frequently, it is advisable to ask all stutterers to over-emphasize the breathiness in the beginning stages of the clinical work, so that they will understand the action of the speech mechanism and perceive the feeling of the pouring out of the breath. Also, the average stutterer will tend to compromise on the amount of breathiness he uses in speech in outside situations. The exaggeration in the clinic allows for this anticipated com-

> promise. One advantage in advocating the breathy tone is that the stutterer is given something specific and tangible to do, an action well within his field of understanding and obvious in execution to the visual, auditory, and kinaesthetic senses. One factor which helps to mitigate the unnaturalness in the use of the pattern is that the inflections of normal speech are required (Hahn, 1941, pp.31-33).

Perhaps the most fascinating point about these early "prolonged speech" treatments is that they almost disappeared from the treatment literature. Very few texts of the 1950s and 1960s refer to them; when they do, it is usually a slighting reference. The promising efforts of Hahn passed with his untimely death in the early 1940s, but they were probably pushed aside with equal effect by the overpowering influence of the Iowa School on therapy practice. In any event, Hahn's work has received virtually no recognition by recent advocates of prolonged speech and its variants. What little recognition it has received is usually a part of an account of discarded methods (for example, Van Riper, 1973).

There are probably many other reasons for the demise of the early speech pattern procedures—though it is unlikely that it was because they were replaced by more effective treatments. One fairly logical possibility is that they relied on producing a speech pattern which was as undesirable as stuttering. For there is little indication that any of these treatments was designed to restore normal-sounding speech. Moreover, while they involved a means to modify stuttering, there is every indication that their successful implementation must have depended on vaguely prescribed clinician-managed and self-managed skills.

One of the ironies of stuttering therapy is the great similarity between procedures used by those described as "traditionalist" and those found among the behavior therapies. One especially vivid example is the resemblance between some techniques promoted by the behavioral preparadigm's most eloguent critic, Charles Van Riper, and those used in many allegedly behavioral treatments. In 1954, for example, Van Riper outlined a range of methods that stutterers could be trained to use as "preparatory sets"—means of changing their stutterings into less debilitating events. These included "carefully initiating the air flow or voice flow with [the] speech attempt" (Van Riper, 1954, p.438), as well as light articulatory contacts in conjunction with a "smooth-prolongation pattern." These techniques were (and are) taught in Van Riper's therapy approach primarily to help the speaker reduce the severity of a stutter, but there is no expectation that such techniques will lead to the removal of stuttering. They have been used in many western countries to help both adults and children to produce, for example, "easy stammering" (Irwin, 1980). In many respects, as will be seen, the only difference between this technique and those that Guitar and Peters (1980), among others, refer to as "fluency shaping" is the technique's purpose. In the case of Van Riper's procedure, the "preparatory set" is employed on words that the speaker anticipates stuttering. The "fluency shaping" aspect in this technique requires the speaker to constantly adopt this altered manner of speech, after the fashion described by Hahn (1941). Of course, those who claim to be employing this procedure within the context of a behavioral framework would argue that the speech pattern is embedded within a schedule of speaking tasks, which systematizes the method and helps to sustain and generalize its benefits. But this difference often turns out to be more a matter of semantics.

Murray (1958) has provided an interesting example of a speech-pattern therapy which resembles many behavioral treatments, and also serves to illustrate the variegated background of "prolonged speech." In his report on Japanese speech-therapy programs, Murray described a therapy school in Tokyo, directed by one Masayuki Hamamoto. In this therapy class

> emphasis is put on replacing the customary pattern of speech with a new one along the lines of sing-song, controlled phrasing, slow rate, and rhythmical breathing. With regard to the latter, it was noted that the speakers learned to inhale deeply and to commence to emit a light vowel sound before gliding into the beginning of the sentence. The mouth movements are exaggerated, perhaps due to the intensive exercises dealing with mouth positions for forming words. (p.244).

This procedure was used in a group-treatment setting with children who were eventually graduated in the expectation that they would then remain fluent. Unhappily, no information is available as to whether they maintained their graduate status. Nevertheless, the procedure certainly contains the ingredients of practices used in many recently described treatments.

The recent and not-so-recent, history of stuttering therapy contains ample evidence that emphasized vocalization and de-emphasized articulatory gestures have been used extensively in therapy over the years. They were certainly used well before DAF was introduced to clinical practice in order to either "prevent" stuttering or provide a "fluent speech pattern," although they usually accompanied other activities. Wherever it is possible to learn exactly how these techniques were used, it would seem evident that unspecified clinician judgments were a prominent part of their use in treatment. In the course of the rest of this chapter, it will be seen that such judgments continue to be integral to therapies that use these techniques under the "behavior therapy" label.

DAF and the Prolonged-Speech Revival

It is often stated that theorizing dominates the field of stuttering. But it has never managed to completely obliterate expediency. For whatever is reported—formally or informally—to reduce stuttering eventually finds its way into clinical practice. Thus, it was almost inevitable that the modifying effects of DAF would be thought to have therapeutic possibilities. Actually one of the few exceptions to the expediency rule has been Geniesse's (1935) report that stuttering was reduced when adult stutterers walked on all fours. Probably the only reason that that activity has not been advocated for therapy is because it poses some unappealing difficulties for normal interaction. Yet, many of the unappealing speech characteristics that typified DAF-induced fluency were largely ignored by those keen to promote this twentieth century contribution to stuttering therapy: a machine-produced and controlled fluency. In their zeal, most of these advocates also failed to realize that the machine's effects were not reliable.

The previous review of DAF's effects on stuttering has referred to some of the procedure's rather basic problems that inevitably beset its use in treatment. Perhaps the most obvious is the great variability in the reponse pattern: DAF's ameliorative effects appear to fluctuate with time, speaker attention, speech rate, and, far more significantly, experimenter instruction—hardly the ingredients of a technological breakthrough for treatment. Most of these problems were apparently less significant than the more spectacular finding that, during DAF, nonstutterers seemed to stutter. Yet, some stutterers appeared to become fluent; it was therefore tempting to believe that DAF contained some unique properties for treatment. But, inevitably, the problems with DAF grew in magnitude when it was used more extensively within a behavior-therapy context.

The initial reports on the use of DAF stuttering therapy were flimsy in detail and data. Adamczyk (1959) briefly described the use of an unspecified amount of DAF in the treatment of 15 adults subjects. Their treatment lasted 2 to 3 months, and 13 achieved "great improvement in speaking; in two cases, the improvement was slight" (p.218). Adamczyk (1963) also initiated one of the most imaginative clinical applications of DAF. He arranged a telephone system with built-in DAF for use in conjunction with clinical facilities in the Polish city of Lublin: subjects could phone the central clinic and obtain DAF speech practice while supervised by their clinician. Sixty percent of subjects (n=60) were informally reported markedly improved, or better, as a result of this method. In later reports, Adamczyk (1969) has described using 100-300 msec DAF, or "echo method," in a program involving clinic practice followed by home and demanding-speech-situation tasks. An Italian report by Zerneri (1966) also gave a brief account of DAF use in stuttering therapy. But the reports by both clinicians are far too cursory to adequately judge the therapy benefits. This was largely true also in a DAF study by Cohen and Edwards (1965) with five adult stutterers. These subjects experienced random intervals of either synchronous or 300 msec DAF for 15 hours over 3 weeks. It was claimed that their "secondary stutterings" were replaced by primary, or repetitive, stuttering. Cohen and Edwards also claimed that this presumably beneficial effect carried over to beyond-clinic situations during and after treatment. But this claim was also made without the benefit of data.

Undoubtedly, the most influential behavior therapy research with DAF was reported by Goldiamond (1965). It was influential for numerous reasons, not the least being that it was the first to outline a methodology designed to establish normal-sounding stutter-free speech—a methodology that was copied by numerous other DAF programs. Goldiamond's treatment procedure was a direct extension of the previously described response-contingent experiments using DAF (see Chapter 9). Essentially, subjects passed through a four-stage treatment involving oral reading (mainly) during thrice weekly 50-minute sessions. The program was built on the premise that an "elimination-avoidance" schedule using DAF would replace the stuttering pattern with "some other pattern which does not contain stuttering." The program was described as establishing the new response pattern, altering stimulus control over the new pattern, and shaping it to ostensibly normal speech. Finally, self-control procedures were introduced to sustain beyond-clinic fluency. The subjects were treated individually and began by orally reading at around 25 wpm while experiencing 250 msec DAF, or 10-seconds normal feedback, contingent on self-defined stuttering. An important aspect of this initial phase was that the subject was also *instructed* to use a prolonged speech pattern during DAF conditions. When a stable and generally stutter-free prolonged speech pattern was established, the delay level was reduced by 50 msec and oral-reading rate was increased. Performance-contingent 50 msec reductions in the delay level and an increase in oral-reading rate were continued until the delay was removed. The subject was then said to be speaking at a normal or "supernormal" rate, with little or no stuttering. The concurrent delay reduction and oral-reading-rate increase was claimed to alter stimulus control over the subject's new pattern, and improve its normal-sounding qualities. The self-control procedure was basically counseling aimed at changing the subject's speaking environment in order to aid maintenance. Eight subjects received this form of therapy, though only seven are described in Goldiamond's report. Their within-clinic data trends were generally consistent with treatment condition changes, but the subjects' informally reported improved beyond-clinic performance was not accompanied by data.

Goldiamond (1965) reported that 30 stutterers had been treated by his procedure and "achieved a fluent pattern of reading which is well-articulted, rapid and devoid of blockages" (p.156). But no other information was provided. In spite of the promise of this therapy report—and the very influential effect it has had on current stuttering treatment—it remains the only generally available paper that Goldiamond has written on stuttering treatment. However, some other details on the research program occur within a grant report prepared by Goldiamond (1967). Included there was evidence that neither the contingency schedule nor DAF may have been relevant to the effects produced by the treatment; some subjects were able to produce the desired response pattern without the benefit of DAF. There was also a report on the development of a portable DAF unit to aid carry-over which, in turn, implies that the treatment required much supplementation.

In spite of the many contentious features in Goldiamond's (1965) report, there can be little doubt about its impact on stuttering treatment. The treatment schedule Goldiamond used to instate stutter-free speech has been employed with surprisingly little variation in many stuttering therapy programs. Yet, it is also possible to detect within Goldiamond's report the seeds of many of the problems found in treatments that it spawned. One problem concerns the operational status of the method used to procure both prolonged speech and its presumed normal-sounding derivative. The fact that prolonged speech was not a necessary byproduct of DAF, but relied on clinician instructions and judgment for its appearance, immediately weakened that status. That weakness was compounded by the apparently superfluous role of DAF. Consequently, what at first glance appeared to be a replicable operation described in stimulus-control terms ultimately emerged as a vaguely defined speech pattern produced by relatively ambiguous procedures. Another problem was the absence of carry-over data. Goldiamond suggested that the self-control procedures would enable the subject to "change his environment in a manner likely to optimize the desired changes in his behavior" (1965, p.142), yet no data ever emerged to show that these methods would ensure that subjects sustained their fluency. The fluency-instatement procedure also contained a number of untested characteristics. For example, no data were ever supplied to demonstrate the necessity (or otherwise) of the delay schedule, the performance criteria in the schedule, nor the contribution of speech rate control.[11]

The Initial Mutations of Goldiamond's Procedure

Shortly after Goldiamond's (1965) ground-breaking program appeared, four different groups of clinical researchers produced mutations of his procedure. Each of these research groups has developed otherwise-unique therapy approaches, primarily for adult stutterers, that have also influenced a substantial amount of current stuttering therapy. The features and findings of these programs will now be described.

The Hollins Program

The first of these programs was developed by Ronald Webster at Hollins College in Virginia. This therapy program has undergone a large number of developments since it was initiated by Webster and Lubker in 1968, including the abandonment of DAF. Its initial format differed from Goldiamond's mainly to the extent that continuous, rather than response-contingent, DAF was used with oral reading. When used with 14 stutterers, it was claimed to be "effective in producing fluent speech which transfers to conversational setting outside the laboratory" (p.764). Four of these subjects, who had "strong anticipatory struggle responses," also required instructions to speak without struggle before DAF could be used to sustain their fluency. No speech performance data were provided for any subject, however. But a subsequent development of this program by Webster (1970) (acccompanied by the ambitious title "Stuttering: A Way to Eliminate It...") did provide some performance data. It described a 10-40 hour treatment for eight severe stutterers aged 15 to 47 years. This five-step treatment was the first to be described as a "Fluency Shaping Program," a label that has become synonymous with many programs using prolonged speech and speech-rate control. After training to self-define stutterings, subjects then orally read under continuous 200 msec DAF conditions. At this time, each subject "was instructed to prolong his speech." The DAF volume was faded until the subject maintained fluent speech at 30-35 wpm. Then followed a "smoothing operation," in which the subject was instructed to "decrease the speed and amplitude with

[11] In different places, mention has been made of variations that Goldiamond has introduced to the treatment described in his 1965 publication. Soderberg (1968) refers to a personal communication with Goldiamond which indicated the treatment program was altered to 1 week of intensive therapy. Another personal communication with Goldiamond by Azrin and Nunn (1974) has indicated that subjects are now required to use "juncturing" or speaking in phrases of specified duration during treatment. Presumably, this treatment also includes DAF.

which he made consonant sounds, while simultaneously prolonging vowel sounds. In addition, subjects were instructed to make smooth transitions from one speech sound to another within a word'' (Webster, 1970, p.158). After a clinician judged that this target had been reached, the oral-reading rate was increased to around 80-100 wpm. If stuttering reappeared, then the subject was instructed to smooth or slow his speech rate. Then followed rate-discrimination training, in which the subject learned to vary his rate within certain speech-rate ranges. Only then was the conversational speech introduced, plus instructions to use the ''new fluent speech pattern'' in the home for short periods. The instructions also emphasized the use of a self-control strategy; the subject was required to either reintroduce the new pattern or return to the old pattern if stuttering reappeared.

Webster (1970) claimed that the fluency generated by this program persisted for approximately 10 months (the time at which the report was written), and only one subject reported recurrence of stuttering. However, the criterion for releasing subjects from treatment was that ''they had less than five blocks a day,'' though no data accompanied the claimed carry-over effects. The reported performance data are also somewhat misleading, since they refer to base-line and within-treatment conditions without details on the oral-reading intervals in each condition. Furthermore, although these data show reduced stuttering in treatment, no reliability or speech-rate data were included. It is also evident in Webster's later writings that the program's clinical benefits were less than satisfactory. For instance, in 1974, Webster claimed that 16 subjects had been treated by this program and all were ''markedly improved,'' but with the following rider: ''Most of the subjects reported that they could maintain good speech fluency; however, they reported that great concentration was required on their part and that even then they were not able to maintain good fluency at all times'' (Webster, 1974a, p.32). In later treatment programs, Webster has placed more emphasis on training speakers to produce different classes of speech sounds in a manner derived from the prolonged speech pattern; DAF was dispensed with completely. But these earlier treatments relied heavily on clinician judgments to train and assess target behaviors, and like many related programs, they were not accompanied by information that would enable reasonable replication of their operations.

The Curlee and Perkins Program

Another variation on Goldiamond's program was Curlee and Perkins's (1969) ''Conversational Rate Control Therapy.'' Their principal variation was replacement of oral reading with conversation, plus the use of continuous rather than response-contingent DAF. They also introduced strategies to sustain some of the DAF-established behaviors and shift the assumed stimulus-control properties of the clinic to typical beyond-clinic situations.

Upon closer examination, it becomes clear that Curlee and Perkins made some interesting modifications to Goldiamond's method of using DAF that actually reduced, rather than emphasized, speech-rate control. Initially, their subjects conversed for two 15-minute intervals at 250 msec DAF, with less than two stutterings per 5 minutes. Then, in subsequent steps, the delay level was reduced in 50 msec units while the subject endeavored to sustain the 250 msec delay rate (30-35 wpm). After 0 msec delay was reached, DAF was systematically withdrawn. In following steps, the 200, 150, 100, 50 and 0 msec speech rates were established. However, at no point was direct control established over the speaking rate that subjects used at each delay level. Presumably, this depended on clinician judgment, since the subject was only "instructed to slow down his speaking rate by prolonging syllables so that his utterances coincide with the delayed feedback" (Curlee & Perkins, 1969, p.246). In the rest of this program, time-out was used as a contingency on "sticky" speech quality, excessively fast speech rate, or phrases that were "too long." A transfer procedure that followed required speech in prescribed and subject-selected situations. The total time of this program was specified as 90 hours.

Curlee and Perkins provided some preliminary treatment-results information in their 1969 publication. This indicated that 15 adolescent and adult subjects received some or all of this program, and those who completed the treatment "estimated that their stuttering had decreased 75%-95% in those situations not easily available to observation by the clinician" (p.249). In a later paper, Curlee and Perkins (1973) provided some group data from the treatment of 30 stutterers (13-52 years). They were divided into two treatment schedules (15 hours weekly for 6 weeks, or 3 hours weekly for 30 weeks), and data were obtained from 27 subjects before and after treatment. They found that "percentage of words stuttered was reduced in the clinic from a mean of 17.0 to 0.2% and in outside situations from 16.0 to 1.3%" (pp.399-400). But this was the only measurement information; no data were provided on speech rate, measurement reliability, sample size, or posttreatment performance (although this can be derived from a 1974 report by Perkins, Rudas, Johnson, Michael, and Curlee which will be referred to later). More importantly, it was recorded that on "several chance meetings, clients were observed to be stuttering more than their tape recordings represent" (Curlee & Perkins, 1973, p.400), and that all subjects believed they needed additional assistance with their speech. In general, this treatment procedure certainly appeared to produce marked short-term improvements, but Curlee and Perkins obviously regarded these benefits with some diffidence.

The Ryan Program

The third variation of Goldiamond's procedure formed part of a previously reviewed therapy strategy developed by Bruce Ryan, and subsequently extended by the husband-and-wife team of Ryan and Van Kirk. Ryan's main variation was to integrate Goldiamond's DAF schedule with a programmed set of speaking exercises designed to establish, transfer, and maintain target levels of preformance. This schedule has already been described extensively (Chapter 9). During the establishment phase, one of the treatment options was Goldiamond's DAF schedule; this was used in conjunction with oral reading, monologues, and conversational tasks.

Ryan's first description of a DAF therapy program occurs in an account (Ryan,

1971) of the treatment of five children. One child, an 8-year-old male, orally read, monologued, and conversed during continuous DAF, using the 250, 200, 150, 100, 50, and 0 msec delay schedule. He was instructed to prolong each word and speak fluently for 10 minutes at each step. This was accompanied by verbal and token reinforcement for target behaviors, although it was not clear exactly which behavior received these contingencies. This treatment schedule was claimed to reduce the child's stuttering from 10 to less than 0.5 occasions per minute. A transfer procedure was not used because the child's "mother, teacher and school clinician all reported spontaneous transfer of fluent speech to his home and school" (1971, p.267). But this improvement failed to stabilize; 3 months later, during conversational speech, he was recorded at 11.5 stuttered words per minute (SW/M). Thereafter, the subject received a vaguely described program in which the clinician simply instructed the child "to speak slowly and fluently." Then his class peers and teacher were taught to count his stutterings and instruct him to "speak fluently in a prolonged manner if he stuttered." Fifteen months after the start of treatment, it was reported that the child could achieve "0.4 SW/M or less if given appropriate instructions." Unfortunately, Ryan's report on this treatment has questionable clinical value for many reasons. To begin with, it suggests that the treatment procedure was beneficial, but it either omits or inadequately specifies some quite fundamental aspects for evaluating a stuttering treatment. For example, no reliability or generalization data were gathered, and it is not at all clear that the therapy gains were ever independent of "clinical"control (albeit classmates or teacher). It is also difficult to decide from the report whether these gains could be attributed to the treatment. Furthermore, in the absence of speech-rate data, it is quite possible that any improved fluency emerged at the cost of a slow speech rate. In fact, the emphasis placed on slowing and prolonging during the second therapy phase implies that the treatment was not designed to replace prolonged speech with normal speech.

The next account of Ryan's DAF treatment procedure occurs in a study reported by Van Kirk (1972) (for which Ryan served as principal consultant). This program used the format described in Ryan's 1971 publication. Group data were provided for 18 subjects (4-60 years, mean 17.6 years) who passed through briefly described establishment, transfer, and maintenance procedures. The establishment phase included either the DAF schedule described by Ryan (1971) or the GILCU procedure (see Chapter 9), which, therefore, makes it impossible to isolate the DAF procedure's findings. It was reported that before treatment, the group's mean stuttering frequency range was 6.0-11.44 words per minute, depending on the speaking task. After a mean of 14.3 treatment hours in the first two phases, the maintenance contacts extended for between 2 and 20 months (mean 9 months). Over this last phase, the group averaged 0.8 SW/M. However, no information was provided on the origin or reliability for these scores, nor their speech rate. It was also mentioned that "in all the people [involved] there has been only one breakdown in fluency" (Van Kirk, 1972, p.108)—an 8-year-old whose improved performance had maintained for 6 months. Presumably, therefore, either this subject's scores produced the 0.8 SW/M mean score during maintenance, or any other occurrence of stuttering was not regarded as a "breakdown in fluency."

Ryan (1974) subsequently provided an account of the treatment of a number of subjects who experienced the DAF establishment phase of his program. Twenty-eight subjects (ages 8-45 years) received between 2 and 177.2 hours of treatment in this phase, and reached between 0.6 and 0.4 mean SW/M on the Criterion Test (Chapter 9) which was given after each subject completed this phase. Their pretreatment Criterion Test data produced a 12.8 to 9.2 mean SW/M range of scores. A feature of the treatment was that the subjects were free to choose their own speech rates. If a subject repeatedly failed a DAF step, then a branch program was introduced involving prolongation on anticipated stutterings, similar to the preparatory set procedure described by Van Riper (1954). Some consideration was also given to speech quality: "one early result we noticed was that the super-fluent speaker sounding almost like an automaton. To avoid this, we cut down on the instructions to prolong and permitted occasional pausing and other normal dysfluencies" (Ryan, 1974, p.79). Other than this description, the only procedural instructions relating to prolonged speech was guidance for speakers to stretch out their vowels and consonants (p.75). The subjects were permitted to complete the DAF schedule at relatively slow speech rates which were subsequently increased (with or without guidance).

From the original 28 subjects that Ryan (1974) reported receiving the DAF schedule during the establishment phase, only 12 were followed up (1 to 20 months later). Some subjects did not enter the transfer or maintenance phases, and others received either the transfer or maintenance schedules. Actually, only two subjects received the complete transfer and maintenance phases. But both did show more evidence of improvement than their counterparts during the follow-up Criterion Test—they had 8.8 and 3.4 SW/M before treatment and produced less than 0.1 SW/M at both 10 and 3 months follow-up. Unfortunately, the large subject attrition and limited follow-up data in this study make it difficult to even estimate the treatment's contribution to this finding. The durability of the therapy's benefits are also brought into question by some information that Ryan provided on a 21-year-old known as Don (one of the two last-mentioned subjects): "Although Don demonstrated normal fluency, he still thought of himself as a stutterer. Follow-up indicated an additional six months of fluency before a gradual relapse over the next three years" (p.123).

Ryan and Van Kirk (1974) reported treating 50 stutterers (9-66 years) with the same program as that described by Ryan (1974). Forty-nine completed the DAF-scheduled establishment phase, though only 30 proceeded through the transfer and maintenance phases. The conversational-speech data (probably the more clinically relevant speaking data) from all subjects show their mean stuttering decreased from 8.0 to 0.5 SW/M, but their speech rate also declined from 128 to 83.7 words spoken per minute (WS/M). The 30 subjects who completed the transfer phase had a mean of 0.2 SW/M at 135.3 WS/M during conversation on the Criterion Test (the oral reading and monologue means were quite similar). These data imply that the subjects sustained markedly slow speech during the establishment phase, and achieved more normal rates following the transfer phase.

However, the loss of almost 40% of subjects after the establishment phase makes it impossible to decide whether the remaining subject's performance truly reflects the program's benefits. Their data did have the advantages of reliability assessment, plus collection outside the treatment schedule, but they have the disadvantage of being within-clinic measures. Some maintenance data collected on the 30 subjects indicate that over a mean of 5.1 months they received 1.1 hours of therapy, and produced 0.1 SW/M. During this period, "causal observations" indicated "that they are continuing to speak fluently, in a wide variety of settings."

One interesting patient view of Ryan's therapy program appears in a commentary by McCabe and McCollum (1972) from a quite mild adult stutterer, who was treated by the DAF-establishment schedule. Despite the subject's obvious antagonism towards this type of treatment, he apparently achieved self-satisfying benefits that were generally sustained throughout the maintenance schedule. He attributed the continuing benefit of the treatment, though, to monthly telephone contacts with the clinician—which, presumably, formed part of his clinician's version of Ryan's procedure.

The most striking characteristic of Ryan's reports has been the remarkable consistency with which positive findings are reported. Across a large age range, and with subjects who display wide ranges of stuttering, there is every indication that the procedures are invulnerable to age differences (at least, within the range 8-66 years) or frequency and, probably, severity of stuttering. The orderly sequence of treatment steps were also outlined in much more detail than is the case in the two previous research programs. But these virtues are offset by the questionable clinical sifgnificance of the data and the uncertain replicability of much of the treatment methodology. Most data were obtained under treatment or clinic conditions, and accompanied by comments indicating that subjects had to use "speech pattern controls" to retain their improved fluency. The subject attrition rate is also a concern; up to 50% of subjects failed to proceed with treatment (indeed, this could reflect the treatment's true failure rate). Of equal concern is the extensive use of clinician instruction and judgments; speech rate and prolongation play critical roles in much of this treatment, yet the procedures used to measure these variables are generally unspecified. In fact, literally no convincing evidence is provided to show that the treatment operations were actually responsible for therapy benefits.

The Ingham and Andrews Program

The fourth development of Goldiamond's program was an intensive group treatment procedure designed by this writer in Australia during the late 1960s. It was evaluated in a series of treatment studies conducted in collaboration with Gavin Andrews.[12] This program has undergone a number of modifications that

[12] In various publications (for example, Bloodstein, 1975; 1981; Yates, 1975), this program is attributed to "Andrews and Ingham." Since this program was designed and researched by this writer as his PhD thesis (Ingham, 1972), and further developed in postdoctoral studies, that authorship sequence does not reflect that responsibility. Gavin Andrews served as nominal advisor to this program, and assisted in writing up some of the studies that were produced for the writer's doctoral thesis.

will be described later. In its original form (Ingham, 1975a), it was designed to provide conditions that might maximize the possibilities of replacing the stuttering speech pattern with a new stutter-free pattern derived from DAF-instated prolonged speech. To achieve this, a variation of Goldiamond's DAF schedule was integrated with a token economy (Ayllon & Arzin, 1965) in a hospital setting, where every attempt was made to monitor each subject's speech during all nonsleeping periods. The subjects, adults and adolescents, were hospitalized in groups of four, for up to 3 weeks. During this time all food, drinks, and most luxury items were purchased by tokens that were earned or lost via speech behavior. The earning intervals occurred during 45-minute "rating sessions" which were conducted 10-12 times daily, from 7:00 a.m. to 10:00 p.m. In these sessions, subjects spoke a specified number of syllables and earned tokens for stutter-free speech within prescribed speech-rate ranges during a DAF-establishment phase and a following transfer phase. Tokens were lost for failure to achieve the speech performance criteria. They could also be lost for clinician-judged departures from the target speech quality, stutterings, or extended sounds during intervals between rating sessions. This tight control over speech behavior was maintained during the establishment phase, but was systematically withdrawn as the subject proceeded through the transfer phase. During this phase, most within-clinic rating sessions were replaced by speech-situation tasks, in which subjects recorded themselves speaking a prescribed number of syllables. Passage through the establishment and transfer stages was contingent on achieving sequences of sessions in which the target behavior was maintained.

The DAF schedule used in the initial Ingham and Andrews studies was similar to Goldiamond's, except that continuous DAF and conversational speech were used in conjunction with a speech-rate schedule. This schedule was designed to systematically increase speech while DAF was decreased, until a criterion of normal speech rate—180-220 syllables per minute (SPM) and zero stuttering—was reached at 0 msec DAF. Another variation was that subjects were required to achieve completely stutter-free speech at each DAF level before proceeding to the next level. Also, at each level, two sessions were completed with DAF and two without DAF. Clinicians were trained to count syllables and stutterings on-line, which were then converted to percentage of syllables stuttered (%SS) and SPM scores at the end of a rating session (in later programs, electronic counters with displays were used so that subjects could track their speech rate during the establishment-phase rating sessions). Like the other DAF treatment programs, the prolonged speech pattern was partially instated by clinician instructions to speak "with prolonged vowel sounds and smooth transitions between each speech sound" (Ingham & Andrews, 1973a, p.221). If the clinician judged the subject had ceased using the required speech pattern during a rating session, then speech rating ceased and the clinician instructed the subject to begin again in the required pattern. However, the reliability with which the clinician made such judgments was not established.

An overlooked feature of the initial Ingham and Andrews's treatment programs was that they were not simply therapy programs. Each therapy group was also involved in a variety of experiments during the establishment and transfer phases designed to isolate certain treatment variables. In one experiment (Ingham & Andrews, 1973a), a comparison was made between the number of rating sessions that subjects needed to complete the DAF schedule when tokens were administered contingent on speech performance or were not contingent on speech performance. This showed that a composite group (n=11) receiving contingent tokens required significantly fewer sessions than another matched group (n=11) that received noncontingent tokens. There was considerable overlap, though, between individual performances in both groups. Another study (Ingham & Andrews, 1971) compared "speech quality" near the end of the transfer phase by subjects treated with the DAF schedule and others treated by Syllable-Timed (ST) speech during the establishment phase. Both groups (n=10) were closely matched before and towards the end of the treatment program on %SS scores, but their stutterings were categorized in sound and syllable repetitions and other types of stutterings (it was assumed that the first category would contain "milder" stutterings, while the latter would include blocks and prolongations). The groups were almost identical in their mean percentage of sound and syllable repetitions before treatment, but over the last five rating sessions, the DAF treated group had 93.2% of their stutterings in the first category, while the ST treated group had only 37.9% stutterings in the same category. These groups also differed in their speech rate over final rating sessions; during stutter-free sessions, the DAF treated group spoke at a significantly faster rate than during sessions in which stutterings were recorded. However, the ST groups spoke much faster during their "stuttered" sessions, while the DAF group reduced their speech rates only slightly during these sessions. In other words, these data suggested that the ST-treated subjects had to reduce their rate in order to achieve stutter-free speech, but this restriction was not prominent among DAF-treated subjects. A series of experiments on the effects of the token system on telephone performance and on syllables spoken between sessions (Inghan, 1975a; Martin & Ingham, 1973) also showed that a portion of their improved performance during the transfer phase remained under token control.

The outcome evaluations of the token-economy therapy program were derived from within- and between-group comparisons of speech performance and self-ratings made 6 months before treatment, immediately before and after treatment, and at 3 month intervals for 9 months following treatment. Thirty-nine subjects (18-50 years) were treated within the token economy experimental programs: 16 with syllable-timed (ST) speech and 23 with DAF-instated prolonged speech during the establishment phase. A three-mode factor-analysis procedure showed that most of the questionnaire data (personality, neuroticism, and anxiety scale scores) were unchanged over the 16 months of assessment, but the self-ratings of speech performance and the objective speech performance data were markedly altered by the treatment interval. A "fluency factor" improved during the treatment period and remained close to the posttreatment level over the subsequent 9 months (Ingham, 1975a, p.373). Of more relevance was the speech performance of both subject groups before and after treatment. These scores are shown in Table 10.2. However, a more clinically meaningful basis of comparison between both groups is the number of subjects who were stutter-free and within the target speech rate range: 9 months after treatment the ST group had nine of its 16 subjects in that category (56.2%), while 15 of the 23 subjects (65.2%) in the DAF-prolonged speech group achieved the same status.

On the face of it, the token-economy program's use of DAF was promising. The data trends suggested that the prolonged speech procedure yielded more beneficial effects than a reasonably proximate treatment control using an alternative

Table 10.2
Mean percentage of syllables stuttered (%SS) and syllables spoken per minute (SPM) of subjects treated by either syllable-timed speech (n=16) or prolonged speech (n=23) on each treatment outcome assessment occasion.*

	Syllable-Timed Speech Group		*Prolonged Speech Group*	
Assessment occasions	***%SS***	***SPM***	***%SS***	***SPM***
1	13.80	113.7	18.16	93.6
2	13.57	111.6	16.41	91.3
3	0.77	204.4	0.11	206.7
4	3.17	186.5	1.80	204.6
5	2.92	189.7	0.58	208.0
6	2.07	191.7	0.50	204.8

*(from Ingham, 1975a, p.374).

speech pattern (syllable-timed speech). Moreover, these effects appeared to be durable over time. But it was almost inevitable that these data would provide only a facile account of therapy effects; they were collected within a clinic, during conversation with a clinician, and without the accompaniment of data attesting to their external validity. There is also no indication in a "0%SS at 180-220 SPM" score that the subjects' speech quality was related to normal fluency. At best, it could be claimed that a majority of subjects were capable of attaining stutter-free speech, at relatively normal speech rates, during 1000-syllable conversations with a clinician at intervals over 9 months—hardly clinically meaningful information. The limitations of this finding were partly evident when some of these subjects were covertly recorded during a conversation and monologue with a female research assistant 9 months after the last assessment occasion (Andrews & Ingham, 1972). During this assessment, 17 of the 23 subjects produced a mean of 7.8%SS at 152 SPM, and only 2 were stutter-free.

The four treatment programs described above formed the first wave of behaviorally oriented treatments that appeared in the wake of Goldiamond's report. But they were not the only clinical programs that reported using this approach. Soderberg (1969) described a treatment study presented at an ASHA convention by Gross and Nathanson, which reportedly used Goldiamond's procedure with some measure of benefit. Also Watts (1971) described an 11-day (2 hours per day) program with 8 stutterers in which the subjects used DAF in the first treatment session to establish fluency. Thereafter the subjects were instructed "to speak slowly with elongated vowels." Ratings of speech performance showed improvement within treatment sessions, and some evidence of relapse within and outside of these sessions 4 months after treatment. But neither of these treatments introduced procedures that have influenced stuttering therapy practices or research.

From the vantage point of the present, these initial DAF-treatment studies appeared to initiate a large amount of therapy research. But, for many who were working in the area at this time, including this writer, they also initiated a great deal of concern about the efficacy of these treatments, and about the validity of measurement methodologies that were available to evaluate therapy. From the preceding review, it should be clear that there was often a striking gap between the type of data used to evaluate treatment and some incidentally gathered information that described the subjects' speech away from assessment conditions. That concern was also shared by many of the critics of these behavioral treatments (Boehmler, 1970; Sheehan, 1970; Van Riper, 1970; 1973) who were, justifiably, unimpressed by some of the excessive and unwarranted publicity these treatments received during the early 1970s.

If the aim of these treatments was to produce a normally fluent speaker, then the performance data they used was certainly inadequate to the task of measuring for that objective—or even proximity to that objective. Although, in defense of these therapies, their measurement methods were often vast improvements on past methods. The reports from the first wave of DAF treatments suggest that they generally produced a form of fluency which did not always resemble normal-sounding speech, and often depended on the speaker constantly "managing" the process of speaking to sustain that "fluency." There was also an uncertain association between the procedures employed in these programs and behavior therapy. The procedures depended on ill-defined speech parameters, monitored by clinicians who were required to use unspecified judgments, and with questionable (certainly nonestablished) reliability. In short, the methodologies of these therapies almost made a mockery of the notion that the treatments were examples of behavior therapy. That is not to say that these parameters could not be operationalized. Yet, surprisingly, even now, there is virtually no attempt to establish the reliability of the central methods employed in these therapies. Indeed, as will be seen, this oversight continues to plague many of the therapies that followed this first wave.

The Move Away from DAF

The next stage in the development of the DAF-based therapies was, ironically, the large-scale abandonment of DAF. It was replaced, in most cases, by training subjects to imitate the prolonged speech pattern. That is, stutterers were trained to prolong their vowel sounds, use gentle articulatory contacts, and reduce speech rate. In addition, some emphasis was placed on modifying breathing and using short phrases. The result, in many cases, was that the resemblance between these techniques and those used by earlier workers became almost complete. Nevertheless, one interesting development was the growth of investigations into treatment evaluation techniques, as well as procedures designed to generalize and maintain treatment gains. Most of these investigations accompanied the developments that occurred in at least three of the four major mutations from Goldiamond's procedure. These developments, and the accompanying research, are traced in the following sections.

Developments in the Hollins Program

Of all the therapy programs reviewed in this book, none has provoked more publicity than Webster's program at Hollins College. This is one of the most advertised treatment programs in the United States, and receives patients from all over the country (and beyond) for a 3-week residential treatment program (Webster, 1980). The publicity this program has received has also been a source of some controversy. That controversy stems partly from the program's inordinate publicity on the basis of quite scant treatment-evaluation data. On the other hand, this program incorporates some extremely inventive treatment techniques that have served to operationalize much of the therapy process.

The development in the Hollins College "Fluency Shaping Program" has been outlined in two principal publications (Webster, 1974a; 1980). The initial publication describes the emergence of a treatment based on the premise that "stutterers make the sounds of speech incorrectly" (1974a, p.35). To correct this problem, a programmed text was developed by Webster to assist stutterers in learning three basic skills:

> (1) the gentle initiation of phonation (or, more precisely, how to produce speech which had "correct" amplitude versus time contours rather than the "incorrect" amplitude versus time contours of disfluent speech); (2) how to produce unvoiced consonants in such a way that the "correct" phonatory activity could occur following those sounds; and (3) how to slightly increase the duration of most speech sounds (1974, p.35).

The therapist checked the subject's self-definition of correct or incorrect productions of the main classes of speech sounds (vowel, vowel-like consonants, fricatives, stop consonants) via a programmed text. Additional assistance was provided from tape recordings that illustrated target speech sounds at different stages. The subject's target in the program is to produce stutter-free sentences at 100-130 words per minute. One unusual feature is that transfer procedures are introduced throughout the fluency-establishment phase. The transfer procedure required increased amounts of speaking in various situations, but it is not clear whether they are programmed in the same fashion as the establishment procedures.

The evaluation of the Hollins treatment program is its principal weakness. Thus far, no information has been provided to demonstrate the efficacy of the within-treatment procedures, while the outcome evaluation has been unsatisfactory and often confusing. In the 1974 accounts of this program (Webster, 1974a), there is an evaluation of 20 randomly selected subjects (8-52 years). They were treated by different forms of this program and assessed on an unspecified oral-reading task immediately before treatment, and at a median interval of 25 months after treatment on an oral-reading and conversational task (both of unspecified duration). The subjects also provided self-reports on their speech quality and fluency, and completed the Perceptions of Stuttering Inventory (PSI) (Woolf, 1967). The speech-performance data show some evidence of improvement (at least on the oral-reading task). Nine of the 20 subjects produced fewer than 1% "disfluencies" on the posttreatment conversational task, but no subject had zero disfluencies on both speech tasks at follow-up. All but one subject believed speech quality was better at follow-up, when compared with before-treatment, and 12 were satisfied with their current level of fluency.The PSI scores for *another* group of 19 subjects were also consistent with performance improvement resulting from treatment. However, in the absence of reliability data, sample-size information, speech-rate data, and beyond-clinic data, it is difficult to estimate the value of these findings.

There is much that is paradoxical in Webster's approach to treatment research. This is exemplified in some descriptions accompanying his later therapy programs. For instance, Webster (1977a) has described the essence of his more recent treatment as one that "is substantially more detailed and specific in the response with which it is concerned ... [and involving] ... procedures that are tailored to the establishment and overlearning of new responses and ... transfer training" (p.73). To achieve part of this process, he has also developed a "Voice Monitor" unit—a miniature computer-programmed unit designed to "shape" the speed and amplitude gradient of voice onsets. In other words, it provides an operationalized method for procuring one primary target behavior—gentle onsets. It was also supplemented by training subjects to time their syllable durations. But, for some reason, no data have ever been produced to demonstrate the effectiveness of these methods. This concern for specificity along with a lack of concern for evaluation colors many reports on the Hollins Fluency Shaping Program (Webster, 1979; 1980).

The most recently described Hollins program (Webster, 1980) contains three phases. Initially, the subject learns to co-ordinate diaphragmatic breathing for "slow-motion speech flow," followed by training in gentle voice productions. Secondly, these skills are then practiced with increasingly larger amounts of speech. Finally, the subject completes a series of "personal contacts" and telephone calls that form the transfer stage (although transfer strategies also accompany the first two phases). In addition, a week's home-practice program is provided. The total program time is 100 hours spread over 3 weeks. The program has been evaluated in roughly the same manner as previous programs, although there have been some improvements in the method of evaluation. To begin with, its evaluation is distinguished by the largest number of subjects reported in a recent stuttering therapy report; 200 subjects were randomly selected from approximately 1000 who have received this treatment. Assessments were made before and after treatment, and then (on average) 10 months later via a 500-word oral-reading task and a 300-500 word conversation. An additional improvement in evaluation is that the follow-up assessment was obtained from a surprise telephone call. The results of this evaluation are shown in Table 10.3. It was also reported that the group's mean PSI scores showed an improvement trend which paralleled that found in the speech-performance data. The method used to evaluate this treatment is obviously a vast improvement on methods previously employed in the Hollins program. But, yet again, these data are not accompanied by either reliability data, information on the group's speech performance away

Table 10.3
Summary of results of assessment of 200 subjects treated by the Hollins Fluency Shaping Program* as reported by Webster (1980).

	Pretreatment	*Posttreatment*	*Follow-up*
Mean percent disfluent words	15.2	1.3	3.2
Percent of cases with disfluency scores at or below 3%	3.0	92.0	80.0

* from Webster (1980, p.317)

from a formal testing situation,[13] or speech-rate data. The high percentage of improved cases within such a large subject population may reflect the treatment's efficacy, but in the absence of other relevant data it simply craves questions about the population's overall performance.

There have been two reports on applications of the Hollins program that have not emerged from that institution. The first was a nonintensive application of one Hollins program by D. Schwartz and M. Webster (1977a; 1977b). This program used the manuals and equipment from the Hollins Program for therapy conducted over a minimum of 6 hours a week for 3 months. Schwartz and Webster treated 29 subjects (9-50 years), but provided pretreatment, posttreatment, and 45-day follow-up assessment data on only 8 subjects. Oral-reading (500 words) and conversational-speech (unspecified length) data were collected, along with some rating-scale scores on each assessment occasion. The 8 subjects' data show that all improved their immediate posttreatment "dysfluency" frequency scores on the oral-reading task (except 1 subject who was not dysfluent during any oral-reading assessment) and conversational task, though only 4 subjects remained improved on both tasks over the follow-up period. Furthermore, only 1 of these 4 subjects was stutter-free on both follow-up tasks.[14] It is quite difficult to estimate the clinical value of these data, since they emerged from within-clinic measures made over one of the shortest follow-up periods reported in a stuttering-therapy study. At best, the data show that this nonintensive application of Webster's procedure may achieve some within-clinic improvement, but they fail to show the treatment's responsibility for these effects. Moreover, the absence of speech-rate data introduces the possibility that these gains were at the cost of unusually slow speech.

[13] The surprise follow-up telephone assessment is not necessarily indicative of beyond-clinic performance. The call was made by a member of the clinic staff and could thereby share much in common with the telephone tasks that formed part of the therapy program.

[14] There are some slight discrepancies between the data reported for these subjects in the 1977a and 1977b reports.

The second report was Mallard and Kelley's (1982) account of the use of Webster's (1980) procedure in a 3-week intensive therapy program. Fifty stutterers (41 males and nine females; 14-50 years) were treated mainly in groups of two or four for 6.5 hours daily. They were assessed from a conversational response (unspecified length) to a questionnaire, and an oral reading (500 words) before and after therapy. Only 28 of the subjects were assessed "at least" 6 months later. Mallard and Kelley's findings are unimpressive for a number of reasons. After therapy, the group's mean percentage of "disfluencies" on both speech tasks was reduced by 85-90%, but at follow-up, the mean reduction on the conversational task had risen to just over 50%—and this figure omits the 22 subjects who were not followed up. However, even this finding has dubious clinical significance. The data were not assessed for reliability and they were derived from clinic conditions. In fact, their questionable clinical value was acknowledged by Mallard and Kelley: "These follow-up data represent how well the client could speak, not necessarily how well he or she spoke on a consistent basis" (1982, p.293).

Webster's overall approach to the investigation and modification of his stuttering therapy program is puzzling. On the one hand, it has produced some very inventive and useful treatment methods. Also, the methods used in the clinical process, particularly in recent programs, have greatly improved the replicability of the treatment procedure. On the other hand, the approaches used to investigate and conduct this therapy program makes it as relevant to stuttering therapy as, say, the Weight Watchers system is to the treatment of obesity. That is not meant to damn its virtues with faint praise, for this form of therapy may be an expedient way of benefiting a large number of people. But this very expediency militates against devising an appropriate treatment format for an individual. Like many "standardized" behavior therapies, it probably incorporates some extremely effective treatment agents. Yet, to date, any justification for the program's structure and the therapeutic strength of any of its procedures has almost relied on anecdotal evidence. It is quite possible, for example, that the combination of speaking practice, group support, an adequate therapy fee, and the expectations associated with attending a prestigious therapy program are its most significant treatment agents.[15] That is not meant to suggest that these *are* its treatment agents, but in the absence of clarifying research, they have as much claim to the treatment's effects as any of the reported therapy activities. Ironically, Webster has expressed considerable concern about such issues in stuttering therapy. For instance, in writing about stuttering research he has made the following pertinent observation:

> The basic thrust of our work should be to establish reliable, functional relationships between objectively specifiable stimulus and response events....As a data base is created we should search for relationships among data that lead inductively to the organization of information and to the derivation of straightforward, testable, empirical hypotheses (Webster, 1977b, p.71).

[15] Similar variables may be influential in many other therapy programs reported in this chapter.

It is difficult to understand why the same concern is not reflected in therapy investigations on the Hollins program.

Developments in the Curlee and Perkins Program

The main extensions to the Curlee and Perkins (1969; 1973) treatment program have been made by Perkins. In many respects the nature of these extensions mirrors some of the diffidence that Curlee and Perkins have expressed over their early therapy efforts. These extensions also form a perfect contrast to Webster's development of a motor skill-control approach with limited emphasis on peripheral strategies. Perkins's contribution has been to move the Curlee and Perkins treatment towards a less specified approach. That movement has been consistent with his following comments on stuttering therapy:

> Having devoted quite a few years to the treatment of stuttering within the framework of psychoanalytic theory, operant conditioning, and a motor skill theory, I can attest to the fact that each is applicable to a part of the stutterer's problem, but none alone is adequate to cope with the person who stutters as a whole (Perkins, 1974, p.107).

Perkins's quite eclectic approach to treatment is evident in a series of publications in the early 1970s (Perkins, 1973a; 1973b; Perkins, Rudas, Johnson, Michael, & Curlee, 1974) that described the most recent development in the Curlee and Perkins program. This program included a number of features aimed at providing "indiginous satisfactions" that would assist maintenance of fluency: "The ingredients that appear necessary and sufficient to shape normal speech include fluency, rate, breathstream management, prosody and self-confidence" (Perkins, 1973a, p.286). To achieve this, Perkins (1973b) described a partially programmed therapy which required subjects to achieve a series of goals that varied in their specificity, but they also depended heavily on clinician judgments. The subject had to achieve a criterion of stutter-free prolonged speech followed by "breath flow," "prosody," self-responsibility for progress, "slow-normal speech," "psychotherapy" (involving Shames, Egolf, and Rhodes's thematic content-modification procedure), normal speech rate, non-DAF-controlled speech rate, and "clear voice." These were succeeded by a series of relatively unspecified procedures designed to assist generalization. They involved self-assessed speech-quality training, planned speaking tasks, and counseling, along with systematic withdrawal of clinician contact. Unfortunately, none of these procedures incorporated the specifications needed for replication, and for the most part they relied upon a combination of clinician ratings and client judgments as to when a procedural goal was reached.

Perkins, Rudas, Johnson, Michael, and Curlee (1974) reported a study aimed at assessing the therapy benefits of Perkins's (1973b) treatment program. This was made by comparing the performance of the 27 subjects (12-52 years) who were treated in the original Curlee and Perkins (1973) program (Group 1), and 17 subjects (19-51 years) treated by Perkins's (1973b) procedure (Group 2). Comparisons were made on %SS and SPM scores obtained before and after treatment, then 3 and 6 months later. At the end of the treatment phase, listener ratings of speech quality were also obtained. In general terms, the findings show that 70% of all subjects reduced their %SS scores by 85%, or more, at the cessation of treatment, but only 30% of Group 1 and 53% of Group 2 retained that level 6 months later. The treatment included a target normal-speech rate of 225 (+ or − 20) SPM, [16] but it was not made clear how many subjects actually achieved that rate 6 months after treatment. The subjects' rate, prosody, and fluency were assessed for normalcy by comparisons between listener judgments on their speech samples and those obtained from normal speakers. Essentially, these judgment data show that 6 months after treatment, Group 1 was slower and less expressive than the normal speakers, while Group 2 was rated more fluent, but slower than the normals. Beyond-clinic data from unspecified "generalization situations," were only related to within-clinic data via correlation coefficients. These showed the %SS scores in both conditions correlated 0.94 before treatment, 0.76 at the end of treatment, and 0.91 6 months later. However, Perkins et al. (1974) acknowledged that the "the client's typical speaking behavior cannot be determined from our results" (p.425).

The Perkins et al. (1974) report carries many suggestions that the variations made to Curlee and Perkins's program had improved the probability that the treatment would produce durable and normal-sounding speech. The revisions certainly introduced some procedures that could be useful for shaping speech quality and aiding generalization. In fact, numerous reports from other clinicians have mentioned that they used Perkins's procedure for just that purpose. But there are two main reasons why it is simply impossible to determine from these data if this therapy program does improve outcome. The first reason concerns the descriptions that accompany these treatment techniques. Like many similar treatment reports, it is difficult to learn exactly how the treatment "works" from the limited information on the procedures. For instance, it is not clear just what criteria were used to determine how subjects progress through, or even complete, treatment. The second reason is that any improvements that might be attributed to the program from Group 2's performance may be due to many factors other than the treatment methodology. A most obvious factor is therapy time. Group 1 received exactly 90 hours of treatment while Group 2 was, presumably, on some form of performance-contingent schedule and received between 91 and 184 hours of treatment. In short, this difference alone could explain the better result from Group 2. Perkins et al. even acknowledged that these data "suggested that fluency improved with longer treatment" (1974, p. 421). Another important factor is that before treatment, Group 2's mean-stuttering frequency was just over half the mean frequency for Group 1. It is entirely possible, therefore, that these differences alone were sufficient to give the edge to Group 2's therapy outcome result.

Helps and Dalton (1979) investigated a therapy program which claimed to have used Perkins's (1973b) procedures. They used occasional DAF and a speech-rate

[16] Perkins et al. (1974) incorrectly attribute this SPM range to Andrews and Ingham (1972). In fact, the rate that Andrews and Ingham suggested was 200 (+ or − 20) SPM.

schedule in a fixed-duration therapy program (20 hours a week for 3 weeks, then another week of therapy a month later). Their procedure used an establishment phase (mainly clinician and tape models to help train prolonged speaking during oral-reading and conversational tasks), a within- and outside-clinic assignment-transfer phase, and a self-managed maintenance schedule involving daily practice. Some of their subjects were also assigned to a follow-up program containing 2-hour weekly sessions for 6 months. Unhappily, the procedural descriptions accompanying this program are far too vague to gauge its content, let alone the criteria used for therapy progress. The findings also suffer from the absence of reliability assessment data. Consequently, it is virtually impossible to ascertain the program's contribution to outcome. The reported percent-words-stuttered and word-per-minute scores for 44 subjects (18-43 years) show that the treatment may have achieved some benefits. Six months after treatment the group had increased its speech rate and retained a 61% reduction in stuttering frequency. And 12 months after treatment, 19 of the 29 subjects had reduced their frequency of stuttering by 60% or more. But even these data are deceptive, for most of these subjects were also involved in weekly therapy sessions throughout 6 months of the follow-up period. When the subjects were partitioned into "follow-up" and "non-follow-up" therapy, there is some indication that the former group was better off when assessed 6 months later, but this finding is offset by substantial subject attrition. A comparison was made with a group of subjects who were treated by syllable-timed speech within the same therapy and assessment time-frame. The somewhat suspect data suggested that the prolonged speech treatment produced a better outcome. But, in view of the numerous inadequacies in this study, it would be unfair to invest any importance in this finding.

A single case study by Turnbaugh and Guitar (1981) provides a useful example of how Perkins's procedures may be applied in a public school setting. A 12-year-old male stutterer received two to three 20-minute treatment sessions a week for 8 months except for an intensive treatment of 5.5 hours per day on 2 consecutive days during the 6th month. During the period before the intensive treatment, their therapy was described as attitude modification using "Van Riperian methodology." At the beginning of this phase, the subject's speech was assessed (in an unspecified way) at 10.47% SS and 183 SPM. Immediately before the intensive treatment, a 2.5 minute sample of conversation with the clinician produced 5.6% SS at 171 SPM. Meanwhile, his communication attitude score, derived from the abridged Erickson Scale of Communication attitudes (Andrews & Cutler, 1974; Erickson, 1969), went from 17 to 6 (within an assumed "normal" communication-attitude-score range for 12-year-olds). The intensive program used a slightly modified version of Perkins's (1973b) schedule (using DAF, excluding psychotherapy, and interposing 3-minute performance criteria for passing each step) and showed a postintensive phase assessment of 0.28% at 103 SPM. At the end of the 8-month period, the subject continued to have a low stuttering rate, but also a low speech rate. Four months later, during a conversation with the clinician, he produced 2.2%SS at 198 SPM, and so a maintenance treatment was instituted. After another 4 months, a 3-minute speech sample produced 1.61%SS at 207 SPM (though this was accompanied by a relatively low interrater agreement of 82% for the %SS scores). In many ways this report is a useful example of how a group treatment procedure may be adapted to a common clinical circumstance. In this instance, though, the treatment result may be equally interpreted as reflecting either the benefits of prior "Van Riperian methodology" or the need for additional therapy.

One interesting variation on the therapy activities that Perkins (1981) and his co-workers (Johnson, 1980a) have promoted is parent use of breathstream management to modify stuttering in preschool children. The procedure involves training parents to

> speak at a slowed speech rate of 160 to 190 syllables per minute while maintaining an effortless, smooth, continuous breath flow and short five- to six-word phrases to help maintain the slower rate. They are also taught to selectively attend to their child's fluency....After determining how the parents are reacting at present, the clinician instructs them to eliminate all attending responses to abnormally disfluent utterances and to increase attention to fluency (Johnson, 1980a, p. 303.

Johnson (1980a) reported some limited data from use of this modeling technique with seven children (3-6 years). Recordings obtained on the children after various periods (3 months to 6 years) show that five children retained a reduced percentage of disfluent syllables. The parents of four children also judged their child to be normally fluent after treatment. However, these data are not sufficient to determine whether there was any association between the treatment and outcome.

Gregory (1973) and, more recently, Gregory and Hill (1980) have described a similar method among the approaches they have used in treating young children. Across a hierarchy of increasingly complex speaking tasks the clinician provides a model of "easy, relaxed speech with smooth movements." The program is reported to have resulted in "normal fluency that is maintained following 9 to 18 months" of this therapy for 70% of the children they have treated. But no other data are reported.

In some ways there is a parallel between the developments that have taken place in the Curlee and Perkins procedure and the Hollins program. Both have introduced a variety of seemingly useful therapy practices, but the constituent parts of both programs have not been clearly demonstrated as responsible for improving the prospects of therapy outcome. To be sure, the reported data from Perkins's (1973b) procedure show that stutterers have yielded gains from this treatment, although it is less certain that these have been sustained n clinically meaningful circumstances. It is also not clear that this therapy process should be described as behaviorally oriented since, increasingly (see Perkins, 1973a; 1974; 1981), Perkins regards nonbehavioral methods as integrall to this treatment. Nevertheless, over the past decade Perkins has produced a largely pragmatic and extremely influential approach to stuttering treatment.

Developments in the Ingham and Andrews Program

The early Ingham and Andrews experimental therapy programs highlighted the need for a number of modifications to their token-economy-based procedures in order to improve outcome and clinical viability. To some extent the original program's viability is demonstrated by its use in many different treatment settings and in different countries. Perhaps the main modifications have been, ironically, the abandonment of much of the token system, the attachment of various maintenance strategies, and replacement of DAF with therapist and tape model controls. Much of this is reflected in a revised format outlined by Ingham and Andrews (1973c), which has also become the basis of a quite vigorous program of stuttering therapy research in Australia and, to some extent, in Canada. This research has been directed towards various areas of treatment including assessment methods, maintenance techniques, and the role of attitudinal factors.

The Ingham and Andrews (1973c) treatment schedule used an almost completely performance-contingent schedule of procedures. It was also based on an intensive treatment establishment and transfer stage, followed by a maintenance schedule which reduced the frequency of performance assessments contingent on maintained target behaviors. In most respects the establishment and transfer schedules resembled those described for the earlier treatment program, except that the amount of target speecn behavior required at each step was increased by 50%. Also, subjects trained with tape-recorded models of the target behavior, in order to complete the establishment-phase requirements. Thereafter, they shaped their own speech quality, while meeting rating-session requirements, until they achieved a target rate of 170-210 SPM and zero stuttering during each 1300-syllable speaking task was achieved. Identical requirements obtained throughout the transfer phase and into a maintenance phase which required a minimum of 128 weeks to complete.

Perhaps the program's main characteristic is the relatively standardized hierarchy of speech tasks and the strict criteria used for passage through the program. Unlike related programs, this passage depends upon complete absence of observed stuttering at each level, with intermittent assessments in order to ensure that these criteria are sustained. But it also suffers from a procedural weakness common to related programs—the lack of a reliable procedure for measuring the prolonged speech pattern characteristics at each step in the establishment phase. It is also weakened by a "break" in the hierarchy between the transfer and maintenance phases; that is, if subjects fail the maintenance-phase requirements, they cannot return to the transfer phase.[17]

At the time of writing, no large-scale-outcome-evaluation has been conducted on this treatment program, however it has been used in five experimental studies designed to evaluate assessment and maintenance strategies.

One of the first investigations in the Ingham and Andrews (1973c) program concerned the validity of the maintenance-phase assessments. Ingham (1975b) compared a series of covertly and overtly recorded assessments for nine stutterers (17-42 years), 3 and 6 months following the transfer phase. Recordings

[17] Of course, this might be possible in certain clinical facilities, but the manner in which this program is usually organized precludes this option.

were obtained across three situations (talking to a stranger, to a nonstranger, and telephone conversations), with and without the subject's awareness. However, only marginal differences appeared between the subjects' mean %SS scores in both assessment conditions (although their mean speech rate scores in the covert conditions were significantly slower). Quite substantial individual differences appeared in the %SS scores of some subjects on the covert assessments when compared with their counterpart overt assessments. These indicated that an apparently acceptable level of performance in overt assessments may not resemble assessments made under—presumably—more clinically valid circumstances.

The role of covert assessment emerged as an important consideration in three subsequent studies designed to assess the efficacy and content of the performance-contingent maintenance procedure. In the first of these (Ingham, 1980), nine stutterers (9-23 years) entered either an ABA or BAB maintenance-phase program in which the B condition was the performance-contingent maintenance schedule and the A condition was an equivalent nonperformance-contingent schedule. Regular within- and beyond-clinic assessments were supplemented by irregular covert assessments via telephone. The data from these subjects, collected over a 96-week period, indicated that the performance-contingent schedule was associated with a pattern of maintained and generalized reductions in stuttering. The clinical value of the procedure was demonstrated by the complete absence of stuttering in six subjects across all assessment conditions at the final assessment. However, for two subjects, the covert recordings at the final assessment revealed that considerable amounts of stuttering still occurred during telephone conversations. One method of treating beyond-clinic performance deterioration was described in a single subject study (Ingham, 1981a) with a 15-year-old female stutterer. She had achieved criterion-performance during within-clinic conditions, yet recordings made with her family, friends, and at school showed that her stuttering continued. When these recordings were integrated with the performance-contingent maintenance schedule in a multiple-baseline experimental design it was shown that her stuttering reduced almost immediately and remained close to zero over a 30-week period. The clinical validity of these overt recordings was supplemented by two covert recordings made in the family setting. Another study (Ingham, 1982b) was conducted with two male stutterers (18 and 20 years) in order to assess the efficacy of a self-evaluation procedure (Wood & Flynn, 1978) on maintenance. The general purpose of this study was to gauge the viability of replacing the clinician-managed maintenance schedule with a self-managed maintenance schedule. Both subjects were routinely recorded, overtly and covertly, while speaking with parents over the telephone (in one case, while talking with a relative). Eventually the overt recordings were evaluated by the subject after each had demonstrated agreement with the clinician's stuttering- and speech-rate-range scores. Each subject managed a performance-contingent maintenance schedule built around recorded telephone conversations and conversations with family members. Whenever the self-evaluation procedure was introduced, it was associated with obvious reductions in stuttering across the overt *and* covert recordings. In both cases, and across a total of five speaking situations, stuttering remained at virtually zero throughout the 6-month period following self-evaluation training. The clinical value of this finding will be discussed later, but the important procedural result of these studies was that both maintenance and generalization were demonstrated to be modifiable by a clinician-managed—or largely self-managed—performance-contingent schedule. Moreover, the procedure's external validity was generally evident in data obtained from systematic covert recordings from both subjects.

Another assessment issue, relevant to all therapies that use speech pattern techniques, is the perceived quality or normalcy of posttreatment speech. It will be recalled that both Jones and Azrin (1969) and Perkins et al. (1974) used listener ratings. In a partial evaluation of these ratings, Ingham and Packman (1978) had listeners try to identify stutterers (n=9; 13-24 years), who had completed the transfer phase of Ingham and Andrews's (1973c) program, from normally fluent counterparts via 1-minute speech samples. Although the stutterers were generally rated acceptably normal via the Jones and Azrin, and the Perkins et al. procedure, they were still identified as stutterers more often than their counterparts. When listeners were forced to choose "the stutterer" within sample pairs, however, then seven of the nine stutterers were not confidently identified as either a "stutterer" or a "non-stutterer." An interesting incidental finding related to the treatment target measures; some subjects had zero stuttering at 170-210 sysllables per minute, but this was not sufficient for their speech to be judged as normal sounding. Rather predictably, this confirmed Perkins's (1973a) claim that other parameters are equally important in producing normal fluency. The method used in this investigation is one way of determining whether a treatment produces perceptually normal speech, although its most obvious limitation is that it is an after-the-event assessment which is somewhat impractical for treatment control purposes.

One result of these experimental studies was the development of a treatment program (Ingham, 1981b) built upon "hierarchy control," rather than a token economy. Hence, the subject's success at moving through the speaking task hierarchy is assumed to control performance. The structure of the program is similar to the Ingham and Andrews (1973c) format, except that a self-evaluation-training procedure overlaps the transfer and maintenance phases with a variety of "branch" maintenance strategies (Ingham, in press). But the long-term benefits of this program are yet to be established.

Some variations on the Ingham and Andrews (1973c) treatment procedure have also been introduced by a number of other researchers. One of the first was introduced by Andrews (1973), and led to establishment of an adult group treatment program which is conducted under conditions similar to those outlined in the earlier Ingham and Andrews treatment studies. In an initial investigation with an adult mild stutterer, Andrews (1973) described the use of the Ingham and Andrews procedure for individual treatment. A main variation was the introduction of small changes in target speech rate (five syllables per minute) throughout the establishment phase. The subject was reported to have achieved stutter-free speech, although it was also stated that he "still stutters occasionally." Ultimately, this treatment was used in a group setting and became known as the "Prince Henry Programme," because of its location in a like-named Australian hospital. The evolved program (Prince Henry Hospital, 1976) has been described in reports by Howie, Andrews, and Tanner (1978) and Howie, Tanner, and Andrews (1981). During the establishment and transfer stages, it differs in some important ways from the Ingham and Andrews (1973c) procedure.[18] The most important is that daily targets of performance are set, and subjects are obliged to complete the entire establishment, or Instatement Phase, within 5 days. The Transfer Phase is then automatically introduced for 2 weeks, and patients are treated on relatively less-controlled outpatient arrangements. The Maintenance Phase also involves a variety of formal and informal activities which include beyond-clinic speech practice, "follow-up clinics" at 3, 6, 9, and 24 weeks after the transfer phase, and attendance at meetings of previously treated stutterers via an organization known as the "Speakeasy Club."

One of the obvious problems in evaluating the effects of long and informally managed maintenance procedures, such as that described by Howie, Tanner, and Andrews (1981), is that it is difficult to determine the point at which the treatment process actually ceases. This is especially evident in therapies in which subjects join groups designed to help them sustain treatment gains. The point is well illustrated in the Howie et al. (1981) study, which is titled "Short- and Long-term Outcome in an Intensive Treatment Program for Adult Stutterers." Yet, within this report they acknowledge that "assessing the final outcome of treatment was not possible; rather we describe the progress of groups of clients at various points in their progress through the program" (p.105).

Nevertheless, Howie et al's data are interesting because they show, convincingly, that treatment gains were maintained at around two months, and then again at 12 to 18 months following the transfer phase. One group of 36 adult stutterers was evaluated from overt 3-minute telephone calls made immediately before and after the intensive part of treatment (establishment and transfer phases), and then 3 to 9 weeks later. At pretreatment they produced mean scores of 14.6%SS at 138.4 SPM, but, at the final assessment, they were 2.2%SS at 204.9 SPM. There was also no significant difference between the postintensive treatment assessment and the final assessment, although the %SS standard deviation scores went from 0.2%SS to 6.5%SS, indicating some performance deterioration. In another group, containing 43 adult stutterers, 3-minute telephone call assessments were obtained immediately before and after the intensive part of treatment, and then again 12 to 18 months later. These were ostensibly sup-

[18]Howie et al. (1978; 1981) refer to the speech pattern they used in the establishment phase as "smooth-motion speech" in order to distinguish it from "prolonged speech." Its characteristic features are "slow onset of phonation, continuous airflow and movement of articulators throughout each utterance, and extension of vowel and consonant duration" (1981, p.104). Of course, in the absence of replicable and reliable measures that distinguish "smooth-motion speech" from "prolonged speech," it is futile to claim that such differences are meaningful.

plemented by covertly recorded telephone calls[19] made to 23 subjects shortly before their final assessment. The telephone data were supplemented by a questionnaire and a shortened version of the Erickson Scale of Communication Attitudes (Andrews & Cutler,1974). Pretreatment mean counts of 13.0%SS at 140.2 SPM on the overt calls improved to 3.9%SS at 207.1 SPM, 12 to 18 months later. There was also no significant difference between the covert and overt %SS mean scores for 23 subjects at the final assessment (although, not surprisingly, their speech rate was significantly slower in the covert condition). The Erickson Scale mean scores showed a significant reduction from pre- to posttreatment which, as will be discussed, is to be expected from a scale that is responsive to changes in %SS scores (Andrews & Cutler, 1974; Guitar & Bass, 1978). Client satisfaction with this treatment was mixed: on a self-rating form (originally developed by Webster, 1974b), 70.3% of the 43 subjects indicated they were "very much/substantially improved," although 56% reported they were "not satisfied" with their present speech. The treatment may have been responsible for their sustained improvement, though that is very difficult to judge. For example, many subjects were members of speaking-practice clubs, which suggests that their "treatment" was probably continued within a different format. This may be reflected in the finding that almost 25% of the subjects admitted "attending to the act of speaking fluently. ... 100% of the time" at the time of their final assessment. The speech performance data in this study also leave a lot to be desired; a 3-minute telephone conversation, mainly within a clinic, and containing an unspecified amount of speech, is not likely to be indicative of beyond-clinic speech performance.

A number of experimental investigations have been carried out by Andrews and colleagues that relate to treatment assessment methods and the efficacy of the Prince Henry program. A study by Andrews and Harvey (1981) investigated whether immediate pretreatment behavior may be part of a "regression to the mean" brought on by client-expectation effects. Across a number of therapy studies, they showed there were marginal reductions in the stuttering frequency over a 3- to 20-month period prior to treatment intervention. They also reported on 128 stutterers who were assessed 2 to 90 weeks prior to treatment on a monologue and self-rating questionnaire. This showed there was a significant—though clinically unimportant—change in their mean %SS and SPM scores. They did find though that in "a few subjects stuttering had improved considerably, but they were the exceptions" (p.206)—but perhaps not unimportant exceptions, who clearly vindicate the need for base-rate data. An investigation by Andrews and Craig (1982) actually illustrates some of the problems in drawing important clinical decisions from group data. They organized covert and overt telephone assessments of 56 subjects (19-59 years), 4 to 34 months after treatment

[19] It seems improbable that these covert calls were free of "assessment" stimuli: "A psychologist contacted each subject, introducing him/herself as a 'university researcher' and invited the subject to attend an assessment session so that the effectiveness of the program could be evaluated" (Howie et al., 1981, p.106). It is also interesting to speculate on the impact that this forewarning may have had on the subsequent overt assessment.

(presumably after the intensive period) in order to determine the "importance of covert assessment for evaluating the outcome of therapy." Telephone conversations, of unspecified duration, were made by a therapy patient who covertly recorded the subject's speech after stating that "the call was part of his transfer assignment" (a dubiously unobtrusive procedure). But, for 20 subjects, the covert call was disguised as part of a public-opinion survey. The group pretreatment mean %SS score of 16.9 was reduced at posttreatment to 1.71 on overt calls and 1.82 on the covert calls (the subgroup of 20 had a mean of 1.94 %SS). The covert and overt %SS mean scores were not significantly different, though they were also poorly correlated, particularly for the subgroup. Consequently, while the data may suggest that a group's treatment effect is not substantially influenced by overt assessment, the clinical value of this finding is questionable. This is well illustrated in the previously mentioned studies by this writer (Ingham, 1980; 1981a; 1982b) that dealt with individual stutterers. Actually, the artificial nature of Andrews and Craig's telephone assessment even limits its value for group studies.

The last-mentioned point is particularly relevant in any consideration of findings from the Prince Henry program. For, while the Howie et al. (1981) and Andrews and Craig (1982) data show extremely impressive trends, they are derived entirely from brief telephone conversations containing an unspecified amount of speech. It remains to be seen whether these admittedly useful and clinically pertinent data represent their subjects' general speech behavior. There is certainly ample individual-subject data from other studies to show that this is not always true.

Most recently, Howie and Woods (1982) have described three experiments which assessed the effect of the Prince Henry program's token-reinforcement system on passage through that program's Instatement Phase. They reported no differences between the number of rating sessions required to complete this phase by subjects treated by contingent-token reinforcement and subjects treated by either noncontingent or "no token reinforcement." It is claimed that the study failed to replicate a similar experiment by Ingham and Andrews (1973a), but it is difficult to interpret these findings in the light of differences in the Prince Henry program. One reasonable interpretation (Ingham, in press) is that the finding actually demonstrates the ineffectiveness of the modifications introduced to Ingham and Andrews's (1973c) token-reinforcement system by the Prince Henry program (Prince Henry Hospital, 1976). These modifications include an initial substantial donation of tokens, opportunities to pass a rating session independently of the token system, plus additional unspecified clinician assistance to ensure completion of the instatement phase within 5 days. In short, these modifications may have nullified any opportunities for the token system to control speech performance. The data from Howie and Woods's study are also of questionable value, since they are unsupported by reliability assessment.

Another application of the Ingham and Andrews therapy format was reported by Boberg (1976; 1980) in a program which also employed the "traditional" prolongation and cancellation techniques, plus attitude discussions. Initially, four groups of stutterers (n=21; 17-44 years) were treated for 3 weeks (7 hours a day) in a five-phase program embracing the establishment[20] and transfer operations of the Ingham and Andrews procedure. "Succesful" rating sessions were rewarded with money. Also, subjects were taught to accurately count their own stutterings. In the transfer phase, clinicians accompanied subjects into situations in which they completed self-selected situation tasks. The mean stuttering scores for the group were derived from conversations and oral readings, and revealed a pre-post treatment shift from 21-23%SS to 1.3-1.0%SS, which was also reflected across nine speaking tasks. All but two subjects showed increased speech rate in their posttreatment assessment. Only one subject was stutter-free on all the final assessment tasks, however, which is probably not surprising in view of the nonstringent criterion for passage through treatment. Subsequently, Boberg and Sawyer (1977) reported treatment-follow-up data from 13 subjects (eight of whom appear to be included in Boberg's 1976 paper). These subjects were also engaged in a maintenance procedure involving self-managed daily practice and a clinic report on a prearranged (but unspecified) schedule. Six to 24 months after the end of the transfer phase, they were assessed from conversations, reading, and telephone tasks, and all had increased their frequency of stuttering on most tasks. A "refresher weekend," mainly involving prolonged speech practice, was provided for five subjects. Six months later, it was reported that these subjects reversed "the trend toward relapse"—although their data show this was true on all assessment tasks for only one of the five subjects. Actually, the group's data suggest that the treatment produced sustained inprovement in 11 of the 13 subjects.

In a later report, Boberg (1980) introduced more specificity to the treatment schedule, including recorded rather than self-rated assignment sessions during the transfer phase, and reduced overall treatment time. Also the percentage of stuttering permissible to pass from the establishment to the transfer phase was reduced to 1%SS. Data from 12 subjects again show more than a 95% reduction in stuttering from the beginning to the end of the 3-week intensive-treatment phase. In another publication, Boberg (1981) provides an account of the postintensive-treatment performance of these subjects. In this case a variation of Ingham and Andrews's (1973c) performance-contingent maintenance schedule was used with 16 subjects who were compared with a "control group" 12 and 24 months following the intensive treatment. Subject attrition and differences in assessment frequency make it virtually impossible to identify the maintenance procedure's effects. Nevertheless, most of the subjects (n=8) who survived in the maintenance group appeared to sustain proportionately lower percentages of stuttering than the control group subjects. The best interpretation that can be given to these data is that frequent clinician contact during the postintensive-treatment phase retains some measure of control over stuttering. But it is not clear what components of Boberg's program—within either the intensive *or* the maintenance phase—are responsible for the improved performance of his subjects.

[20]The establishment phase differed from Ingham and Andrews's procedure. It involved training in prolonged speech and cancellations (fluently repeating a word on which "struggle" occurred) and used a target of 2%SS (or less) at 140-200 SPM.

Boberg and Fong (1980) have also reported an attempt to employ variations on his treatment procedure with two groups of mentally retarded subjects. The first group was composed of three older-aged subjects (13-19 years; WISC/WAIS IQ 52-79), who were treated for 1 hour each day over 2, 2-week periods, separated by 3 months. The second group also included three subjects, aged 9 or 10 years, whose IQs ranged from 43 down to an untestable level. They were treated for an hour per day for 2 weeks, and then 2 hours a day for another 2 weeks (the time between these treatments was not specified). Only pre- and posttreatment data collected within the clinic are provided, and these show only modest reductions in stuttering—which is probably not surprising considering their limited therapy time. But this is an interesting attempt at modifying this treatment format for a class of stutterers who surely form the largest potential patient group.

The Ingham and Andrews (1973c) treatment procedure, and *its* variants, have introduced some further options to the familiar establishment, transfer, maintenance therapy format. There is reasonably consistent evidence that the principal components of this format have benefited a large number of mainly adult stutterers, and that these benefits have been maintained for periods of 6 to 24 months. By a combination of repeated and occasional unobtrusive measurements across situations and over extensive periods, it is evident that the treatment's benefits are not always clinic-bound. At the same time, it is not at all clear that the reported treatment outcome data are free of treatment control; almost all these data have overlapped either formal or informal maintenance programs that may have influenced treatment evaluation. Possibly the main contribution that Ingham and Andrews's procedure has made to treatment has been its emphasis on measurement and maintenance. The procedure still suffers from its dependence on clinician-judged methods, although with each development the magnitude of this weakness has diminished. The same is true with respect to outcome evaluation methods. Probably the most vivid expression of this issue is this writer's experience with the treatment: for, in spite of the help it has provided many stutterers, and evidence of seemingly durable stutter-free (or improved) speech, not one adult subject treated in this program could be described as becoming an unquestionably normal speaker. In the very best outcomes the gains still appear to depend upon intermittent self-monitoring or "managed fluency."

There is another aspect in the development of this therapy program (and presumably similar programs) that is rarely discussed in the treatment literature. That aspect is the way in which such procedures are translated into general clinical practice. The Australian experience with the Ingham and Andrews procedure may illustrate how behavior therapies occasionally emerge "in the field." This treatment received considerable publicity in Australia during the 1970s, and has become quite popular as an expedient way to treat children, adolescents, and adults in hospitals and community health centers. While this might be considered a desirable byproduct of any published treatment research, the field applications of the treatment have frequently been haphazard and, occasionally, almost calamitous.

The seemingly standardized format of the Ingham and Andrews program (partly because of its use with groups) may also contribute to its misapplication. In one sense, that format implies that subjects must fit the treatment rather than the treatment fit the subject. One interesting attempt to vary that format was reported by Spencer (1976), who endeavored to treat a family containing five adolescent and adult stutterers. Unfortunately, her endeavor included little evidence of either systematic or data-based treatment. Only group data were obtained over a 4-month period, although they did indicate substantial improvement within the family setting. However, a report by Franck (1980) describes a less desirable development in the more "standardized" version of this treatment. Franck's report actually included two versions of Ingham and Andrews's program. The first version required subjects to attend once a week (or every 2 weeks) for mainly self-managed practice in prolonged speech at different speech rates. This was followed by weekly group meetings involving relaxation, plus a within-clinic transfer program based on discussions and various speaking tasks. Fluency was "demanded at all times except during the coffee break." In these 2½-hour sessions, 30 to 70 subjects were somehow managed by two clinicians. This phase continued without specified performance criteria for up to 6 months. Not surprisingly, 50% of Franck's subjects were reported to have dropped out of treatment during this phase. In a third phase (after waiting up to 18 months), groups of four subjects entered a 5-day, 12-hour-per-day program based on the instatement and transfer phases in Ingham and Andrews's (1973c) program. Then followed a fixed 12-month "maintenance" schedule of decreasingly frequent clinic sessions supplemented by extra-clinic patient-group meetings. No evidence was given that passage through treatment was related to performance and, quite predictably, "most patients complain their speech is much more dysfluent outside the clinic" (Franck, 1980, p.10) during the maintenance phase. In one sense, the treatment's patients expressed their confidence in this treatment with their feet: "441 stutterers presented to the department for treatment [but] only 124 remained with the program" (Franck, 1980, p.12). In short, whatever else this treatment offered, it certainly provides a depressing example of how patients may be forced to fit a treatment, rather than vice versa, and a disastrous misapplication of treatment principles.

Some current developments in the therapy procedures developed by this writer may be of some passing interest. At present, much of the establishment and transfer phase is being transformed by the introduction of computer technology in order to operationalize prolonged speech. Procedures are being developed to identify individualized minimal changes in phonatory behavior that are necessary to instate stutter-free speech. Subjects are then trained to self-measure this behavior as a basis for using self-evaluation procedures along the lines described in a recent study (Ingham, Montgomery, & Ulliana, 1983). It is hoped that this will operationalize much of the treatment process and serve to remove the undesirable "standardized" nature of the treatment's current format (Ingham, 1981b).

Other Therapy Approaches Utilizing Prolonged Speech and Its Variants

One of the most publicized current treatments employing a variant of prolonged speech is Shames and Florance's (1980) "Stutter-Free Speech Program" for children and adults. The distinguishing feature of this treatment is its endeavor to come to terms with a common complaint about therapies using prolonged speech: subjects have to monitor their speech to an abnormal extent in order to sustain fluency. Presumably, the effect involved in "monitoring" is not always compensated by the benefits of reduced stuttering. Shames and Florance (1980) described a five-phase treatment format in which the familiar Goldiamond-derived DAF schedule is used to establish stutter-free speech at between 30 and 90 WPM with clinician-judged control over prosody and inflections. The next critical phase aims to train the speaker to monitor accurately target-fluent speech (clinician-judged) at different speech rates. This is "reinforced" by permitting the subject a period of "unmonitored speech." During the transfer phase, the subject uses monitored and unmonitored speech in the clinic, plus client-determined situations. Comparisons are then made between monitored and unmonitored speech. In the final clinician-managed phase the client systematically increases the daily portions of unmonitored speaking time. Follow-up contact with the clinic is systematically decreased, and evaluations are planned over a 5-year period. A variation of the therapy protocol is also used to treat children.

It is difficult to equate the extensive publicity surrounding the Shames and Florance program with the quality of data used to justify its operations or its efficacy. To date, Shames and Florance have not provided any data which show that the introduction of their self-management procedure provides any particular treatment advantages. The idea of using unmonitored speech as a reinforcer for monitored speech is interesting, but its clinical value is unknown. Thus far, no data have shown that this subject-defined response class reinforces any behavior. More significantly, there is no evidence that the overall procedure, whatever it claims to be measuring, serves the therapy process to advantage. The only attempt at data analysis is a report on the "Present Self Concept" of 152 stutterers who were either in therapy or had completed therapy. In the absence of speech-behavior data, or even independent validation of the subjects' self-reports, these data have little value. A later paper by Florance and Shames (1980), which describes transfer and maintenance issues that relate to their program, includes a perceptual-analysis study on the speech of 32 stutterers at different phases in the treatment. Although the stutterers' samples (drawn from phase four) were not distinguishable from the nonstutterers' samples, there is no indication that the samples were drawn from beyond-clinic conditions or represented general speech behavior (this is unlikely since they were only 15-second samples). Recent publicity (Shames, 1982) suggests that this program is now being conducted in a holiday-camp setting under token-economy conditions. This would suggest that the treatment may require additional reinforcers to sustain stutter-free speech. At this time it is obviously premature to evaluate the Shames and Florance program. It contains some interesting ideas, but for the moment these are ideas in search of data.

In recent years, there have been numerous reports of therapy procedures that have used variations of prolonged speech in conjunction with other techniques. However, the treatment formats described in these reports vary greatly in their concern for the methodological detail and measurement. Many incorporate a variety of approaches that, in the main, reflect a continuing search for effective and expedient therapies. Their relevance to behavior therapy is often vague, but they contain a fund of interesting ideas.

One previously mentioned technique involves training of target-speech patterns via tape-recorded models. This has been promoted by a group at Rutgers University headed by Bernard Lee and Maryann Peins. In their procedure, stutterers receive monthly 30-minute tape-recorded speaking lessons in which the principal lesson requires the subject to mime recorded examples of "Legato Style" speech. Lee, McGough, and Peins (1973) described this speech as "characterized by a brief starting of the voice and maintenance of the voice throughout long connected phrases" (p.188). They also emphasize use of slow and gentle articulatory gestures, and encouragement "to speak in long phrases with the voice continuing [unbroken] throughout" (p.191). Peins, McGough, and Lee (1972) compared this treatment procedure with Van Riper's therapy or nontreatment via three groups of 12 stutterers (12-43 years). Severity ratings were made on a 1-minute spontaneous speech sample obtained before therapy, at 3 and 6 months during the 6-month treatment period. Both treatment goups significantly reduced their severity ratings when compared with the control group, but the treatment gains did not differ over the course of these assessments.

Another variation has been Eugene Cooper's endeavor to combine behavioral and nonbehavioral procedures in his "Personalized Fluency Control Therapy" (Cooper, 1976). The so-called behavioral component of this program is built around training in "fluency initiating gestures," which resembles the technique developed by Webster at Hollins College. The treatment has been described in a number of publications (Cooper, 1976; 1977; 1979) but, thus far, without evaluative data.

Another much-publicized therapy, that certainly involves a form of breath-stream management, is Azrin and Nunn's (1974) "regulated breathing" technique. Actually Azrin and Nunn's treatment is a combination of techniques that use incompatible behaviors to treat various problem behaviors (see Azrin & Nunn, 1977). The initial report on their stuttering treatment made the startling claim that "a single counseling session of about 2 hours duration" resulted in stuttering episodes decreasing by "99% during the extended follow-up" (1974, p.279). In this brief period of counseling, subjects are taught (among many other things) relaxation training and incompatible activities for stuttering. The most recent account of this incompatibility training (Azrin, Nunn, & Frantz, 1979) stipulates teaching the subject

> to breathe smoothly during speech by beginning exhalation before speaking, to blend words into the exhalation pattern, and even to continue the smooth exhalation slightly past the last speech sound. Before speaking, the client paused to formulate the content of the speech and inhaled smoothly. ... When a speech block occurred, the client was taught to stop speaking immediately at the first sign of the block, to relax the body and especially the chest muscles, formulate thoughts, to inhale fairly deeply if insufficient air remained in the lungs, to exhale briefly before speaking, and to speak in shorter junctured phrases until the speech blocks seemed unlikely" (1979, p.334).

The client was also taught to organize his environment, and was assisted by close relatives, to aid training and posttreatment practice. In Azrin and Nunn's (1974) report 14 stutterers (4-67 years) counted their "stuttering episodes" per day before treatment (these ranged from 1000 to two). Then, following 2 hours counseling, they counted their episodes during telephone calls (which also included counseling) made throughout 1 week, then once a week for 2 weeks, and finally during four monthly contacts. These counts were reported to have been cross-validated by contact with relatives (no details were provided), and counts made during a follow-up telephone call with the clinician. The data from these "assessments" led to the conclusion that there was a 99% reduction in stuttering episodes. But, absolutely no objectively collected speech behavior data were obtained, nor was any consideration given to the resemblance between normal speech quality and that which was achieved by these subjects. The questionable basis on which remarkable claims were made for this therapy are all the more surprising and disappointing because they come from one of the "founding fathers" of behavior therapy.

Virtually the same treatment and assessment method was used by Azrin, Nunn, and Frantz (1979) in a comparison between regulated breathing and equivalent periods of abbreviated desensitization. In this study clients were seen for one or two 2-3 hour counseling sessions. Thereafter an unspecified number of "treatment" telephone calls were made to clients up to 3 months following treatment; a procedure which, in all likelihood, extended treatment conditions well beyond the two counseling sessions. This is also suggested in their report "that stuttering continued to decrease to a 1 to 2% level during the 3 to 4 month follow-up as long as occasional phone contact advice was available. But when such contact was not scheduled or easily available ... some clients began stuttering again" (1979, p.337). Twenty-one subjects (4-65 years) were treated by "regulated breathing," 14 were assessed after 3 months, and 11 assessed 13 months later. A 97% decrease in episodes was reported at 3 months and a slightly less impressive 79% at 16 months. It is not clear, of course, whether the subjects' "follow-up" ratings represented the performance of the whole group, or whether they even reflected actual speech behavior. However, since the regulated breathing group's ratings emerged as superior to those from the abbreviated desensitization group, it is likely that the treatment was at least more beneficial than a plausible control procedure.

A number of "regulated breathing treatment" reports have appeared recently that go some distance towards clarifying the clinical value of Azrin and Nunn's procedure. A brief report by Small (1975) on the treatment of a 19-year-old male who "stuttered or repeated almost every third word" used elements of the procedure. The subject received 13 consecutive daily sessions of treatment, which included regulated breathing, within and beyond clinic transfer tasks, and behavioral rehearsal under hypnosis. The subject considered himself "cured" at the end of the final session and was discharged, but without any record of his speech performance. Hee and Holms (1976) treated a 10-year-old female in a 1.5-hour counseling session, and then via 5-minute recorded practice sessions conducted by the child's mother over a 12-week "follow-up" period. Stuttering counts [21] from these recordings showed a 98% reduction by the end of that period. Other sources reported, informally, that the girl's speech was improved beyond the recorded setting. Poppen, Nunn, and Hook (1977), in their previously reported multi-treatment study on a 22-year-old severe stutterer, used Azrin and Nunn's (1974) treatment as their last offering. The subject received 2 hours of regulated breathing practice within a total of six 30-minute sessions. The treatment produced the greatest reduction in stuttering when compared with other treatments: from 4% down to 0.9%. However, regulated breathing was preceded by at least four other treatments. The subject's improved performance was reported to have been sustained at an 8-month follow-up, though no systematically gathered data were used to support this claim. Rustin (1978) has also reported using Azrin and Nunn's procedure in a treatment for teen-age subjects, but she has yet to report any treatment benefits.

Other reports of Azrin and Nunn's (1974) treatment procedure have not yielded comparable benefits. They have provided some information on the quality of speech that may emerge from this method, however. Jones (1981) gave a sketchy account of the treatment of a 19-year-old female stutterer who failed to respond to regulated breathing after five sessions of unspecified duration. EMG feedback of masseter muscle tension was then introduced to relax "muscles relevant to speech." This was followed by "practice in speaking on a smooth outflow of breath, remaining relaxed throughout and blending syllables together very gently" (p.130). This procedure was claimed to produce about 90% reduction in percentage of syllables stuttered (%SS), which maintained and generalized over 3 months.

More extensive data have been collected in studies by Ladouceur and colleagues. Ladouceur, Boudreau, and Theberge (1981) compared two groups of eight stutterers (15-47 years) treated by two different versions of Azrin and Nunn's procedure. Both groups received one 90-minute evaluation session followed by a 2-hour treatment session. One group received "awareness training" until each subject counted 80% of clinician-identified stutterings (a procedure that Azrin and Nunn claimed to have used, but, apparently, without specifying success criteria). Both groups then received regulated breathing treatment and

[21] The stuttering counts may have been influenced by counts of repetitions: "A repeated sound repetition, e.g. b-b-block, counted as two instances of stuttering" (Hee & Holmes, 1976, p.41).

were followed for a month. Assessments of speech rate and %SS during conversational speech were made on five occasions throughout this study. Essentially, the groups did not differ in their amounts of stuttering by the final assesssment, and they showed no significant changes in speech rate. More importantly, only about 50% reduction in stuttering occurred between the pre- and posttreatment assessments (approximately 8-9% to 4-5%). However, this less-impressive result may not necessarily reflect the full effect of Azrin and Nunn's treatment, since the systematic follow-up telephone-contact procedure was not used by Ladouceur et al. The same problem appears to have also occurred in a group study by Cote and Ladouceur (1982). They compared %SS and rate-of-speech scores by three groups of eight adult stutterers (18-24 years) over assessments made before and after a treatment phase, and then 2.5 and 6 months later. One group received three 1.5-hour sessions of regulated breathing treatment, another received the same treatment, "but in the presence of a significant other," while the third was an untreated control group. This abbreviated report indicated that the groups did not have significantly different %SS scores (obtained obtrusively and unobtrusively from laboratory and telephone assessments) over the course of all common assessments (the control group was not assessed at the 6-month follow-up). But there is also no evidence that Azrin and Nunn's extensive follow-up telephone-contact procedure formed part of this treatment.

A recent study by Williamson, Epstein, and Coburn (1981) does go some distance towards adequately evaluating an application of Azrin and Nunn's procedure. They used the regulated breathing treatment for a 39-year-old male stutterer within a multiple base-line design, which incorporated speech, EMG, and "social validation" measures. Base-rate and treatment data were derived from once- or twice-weekly sessons (45-60 minutes), in which the subject was recorded orally reading, conversing, role-playing a social situation, and "telephoning" a clinician over an office intercom. Over six base-rate sessions, the subject's percentage of words "dysfluent" ranged from 16 to 46% with a mean-word-per-minute rate of 24.6. The regulated breathing treatment was used in all following sessions; initially, during oral reading and conversation and finally during the role-playing and telephoning tasks. The percentage of "dysfluencies" decreased with each introduction of the treatment, and remained at less than 10%. But the subject's speech rate improved only to around 45 words per minute. The treatment was extended to home practice with the subject's wife (who also used regulated breathing), but was accompanied by clinic sessions over the next 3 months. Thirty-minute home recordings revealed some variation in "dysfluencies" over this period, and a final rating of 2% words "dysfluent." The EMG data showed reductions consistent with the introduction of treatment. The social validation ratings (made by listener judgments of 5-minute speech samples) showed the subject's posttreatment speech was generally understandable, produced by a person with whom the listener would interact, and socially acceptable. But none of these ratings was directed to speech quality, which must have sounded rather unusual: his 33.2-words-per-minute speech rate is roughly one-third the normal speech rate, and close to the level used in the initial phases of DAF treatments.

Andrews & Tanner (1982) produced a rather peculiar "replication" of Azrin and Nunn's procedure with six adult stutterers. Each was assessed from recordings (3 minutes) of conversations and telephone calls made 8 months before and immediately prior to treatment, plus 14, 28, and 100 days after the initial treatment day. The subjects were treated by regulated breathing, and adjuvants recommended by Azrin and Nunn, during 2 hours of individual therapy and (perhaps) via 10 hours observation of other members' therapy.[22] Only four subjects completed the treatment and assessment schedule, and none was reported to have achieved the 99% or 97% reduction in stuttering reported by Azrin and colleagues. Andrews and Tanner (1982) claim their findings were "clinically disappointing," but it is not evident that this reflects directly on Azrin and Nunn's procedure. Admittedly, this procedure does not readily lend itself to replication; however, it does include at least one replicable procedure known to modify stuttering which was not used by Andrews and Tanner—self-recording of stutterings (LaCroix, 1973). There is also some indication in Andrews and Tanner's data that one subject probably benefited substantially from the overall treatment. From Day 1 to Day 100, that particular subject increased his speech rate and reduced stuttering by approximately 50% on one of these assessment conditions over the same period. In short, even though this study only partially replicated Azrin and Nunn's procedure, it still may have yielded some worthwhile gains for some subjects.

The initial promise of Azrin and Nunn's treatment is yet to be substantiated by credible treatment evaluation studies. The procedure probably reduces stuttering, but in all likelihood these reductions occur at the expense of normal-sounding speech. The most substantial treatment effects may turn out to be the artifactual byproducts of subjective ratings made while the subject uses a highly regulated manner of speaking. It is also impossible to identify exactly what treatment, or combination of treatments, may be responsible for any of its benefits. They may all contribute something, for as Johnson (1980b) has noted, the program includes a variety of techniques that are well-known modifiers of stuttering. For example, even the regulated breathing component bears a striking resemblance to the "sigh principle" method used by Gifford (1939) in the 1930s. But almost all of these techniques appear to depend on a more complex therapy schedule than the one described by Azrin and Nunn. At this stage, the growing number of treatment studies on regulated breathing suggests that whenever reasonably objective data have been collected, the results turn out to be far less impressive than those reported by Azrin and Nunn (1974) or Azrin, Nunn, and Frantz (1979).

[22] It is not clear how this treatment was distributed. Subjects attended for 6 hours on Day 1 and another 6 hours on Day 14 when they received "a replication and reinforcement of the instructions" (1982, p.138). This may mean they received an hour of individual therapy and observed therapy for 5 hours on both days. In this event, the very brief individual treatment time that Azrin and colleagues offered subjects during their initial clinic visit may have been divided in two by Andrews and Tanner and offered at intervals separated by 2 weeks. This certainly departs from the procedure recommended by Azrin and Nunn.

Weiner (1978) has promoted another breathstream-regulation approach known as Vocal Control Therapy which is claimed (Weiner, 1981) to incorporate a quite distinctive speech-modification method. The approach is based on the premise that stuttering is reduced by the "proper use of the voice mechanism." The actual treatment procedure has been only vaguely described as involving breathing and voice exercises aimed at achieving adequate airflow and resonant voicing. In addition, easy onset of vocalization, biofeedback, covert positive reinforcement, systematic desensitization, and assertive training may also be used. Transfer and maintenance procedures are incorporated, but like the establishment phase, they are neither systematized nor operationalized. Some pre- and posttreatment data for 12 adult stutterers, who completed this program, show their mean "stuttering events per minute" went from 10.8 to 0.43 on a variety of speaking tasks. These gains were not supplemented by speech-rate data. Follow-up assessment by mail and telephone over a 6- to 48-month period found that nine subjects had retained 80% to 98% fluency (presumably by self-ratings). Despite Weiner's (1981) claim, there is little evidence that this treatment procedure differs in any meaningful way from many of the previously mentioned treatments. Certainly the therapy's descriptions, or the reported speech performance measures, are not sufficient to test that claim.

A similar issue arises in connection with a study by Resick, Wendiggensen, Ames, and Meyer (1978), which evaluated a treatment based on systematic slowing of speech and anxiety management. Their method was also claimed to be "a new treatment for stuttering." Ten daily 1-hour sessions (for two subjects at a time) formed this fixed-duration program. In the first week, subjects were taught relaxation training and anxiety management, with assistance from GSR biofeedback, during the first half-hour. In the second half-hour, they were instructed to orally read and speak using controlled slowed speech. This began at 50 wpm and, contingent on absence of stuttering and anxiety, was increased in steps to 90 wpm. In the final week, subjects learned to practice speaking at 50, 70, and 90 wpm, as well as to speak at 90 wpm in "comfortable" situations. They were not only taught to speak slowly: "Participants were discouraged from developing a rhythmic pattern or relying on long pauses. They were encouraged to prolong the words instead." (1978, p.163). Six stutterers (21-36 years), who received this treatment, were assessed on conversations with a stranger, oral reading, and telephone conversations prior to, immediately following, and 1, 3, and 6 months after treatment. Most of the within-clinic assessments were based on 1-minute speech samples from each situation. These showed that by the final assessment, subjects were virtually stutter-free on the oral reading task, but were only marginally improved on the conversational and telephone tasks—in fact, their performance on these tasks deteriorated throughout the follow-up period. Significantly, the speech rate scores on both of these tasks for four subjects was also well above the target of 90 wpm. This is hardly a promising result for a new treatment, though the report does contain some interesting aspects. In all probability, it actually describes yet another variation on prolonged speech, supplemented by relaxation techniques. It may, therefore, turn out to demonstrate the performance pattern which follows a prolonged speech treatment that *fails* to include planned transfer or maintenance procedures. This possibility is evident in their subjects' consistently poorer performance on telephone conversations, a speech task that was deliberately excluded from the treatment program.

A variation on the Resick et al. (1978) procedure was reported by Turkat, Pomeranz, and Bruch (1981) in the treatment of a 26-year-old female stutterer. They relied upon the use of controlled slow speaking during clinic and beyond-clinic speaking situations. The subject was reported to have benefited from a treatment involving oral reading and speaking at 50 WPM, then 70-75 WPM, and finally 90-95 WPM. But this was an informal and virtually data-less report, using only self-reports to verify treatment effects.

To a large extent, some recent treatment recommendations by Adams and Runyan (1981) virtually amount to changing the subject's speech pattern towards features associated with prolonged speech and its variants. For some time, Adams (1975b; 1980) has advocated careful analysis of respiration and phonation in order to formulate a stuttering therapy—particularly with children. For example, he has suggested that part-word repetitions and sound prolongations point to the need for procedures similar to Perkins's (1973c) breathstream management in order to co-ordinate voicing and articulation (Adams, 1980). Stuttering children without voicing problems, and whose stuttering derives "exclusively from slowness and uncertainty in the operation of various aspects of the language encoding process" (Adams, 1980, p.293), may benefit from rate control and the GILCU approach (Ryan, 1974). Recently, Adams and Runyan (1981) have described subjects who had either "inappropriately timed pauses and hesitations," "low vocal intensity," or "slow VOT of voiced stops," and were treated successfully by individually tailored techniques. Bewilderingly, they provided absolutely no data to support these claims. (Ingham, 1982a).

The current impact of the prolonged speech treatments on stuttering therapy is such that hardly a month passes without the appearance of yet another therapy package based on this procedure. One of the latest is Shine's (1980; 1981) Systematic Fluency Training for Young Children. In this program children are treated individually within the clinic and via a "significant other" (parent, teacher, relative, peer, sibling) who is taught to count stutterings. In clinic conditions, children are taught to use an "easy speaking voice" which includes reduced rate and intensity. Whispering may be used, but generally their speech pattern is described as prolonged speech. Increasingly complex speaking tasks are introduced, while the speaking pattern is retained with the assistance of clinician modeling and token reinforcement. Transfer programs are instituted using within- and beyond-clinic procedures similar to those employed in the establishment phase. And decreasingly frequent assessment sessions are conducted over the following 12 months to form a maintenance phase. The program therefore incorporates many of the procedures used by Ryan (1974). Unhappily, the data-base to Shine's program gives no indicataion that any of the procedures were responsible for the benefits claimed for this treatment. Shine (1980) reports that 20 children (3 to 8 years) were treated by this procedure for between 12 and 133 sessions (50 minutes). Their stuttering ranged from 6.4 to 35.1 stuttered words per minute (SW/M) before treatment and 0.0 to 8.4 SW/M after treatment. Ten children, "who achieved fluency" in treatment, were followed for 6 months to 5 years and had a mean of 0.41 SW/M at follow-up. But absolutely no details are provided on how these data were collected, nor on their representativeness or reliability.

The virtual disdain shown towards systematically gathered speech-behavior data in many treatments means, at best, that their clinical value can only be a matter of conjecture. At worst, it signals a move towards clinical practices that share much in common with quackery. Indeed, when unsubstantiated claims are made for any form of treatment in this day and age, there is good reason to suspect the motives and qualifications of the claimant. Such is the situation with an increasing number of stuttering treatment reports. This is best exemplified in the now notorious claims of Martin Schwartz (1976) in his book "Stuttering Solved." This book describes an "airflow technique" of therapy which depends on speech with "passive flow, soft and slow." Following an intensive-therapy phase, Schwartz recommends a variety of strategies to aid the continuation of slightly exaggerated air flow during speech. The procedure is far from unique and is obviously similar to those described earlier in this chapter. "The results with approximately 185 patients were that 89% of them were completely symptom free in all situations within the week." (Schwartz, 1976, p.93). These subjects then engaged in a year of daily practice, which was partly recorded and sent to Schwartz for evaluation. He then concludes as follows: "Long term follow-up indicates that 83% of my patients have remained symptom-free after one year" (p.94). The outrageousness of this unverified and data-less claim is obvious. Nevertheless, it should be recognized that unverified and data-less claims are, unfortunately, not uncommon among treatment reports reviewed in this chapter.

Schwartz's treatment procedure has been described in at least three other therapy reports. Lee (1976) provided a vague description of Schwartz's treatment with 31 adult stutterers, and accompanied it with yet another unsubstantiated claim: "the patients [had] shown continuous improvement, with 46% being essentially symptom-free in all routine speaking situations" (p.134). Burns and Brady (1980) also reported that airflow therapy was successful as an "adjunctive technique." But they too failed to provide supportive data. The only investigation of airflow therapy that has involved the collection of speech-performance data was reported by Falkowski, Guilford, and Sandler (1982). They described an experimental study of the contribution of the airflow and the "elongation component" in the treatment of two adult stutterers. The subjects' "percentage of disfluencies" and words-per-minute scores were obtained from oral readings and monologues made preceding and during the course of their 4-week (30 hour) treatment, and then 10 weeks later. Both subjects substantially reduced their disfluencies during oral reading tasks, but they failed to show sustained improvement during spontaneous speech. The virtues of this study are marred by its failure to include any details on how the treatment procedures were implemented. There is every likelihood that Schwartz's technique does modify stuttering, but whatever relevance this may have to the achievement of maintained and generalized stutter-free normal-sounding speech is yet to be demonstrated in a suitable study.

Conclusions

The most obvious conclusion that can be drawn from this review is that treatments employing prolonged speech or its variants have accounted for more published reports of stuttering therapy in the past decade than any other procedure. The extent to which these procedures have dominated stuttering therapy in recent years is such that there is even a real risk that they are coming to be regarded as essential to the treatment of this disorder (see, for example, Conture, 1982; Cooper, 1980). One illustration of this dominance is in the author's country, Australia, where it is fair to claim that the publicity given to these treatment procedures has meant that most young clinicians are now virtually unfamiliar with any other therapy procedure. But do the results of these treatments justify this enthusiasm?

The first concern about drawing any conclusions from this treatment review is that it still remains unclear as to whether all of the reviewed treatments share enough in common to warrant considering them together. The only justification at this time is that the "DAF speech pattern" has yet to be reliably distinguished from patterns that derive from methods which use modified voicing, speech rate control, and/or de-emphasized articulatory gestures. What is clear, however, is that together they now form the most publicized "behavioral" treatment for stuttering. As a group, they have probably produced as many claims for therapy success as any other treatment technique used in this century. In the process, in all probability, they have wrested the mantle of therapy controversy away from response-contingent treatments. Certainly, the numerous therapy-success claims of the prolonged speech treatments have been accompanied by increasing skepticism, especially over their relevance to durable and normally fluent speech (Sheehan, 1980; Van Riper, 1979).

Actually, the proponents of many of these treatments have championed much of the skepticism about their effects (Ingham & Andrews, 1973b; Perkins, 1973a). Even the increasingly complex structure of these treatments, particularly their detailed transfer and maintenance procedures, is testimony to the concern shown over the "successful outcomes" from the initial prolonged speech treatments (a factor which also makes it increasingly difficult to identify the principal source of their treatment benefits). But this skepticism has had some benefits; it has encouraged the development of more sophisticated methods of evaluation and more viable treatment strategies which must ultimately benefit all therapy methods.

Much of the debate over the value of these treatments stems from the questionable adequacy (or more precisely the construct validity) of the measurement techniques used to assess stuttering treatments. Andrews and Ingham (1972) made one attempt to come to terms with this problem by describing some necessary components in stuttering-treatment evaluation. Essentially they recommended (1) repeated measurement to determine the trend of stuttering and speech rate before, during, and after treatment; (2) some evidence that treatment effects are not clinic-bound, and (3) the use of unobtrusive measurement as a control over assessment reactivity. But it is now clear that much more is needed to establish internal and external validity in stuttering-treatment research, particularly when the treatment involves a speech-pattern technique.

The most obvious weakness in Andrews and Ingham's (1972) recommendations was their failure to specify measurement techniques that would reflect the peculiarities of prolonged speech or its variants. It was obvious to all who used this method that a treatment target of stutter-free speech at normal speaking rate was insufficient to either gauge treatment success or provide adequate measurement dimensions for incorporation in a treatment. This was confirmed in the perceptual analysis study of Ingham and Packman (1978), which found that treated subjects who had met a target criterion of stutter-free speech at prescribed normal speech rates were still identified by listeners as stutterers. Some related and more controversial findings were obtained by Runyan and Adams (1978; 1979). They obtained audiotapes of the speech of stutterers who had been "successfully therapeutized" by a variety of treatments, including those actually directed by Ryan, Webster, and Perkins. After mixing fluent samples from each group with normal-speaker samples they found that the stutterers' samples from *any* of these treatments were still distinguishable from the normal speakers' samples at levels well beyond chance. What was needed, therefore, was a means to measure and utilize dimensions that would assist stutterers to alter a slow and unnatural type of speech into normally fluent speech. At the very least there was a need for clinicians to be able to determine whether or not that goal had been reached.

What, therefore, do normal speakers do that is convertible to clinically useful measurements? A solution to this problem is yet to be found. Starkweather (1980), for example, recently reviewed research pertaining to this issue and provided some idea of the size of the problem. He concluded that "it is the quality of speech that includes rapid and easy as well as smooth production" (p.195). Starkweather's reference to rate meant normal-sound durations, pause durations, coarticulation, and rate of syllable production. He related "ease of speech" to "muscular and mental" factors. The expression of effort must be such that syllables are stressed at varying levels and at different rates, clearly a difficult dimension to program. And it is certainly unclear how mental effort or monitored control over speech can be measured to anyone's satisfaction. Smoothness is also a perplexing dimension, since normally fluent speakers have many pauses, hesitations, and interjections. So it must mean partially smooth speech. In short, normally fluent speech is so multi- and interdimensional that, for the present, at least, it seems unlikely that it will yield acoustic measures of separate or combined dimensions which permit programmed "construction" of normally fluent speech. In the short term, we are forced back to the inexactitude and clinically cumbersome technique of perceptual judgments by listeners. But there are promising possibilities. The technology for measuring vocal intensity, pauses, and voicing durations has been developed to the point where acoustic, physiologic, and aerodynamic analyses (Adams, 1981) may yet produce some limited quantitative dimensions of normalcy. Perhaps the most interesting possibility is a procedure being developed by Martin (1982), which has been based on the proposition that natural speech quality might be a response class that is manipulable via feedback to the speaker from on-line clinician ratings of naturalness. If this should prove true, then it might provide a much simpler and clinically viable solution to this issue.

The urgent need for viable measures of speech quality also has implications for the status of prolonged speech techniques within a behavior-therapy context. A recurring theme throughout this chapter has been the contrast between the zeal with which many clinicians advocate certain speech-pattern manipulations and their failure to describe the exact form of these manipulations. There is literally no evidence that any of the various prolonged speech treatments produce fundamentally different forms of speech behavior, except, perhaps, in terms of utterance rate. Also, while emphases have been given to different dimensions of the vocal/motor aspects of speech, not one attempt has been made to determine the reliability with which such emphases are managed within a therapy context. That is not to deny the possibility that this could be done. Indeed, listener judgments of these dimensions may turn out to be just as reliable as, say, judgments of stuttering. Also, some treatments have used specialized equipment to teach "easy-onsets" (Agnello, 1975; Webster, 1974a), yet even the efficacy of this equipment has not been documented.

The evidence that many of the improvements produced by the reviewed studies may be clinic-bound is quite plentiful. It appears in incidental reports (Curlee & Perkins, 1973; Ryan, 1974); Webster, 1974a) and has been systematically documented by this author (Ingham, 1981a; 1982b). These accounts show that even when nonclinic data are collected, the assessment process, as such, may bias these data. For example, there is now ample evidence from covert assessment investigations that poorer speech performance may typify the customary beyond-clinic assessment situations. This is not a consistent effect with all subjects (Andrews & Craig, 1982; Ingham, 1981a), but it occurs often enough to threaten the external validity of many treatment-outcome studies. The issue is particularly bothersome because even the situations chosen to compare overt and covert assessment, such as telephone calls (Andrews & Craig, 1982), may not adequately sample beyond-clinic speaking conditions.

At the very least those treatment studies that fail to incorporate recorded speech samples in typical beyond-clinic conditions must be regarded as dubious demonstrations of a therapy benefit. There is even less justification for granting credence to studies that merely assess outcome via self reports without corroborative speech data. This issue will be discussed later.

In light of this review, it is interesting to consider the studies that Andrews, Guitar, and Howie (1980) used to conclude "that treatments based on training a stutterer in prolonged speech and gentle onset techniques are superior to other types of treatments" (p.305). Their review employed Smith and Glass's (1977) meta-analysis technique, which compares groups of treatments on their relative contributions to an overall treatment-effect size. For reasons that should be apparent by now, this is a hazardous strategy, especially if it relies on the dubious outcome-data typically used in treatment reports. And, unfortunately, it does just that. It is also unwise to reach general conclusions when they are based upon treatments that are vaguely described and when examples of many treatments are excluded. Unhappily this also happens. For example, the Andrews et al. (1980) analysis, by necessity, excluded all single subject(s) studies including those that only used response-contingent techniques. [23] In the case of prolonged speech and its variants, the calculations were largely based upon within-clinic data, or data obtained during the course of uncontrolled maintenance programs. The four "gentle onset" studies included an unpublished paper and reports by Ronald Webster (1974a; 1979), and Dianne Schwartz and Michael Webster (1977a). In the latter study the outcome data were within-clinic assessments made only 45 days after treatment ceased. The 1974 Webster study was also based on unspecified within-clinic oral reading and conversational tasks. However, the 1979 Webster study used beyond-clinic data obtained 2 years after treatment—albeit via a surprise telephone call of unstated duration. Five of the 12 "Prolonged Speech" studies (Andrews & Ingham, 1972; Boberg & Sawyer, 1977; Frayne, Coates, & Marriner, 1977; Helps & Dalton, 1979; Ryan, 1974) contained data from within-clinic conditions, or were highly confounded by maintenance-phase activities. In Ryan's (1974) study, for example, a host of treatment strategies were introduced during the maintenance phase, including (in the case of seven subjects) enrollment in additional unspecified therapy (p.108). Moreover, the pertinent follow-up data in Ryan's report were virtually chosen by the subject. The only "prolonged speech technique" studies that definitely used nonclinic data were by Perkins, Rudas, Johnson, Michael & Curlee (1979)[24] and Howie, Tanner, and Andrews (1981). In the former study the data were also subject-recorded in subject-chosen situations which, of course, raises concerns about the representativeness of the obtained samples. The Howie et al. (1981) study had the advantage of beyond-clinic telephone-call data (although of an unspecified amount) supplemented, in part, by ostensibly covert telephone calls; but the outcome data in this case were confounded by an extensive and uncontrolled maintenance program. In short, it is impossible to accept that the data entered in the Andrews et al. (1980) meta-analysis adequately assessed treatment outcome —certainly not in a fashion which would justify the outright superiority of these treatments.

So, what is a suitable alternative method for estimating the efficacy of these treatments? A straightforward answer is almost impossible, since most of the reported treatments intermix many potentially effective treatment agents. In general terms, at least, it is probable that numerous subjects who have passed through these treatment programs have gained markedly improved speech that generalized to nonclinic situations over about 2 years. But their speech is not necessarily equatable with normal-sounding speech, and, in many instances, it is

[23] For some reason, Martin and Haroldson's (1969) study on the effect of time-out (incorrectly described as an example of "reinforcement") was included, even though it was an experimental study without therapeutic purpose.

[24] Andrews et al. (1980) used a grant report by Perkins to obtain the beyond-clinic data they, presumably, included in their meta-analysis.

probably retained at the cost of constant attention to speech production. However, there is an additional issue: a clear picture of treatment efficacy is almost impossible to derive from group studies where it is usually impractical (even invalid) to relate the multitude of implicated variables to treatment effects (Hersen & Barlow, 1976). In planned single-subject(s) experimental studies at least some of these variables can be controlled. Repeated measurement and supplemental recording of speech across treatment and outcome phases certainly permits a more clinically relevant account of treatment effects, and also serves to stave off threats to the study's internal and external validity. At present, it is far from clear which treatment component(s) is necessary either to establish improved speech or to transfer and maintain treatment effects.

Part of the search for sources of maintained treatment effects in many of the prolonged speech therapies requires some evaluation of the role of speech-pattern variables within the maintenance strategies used to sustain their benefits. If the "fluency" or "partial fluency" that emerges from the "establishment/transfer" phases in these therapies rests on a scaffold of controlled speech rate, modified breathstream activity, or any other byproduct of prolonged speech treatment, then it should be stated that the maintenance strategy is designed (or not designed) to retain these speech pattern varibles. This is rarely the case. There are some maintenance strategies that explicitly incorporate these variables, and thereby make it clear that the subject's improved speech will only partially resemble normal-sounding fluent speech. In effect, the retained fluency may depend as much on the sustained speech pattern variables as it does on the maintenance strategy format. One example of this type of maintenance strategy is Boberg and Sawyer's (1977) "booster system" which incorporates intensive practice in the use of prolonged speech variables.

Other maintenance strategies link up with establishment and transfer phases which are designed to produce fluency that does approximate normal speech. In such cases, only stutter-free speech (perhaps within normal speech-rate ranges) is the principal target behavior incorporated within such strategies; the prolonged speech variables are de-emphasized in anticipation that they will eventually become part of normal-sounding speech. This approach is demonstrated in the maintenance programs developed by this writer (Ingham, 1980; 1982b). These strategies are based on the assumption that stutter-free speech is a trained skill that can be evoked under planned discriminable and indiscriminable contingency schedules (Ingham, 1982c). The strategies do not incorporate the planned use of speech-pattern variables which would thereby make them necessary and significant for any maintained speech performance. In general, therefore, any effort to identify the efficacy of the prolonged speech treatments will need to recognize the array of variables implicated, by design or otherwise, in their maintenance phases.

In recent years, one variable that some authorities have regarded as important for sustaining the benefits of prolonged speech treatments is the stutterer's attitude towards communication. The relevance of this factor first emerged in a study by Andrews and Cutler (1974) which found that an amended version of

Erickson's (1969) communication-attitudes questionnaire (the S24) reflected changes in speech performance over the course of the establishment and transfer phase of Ingham and Andrews's (1973a) treatment program. The importance of communication attitudes to sustained posttreatment performance was ostensibly bolstered by evidence from a study by Guitar and Bass (1978), which showed that subjects who failed to "normalize" such attitudes by the end of the transfer phase in Ingham and Andrews's program were more likely to perform poorly a year later. However, the validity of this finding is extremely doubtful since an alternative analysis of these data (Guitar, 1981; Ingham, 1979) revealed that the "non-normalized" subjects did *not* have significantly poorer speech performance than their "normalized" counter-parts. Moreover, since the S24 Scale was actually designed (Andrews & Cutler, 1974) to reflect changes in speech behavior, it is quite possible that the Scale's scores are influenced by speech performance rather than attitudes. So, for the present, it seems unlikely that the type of "attitudes" measured by the S24 provide better predictions of posttreatment performance than would be derived from adequately sampled speech behavior.

One final consideration is the relationship between the concept of a speech-pattern technique and a therapy format. One of the most obvious trends among therapies using prolonged speech and its variants has been the move towards intensive intervention, particularly with adults. There exists some admittedly less-than-ideal evidence that intensive treatments produce better results than similar nonintensive treatments (Ingham, 1975a; Perkins et al., 1974). One reason for this trend towards intensive treatment may be expediency, but it may also be recognition of therapy principles that are more appropriate for achieving the complete behavior change required for a "new fluent speech pattern." For, if the purpose in this type of treatment is to *replace* one behavior with another (Goldiamond, 1965), then it does not make intuitive sense to permit jeopardy of the replacement process by retention of the original behavior. In an intensive setting, it is more likely that this replacement process will be under greater control, thereby increasing the probability that the new behavior is constantly present. This is not to suggest that degrees of intensiveness necessarily correlate with treatment success, but growing recognition of this principle could explain the increasing prevelance of intensive prolonged speech treatments.

There is little doubt that prolonged-speech-treatment research has begun to generate procedures which improve the chance that stutterers may achieve generalized and maintained improved speech. The arguments over treatment efficacy have also contributed much to the development of a generalization technology (Stokes & Baer, 1977) for stuttering treatments as well as more credible outcome-evaluation procedures. At the same time, these therapies seem to have stimulated the revival of practices that share more in common with "stuttering schools" (Clark, 1964) of the 1920s and 1930s than with behavior therapy. There is reason to speculate that the cause of this is the continuing failure to adequately operationalize the prolonged-speech-treatment process. The sooner this is corrected, the sooner there might emerge a treatment method that clinicians may choose with justifiable confidence.

References

Adamczyk, B. Anwendung des apparates fur die erzeugung von kunstlichen widerhall bei der behandlung des stotterns. *Folia Phoniatricia*, 1959, *11*, 216-218.

Adamczyk, B. Correction of speech in stutterers by means of a telephone with the use of an artificial echo. *Otolaryngologia Polska*, 1963, *17*, 482-484.

Adamczyk, B. Psychotherapeutische faktoren der behandlung des stotterns mit der "Echomethods." *Folia Phoniatrica*, 1969, *21*, 300-306.

Adams, M.R. A physiologic and aerodynamic interpretation of fluent and stuttered speech. *Journal of Fluency Disorders*, 1974, *1*, 35-47.

Adams, M.R. Vocal tract dynamics in fluency and stuttering: A review and interpretation of past research. In L.M. Webster & L.C. Furst (Eds.), *Proceedings of the First Annual Hayes Martin Conference on Vocal Tract Dynamics*. New York: Speech & Hearing Institute, New York, 1975(a).

Adams, M.R. Clinical interpretations and applications. In L.M. Webster & L.C. Furst (Eds.), *Proceedings of the First Annual Hayes Martin Conference on Vocal Tract Dynamics*. New York: Speech & Hearing Institute, New York, 1975(b).

Adams, M.R. Comments on Schwartz's: "The core of the stuttering block." *Journal of Speech and Hearing Disorders*, 1975, *40*, 136. (c)

Adams, M.R. The young stutterer: Diagnosis, treatment and assessment of progress. *Seminars in Speech, Language and Hearing*, 1980, *1*, 289-299.

Adams, M.R. The speech production abilities of stutterers: Recent, ongoing, and future research. *Journal of Fluency Disorders*, 1981, *6*, 311-326.

Adams, M.R., & Hayden, P. The ability of stutterers and nonstutterers to initiate and terminate phonation during production of an isolated vowel. *Journal of Speech and Hearing Research*, 1976, *19*, 290-296.

Adams, M.R., & Moore, W.H., Jr., The effects of auditory masking on the anxiety level, frequency of dysfluency, and selected vocal characteristics of stutterers. *Journal of Speech and Hearing Research*, 1972, *15*, 572-578.

Adams, M.R. & Ramig, P. Vocal characteristics of normal speakers and stutterers during choral reading. *Journal of Speech and Hearing Research*, 1980, *23*, 457-469.

Adams, M.R., & Reis, R. The influence of the onset of phonation on the frequency of stuttering. *Journal of Speech and Hearing Research*, 1971, *14*, 639-644.

Adams, M.R., & Reis, R. Influence of the onset of phonation on the frequency of stuttering: A replication and reevaluation. *Journal of Speech and Hearing Research*, 1974, *17*, 752-754.

Adams, M.R., & Reis, R. A reply to Martin Young. *Journal of Speech and Hearing Research*, 1975, *18*, 603-605.

Adams, M.R., Riemenschneider, S., Metz, D., & Conture, E. Voice onset and articulatory constriction requirements in a speech segment and their relation to the amount of stuttering adaptation. *Journal of Fluency Disorders*, 1975, *1*, 24-31.

Adams, M.R., & Runyan, C.M. Stuttering and fluency: Exclusive events or points on a continuum? *Journal of Fluency Disorders*, 1981, *6*, 197-218.

Adams, M.R., Runyan, C., & Mallard, A.R. Air flow characteristics of the speech of stutterers and nonstutterers. *Journal of Fluency Disorders*, 1975, *1*, 4-12.

Agnello, J.G. Voice onset and voice termination features of stutterers. In L.M. Webster & L.C Furst (Eds.), *Proceedings of the First Annual Hayes Martin Conference on Vocal Tract Dynamics*. New York: Speech & Hearing Institute, New York, 1975.

Agnello, J.G., & Wingate, M.E. Some acoustical and physiological aspects of stuttered speech. Paper read to American Speech & Hearing Association Convention, San Francisco, 1972.

Andrews, G. Stuttering therapy. How simple can an effective treatment programme become? *Australian Journal of Human Communication Disorders*, 1973, *1*, 44-46.

Andrews, G., & Craig, A. Stuttering: Overt and covert measurement of the speech of treated subjects. *Journal of Speech and Hearing Disorders*, 1982, *47*, 96-99.

Andrews, G., & Cutler, J. Stuttering therapy: The relation between changes in symptom level and attitudes. *Journal of Speech and Hearing Disorders*, 1974, *39*, 312-319.

Andrews, G., Guitar, B., & Howie, P. Meta-analysis of the effects of stuttering treatment. *Journal of Speech and Hearing Disorders*, 1980, *45*, 287-307.

Andrews, G., & Harvey, R. Regression to the mean in pretreatment measures of stuttering. *Journal of Speech and Hearing Disorders*, 1981, *46*, 204-207.

Andrews, G., Howie, P.M., Dozsa, M., & Guitar, B.E. Stuttering: Speech pattern characteristics under fluency-inducing conditions. *Journal of Speech and Hearing Research*, 1982, *25*, 208-216.

Andrews, G., & Ingham, R.J. An approach to the evaluation of stuttering therapy. *Journal of Speech and Hearing Research*, 1972, *15*, 296-302.

Andrews, G., & Tanner, S. Stuttering treatment: An attempt to replicate the regulated-breathing method. *Journal of Speech and Hearing Disorders*, 1982, *47*, 138-140.

Anonymous. *The causes, prevention and treatment of stammering and stuttering.* New York: Excelsior,1870.

Arens, C.J., & Popplestone, J.A. Verbal facility and delayed speech feedback. *Perceptual and Motor Skills*, 1959, *9*, 270.

Atkinson, C.J. Adaptation to delayed side-tone. *Journal of Speech and Hearing Disorders*, 1953, *18*, 386-391.

Atkinson, C.J. Some effects on intelligibility as the sidetone level and the amount of sidetone delay are changed. *Proceedings of the Iowa Academy of Science*, 1954, *61*, 334-340.

Ayllon, T., & Azrin, N.H. The measurement and reinforcement of behavior of psychotics. *Journal of the Experimental Analysis of Behavior*, 1965, *8*, 357-383.

Azrin, N.H., & Nunn, R.G. A rapid method of eliminating stuttering by a regulated breathing approach. *Behaviour Research and Therapy*, 1974, *12*, 279-286.

Azrin, N.H., & Nunn, R.G. *Habit control: Stuttering, nailbiting and other nervous habits.* New York: Simon & Schuster, 1977.

Azrin, N.H., Nunn, R.G., & Frantz, S.E. Comparison of regulated-breathing versus abbreviated desensitization on reported stuttering episodes. *Journal of Speech and Hearing Disorders*, 1979, *44*, 331-339.

Azzi, A., & Invernizzi, M. La prova della voce ritardata come mezzo diagnostico nelle sordita psicogene. *Rivista Oto-Neuro-Oftalmologica*, 1951, *24*, 1-5.

Bachrach, D.L. Sex differences in reactions to delayed auditory feedback. *Perceptual and Motor Skills*, 1964, *19*, 81-82.

Beaumont, J.T., & Foss, B.M. Individual differences in reacting to delayed auditory feedback. *British Journal of Psychology*, 1957, *48*, 85-89.

Bell, A.M. *The faults of speech.* Washington: The Volta Bureau, 1904.

Bender, J.F., & Kleinfield, V.M. *Principles and practices of speech corection.* New York: Pitman, 1938.

Besozzi, T.E., & Adams, M.R. The influence of prosody on stuttering adaptation. *Journal of Speech and Hearing Research*, 1969, *12*, 818-824.

Bills, A.G. The relation of stuttering to mental fatigue. *Journal of Experimental Psychology*, 1934, *17*, 574-584.

Black, J.W. The effect of room characteristics upon vocal intensity and rate. *Journal of the Acoustical Society of America*, 1950, *21*, 174-176.

Black, J.W. The effect of delayed side-tone upon vocal rate and intensity. *Journal of Speech and Hearing Disorders*, 1951, *16*, 56-60.

Bloodstein, O. A rating scale study of conditions under which stuttering is reduced or absent. *Journal of Speech and Hearing Disorders*, 1950, *15*, 29-36.

Bloodstein, 0. *A handbook on stuttering.* (2nd ed.) Chicago: National Easter Seal Society, 1975.

Bloodstein, O. *A handbook on stuttering.* (3rd ed.) Chicago: National Easter Seal Society, 1981.

Boberg, E. Intensive group therapy program for stutterers. *Human Communication*, 1976, *1*, 29-42.

Boberg, E. Intensive adult therapy program. *Seminars in Speech, Language and Hearing*, 1980, *1*, 365-373.

Boberg, E. Maintenance of fluency: An experimental program. In E. Boberg (Ed.), *Maintenance of fluency*. New York: Elsevier, 1981.

Boberg, E., & Fong, L. Therapy program for young retarded stutterers. *Human Communication*, 1980, *5*, 95-102.

Boberg, E., & Sawyer, L. Maintenance of fluency following intensive therapy. *Human Communication*, 1977, *2*, 21-28.

Boehmler, R.M. An evaluation of behavior modification in the treatment of stuttering. In Speech Foundation of America, Publication No. 7, *Conditioning in stuttering therapy*, Memphis: Speech Foundation of America, 1970.

Borman, E.G. "Ephphatha, or, some advice to stammerers." *Journal of Speech and Hearing Research*, 1969, *12*, 453-461.

Bradshaw, J.L., Nettleton, N.C., & Geffen, G. Ear asymmetry and delayed auditory feedback: Effects of task requirements and competitive stimulation. *Journal of Experimental Psychology*, 1972, *94*, 296-275.

Brayton, E.R., & Conture, E.G. Effects of noise and rhythmic stimulation on the speech of stutterers. *Journal of Speech and Hearing Research*, 1978, *21*, 285-294.

Brenner, N.C., Perkins, W.H., & Soderberg, G.A. The effect of rehearsal on frequency of stuttering. *Journal of Speech and Hearing Research*, 1972, *15*, 483-486.

Brokaw, S.P., Singh, S., & Black, J.W. The duration of speech in conditions of delayed side tone. *Speech Monographs*, 1966, *33*, 452-456.

Bruce, M.C., & Adams, M.R. Effects of two types of motor practice on stuttering adaptation. *Journal of Speech and Hearing Research*, 1978, *21*, 421-428.

Burke, B.D. Susceptibility to delayed auditory feedback and dependence on auditory or oral sensory feedback. *Journal of Communication Disorders*, 1975, *8*, 75-96. (a)

Burke, B.D. Variables affecting stutterer's initial reactions to delayed auditory feedback. *Journal of Communication Disorders*, 1975, *8*, 141-155. (b)

Burns, D., & Brady, J.P. The treatment of stuttering. In A. Goldstein & E.B. Foa (Eds.), *Handbook of behavioral interventions.* New York: Wiley, 1980.

Butler, B.R., & Stanley, P.E. The stuttering problem considered from an automatic control point of view. *Folia Phoniatrica*, 1966, *18*, 33-44.

Butler, R.A., & Galloway, F.T. Factorial analysis of the delayed speech feedback phenomenon. *Journal of the Acoustical Society of America*, 1975, *29*, 632-635.

Chase, R.A. Effect of delayed auditory feedback on the repetition of speech sounds. *Journal of Speech and Hearing Disorders*, 1958, *23*, 583-590.

Chase, R.A., & Guilfoyle, G. Effect of simultaneous delayed and undelayed auditory feedback on speech. *Journal of Speech and Hearing Research*, 1962, *5*, 141-151.

Chase, R.A., Sutton, S., First, D., & Zubin, J. A developmental study of changes in behavior under delayed auditory feedback. *Journal of Genetic Psychology*, 1961, *99*, 101-112.

Chase, R.A., Sutton, S., & Rapin, I. Sensory feedback influences on motor performance. *Journal of Auditory Research*, 1961, *1*, 212-223.

Cherry, C., & Sayers, B.McA. Experiments upon the total inhibition of stammering by external control and some clinical results. *Journal of Psychosomatic Research*, 1956, *1*, 233-246.

Chevrie-Muller, C. A study of laryngeal function in stutterers by the glottographic method. In *Proceedings VII Congress de la Societé Francaise de Medicine de la Voix et de la Parole*. Paris: 1963.

Clark, R.M. Our enterprising predecessors and Charles Sydney Bluemel. *Asha*, 1964, *6*, 107-114.

Cohen, J.G., & Edwards, A.E. The extraexperimental effects of random sidetones. *Proceedings of the American Psychological Association*, 1965, 211-212.

Colcord, R.D., & Adams, M.R. Voicing duration and vocal SPL changes associated with stuttering reduction during singing. *Journal of Speech and Hearing Research*, 1979, *22*, 468-479.

Commodore, R.W., & Cooper, E.B. Communicative stress and stuttering frequency during normal, whispered, and articulation-without-phonation speech modes. *Journal of Fluency Disorders*, 1978, *3*, 1-12.

Conture, E.G. Some effects of noise on the speaking behavior of stutterers. *Journal of Speech and Hearing Research*, 1974, *17*, 714-723.

Conture, E.G. *Stuttering*. Englewood Cliffs, NJ: Prentice-Hall, 1982

Conture, E.G., McCall, G.N., & Brewer, D.W. Laryngeal behavior during stuttering. *Journal of Speech and Hearing Research*, 1977, *20*, 661-668.

Cooper, E.B. *Personalized fluency control therapy*. Boston: Teaching Resources, 1976.

Cooper, E.B. Controversies about stuttering therapy. *Journal of Fluency Disorders*, 1977, *2*, 75-86.

Cooper, E.B. Intervention procedures for the young stutterer. In H.H. Gregory (Ed.), *Controversies about stuttering therapy*. Baltimore: University Park Press, 1979.

Cooper, E.B. Etiology and treatment of stuttering. *Ear, Nose, and Throat Journal*, 1980, *59*, 60-76.

Cooper, M.H., & Allen, G.D. Timing control accuracy in normal speakers and stutterers. *Journal of Speech and Hearing Research*, 1977, *20*, 55-71.

Cooper, Jr., W.A., Strockinger, T.E., & Billings, B.L. Pure tone delayed auditory feedback: Development of criteria of performance deterioration. *Journal of the American Audiology Society*, 1976, *1*, 192-196.

Cote, C., & Ladouceur, R. Effects of social aids and the regulated breathing method in the treatment of stutterers. *Journal of Consulting and Clinical Psychology*, 1982, *50*, 450.

Cross, D.E., & Luper, H.L. Voice reaction time of stuttering and nonstuttering children and adults. *Journal of Fluency Disorders*, 1979, 4, 59-77.

Cross, D.E., Shadden, BB., & Luper, H.L. Effects of stimulus ear presentation on the voice reaction time of adult stutterers and nonstutterers. *Journal of Fluency Disorders*, 1979, 4, 45-58.

Cross, H.M. The motor capacities of stutterers. *Archives of Speech*, 1936, 7, 112-132.

Cullen, Jr., J.K., Fargo, N., Chase, R.A., & Baker, P. The development of auditory feedback monitoring. 1. Delayed auditory feedback studies on infant cry. *Journal of Speech and Hearing Research*, 1968, *11*, 85-93.

Culligan, W.L., & Springer, M.T. Voice initiation and termination times in stuttering and nonstuttering children. *Journal of Speech and Hearing Research*, 1980, *23*, 344-360.

Curlee, R.F., & Perkins, W.H. Conversational rate control therapy for stuttering. *Journal of Speech and Hearing Disorders*, 1969, *34*, 245-250.

Curlee, R.F. & Perkins, W.H. Effectiveness of a DAF conditioning program for adolescent and adult stutterers. *Behaviour Research and Therapy*, 1973, *11*, 395-401.

Davidson, G.D. Sidetone delay and reading rate, articulation, and pitch. *Journal of Speech and Hearing Research*, 1959, *2*, 266-270.

Delaney, C.M. The function of the middle ear muscles in stuttering. *The South African Journal of Communication Disorders*, 1979, *26*, 20-34.

Di Simoni, F.G. Preliminary study of certain timing relationships in the speech of stutterers. *Journal of the Acoustical Society of America*, 1974, *56*, 695-696.

Doms, M.C., & Lissens, D. Stuttering and the laryngectomee. In Y. Lebrun & R. Hoops (Eds.), *Neurolinguistic approaches to stuttering.* The Hague: Mouton, 1973.

Draegert, G.L. Relationships between voice variables and speech intelligibility in high level noise. *Speech Monographs*, 1951, *18*, 272-278.

Erickson, R. Assessing communication attitudes among stutterers. *Journal of Speech and Hearing Research*, 1969, *12*, 711-724.

Fairbanks, G. Systematic research in experimental phonetics: 1. A theory of the speech mechanism as a servosystem. *Journal of Speech and Hearing Disorders*, 1954, *19*, 133-139.

Fairbanks, G. Selective vocal effects of delayed auditory feedback. *Journal of Speech and Hearing Disorders*, 1955, *20*, 333-346.

Fairbanks, G., & Guttman, N. Effects of delayed auditory feedback upon articulation. *Journal of Speech and Hearing Research*, 1958, *1*, 12-22.

Falkowski, G.L., Guilford, A.M., & Sandler, J. Effectiveness of a modified version of airflow therapy: Case studies. *Journal of Speech and Hearing Disorders*, 1982, *47*, 160-164.

Few, L.R., & Lingwall, J.B. A further analysis of fluency within stuttered speech. *Journal of Speech and Hearing Research*, 1972, *15*, 356-363.

Fillenbaum, S. Adaptation with constant and variable delay in auditory feedback. *Psychonomic Science*, 1965, *3*, 45-46.

Florance, C.L., & Shames, G.H. Stuttering treatment: Issues in transfer and maintenance. *Seminars in Speech, Language and Hearing*, 1980, *1*, 375-388.

Fonagy, I. & Fonagy, J. Sound pressure level and duration. *Phonetica*, 1966, *15*, 14-21.

Franck, R. Integration of an intensive program for stutterers within the normal activities of a major acute hospital. *Australian Journal of Human Communication Disorders*, 1980, *8*, 4-15.

Frayne, H., Coates, S.F., & Marriner, N.A. Evaluation of posttreatment fluency by naive subjects. *Australian Journal of Human Communication Disorders*, 1977, *5*, 48-54.

Freeman, F.J., Phonation and fluency. In L.M. Webster & L.C. Furst (Eds.), *Proceedings of the First Annual Hayes Martin Conference on Vocal Tract Dynamics*. New York: Speech & Hearing Institute, New York, 1975.

Freeman, F.J. Phonation in stuttering: A review of current research. *Journal of Fluency Disorders*, 1979, *4*, 79-89.

Freeman, F.J., & Rosenfield, D.B. "Source" in dysfluency. *Journal of Fluency Disorders*, 1982, *7*, 295-296.

Freeman, F.J., & Ushijima, T. Laryngeal activity accompanying the moment of stuttering: A preliminary report of EMG investigations. *Journal of Fluency Disorders*, 1975, *1*, 36-45.

Freeman, F.J., & Ushijima, T. Laryngeal muscle activity during stuttering. *Journal of Speech and Hearing Research*, 1978, *21*, 538-562.

Freeman, F.J., Ushijima, T., & Hirose, H. Reply to Schwartz's "The core of the stuttering block." *Journal of Speech and Hearing Disorders*, 1975, *40*, 137-139.

Fujita, K. Pathophysiology of the larynx from the viewpoint of phonation. *Journal of the Japanese Society of Otorhinolaryngology*, 1966, *69*, 459.

Garber, S.F., & Martin, R.R. Effects of noise and increased vocal intensity on stuttering. *Journal of Speech and Hearing Research,* 1977, *20,* 233-240.

Garber, S.R., & Siegel, G.M. Feedback and motor control in stuttering. Unpublished manuscript, 1981.

Gautheron, B., Liorzou, A., Even, C., & Vallancien, B. The role of the larynx in stuttering. In Y. Lebrun & R. Hoops (Eds.), *Neurolinguistic approaches to stuttering.* The Hague: Mouton, 1973.

Geniesse, H. Stuttering. *Science,* 1935, *82,* 518.

Gibbons, E.W., Winchester, R.A. & Krebs, D.F. The variability of oral reading rate. *Journal of Speech and Hearing Disorders,* 1958, *23,* 591-593.

Gibney, N. Delayed auditory feedback: Changes in the volume intensity and the delay interval as variables affecting the fluency of stutterers' speech. *British Journal of Psychology,* 1973, *64,* 55-63.

Gifford, M.F. *Correcting nervous speech disorders.* New York: Prentice-Hall, 1939.

Gifford, M.F. *How to overcome stammering.* New York: Prentice-Hall,1940.

Goldiamond, I. The maintenance of ongoing fluent behavior and stuttering. *Journal of Mathetics,* 1962, *1,* 57-95.

Goldiamond, I. Stuttering and fluency as manipulatable operant response classes. In L. Krasner & L.P. Ullmann (Eds.), *Research in behavior modification.* New York: Holt, Rinehart & Winston, 1965.

Goldiamond, I. Supplementary statement to operant analysis control of fluent and nonfluent verbal behavior. Report to Department of Health, Education, and Welfare. Public Health Service Application No.MH-8876-03, 1967.

Goldiamond, I., Atkinson, C.J., & Bilger, R.C. Stabilization of behavior and prolonged exposure to delayed auditory feedback. *Science,* 1962, *135,* 437-438.

Gregory, H.H. Modeling procedures in the treatment of elementary school children who stutter. *Journal of Fluency Disorders,* 1973, *1,* 58-63.

Gregory, H.H. Review of Stuttering Solved by Martin F. Schwartz. *Rehabilitation Literature,* 1977, *38,* 157-159.

Gregory, H.H. The controversies: Analysis and current status. In H.H. Gregory (Ed.), *Controversies about stuttering therapy.* Baltimore: University Park Press, 1979.

Gregory, H.H. & Hill, D. Stuttering therapy for children. *Seminars in Speech, Language and Hearing.* 1980, *1,* 351-363.

Gruber, L. Sensory feedback and stuttering. *Journal of Speech and Hearing Disorders,* 1965, *30,* 378-380.

Gruber, L. Reply to "A feedback model of the stuttering problem—an engineer's view." *Journal of Speech and Hearing Disorders,* 1970, *35,* 309-310.

Guitar, B.E. A correction to "A response to Ingham's critique." *Journal of Speech and Hearing Disorders,* 1981, *46,* 440.

Guitar, B., & Bass, C. Stuttering therapy: The relation between attitude change and long-term outcome. *Journal of Speech and Hearing Disorders,* 1978, *43,* 392-400.

Guitar, B., & Peters, T.J. *Stuttering: An integration of contemporary therapies.* Memphis: Speech Foundation of America, 1980.

Hahn, E.F. A study of the effect of remedial treatment on the frequency of stuttering in oral reading. *Journal of Speech Disorders,* 1941, *6,* 29-38.

Ham, R., & Steer, M.D. Certain effects of alterations in auditory feedback. *Folia Phoniatrica,* 1967, *19,* 53-62.

Hanley, C.N., & Tiffany, W.R. An investigation into the use of electro-mechanically delayed side tone in auditory testing. *Journal of Speech and Hearing Disorders,* 1954, *19,* 367-374. (a)

Hanley, C.N., & Tiffany, W.R. Auditory malingering and psychogenic deafness. *Archives of Otolaryngology*, 1954, *60*, 197-201. (b)

Hanley, C.N., Tiffany, W.R., & Brungard, J.M. Skin resistance changes accompanying the sidetone test for auditory malingering. *Journal of Speech and Hearing Research*, 1958, *1*, 286-293.

Hanley, T.D. Comparative responses to delayed auditory feedback among speakers of four languages. *Phonetica*, 1968, *18*, 46-54.

Hayden, P.A., Scott, D.A., & Addicott,J. The effects of delayed auditory feedback on the overt behaviors of stutterers. *Journal of Fluency Disorders*, 1977, *2*, 235-246.

Healey, E.C., & Adams, M.R. Rate reduction strategies used by normally fluent and stuttering children and adults. *Journal of Fluency Disorders*, 1981, *6*, 1-14. (a)

Healey, E.C., & Adams, M.R. Speech timing skills of normally fluent and stuttering children and adults. *Journal of Fluency Disorders*, 1981, *6*, 233-246. (b)

Healey, E.C., Mallard, A.R., & Adams, M.R. Factors contributing to the reduction of stuttering during singing. *Journal of Speech and Hearing Research*, 1976, *19*, 475-480.

Healey, E.C., & Turton, L.J. Comments on laryngeal behavior during stuttering. *Journal of Speech and Hearing Research*, 1979, *22*, 412-413.

Hee, J.C., & Holmes, P.A. Elimination of stuttering by a regulated breathing approach. *Journal of Communication Pathology*, 1976, *8*, 40-44.

Helps, R., & Dalton, P. The effectiveness of an intensive group speech therapy programme for adult stammerers. *British Journal of Disorders of Communication*, 1979, *14*, 17-30.

Hersen, M., & Barlow, D.H. *Single case experimental designs: Strategies for studying behavior change*. New York: Pergamon, 1976.

Hillman, R.E., & Gilbert, H.R. Voice onset time for voiceless stop consonants in the fluent reading of stutterers and nonstutterers. *Journal of the Acoustical Society of America*, 1977, *61*, 610-611.

Homann, H.W.W. Experimentally induced blockage of a sustained vowel by nonlinear distortion of sidetone. *Speech Monographs*, 1964, *31*, 233.

Horovitz, L., Johnson, S., Pearlman, R., Schaffer, E., & Hedin, A. Stapedial reflex and anxiety in fluent and disfluent speakers. *Journal of Speech and Hearing Research*, 1978, *21*, 762-767.

Howie, P., Andrews, G., & Tanner, S. An intensive behaviour modification programme for the treatment of stutterers. *Australian Behaviour Therapist*, 1978, *5*, 17-19.

Howie, P.M., Tanner, S., & Andrews, G. Short- and long-term outcome in an intensive treatment program for adult stutterers. *Journal of Speech and Hearing Disorders*, 1981, *46*, 104-109.

Howie, P.M., & Woods, C.L. Token reinforcement during the instatement and shaping of fluency in the treatment of stuttering. *Journal of Applied Behavior Analysis*, 1982, *15*, 55-64.

Hutchinson, J.M., & Brown, D. The Adams and Reis observations revisited. *Journal of Fluency Disorders*, 1978, *3*, 149-154.

Hutchinson, J.M., & Navarre, B.M. The effect of metronome pacing on selected aerodynamic patterns of stuttered speech: Some preliminary observations and interpretations. *Journal of Fluency Disorders*, 1977, *2*, 189-204.

Hutchinson, J., & Norris, G. The differential effect of three auditory stimuli on the frequency of stuttering behaviors. *Journal of Fluency Disorders*, 1977, *2*, 283-293.

Ingham, R.J. The development, application and analysis of a token system for the treatment of adult stutterers. Unpublished doctoral dissertation, University of New South Wales, 1972.

Ingham, R.J. Operant methodology in stuttering therapy. In J. Eisenson (Ed.), *Stuttering: A second symposium*. New York: Harper & Row, 1975. (a)

Ingham, R.J. A comparison of covert and overt assessment procedures in stuttering therapy outcome evaluation. *Journal of Speech and Hearing Research,* 1975, *18,* 346-354. (b)

Ingham, R.J. Comment on "stuttering therapy: The relation between attitude change and long-term outcome." *Journal of Speech and Hearing Disorders,* 1979, *44,* 397-400.

Ingham, R.J. Modification of maintenance and generalization during stuttering treatment. *Journal of Speech and Hearing Research,* 1980, *23,* 732-745.

Ingham, R.J. Evaluation and maintenance in stuttering treatment: A search for ecstasy with nothing but agony. In E. Boberg (Ed.), *Maintenance of fluency.* New York: Elsevier, 1981, (a).

Ingham, R.J. *Stuttering therapy manual: Hierarchy control schedule.* Sydney, Australia: Cumberland College Press, 1981, (b).

Ingham, R.J. Some comments on "Stuttering and fluency: Exclusive events or points on a continuum?" *Journal of Fluency Disorders,* 1982, *7,* 303-307. (a)

Ingham, R.J. The effects of self-evaluation training on maintenance and generalization during stuttering treatment. *Journal of Speech and Hearing Disorders,* 1982, *47,* 271-280. (b)

Ingham, R.J. Stuttering therapy maintenance procedures. In W.H. Perkins (Ed.), *Current therapy of communication disorders.* New York: Thieme-Stratton, in press.

Ingham, R.J. On taken reinforcement and stuttering therapy: Another view on findings reported by Howie and Woods (1982). *Journal of Applied Behavior Analysis,* in press.

Ingham, R.J., & Andrews, G. Stuttering: The quality of fluency after treatment. *Journal of Communication Disorders,* 1971, *4,* 279-288.

Ingham, R.J., & Andrews, G. An analysis of a token economy in stuttering therapy. *Journal of Applied Behavior Analysis,* 1973, *6,* 219-229. (a)

Ingham, R.J., & Andrews, G. Behavior therapy and stuttering: A review. *Journal of Speech and Hearing Disorders,* 1973, *38,* 405-441. (b)

Ingham, R.J., & Andrews, G. Details of a token economy stuttering therapy programme for adults. *Australian Journal of Human Communication Disorders,* 1973, *1,* 13-20. (c)

Ingham, R.J., & Carroll, P.J. Listener judgment of differences in stutterers' nonstuttered speech during chorus- and nonchorus-reading conditions. *Journal of Speech and Hearing Research,* 1977, *20,* 293-302.

Ingham, R.J., Montgomery, J., & Ulliana, L. An investigation on the effect of manipulating phonation duration on stuttering. *Journal of Speech and Hearing Research,* in press.

Ingham, R.J., & Packman, A.C. Perceptual assessment of normalcy of speech following stuttering therapy. *Journal of Speech and Hearing Research,* 1978, *21,* 63-73.

Ingham, R.J., & Packman, A.C. A further evaluation of the speech of stutterers during chorus- and nonchorus-reading conditions. *Journal of Speech and Hearing Research,* 1979, *22,* 748-793.

Irving, R.W., & Webb, M.W. Teaching esophageal speech to a pre-operative severe stutterer. *Annals of Otology, Rhinology and Laryngology,* 1961, *70,* 1069-1079.

Irwin, A. *Stammering: Practical help for all ages.* Harmondsworth: Penguin, 1980.

Jensen, P., Sheehan, J., Williams, W., & LaPointe, L. Oral sensory-perceptual integrity of stutterers. *Folia Phoniatrica,* 1975, *27,* 38-45.

Johnson, L.J. Facilitating parental involvement in therapy of the disfluent child. *Seminars in Speech, Language and Hearing,* 1980, *1,* 301-309.

Johnson, L. Response to Azrin et al. *Journal of Speech and Hearing Disorders,* 1980, *40,* 426-427. (b)

Johnson, W., & Brown, S.F. Stuttering in relation to various speech sounds. *Quarterly Journal of Speech,* 1935, *21,* 481-496.

Johnson, W., & Rosen, L. Studies in the psychology of stuttering: VII. Effect of certain changes in speech pattern upon frequency of stuttering, *Journal of Speech Disorders,* 1937, *2,* 105-109.

Jones, B.A. Modified regulated-breathing in treatment of a single case of stuttering. *Perceptual and Motor Skills,* 1981, *52,* 130.

Jones, R.J., & Azrin, N.H. Behavioral engineering: Stuttering as a function of stimulus duration during speech synchronization. *Journal of Applied Behavior Analysis,* 1969, *2,* 223-229.

Kenyon, E.L. The etiology of stammering: The psychophysiologic facts which concern the production of speech sounds and of stammering. *Journal of Speech Disorders,* 1943, *8,* 337-348.

Kodman, F. Controlled reading rate under delayed speech feedback. *Journal of Auditory Research,* 1961, *3,* 186-194.

Krombholz, H., & Rubeling, H. Long-term effect of delayed auditory feedback on speech. *Folia Phoniatrica,* 1974, *26,* 339-361.

LaCroix, Z.E. Management of disfluent speech through self-recording procedures. *Journal of Speech and Hearing Disorders,* 1973, *38,* 272-274.

Ladouceur, R., Boudreau, L., & Theberge, S. Awareness training and regulated-breathing method in modification of stuttering. *Perceptual and Motor Skills,* 1981, *53,* 187-194.

Lane, H., & Tranel, B. The Lombard sign and the role of hearing in speech. *Journal of Speech and Hearing Research,* 1971, *14,* 677-709.

Langova, J., Moravek, M., Novak, A., & Petrik, M. Experimental interference with auditory feedback. *Folia Phoniatrica,* 1970, *22,* 191-196.

Lechner, B.N. The effects of delayed auditory feedback and masking on the fundamental frequency of stutterers and nonstutterers. *Journal of Speech and Hearing Research,* 1979, *22,* 343-353.

Lee, B. Some effects of sidetone delay. *Journal of the Acoustical Society of America,* 1950, *22,* 639-640. (a)

Lee, B. Effects of delayed speech feedback. *Journal of the Acoustical Society of America,* 1950, *22,* 824-826. (b)

Lee, B. Artificial stutter. *Journal of Speech and Hearing Disorders,* 1951, *16,* 53-55.

Lee, B.S., McGough, W.E., & Peins, M. A new method for stutter therapy. *Folia Phoniatrica,* 1973, *25,* 186-195.

Lee, J. Application of Martin Schwartz's airflow technique in the treatment of stuttering. *Journal of Speech and Hearing Disorders,* 1976, *41,* 133-134.

Lotzman, G. Zur anwendung variierter verzogerungszeiten bei balbuties. *Folia Phoniatrica,* 1961, *13,* 276-312.

Love, L.R., & Jeffress, L.A. Identification of brief pauses in the fluent speech of stutterers and nonstutterers. *Journal of Speech and Hearing Research,* 1971, *14,* 229-240.

MacKay, D.G. Metamorphosis of a critical interval: Age-linked changes in the delay in auditory feedback that produces maximal disruption of speech. *Journal of The Acoustical Society of America,* 1968, *43,* 811-821.

MacKay, D.G. To speak with an accent: Effects of nasal distortion on stuttering under delayed auditory feedback. *Perceptual Psychophysics,* 1969, *5,* 183-188.

MacKay, D.G. How does language familiarity influence stuttering under delayed auditory feedback? *Perceptual and Motor Skills,* 1970, *30,* 655-669.

Mahaffey, R., & Stromsta, C.P. The effects of auditory feedback as a function of frequency, intensity, time and sex. *De Therapia Vocis et Loquellae, II,* 1965, 233-235.

Mallard, A.R., Hicks, D.M., & Riggs, D.E. A comparison of stutterers and nonstutterers in a task of controlled voice onset. *Journal of Speech and Hearing Research,* 1982, *25,* 287-290.

Mallard, A.R., & Kelley, J.S. The Precision Fluency Shaping Program: Replication and evaluation. *Journal of Fluency Disorders*, 1982, *7*, 287-294.

Manning, W.H., & Coufal, K.J. The frequency of disfluencies during phonatory transitions in stuttered and nonstuttered speech. *Journal of Communication Disorders*, 1976, *9*, 75-81.

Martin, J.E. The signal detection hypothesis and perceptual defect theory of stuttering. *Journal of Speech and Hearing Disorders*, 1970, *35*, 252-255.

Martin, R.R. Personal communication, 1982.

Martin, R.R., & Haroldson, S.K. The effects of two treatment procedures on stuttering. *Journal of Communication Disorders*, 1969, *2*, 115-125.

Martin, R., & Haroldson, S.K. Effects of five experimental treatments on stuttering. *Journal of Speech and Hearing Research*, 1979, *22*, 132-146.

Martin, R.R., & Ingham, R.J. Stuttering. In B. Lahey (Ed.), *The modification of language behavior*, Springfield, IL: Charles C. Thomas, 1973.

Martin, R.R., Lawrence, B.A., Haroldson, S.K., & Gunderson, D. Stuttering and oral stereognosis. *Perceptual and Motor Skills*, 1981, *53*, 155-162.

May, A.E., & Hackwood, A. Some effects of masking and eliminating low frequency feedback on the speech of stammerers. *Behaviour Research andd Therapy*, 1968, *6*, 219-223.

McCabe, R.B., & McCollum, D. The personal reactions of a stuttering adult to delayed auditory feedback. *Journal of Speech and Hearing Research*, 1972, *37*, 536-541.

McCall, G.N. Spasmodic dysphonia and the stuttering block: Commonalities or possible connections. In L.M. Webster & L.C. Furst (Eds.), *Proceedings of the First Annual Hayes Martin Conference on Vocal Tract Dynamics*. New York: Speech & Hearing Institute, New York, 1975.

McFarlane, S.C., & Prins, D. Neural response time of stutterers and nonstutterers in selected oral motor tasks. *Journal of Speech and Hearing Research*, 1978, *21*, 768-778.

McGee, S.R., Hutchinson, J.M., & Deputy, P.N. The influence of the onset of phonation on the frequency of disfluency among children who stutter. *Journal of Speech and Hearing Research*, 1981, *24*, 269-272.

McLean, A.E., & Cooper, E.B. Electromyographic indications of laryngeal-area activity during stuttering expectancy. *Journal of Fluency Disorders*, 1978, *3*, 205-219.

Metz, D.E., Conture, E.G., & Caruso, A. Voice onset time, frication, and aspiration during stutterers' fluent speech. *Journal of Speech and Hearing Research*, 1979, *22*, 649-656.

Murphy, M., & Baumgartner, J.M. Voice initiation and termination time in stuttering and nonstuttering children. *Journal of Fluency Disorders*, 1981, *6*, 257-264.

Murray, F.P. Observations on therapy for stuttering in Japan. *Journal of Speech and Hearing Disorders*, 1958, *23*, 243-249.

Mysak, E.D. Servo-theory and stuttering. *Journal of Speech and Hearing Disorders*, 1960, *25*, 188-195.

Naylor, R.V. A comparative study of methods of estimating the severity of stuttering. *Journal of Speech and Hearing Disorders*, 1953, *18*, 30-37.

Neelley, J.N. A study of the speech behavior of stutterers and nonstutterers under normal and delayed auditory feedback. *Journal of Speech and Hearing Disorders*, Monograph Supplement No.7, 1961, 63-82.

Nessel, E. Die verzogerte sprachruckkopplung (Lee-effekt) bei stotterern. *Folia Phoniatrica*, 1958, *10*, 199-204.

Netsell, R. The acquisition of speech motor control: A perspective with directions for research. In R. Stark (Ed.), *Language behavior in infancy and early childhood*. New York: Elsevier North-Holland, 1981.

O'Dwyer, N.J., Quinn, P.T., Guitar, B.E., Andrews, G., & Neilson, P.D. Procedures for verification of electrode placement in EMG studies of orofacial and mandibular muscles. *Journal of Speech and Hearing Research*, 1981, *24*, 273-288.

Panconcelli-Calzia, G. Die bedingtheit des Lombardschen versuches in der stimmund sprachheilkunde. *Acta Otolaryngologica*, 1955, *45*, 244-251.

Peins, M., McGough, W.E., & Lee, B.S. Evaluation of a tape-recorded method of stuttering therapy: Improvement in a speaking task. *Journal of Speech and Hearing Research*, 1972, *15*, 364-371.

Perkins, W.H. Physiological studies. In J.G. Sheehan (Ed.), *Stuttering: Research and therapy*, New York: Harper & Row, 1970.

Perkins, W.H. Replacement of stuttering with normal speech: I. Rationale. *Journal of Speech and Hearing Disorders*, 1973, *38*, 283-294. (a)

Perkins, W.H. Replacement of stuttering with normal speech: II. Clinical procedures. *Journal of Speech and Hearing Disorders*, 1973, *38*, 295-303. (b)

Perkins, W.H. Author's response to "comment on 'replacement of stuttering with normal speech.' " *Journal of Speech and Hearing Disorders*, 1974, *39*, 106-107.

Perkins, W.H. Measurement and maintenance of fluency. In E. Boberg (Ed.), *Maintenance of fluency*. New York: Elsevier, 1981.

Perkins, W.H., Bell, J., Johnson, L., & Stocks, J. Phone rate and the effective planning time hypothesis of stuttering. *Journal of Speech and Hearing Research*, 1979, *22*, 747-755.

Perkins, W.H., Rudas, J., Johnson, L., & Bell, J. Stuttering: Discoordination of phonation with articulation and respiration. *Journal of Speech and Hearing Research*, 1976, *19*, 509-522.

Perkins, W.H., Rudas, J., Johnson, L., Michael, W.B., & Curlee, R.F. Replacement of stuttering with normal speech: 111. Clinical effectiveness. *Journal of Speech and Hearing Disorders*, 1974, *39*, 416-428.

Peters, R.W. The effect of changes in side-tone delay and level upon rate of oral reading of normal speakers. *Journal of Speech and Hearing Disorders*, 1956, *19*, 483-490.

Platt, J.R. Strong inference. *Science*, 1964, *146*, 347-353.

Poppen, R., Nunn, R.G., & Hook, S. Effects of several therapies on stuttering in a single case. *Journal of Fluency Disorders*, 1977, *2*, 35-44.

Prince Henry Hospital. *Therapist manual for the stuttering treatment program*. Division of Communication Disorders,1976.

Prosek, R.A., Montgomery, A.E., Walden, B.E., & Schwartz, D.M. Reaction-time measures of stutterers and nonstutterers. *Journal of Flluency Disorders*, 1979, *4*, 269-272.

Prosek, R.A., & Runyan, G.M. Temporal characteristics related to the discrimination of stutterers and nonstutterers' speech samples. *Journal of Speech and Hearing Research*, 1982, *25*, 29-33.

Ramig, P.R., & Adams, M.R. Vocal changes in stutterers and nonstutterers during high- and low-pitched speech. *Journal of Fluency Disorders*, 1981, *6*, 15-33.

Reich, A., Till, J., & Goldsmith, H. Laryngeal and manual reaction times of stuttering and nonstuttering adults. *Journal of Speech and Hearing Research*, 1981, *24*, 192-196.

Reis, R., & Adams, M.R. Comments on "The Adams and Reis observations revisited." *Journal of Fluency Disorders*, 1978, *3*, 299-302.

Resick, P.A., Wendiggensen, P., Ames, S., & Meyer, V. Systematic slowed speech: A new treatment for stuttering. *Behaviour Research and Therapy*, 1978, *16*, 161-167.

Ringel, R.L., & Minifie, F.D. Protensity estimates of stutterers and nonstutterers. *Journal of Speech and Hearing Research*, 1966, *9*, 289-296.

Robinson, G.M. The delayed auditory feedback effect as a function of speech rate. *Journal of Experimental Psychology*, 1972, *95*, 1-5.

Ruhm, H.B., & Cooper, Jr., W.A. Delayed feedback audiometry. *Journal of Speech and Hearing Disorders*, 1964, *29*, 448-455.

Runyan, C.M. & Adams, M.R. Perceptual study of the speech of "successfully therapeutized" stutterers. *Journal of Fluency Disorders*, 1978, *3*, 25-39.

Runyan, C.M., & Adams, M.R. Unsophisticated judges perceptual evaluations of the speech of "successfully treated" stutterers. *Journal of Fluency Disorders*, 1979, *4*, 29-38.

Runyan, C.M., & Bonifant, D.C. A perceptual comparison: All-voiced versus typical reading passage read by children. *Journal of Fluency Disorders*, 1981, *6*, 247-255.

Rustin, L. An intensive group programme for adolescent stammerers. *British Journal of Disorders of Communication*, 1978, *13*, 85-92.

Ryan, B. Operant procedures applied to stuttering therapy for children. *Journal of Speech and Hearing Disorders*, 1971, *36*, 264-280.

Ryan, B.P. *Programmed therapy for stuttering in children and adults*. Springfield, IL: Charles C.Thomas, 1974.

Ryan, B.P., & Van Kirk, B. The establishment, transfer and maintenance of fluent speech in 50 stutterers using delayed auditory feedback and operant procedures. *Journal of Speech and Hearing Disorders*, 1974, *39*, 3-10.

Schmitt, L.A., & Cooper, E.B. Fundamental frequencies in the oral reading behavior of stuttering and nonstuttering male children. *Journal of Communication Disorders*, 1978, *11*, 17-23.

Schwartz, D., & Webster, L.M. A clinical adaptation of the Hollins Precision Fluency Shaping Program through de-intensification. *Journal of Fluency Disorders*, 1977, *2*, 3-10. (a)

Schwartz, D., & Webster, L.M. More on the efficacy of a protracted precision fluency shaping program. *Journal of Fluency Disorders*, 1977, *2*, 205-215. (b)

Schwartz, M.F. Effect of delayed sidetone upon the reading rate of whispered speech. *Speech Monographs*, 1961, *26*, 293-295.

Schwartz, M.F. Syllable duration in oral and whispered speech. *Journal of the Acoustical Society of America*, 1967, *41*, 1367-1369.

Schwartz, M.F. The core of the stuttering block. *Journal of Speech and Hearing Disorders*, 1974, *39*, 169-177.

Schwartz, M.F. *Stuttering solved*. New York: McGraw-Hill, 1976.

Shaffer, G. Measures of jaw movement and phonation in nonstuttered and stuttered production of voiced and voiceless plosives. *Speech Monographs*, 1940, *7*, 85-92.

Shames, G.H. *The stutter-free speech program*. Publicity pamphlet for a treatment program conducted at Camp Challenge, Sorento, FL, August 15-22, 1982.

Shames, G.H., & Florance, C.L. *Stutter-free speech: A goal for therapy*. Columbus: Charles E. Merrill, 1980.

Shapiro, A.I. An electromyographic analysis of the fluent and dysfluent utterances of several types of stutterers. *Journal of Fluency Disorders*, 1980, *5*, 203-231.

Shearer, W.M., & Simmons, F.B. Middle ear activity during speech in normal speakers and stutterers. *Journal of Speech and Hearing Research*, 1965, *8*, 203-207.

Sheehan, J.G. Reflections on the behavioral modification of stuttering. In Speech Foundation of America, Publication No.7, *Conditioning in Stuttering Therapy*, Memphis: Speech Foundation of America, 1970.

Sheehan, J.G. Problems in the evaluation of progress and outcome. *Seminars in Speech, Language and Hearing*, 1980, *1*, 389-401.

Shine, R.E. Direct management of the beginning stutterer. *Seminars in Speech, Language and Hearing*, 1980, *1*, 339-350.

Shine, R.E. *Systematic fluency training for young children*. Tigarad,OR: C.C. Publications, 1981.

Siegel, G.M. Feedback process in speech development and disorder. Paper read to Van Riper Lectures in Speech Pathology and Audiology, Western Michigan University, Kalamazoo, MI, May 1981.

Siegel, G.M., Fehst, C.A., Garber, S.R., & Pick, Jr., H.L. Delayed auditory feedback with children. *Journal of Speech and Hearing Research*, 1980, *23*, 802-813.

Siegel, G.M., & Pick, Jr., H.L. Auditory feedback in the regulation of voice. *Journal of the Acoustical Society of America*, 1974, *56*, 1618-1624.

Sklar, B. A feedback model of the stuttering problem—an engineer's view. *Journal of Speech and Hearing Disorders*, 1969, *34*, 226-230.

Small, M.M. Treatment of stuttering: A case history. *Perceptual and Motor Skills*, 1975, *41*, 812.

Smith, K.U., *Delayed sensory feedback and behavior*. Philadelphia: Saunders, 1966.

Smith, K.U., & Tierney, D. Delayed speech feedback and age. *Journal of Speech and Hearing Research*, 1971, *14*, 214-219.

Smith, M.L., & Glass, G.V. Meta-analysis of psychotherapy outcome studies. *American Psychologist*, 1977, *32*, 752-760.

Soderberg, G.A. A study of the effects of delayed side-tone on four aspects of stutterers' speech during oral reading and spontaneous speech. *Speech Monographs*, 1960, *27*, 252-253.

Soderberg, G.A. Delayed auditory feedback and stuttering. *Journal of Speech and Hearing Disorders*, 1968, *33*, 260-267.

Soderberg, G.A. Delayed auditory feedback and the speech of stutterers: A review of studies. *Journal of Speech and Hearing Research*, 1969, *34*, 20-29.

Spencer, G. The status of environmental and group cohesiveness in the treatment of stuttering. *Australian Journal of Human Communication Disorders*, 1976, *4*, 140-145.

Spilka, B. Some vocal effects of different reading passages and time delays in speech feedback. *Journal of Speech and Hearing Disorders*, 1954, *19*, 37-47.

Spuehler, H.E. Delayed sidetone and auditory flutter. *Journal of Speech and Hearing Research*, 1962, *5*, 124-132.

Starbuck, J., & Steer, M. The adaptation effect in stuttering and its relation to thoracic and abdominal breathing. *Journal of Speech and Hearing Disorders*, 1954, *19*, 440-449.

Starkweather, C.W. Speech fluency and its development in normal children. In N.J. Lass (Ed.), *Speech and language: Advances in basic reserach and practice, Vol 4*. New York: Academic Press, 1980.

Starkweather, C.W., Hirschman, P., & Tannenbaum, R.S. Latency of vocaliztion onset: Stutterers versus non-stutterers. *Journal of Speech and Hearing Research*, 1976, *19*, 481-492.

Starkweather, C.W., & Myers, M. Duration of subsegments within the intervocalic intervals in stutterers and nonstutterers. *Journal of Fluency Disorders*, 1979, *4*, 205-214.

Stephen, S.C.G., & Haggard, M.P. Acoustic properties of masking/delayed feedback in the fluency of stutterers and controls. *Journal of Speech and Hearing Research*, 1980, *23*, 527-538.

Stokes, T.F., & Baer, D.M. An implicit technology of generalization. *Journal of Applied Behavior Analysis*, 1977, *10*, 349-367.

Stromsta, C. Experimental blockage of phonation by distorted sidetone. *Journal of Speech and Hearing Research*, 1959, *2*, 286-301.

Stromsta, C. Delays associated with certain sidetone pathways. *Journal of the Acoustical Society of America* 1962, *34*, 392-396.

Stromsta, C. Interaural phase disparity of stutterers and nonstutterers. *Journal of Speech and Hearing Research*, 1972, *15*, 771-780.

Stromsta, C., & Fibiger, S. Physiological correlates of the core behavior of stuttering. *Proceedings, XVIII International Congress of Logopedics and Phoniatrics*, Washington, 1980.

Sutton, S., & Chase, R.A. White noise and stuttering. *Journal of Speech and Hearing Research*, 1961, *4*, 72.

Tiffany, W.R., & Hanley, C.N. Delayed speech feedback as a test for auditory malingering. *Science*, 1952, *115*, 59-60.

Tiffany, W.R., & Hanley, C.N. Adaptation to delayed sidetone. *Journal of Speech and Hearing Disorders*, 1956, *21*, 164-172.

Timmons, B.A. Sex as a factor influencing sensitivity to delayed auditory feedback. *Perceptual and Motor Skills*, 1971, *32*, 824-826.

Timmons, A., & Boudreau, J.P. Auditory feedback as a major factor in stuttering. *Journal of Speech and Hearing Disorders*, 1972, *37*, 476-484.

Timmons, B.A., & Boudreau, J.P. Age, sex, and delay time as factors affecting reaction to delayed auditory feedback. *Perceptual and Motor Skills*, 1976, *43*, 27-30.

Timmons, B.A., & Boudreau, J.P. Delayed auditory feedback and the speech of stuttering and non-stuttering children. *Perceptual and Motor Skills*, 1978, *46*, 551-555.

Timmons, B.A., & Boudreau, J.P. Speech disfluencies and delayed auditory feedback reactions of stuttering and non-stuttering children. *Perceptual and Motor Skills*, 1978, *47*, 859-862. (b)

Timmons, B.A., & Rankin, R.J. Similarities in reaction of twins to delayed auditory feedback. *Perceptual and Motor Skills*, 1970, *30*, 935-938.

Treon, M., & Tamayo, F.M.V. The separate and combined effects of GSR biofeedback and delayed auditory feedback on stuttering: A preliminary study. *Journal of Fluency Disorders*, 1974, *1*, 3-9.

Tuck, A.E. An alaryngeal stutterer: A case history. *Journal of Fluency Disorders*, 1979, *4*, 239-243.

Turkat, I.D., Pomeranz, J.F., & Bruch, M.H. Rapid treatment of a 22-year stammering problem by slow speech training. *Scandinavian Journal of Behaviour Therapy*, 1981, *10*, 49-53.

Turnbaugh, K.R., & Guitar, B.E. Short-term intensive stuttering treatment in a public school setting. *Language, Speech and Hearing Services in Schools*, 1981, *12*, 107-114.

Van Kirk, B. Operant therapy programs for stuttering conducted in a rehabilitation center. *Rehabilitation Literature*, 1972, *33*, 107-108.

Van Riper, C. Study of the thoracic breathing of stutterers during expectancy and occurrence of stuttering spasms. *Journal of Speech Disorders*, 1936, *1*, 61-72.

Van Riper, C. *Speech therapy: A book of readings*. New York: Prentice-Hall, 1953.

Van Riper, C. *Speech correction: Principles and methods*. Englewood Cliffs, NJ: Prentice-Hall, 1954.

Van Riper, C. Behavior modification: An overview. In Speech Foundation of America, Publication No.7, *Conditioning in stuttering therapy*, Memphis: Speech Foundation of America, 1970.

Van Riper, C. *The treatment of stuttering*. Englewood Cliffs, NJ; Prentice-Hall, 1973.

Van Riper, C. To Banff—with love. *Western Michigan University Journal of Speech, Language and Hearing*, 1979, *15*, 1-3.

Venkatagiri, H.S. The relevance of DAF-induced speech disruption to the understanding of stuttering. *Journal of Fluency Disorders*, 1980, *5*, 87-98.

Venkatagiri, H.S. Reaction time for voiced and whispered /a/ in stutterers and nonstutters. *Journal of Fluency Disorders*, 1981, *6*, 265-271.

Watts, R. The treatment of stammering by the intensive practice of fluent speech. *British Journal of Disorders of Communication*, 1971, *6*, 144-147.

Webster, R.L. Stuttering: A way to eliminate it and a way to explain it. In R. Ulrich, T. Stachnik, & J. Mabry (Eds.), *Control of human behavior Vol. 2* Glenview, IL: Scott, Foresman & Company, 1970.

Webster, R.L. A behavioral analysis of stuttering treatment and theory. In K.S. Calhoun, H.E. Adams, & K.M. Mitchell (Eds.), *Innovative treatment methods in psychopathology*. New York: Wiley, 1974 (a).

Webster, R.L. *The precision fluency shaping program: Speech reconstruction for stutterers*. Roanoke, VA: Hollins Communication Research Institute, 1974 (b).

Webster, R.L. Concept and theory in stuttering: An insufficiency of empiricism. *Journal of Communication Disorders*, 1977, *10*, 65-71. (a)

Webster, R.L. A few observations on the manipulation of speech response characteristics in stutterers. *Journal of Communication Disorders*, 1977, *10*, 73-76. (b)

Webster, R.L. Empirical considerations regarding stuttering therapy. In H.H. Gregory (Ed.), *Controversies about stuttering therapy*. Baltimore: University Park Press, 1979.

Webster, R.L. Evolution of a target-based behavioral therapy for stuttering. *Journal of Fluency Disorders*, 1980, *5*, 303-320.

Webster, R.L., & Lubker, B.B. Interrelationships among fluency producing variables in stuttered speech. *Journal of Speech and Hearing Research*, 1968, *11*, 754-766.

Webster, R.L., Schumacher, S.J., & Lubker, B.B. Changes in stuttering frequency as a function of various intervals of delayed auditory feedback. *Journal of Abnormal Psychology*, 1970, *75*, 45-49.

Weiner, A.E. Vocal control therapy for stutterers: A trial program. *Journal of Fluency Disorders*, 1978, *3*, 115-126.

Weiner, A. Response to Andrews, Guitar and Howie. *Journal of Speech and Hearing Disorders*, 1981, *46*, 335.

Wendahl, R., & Cole, J. Identification of stuttering during relatively fluent speech. *Journal of Speech and Hearing Research*, 1961, *4*, 281-286.

West, R., & Nusbaum, E. A motor test for dysphemia. *Quarterly Journal of Speech*, 1929, *15*, 469-479.

Wiener, N. *Cybernetics: Or control and communication in the animal and the machine*. Cambridge, MA: MIT Press, 1948.

Williamson, D.A., Epstein, L.H., & Coburn, C. Multiple baseline analysis of the regulated breathing procedure for the treatment of stuttering. *Journal of Fluency Disorders*, 1981, *6*, 327-339.

Winchester, R.A., Gibbons, E.W., & Krebs, D.F. Adaptation to sustained delayed sidetone. *Journal of Speech and Hearing Disorders*, 1959, *24*, 25-28.

Wingate, M.E., A standard definition of stuttering. *Journal of Speech and Hearing Disorders*, 1964, *29*, 484-489.

Wingate, M.E. Prosody in stuttering adaptation. *Journal of Speech and Hearing Research*, 1966, *9*, 550-556. (a)

Wingate, M.E. Stuttering adaptation and learning I. The relevance of adaptation studies to stuttering as learned behavior. *Journal of Speech and Hearing Disorders*, 1966, *31*, 148-156. (b)

Wingate, M.E. Stuttering as phonetic transition defect. *Journal of Speech and Hearing Disorders*, 1969, *34*, 107-108. (a)

Wingate, M.E. Sound and pattern in "artificial" fluency. *Journal of Speech and Hearing Research*, 1969, *12*, 677-686. (b)

Wingate, M.E. Effect on stuttering of changes in audition. *Journal of Speech and Hearing Research*, 1970, *13*, 861-873.

Wingate, M.E. *Stuttering: Theory and treatment*. New York: Irvington, 1976.

Wingate, M.E. The immediate source of stuttering: An integration of evidence. *Journal of Communication Disorders*, 1977, *10*, 45-51.

Wingate, M.E. The first three words. *Journal of Speech and Hearing Research*, 1979, *22*, 604-612.

Wingate, M.E. "Vocalization" ≠ phonation. *Journal of Speech and Hearing Research*, 1979, *22*, 667-671. (b)

Wingate, M.E. Sound and pattern in artificial fluency: Spectrographic evidence. *Journal of Fluency Disorders*, 1981, *6*, 95-118. (a)

Wingate, M.E. Questionnaire study of laryngectomee stutterers. *Journal of Fluency Disorders*, 1981, *6*, 273-281. (b)

Wolf, A.A., & Wolf, E.G. Feedback processes in the theory of certain speech disorders. *Speech Pathology and Therapy*, 1959, *2*, 48-55.

Wood, R., & Flynn, J.M. A self-evaluation token system versus an external evaluation token system alone in a residential setting with predelinquent youths. *Journal of Applied Behavior Analysis*, 1978, *4*, 503-512.

Woolf, G. The assessment of stuttering as struggle, avoidance, and expectancy. *British Journal of Disorders of Communication*, 1967, *2*, 158-171.

Wyke, B. Neurological mechanisms in stammering: An hypothesis. *British Journal of Disorders of Communication*, 1970, *5*, 6-15.

Wyke, B. The neurology of stuttering. *Journal of Psychosomatic Research*, 1971, *15*, 423-432.

Wyke, B. Phonatory reflex mechanisms and stammering. *Folia Phoniatrica*, 1974, *25*, 321-338.

Yates, A.J. Recent empirical and theoretical approaches to the experimental manipulation of speech in normal subjects and in stammerers. *Behaviour Research and Therapy*, 1963, *1*, 95-119.

Yates, A.J. Delayed auditory feedback and shadowing. *Quarterly Journal of Experimental Psychology*, 1965, *17*, 125-131.

Yates, A.J. The relationship between theory and therapy in the clinical treatment of stuttering. In B.B. Gray & G. England (Eds.), *Stuttering and the conditioning therapies*. Monterey, CA: Monterey Institute for Speech and Hearing, 1969.

Yates, A.J. *Behavior therapy*. New York: Wiley, 1970.

Yates, A.J. *Theory and practice in behavior therapy*. New York: Wiley, 1975.

Yeni-Komshian, G., Chase, R.A., & Mobley, R.L. The development of auditory feedback monitoring. II. Delayed auditory feedback studies on the speech of children between two and three years of age. *Journal of Speech and Hearing Research*, 1968, *11*, 307-315.

Young, M. Identification of stutterers from recorded samples of their "fluent" speech. *Journal of Speech and Hearing Research*, 1964, *7*, 302-303.

Young, M.A. Comment on "Stuttering frequency and the onset of phonation." *Journal of Speech and Hearing Research*, 1975, *18*, 600-602.

Zalosh, S., & Salzman, L.F. After effects of delayed auditory feedback. *Perceptual and Motor Skills*, 1965, *20*, 817-823.

Zerneri, L. Attempts to use delayed speech feedback in stuttering therapy. *Journal Francais d' Oto-Rhino-Laryngologie et Chirurgie Maxillo-Faciale*, 1966, *15*, 415-418.

Zimmerman, G. Articulatory dynamics of fluent utterances of stutterers and non-stutterers. *Journal of Speech and Hearing Research,* 1980, 23, 95-107. (a)

Zimmerman, G. Articulatory behaviors associated with stuttering: A cinefluorographic analysis. *Journal of Speech and Hearing Research,* 1980, *23,* 108-121.

Zimmerman, G. Stuttering: A disorder of movement. *Journal of Speech and Hearing Research,* 1980, *22,* 122-136. (c)

Zimmerman, G., & Allen, E.L. Questions concerning Schwartz's "The core of the stuttering block." *Journal of Speech and Hearing Disorders,* 1975. *40,* 135-136.

11

Other Approaches to Anxiety-Reduction Treatment of Stuttering

Introduction

This chapter brings together three aproaches to stuttering treatment that have been concerned, in different ways, with the influence of anxiety or stress on the disorder, but which do not fit comfortably with the procedures discussed in Chapter 6. These treatment approaches are biofeedback, hypnosis, and drug therapy. Each approach has little in common with the other, except that their modus operandi derives from the premise that if tension or stress is modified, then stuttering will also be modified. The main reason for reserving their review until this point is because they are more appropriately considered against the backdrop of precedures dealt with in previous chapters. This is especially true of biofeedback. Each approach may eventually warrant more extensive coverage, but, for the present, they mainly represent alternative applications of the anxiety-reduction principle of treatment. This chapter will also differ slightly from previous chapters in that only limited consideration will be given to the experimental foundations of these treatments.

Biofeedback and Stuttering

Introduction

The previous chapters reveal that virtually every behavior therapy development has almost immediately found its way into stuttering therapy. Not surprisingly, therefore, biofeedback, perhaps the most publicized current procedure, was quickly introduced to stuttering therapy. What is surprising, however, is that in spite of its popularity and its apparent suitability for various stuttering treatments, the reports on its use with stutters have been relatively meager—certainly meager in comparison to its widespread use in behavior therapy.

Attempts to identify biofeedback's distinguishing features have caused some minor debates, principally because of its connections with relaxation training (Tarler-Benlolo, 1978) and its procedural resemblance to operant-conditioning methodology (Hatch & Gatchel, 1981; Shapiro & Surwit, 1976). Nonetheless, among many definitions that have been offered for biofeedback, perhaps one offered by Yates (1980) is fairly representative and serves to capture its distinctiveness:

> Biofeedback refers to the display of some aspect of the physiological functioning of the individual with the expectation that observation of the characteristics of the display will enable the individual to attain increased voluntary control over the physiological function being displayed (p.1).

When this procedure has been employed in a clinical context, it has generally involved physiological functions that are not usually under voluntary control, or the regulation of functions that have been impeded by trauma or disease. The biofeedback process depends on the detection and amplification of response characteristics of the physiological function, the processing of the response characteristics of the physiological function, the processing of the response, and, finally, immediate feedback of a form of the response. It will be recognized from the previous chapter that biofeedback therefore incorporates a closed-loop feedback system. It may also be conceptualized as a response-contingent procedure, particularly when the feedback signal is noncontinuous; that is, it occurs only when the function exceeds some level. However, the main point of difference between these procedures probably relates to the almost traditional description of operants as responses that exert control over the external environment. In contrast, biofeedback endeavors to train the subject to be able to exert control over the internal environment.

Another aspect of biofeedback methodology in a clinical context is that it involves physiological functions that are either necessary conditions for the presence of a problem behavior, or *are* the problem behavior. In either case they are not usually controllable unless transduced for feedback display. Certain physiological-response systems are frequently employed in clinical applications of biofeedback in the belief that they have functional relevance for a particular problem, or that they are the problem. Among the more common systems are blood pressure, finger temperature, heart rate, electromyograms (EMG), galvanic skin reponse (GSR), and electroencephalograms (EEG). Thus far only EMG, GSR, and EEG have been used to either assess or treat stutterers: consequently, only these biofeedback systems will be considered in this chapter.

EMG is a response to minute electrochemical changes that occur when a muscle contracts. This can be measured either directly, via implanted electrodes, or by surface electrodes that distinguish changes, invariably in certain groups of muscles, from a general surface "noise" level in other muscle areas. The signal can be transduced so that it reflects the amplitude and frequency of the target muscle(s) activity.

A GSR measure is essentially a recorded variation in the electrical conductance of the skin that normally occurs in response to stimulation or arousal. This response takes the form of activation in the sweat glands and usually corresponds to unusual emotional reactions. The GSR is typically recorded from the subject's hands.

EEG is the transduction of electrical activity from the cerebral cortex. No single cell is involved, but rather, the average pattern of firing from many thousands of neurons that occasionally synchronize to form regular patterns within the EEG. Four major frequency patterns have been identified and each has been associated with some perceived state. For example, the 14-30 Hz, or Beta pattern, is associated with an alert and "thinking" state, while the Alpha pattern (8-13 Hz), is associated with relaxed alertness. The lower frequency patterns, Theta and Delta, normally occur during sleep. The Alpha pattern has been of most interest to biofeedback clinicians, but, as will be seen, it has the awkward characteristic of being influenced by a variety of difficult-to-control conditions.

Most applications of biofeedback in stuttering have involved EMG recording, largely because of its success in controlling and reducing minute muscle activity and, thereby, its apparent suitability for systematic desensitization procedures. The first EMG studies were carried out by Hefferline (1958), Basmajian (1963), and Carlsoo and Edfeldt (1963), and demonstrated the considerable control that humans can have over microvoltage levels of muscle activity. Hefferline's investigations ultimately had some relevance for stuttering, since they showed that normal subjects could manipulate masseter-muscle activity via visual feedback from surface electrodes. Basmajian (1963) demonstrated similar effects from single motor units in hand muscles using implanted electrodes—his subjects could repress one motor unit and recruit another independently, with assistance from aural EMG feedback. In later investigations, Basmajian and Newton (1974) showed that clarinet players could control single motor units in their cheek muscles, and Basmajian and White (1973) found similar effects were possible in the lip muscles of trumpet players. These studies had special relevance to stuttering research, since they demonstrated the remarkable amount of control that humans could exert over many of the muscles that are integral to speech behavior. Subsequently, as Yates (1980) has observed, it became clear that frequency-modified auditory feedback was especially effective in achieving single motor unit control and that it was also possible to maintain this control for lengthy periods without feedback.

Surface EMG muscle activity recording does not give a precise measure of specific muscle action but it does reflect general levels of muscle tension in regions that are proximate to the placement of an EMG electrode. The clinical implications of being able to transduce measures of this tension were considerable since excessive muscle tension had long been regarded as significantly implicated in numerous problem conditions (Jacobson, 1938; Wolpe, 1958). For example, tension headaches had been regarded as related to—and possibly caused by—excessive contractions of the head musculature, particularly the frontalis muscle (Wolff, 1963). This led Budzynski and Stoyva (1969) to speculate that training subjects to control frontalis muscle tension would assist relaxation treatment for tension headaches as well as many other tension-related disorders.

Budzynski and Stoyva's (1969) pioneering biofeedback therapy procedure employed analog audio EMG feedback from surface electrodes located just above both eyebrows. It was assumed that forehead muscle activity, particularly in this region, is dominated by the frontalis muscle activity. They arranged for 15 normal subjects to be randomly allocated to either a no-feedback control, an irrelevant-feedback group (the subjects heard a fixed low tone), and an experimental group that was instructed to try to keep the feedback tone as low as possible (equatable with low muscle tension). All subjects were told to relax deeply, but the experimental group produced the lowest muscle action potential, and retained that low level in a final no-feedback session. This continuous-feedback procedure founded a host of investigations designed to test the procedure's value in treating tension headaches, chronic anxiety (general or specific), insomnia, hyperactivity, drug abuse, and other conditions thought to involve excessive muscle tension. Budzynski and colleagues (Budzynski, Stoyva, & Adler, 1970; Budzynski, Stoyva, Adler, & Mullaney, 1973) later reported that their procedure was superior to relaxation in reducing the frequency of tension headaches. However, much subsequent research (Burish, 1981; Yates, 1980) on this treatment technique has shown that these were not reliable findings. In fact, the results of carefully controlled studies, mainly with the Budzynski et al. procedure, on the treatment of all of the above problems has shown "that even when EMG biofeedback training is effective in treating various stress-related disorders, it is generally no more effective in this regard than other forms of relaxation training" (Burish, 1981, p.417). In other words, the less expensive systematic relaxation and desensitization procedures described in Chapter 6 may be equally effective means of treating stress-related conditions.

The current troubled state of EMG-biofeedback-treatment research may simply reflect the present state of technology. It is possible, for example, that future technical developments will make it possible to identify more specific muscle groups that are either implicated in, or integral to, a particluar problem. But this assumes that the main reason for its use is to train subjects to gain control over such critical muscle systems. This may differ from the assumption that has prompted the use of biofeedback in much therapy practice. Budzynski and Stoyva (1969), for instance, speculated that reducing tension in specific muscle groups with biofeedback might generalize to other unrelated muscle groups. They envisaged that the procedure would thereby turn out to be a more reliable, even more valid, method for use with systematic desensitization. These different treatment assumptions also have significance to the findings and current applications of EMG biofeedback in stuttering treatment.

EMG Measurement and Stuttering

The notion that stutterers experience unusual and uncontrollable muscle actions preceding, or during, an interval of stuttering has had much currency throughout the long history of research and treatment for this disorder. The earlier descriptions of stuttering as a "spasm," for instance, graphically depicts the presumed role of unusual muscle action in the disorder. Much of that research has already been reviewed in Chapters 6 and 10. So in what follows, the main interest will be in research on the types of muscle activities that are implicated in the appearance and variation of stuttering, or activities that may have relevance for biofeedback treatment.

The most obvious places to look for critical muscle activities are those that stutterers describe as tension-filled during stuttering. Snidecor (1955) conducted such a study and found that his respondents described numerous parts of their bodies as tension-ridden during stuttering episodes; predictably, the most common areas were in the oral region, particularly the jaws and front of the throat. With some justification, therefore, many biofeedback investigators have sought to determine whether stutterers exhibit unusual levels of tension in the articulators and the laryngeal zone.

The principal facial muscle group controlling jaw movements are the masseter muscles. These muscles have been an obvious point of interest for those who argue that abnormal muscle activity might be associated with stuttering. This possiblity led Travis (1934) to conduct the very first surface-EMG investigation on the speech musculature of stutterers. He transduced the activity of the left and right side masseter muscles of 24 adult stutterers, plus a matched group of nonstutterers, and reported that only during stutterings were there disharmonious muscle actions from both sides of the jaw. Such disharmony was also described as less evident when these subjects emulated stuttering. But Travis supplied no data in support of these findings. Sheehan and Voas (1954) also obtained surface-EMG measures of masseter-muscle activity during stuttered and fluent single word utterances. Essentially, they found the point of maximum muscle activity occurred at longer intervals after the onset of a stuttered word than after the onset of a fluent word—which is predictable, since the stuttered word usually takes longer to complete. Some of the main methodological problems in these initial EMG investigations were addressed by Williams (1955). He used various methods to quantify EMG activity, but failed to find muscle actions that distinguished between stutterings, other utterances, or jaw movements by either normals (n=15) or stutterers (n=15).

There have been two other EMG studies of masseter-muscle activity in stutterers that purport to demonstrate stutterers have unusual activity levels. Platt and Basili (1973) had three adult stutterers orally read /p/- or /b/-initial words while blocking "in a fashion that was usual for them," and while making similar jaw movements. Masseter and suprahyoid (beneath the chin) muscle actions were derived from surface EMG recordings made during 1400 to 400 msecs prior to each response. Generally, Platt and Basili found that the frequency and amplitude of the signal did not differ during the speech or nonspeech tasks, and that a substantial level of activity preceded each response. This may show that minute tremors precede stuttering or stuttering-like movements. But there are some problems with this study that limit its interpretive value. For example, there was no evidence that the subjects actually stuttered on the target words, and there was no control over the possibility that even the fluent productions by nonstutterers could have produced similar activity patterns. It is also noteworthy that this study failed to include reliability data.

Kalotkin, Manschreck, and O'Brien (1979) reported that a group of stutterers (n=6; 24-33 years) displayed significantly greater masseter-muscle tension, when compared with six matched nonstutterers, during conversational speech, but not during relaxation. However, this study is also flawed by the absence of reliability data, plus the absence of measures of a relationship between their subjects' stuttering and surface-EMG activity. Even if these data were reliable, however, the finding that stutterers have slightly higher EMG scores does not demonstrate a functional association between EMG activity and stuttering (this is made more likely by the subjects' stuttering severity ratings failing to correlate with their EMG scores).

In general, the EMG investigations of masseter muscle activity show that any increments in this activity reflect movements which occur during the interval of stuttering rather than preceding a stuttering. Of course, this may also mean that such heightened activity is antagonistic to the production of fluent utterances. Moreover, the potential clinical value of any measured changes in masseter-muscle activity would appear to be much more substantial if this characteristic preceded, rather than accompanied, a stuttering.

The role of laryngeal muscle activity in stuttering has been the focus of much research in recent years, most of which was discussed in the previous chapter. It will be recalled, for example, that direct EMG recordings (Freeman & Ushijima, 1978) and fluoroscopic analyses (Conture, McCall, & Brewer, 1977) of the activities of certain laryngeal muscle groups, most notably the posterior and anterior cricoarytenoid muscles, have suggested that abnormal abduction-adduction patterns accompany stutterings. Indeed, there is convincing evidence that these abnormal patterns are unlikely to be invariantly related to stuttering (Shapiro, 1980). But of relevance to biofeedback research is lack of evidence that this unusual action actually precedes the moment of stuttering. Like the activities of the masseter muscle, it may emerge that these unusual laryngeal patterns only occur during the extraordinary movements that accompany a stutter. In this event it seems reasonable to speculate that they would have rather limited functional value in feedback arrangements. The point is illustrated in a study by McLean and Cooper (1978). They obtained surface EMG recordings of the larynx of 19 stutterers (14-77 years) during a 10-second interval preceding either an expected stutter or a fluent production. This revealed no significant differences between the levels of muscle activity preceding a stuttered or nonstuttered production, nor between correctly or incorrectly anticipated events. The possibility, though, that variations in laryngeal-muscle activity may accompany variations in stuttering frequency is indirectly suggested in a study of nonstutterers by Moore, Cunko, and Flowers (1979). They reported that EMG activity measures of masseter- and laryngeal-muscle activity showed differential trends with reductions in disfluencies across repeated oral readings: only the laryngeal-muscle-EMG measures tended to decrease along with disfluencies. At best, these findings simply imply that unusual laryngeal-muscle activity may accompany the interval of stuttering; they give no indication that such activity precedes the onset of stuttering.

All of the foregoing studies on EMG measurement with stuttering have demonstrated that variable, but heightened, muscle activity in the masseter and laryngeal areas may accompany stuttering. But these are not the only sites that have been investigated in studies concerned with manipulating feedback from muscle areas in stutterers. Before these studies are reveiwed, however, consideration should be given to findings which highlight the extensive individual differences in principal muscle activities during or preceding stuttering. Myers (1978) obtained eight different measures (respiration, inspiration, expiration, blood volume pulse, tonic and phasic skin conductance via GSR, heart rate, and EMG measures of the laryngeal area) from eight stutterers prior to, or during, stutterings. These measures showed that only one subject's laryngeal-EMG level was substantially correlated with prestuttering or stuttering intervals, while GSR measures tended to correlate with similar events for only one other subject. Overall, Myers's data reveal little evidence of any other association between these measures. The obvious implication from these findings for biofeedback methodology is that they highlight the importance of searching for highly individualized functional relationships between muscle tension and stuttering—certainly, a strategy synonymous with behavior therapy practice.

The previous studies have shown that EMG muscle activity is not usually associated with intervals preceding stuttering. But it could be that the feedback of activity levels accompanying stuttering may be useful in reducing its severity or frequency.This possibility will be considered in the course of the following review of biofeedback modifications and/or treatments of stuttering. Incidentally, unlike most procedures, there is much overlap between the experimental investigations of biofeedback and its use in a therapy context. And it is this blending of experimentation and therapy—all too infrequent in stuttering therapy—which is beginning to yield some reasonably clear indications of biofeedback's treatment value.

EMG Feedback and Stuttering

The initial applications of EMG biofeedback to stutterers appeared in 1975.The first was a report by Hanna, Wilfling, and McNeil (1975), who described a time-series experiment on a 19-year-old male stutterer whose "disfluencies were accompanied by obvious throat and facial tension" (p.270). Surface-EMG recording and feedback from the thyroid prominence occurred during two experimental sessions in which the subject spoke spontaneously about scenes shown on TAT cards. Following a 9-minute baseline period, the subject was taught to modify an audio frequency that increased in proportion to the EMG signal. He was then instructed to keep the tone at a low frequency during subsequent 9-minute feedback sessions. In the first experimental session the "feedback on" conditions were associated with a lower percentage of syllables stuttered than the "feedback off" conditions. The second session included a false feedback condition (the subject was unaware that his EMG feedback signals were actually generated by another person), which showed that part of the effects may have been due to the presence of the tone. The sum findings from this study were not particularly impressive. To begin with, the subject's data were not accompanied by reliability estimates and his speech rate was extremely slow across all conditions. In summary, his percentage of syllables stuttered was generally reduced to slightly below 50% of baseline levels during "feedback on" conditions, and his speech rate went from 47.1 words per minute during the baseline to a maximum of only 57.1 during the true feedback conditions. It was also noted that the EMG levels were consistently reduced during "feedback on" conditions.

Guitar (1975) reported a two-part study which investigated the effects of different types of EMG feedback with four adult stutterers. The first part measured the results of training three stutterers to reduce EMG-activity levels derived from four separate sites; frontalis, lip, chin, and larynx. Comparisons were then made between the percentage of microvoltage reduction from a baseline level of activity at a site, and the percentage of reduced stutterings on a word list which had been paired with feedback conditions. Variable results were reported; one subject showed most reductions as a result of lip-site training, another produced most benefits from the laryngeal-area feedback, and for the third subject, the lip- and larynx-site-feedback conditions were equally related to reduced stuttering. It was also reported, informally, that some generalization of the treatment's gains had been detected in beyond-clinic conditions for two of these subjects. The fourth stutterer, a 32-year-old male, was the subject of a more extensive therapy-oriented study. A pretreatment assessment period showed his conversational speech contained a mean of 17% syllables stuttered (%SS), while telephone conversations over part of this period yielded 19%SS. Pre-utterance EMG levels were compared with those obtained at resting levels in a pretreatment condition, and this led to the choice of a chin site for feedback training. In two 40-minute training sessions, the subject was taught to reduce EMG-feedback-tone levels just before uttering a word he thought he would stutter. These were followed by three 40-minute treatment sessions designed to reduce stuttering only during conversational speech. In the first session, EMG feedback was provided, but in the last two sessions no feedback was provided, and the subject was simply instructed to retain the low EMG levels achieved in earlier sessions. Over these three sessions, the subject's %SS scores were virtually zero. By contrast, he produced a mean of 22%SS during a series of concurrent office-telephone calls. He was then instructed to use his muscle-reduction skills during all telephone calls in his office, and again without the feedback equipment. Telephone calls, of unspecified length, over 10 days showed his stuttering reduced immediately to 2%SS and remained at 0%SS over the final 8 days. A video recording 5 weeks later of the subject conversing with a stranger also revealed no stuttering. Nine months later, the subject sent the experimenter a tape recording of his conversational and telephone speech and, once again, no stuttering was recorded (his speech rate was stated to be normal). The reliability of the stuttering measures was based on .90 agreement between subject's and experimenter's counts during oral reading. In many respects, this is one of the most interesting examples of the application of a behavior therapy procedure in the treatment of stuttering. To some extent it is weakened by the absence of speech-rate data, but it does describe a useful and inventive application of biofeedback methodology in stuttering therapy. As time passes, though, it becomes more interesting for another puzzling reason—as will be seen, it is still the only study to have reported an apparently successful outcome from the exclusive use of biofeedback methodology in stuttering therapy.

The third 1975 study was reported by Legewie, Cleary, and Rackensperger (1975). In this study (which clearly suffers from its English translation), the experimenters described surface-EMG monitoring of various areas of the face for one subject (25 years) and surface-EMG feedback from the submandibular muscle in the treatment of a 24-year-old stutterer. The latter subject was described as hospitalized in a psychiatric ward for "severe stuttering accompanied by neurotic disorder showing depressive anacastic features." From limited descriptive data provided on the first subject, it was claimed that EMG recordings made "it possible to register a 'micro' symptom: short clonic and tonic contractions without manifest stuttering" (p.139). In the second subject, EMG activity was fed back whenever it reached a level "above which smooth syllable-time speech was not possible and gave way to speech blocks" (p.140). It is not made clear whether the subject continued to receive training in the use of rhythmic speech—a procedure the clinicians had previously introduced in conjunction with a metronome-based treatment. The subject was reported to have been able to talk to three or four people "without long speech blocks" over the course of a vaguely described treatment schedule. However, it was also reported that biofeedback's contribution "to the therapy and rehabilitation of the patient was practically nil" (p.141). Unhappily, these experimenters failed to include any speech-performance data in their report.

Another investigation on laryngeal area EMG biofeedback was reported by Cross (1977). Like the Hanna et al. (1975) study, Cross also endeavored to distinguish the effect of false and true feedback, but during oral reading rather than spontaneous speaking conditions. Four young adult stutterers, who had "recently been or ... [were] presently enrolled in stuttering therapy" (Cross, 1977, p.110), orally read a 200-word "adaptation passage," a 500-word-baseline passage, and a 500-word experimental passage, in three sessions over a week. Prior to the experiment, the subjects were informed "that the tension in the laryngeal area during speech had been shown to be positively correlated with their increased stuttering" (p.111), and that the EMG-click-frequency rate would reflect that tension. While the subjects were only told to listen to the click rate in the experimental readings, it is reasonable to assume that they would have endeavored to reduce that rate. The experimental readings involved one of the three conditions that were given in random order across the four subjects: (1) false increase in feedback, (2) false decrease in feedback, and (3) true feedback. Only median percentages of stutterings were reported; these showed that the true feedback condition was associated with a median decrease of 9%, although the false-increase-feedback condition also produced a 5% decrease. By contrast, the false-decrease condition was only associated with a median 1% decrease. But these findings do not show whether this was a consistent trend across all subjects, and their value is weakened by the absence of speech-rate or reliability data.

The contribution to stuttering modification of EMG feedback from areas other than the larynx has been explored in a few other experimental and therapy-oriented studies. With the exception of Guitar's (1975) study, only one research group has investigated the influence of frontalis-muscle-EMG feedback on stuttering.[1] This sole investigation was by Pachman, Oelschlaeger, Hughes, and Hughes (1978), who measured the association between increases and decreases in frontalis-muscle-EMG feedback, and some stuttering behaviors, by two "college age" stutterers. Unfortunately, the behaviors were restricted to part-word repetitions, and the report only summarized the procedure and findings. With training, both subjects were able to increase and lower their EMG-auditory-feedback signal during spontaneous speech, and in subsequent sessions it was found that both of these directional changes in EMG level were associated with unspecified reductions in part-word repetitions. This study had a rather limited perspective, but it does point up some interesting conceptual issues with respect to biofeedback. Almost all investigations of biofeedback have directed their subjects to lower, rather than raise, muscle tension. Consequently, if the Pachman et al. (1978) results are reliable—and they are at least consistent with Cross's (1977) findings—then it is conceivable that heightened muscle tension in some areas could be surprisingly beneficial for some stutterers. The issue will be considered again later in this chapter.

The extensive biofeedback treatment research of Lanyon and colleagues has been based on one of the more typical assumptions underlying EMG feedback in stuttering treatment. This work has involved only masseter-muscle-EMG feedback, and employs "the general hypothesis that excessive muscle tension in areas of the body related to speech is a basic factor in stuttering, through direct interference with normal speech production" (Lanyon, 1977, p.860). Actually, Lanyon, Barrington, and Newman (1976) went even further with this hypothesis and claimed that excessive masseter-muscle tension *is* responsible for maintaining stuttering.

Lanyon's treatment research is reported in a series of publications (Lanyon, 1977; 1978; Lanyon, Barrington, & Newman, 1976) that document the development of his biofeedback-therapy procedure. The initial report outlined a series of preliminary applications of a method which involved visual feedback of masseter-muscle-EMG potentials. These applications were made to eight subjects (17-35) who stuttered on 35% (or more) words during a 300-word oral reading task. The subjects were trained to maniuplate the feedback signal to a criterion level. Then they either counted (two subjects) or orally read word-lists (six subjects) during alternate "feedback on" or "feedback off" conditions in once- or twice-weekly sessions. When 95% of words were stutter-free during feedback-on conditions, the subjects negotiated two-syllable, three-syllable and then four-syllable word-lists contingent on successfully uttering 95% of these words. The data obtained from the subjects who orally read show that their mean numbers of "nonfluent units" were substantially fewer during feedback-on, when compared with feedback-off conditions. It was evident that some subjects improved during the feedback-off

[1] This is somewhat surprising considering the number of treatments of stress-related disorders (Burish, 1981) that have used feedback from the region.

condition, but it is not clear whether this should be attributed to carry-over of the relaxation effect or some other factor. The problem in interpreting the overall result, including the suggested carry-over effect, is that during feedback-off conditions the "subjects were instructed to talk in their normal manner." This could mean that they ignored any beneficial learning from the feedback-on condition or changed their manner of speaking during both conditions. In either case, it is possible that the effects of feedback were confounded by additional differences between the reading conditions.

The same issues arise in Lanyon's (1977) second report on the development of this treatment. This report incorporated three studies, the first of which replicated the Lanyon et al. (1976) oral-reading procedure with seven adult stutterers. All subjects achieved the four-syllable criterion and were reported to be virtually stutter-free during feedback-on conditions. The two additional studies were designed to assess the efficacy of fairly limited generalization strategies. The first continued the above-mentioned procedure with spontaneously spoken single syllables, followed by dual-syllable words and, finally, two-syllable phrases. The subjects, six adult stutterers, were also taught to relax to a criterion EMG level without the aid of visual feedback—the clinician indicated to the subject whenever tension levels were above criterion level. It was reported that stuttering was virtually absent during the feedback-on and feedback-off conditions, but the relaxation levels were lower with the assistance of indirect feedback from the clinician than they were without this aid. In the final study, six adult stutterers received the same training, but extended their spontaneous speech to four-word phrases. Once again, there was virtually no difference in stuttering frequency in those conditions in which relaxation targets were indirectly fed back and the alternative condition. At best, these studies appear to have only incidental relevance to biofeedback principles since they were largely concerned with assessing the consequences of indirect feedback regarding relaxation. And because stuttering was virtually absent throughout the treatment tasks, it is impossible to discern whether relaxation mediated the subjects' stuttering frequency.

Lanyon's most recent report (1978)[2] outlines another attempt to improve the clinical value of his treatment program. He argues (Lanyon, 1977; 1978) that the relaxation training mentioned above was based on the internalization of cues derived from the EMG-feedback training, and that this skill would assist in the transfer of any improved performance to beyond laboratory situations. To this end, four stutterers (ages unspecified) received virtually the same procedure as previously, with the addition of either a hierarchy of spontaneous speech tasks in situations surrounding the laboratory (the clinicians accompanied the subject and monitored a feedback apparatus that was attached to the subject), or home practice with a portable feedback unit. In addition, the visual feedback system

[2]There is a later report by Lanyon and colleagues (Lanyon, Lanyon, & Goldsworthy, 1979) which evaluated 32 stutterers, who were engaged in the EMG feedback program, via MMPI and parts of a stuttering-severitiy scale. But no speech-performance data were provided. There is no indication that the subjects' therapy was distinguishably different from that reported in other studies by Lanyon.

was replaced by auditory feedback. Oral-reading and spontaneous-speech assessments made under varied conditions before treatment, immediately after treatment, and 6 or 18 months later, reflected some sustained improvement in performance. But at follow-up, the maximum gain on the spontaneous speech task was a 66% reduction in disfluencies (accompanied by a substantial improvement in words spoken per minute). The difficulty in interpreting the therapy benefits from so few assessments is that the subjects' performance changes may not have exceeded their untreated performance variability.

Generally, the findings reported by Lanyon are preliminary in nature; it is evidently a treatment procedure that is undergoing a gradual development. Nevertheless, it already incorporates some features which limit both its relevance to biofeedback therapy and its clinical viability. The inclusion of a hierarchy of speaking tasks, which are changed contingent on criterion performance, could mean that any improved performance is attributable to contingency management rather than biofeedback. Similarly, there is no evidence in Lanyon's data that any of the treatment gains included maintained stutter-free speech, except during conditions in which relaxation might have been a source of assistance. At the same time, it is apparent that only part of the development of Lanyon's treatment schedule has been reported. It is a schedule that requires additional features and evaluation before it could be described as clinically viable.

One attempt at extending Lanyon's procedure was reported by Manschreck, Kalotkin, and Jacobson (1980). They devised a treatment for eight stutterers (24-39 years), in which relaxation training preceded practice in modifying masseter-muscle-EMG feedback during half-hour sessions. After completing a hierarchy of tasks (similar to those used by Lanyon) with feedback assistance, the subject had to repeat the hierarchy using relaxation and no feedback. The procedure's benefits were assessed from oral-reading and spontaneous-speaking tasks given prior to and following treatment, plus 3 to 6 months after treatment. But these benefits are difficult to identify because the sole measure of speech performance was "percent time dysfluent" which appears to measure the durations of stutterings, not their frequency. On the basis of this peculiar measure (unsupported by reliability data) there was an inconsistent therapy-outcome pattern. Most subjects reduced their "percent time dysfluent" at follow-up, when compared with their before-treatment scores, though two actually showed deterioration on some tasks. The bulk of the brief reports on each subject's performance testified to some assistance from therapy, but it is not clear how well subjects were able to sustain that assistance. Once again, the findings of this treatment, whatever their value to clinical practice, are probably best interpreted as derivatives of relaxation rather than biofeedback.

Most of the shortcomings in the biofeedback-treatment studies stem from inadequate measurement methodology. One of the most interesting attempts to offset some of these shortcomings occurs in a study reported by Moore (1978), which used either the masseter muscle or a chin site for feedback. The feedback site was chosen by asking the subject to identify an area(s) where muscle tension was highest during stuttering: two subjects nominated the masseter muscle and the other nominated the chin. In three single-subject experimental treatment studies, the subjects (19, 20, and 27 years) were repeatedly assessed for percentages of disfluencies and EMG-microvolt levels during sessions involving oral reading and, in one case, conversational speech. After a base-rate disfluency and EMG level was established, all subjects were exposed to a procedure designed to shape reductions in EMG levels during speech. In what was really a negative reinforcement schedule, any EMG activity *above* a prescribed level activated 65dB white noise. The shaping procedure ceased when the noise remained off for 50% of session time. A task schedule, which resembled that employed by Lanyon (1977; 1978), was used for two subjects; they progressed from single-syllable words through to 5-minute oral readings (it is not clear what criteria were used to determine task progress). The other subject began treatment immediately at the 5-minute oral-reading task and then conversed with one or two people each session. The within- and between-session data for this last subject (gathered over 38 sessions) show that, initially, and for about half of all sessions, the feedback conditions produced reduced EMG levels and were associated with reduced stuttering; but this association was not evident over the last sessions when the frequency of disfluencies always remained near zero. The other two subjects' data are equally ambiguous: in neither subject is it clear that the EMG feedback was associated with reduced stuttering. In fact, in the case of the former subject, Moore acknowledges that

> Clinically significant reductions in disfluency were obtained only after analysis of the data suggested a change in procedure (that is, progressive and systematic manipulation in task complexity). Had these changes not been undertaken, continual use of EMG feedback could not have been justified (1978, p.133).

This adds further support to the contention that the hierarchy schedule, as such, may offer powerful treatment effects that could have overridden the feedback condition. Another significant factor relates to an observation by Moore regarding the strategies that some subjects used to remove the feedback tone:

> It seems apparent that other vocal behaviors are importantly related to EMG amplitude decreases including changes in vocal onset (rapid, abrupt onsets seemed to be replaced with gradual "easy" onsets), intensity (a general decrease in intensity levels), and pitch (a tendency towards monopitch). ... Indeed, enhanced fluency seems to be related to other variables than simply lowering EMG activity (p.136).

As interesting as this observation may seem, it is unsupported by relevant data, or even listener judgments, of changes in speech quality. But the notion that variables other than EMG modification might be implicated in any biofeedback benefit is certainly provocative, and may be added to contingency factors as potential treatment agents in these studies.

St. Louis, Clausell, Thompson, and Rife (1982) reported the only therapy application of EMG feedback with a young child (4.5 years old). The laryngeal area was chosen as a feedback site after assessments of differences between tension levels in various sites during silence and speech. The feedback during treatment sessions was a descending light-signal arrangement and "children's music coming on whenever the criterion level was reached" (p.197). But the before- and after-treatment results were unimpressive—a mere 10% reduction in percentage of words stuttered.

Some other treatment reports have described using EMG feedback within multicomponent-therapy programs. For example, in Beaty's (1980) multimodal-therapy program for a 15-year-old male stutterer, it was reported that EMG-auditory feedback from "electrodes on the vocal sites" was used because of tightening and "locking of jaw" on certain words. Similarly, Weiner (1978) has utilized unspecified biofeedback for "excessive muscle activity" as part of her "Vocal Control Therapy" procedure. In two other previously reviewed studies, Azrin and Nunn's (1974) regulated breathing technique was supplemented by EMG feedback or monitoring from the masseter muscle and Jones's (1981) brief account of therapy for a 19-year-old female stutterer indicated that when EMG feedback was introduced, there was subsequent improvement in the subject's ability to produce what was evidently a variant of prolonged speech. In a more detailed and data-based report, Williamson, Epstein, and Coburn (1981) monitored masseter-muscle-EMG responses during the course of a regulated breathing treatment for a 37-year-old stutterer. Each introduction of the regulated breathing method to different social settings was graphically shown to be usually associated with a concurrent decrease in "percentage of dysfluencies" and EMG counts. This led the researchers to conclude that "elevated facial EMG of stutterers is a result of the 'dysfluent' speech rather than the cause of stuttering" (p.338). But there are other ways of interpretating these data. One strong possibility is that the regulated breathing procedure may have introduced a pattern of behaviors that were more responsible than reduced "dysfluencies" for reducing the EMG scores.

GSR Feedback and Stuttering

Quite a number of studies concerned with the relationship between anxiety and stuttering have also employed GSR measures. For the most part, such measures were used to operationalize state anxiety. The principal studies have already been reviewed in Chapter 6, where, it will be recalled, very little satisfactory evidence was found to show that variations in GSR measures were directly related to the frequency or severity of stuttering. This was particularly evident in studies reported by Gray and England (1972) and Reed and Lingwall (1976; 1980). In each case, reductions in stuttering frequency were certainly not consistently associated with reductions in GSR measures. On this basis, it would seem to follow that variations in GSR would be unlikely to influence variations in stuttering. Nevertheless, this is an empirical issue, and one suitable for consideration via biofeedback research.

To date, only very limited use has been made of GSR feedback in a clinical context. Treon and Tamayo (1974) reported treating two 19-year-old stutterers by a combination of DAF and GSR. In the GSR biofeedback conditions, the subjects were instructed to achieve an unspecified "low wave" level, which was used as a treatment target with and without DAF. Basically, the design of this study makes it impossible to discern whether the manipulations in GSR level during feedback-on and feedback-off conditions had any influence on "stuttering blocks." The experimenters claimed that when GSR biofeedback was combined with DAF it was exceptionally beneficial, but there is little evidence in either subjects' data that would justify any enthusiasm over the treatment. Resick, Wendiggensen, Ames, and Meyer (1978) used audio feedback of GSR levels in their "slow speech" treatment program. The GSR feedback was mainly used in conjunction with relaxation training. However, the effects of this training were not separated from the slow speech procedure, and there is certainly no evidence that the biofeedback procedure provided any treatment benefits. The same is true in a report by Yonovitz, Shepherd, and Garrett (1977). They used GSR feedback to measure the "state of relaxation" during a reciprocal inhibition treatment program for a 13-year-old male stutterer. In this case, it was also not clear whether the GSR measures were used in any direct way to influence the therapy process.

Quite obviously, none of the studies that have reported using GSR biofeedback in a therapy context seriously investigated its efficacy. A reasonably straightforward laboratory study is obviously required in order to ascertain whether GSR-biofeedback training modifies stuttering—particularly by those subjects whose state anxiety is debilitative and is reflected in high GSR indicies.

EEG Feedback and Stuttering

The use of EEG feedback in stuttering treatment is even rarer than the use of GSR feedback. The reasons for this are fairly straightforward, in view of the checkered history of EEG biofeedback (Yates, 1980) and the formidable technical problems involved in identifying feedback effects (Ancoli & Kamiya, 1978). Most applications of EEG biofeedback have been directed towards increasing the presence of alpha waves (usually 8-13Hz) in anticipation that the emotional state regularly correlated with those waves—relaxed alertness—will facilitate performance. The main difficulty in establishing control over alpha waves is that they are now known to be influenced by numerous variables that, in turn, restrict clinical viability. Drowsiness, electrode placement on the scalp, eye movement, and room illumination level are only some variables known to disrupt or regulate alpha waves. Nonetheless, this method gained some favor among many clinicians because it raised the possibility that EEG biofeedback could produce "altered states of consciousness," which might then enable the subject to cope with unusual levels of stress.

Thus far, the only investigation on the effects of EEG biofeedback with a stutterer is a study reported by Moore, Dunster, and Lang (1975). They assessed the effect of feedback training on stuttering frequency from a 651-word oral-reading task (made up of three passages read in random order during the study). After a single baseline session, the subject (a 36-year-old male stutterer) preceded the following 11 sessions with 15 minutes of EEG feedback training.

With his eyes closed, the subject attempted to shut off a tone that was activated if his wave frequency fell outside the 8-12Hz range. The data were evaluted on the basis of the intervals of time in a session that the subject was able to produce alpha waves. For no obvious reason, it was decided to assess the amount of stuttering when the alpha time was either greater or less than 61% of the EEG feedback interval (in the baseline session it was 53.07%). This showed that a mean of 33.14 stutterings (per 651 words) occurred when alpha-wave time exceeded 61%, but the mean was 80.80 stutterings when alpha-wave time was less than 61%. This post hoc analysis of the subject's data is a dubious procedure, particularly when it is not accompanied by a rationale. In any event, the size of the changes in stuttering frequency were certainly not clinically substantial, and there is no clear evidence that the subject actually learned to control the presence of alpha waves.

Conclusions from Biofeedback Studies

In many ways, the contributions of biofeedback principles to stuttering has been a major disappointment. The disappointment is not so much a product of the mediocre clinical results or the methodological inadequacies of many of the studies, but stems from the surprising lack of creativity in the reported biofeedback methodologies. The bulk of the studies have been directed at assessing the effects of muscle-tension feedback in areas that are often pre-determined (Lanyon, 1977; 1978; Manschreck, Kalotkin, & Jacobson, 1980) to be controlling stuttering. Very few studies (Guitar, 1975; Williamson, Epstein, and Coburn, 1981; Moore, 1978) have used some form of assessment to determine the site of electrode placement, and only one student (Guitar, 1975) has provided data justifying a placement. But EMG, EEG, or GSR feedback are only some of many feedback methods that could be suitable for stuttering. Most of these techniques operate on the premise that the stutterer is experiencing either debilitating levels of tension in certain areas of the body (as determined by EMG), or is in a state of anxiety (as determined by GSR or EEG measures). These may be plausible premises in the case of certain individuals, but, as was shown in Chapters 6 and 10, it is unlikely to be a general and functionally important characteristic of stutterers. On the basis of what is known about variables that may control or modify stuttering, it would seem far more appropriate to investigate the effects of feeding back information from characteristics of the voice signal, or perhaps the speaker's breathstream.

It could be that the relatively unimpressive findings from the clinical biofeedback studies is one indicator that the premises for these treatments are shaky. Across the studies that have used biofeedback with therapeutic intent, there are reports on 38 stutterers (this excludes those studies that have used EMG or GSR feedback as a supplementary technique). Yet, only one stutterer is reported to have achieved reasonably sustained stutter-free speech as a result of treatment; that subject was reported in Guitar's (1975) study. The gains reported in other studies are invariably difficult to evaluate because they derive from a within-clinic task or they are reductions in stuttering frequency (or duration) that are well short of stutter-free speech. At the very least, this would suggest that the procedures used thus far cannot be regarded as favored methods of treatment.

A final issue concerns the treatment methodology used in some EMG-biofeedback studies. In many treatment reports, it is almost impossible to identify the contribution of the biofeedback procedure from the contributions of relaxation, or the arrangement of contingencies. In some of Lanyon's studies (Lanyon, 1977), for example, it is possible that relaxation instructions were as effective as feedback in reducing stuttering. While in other feedback studies, for example, those reported by Lanyon (1978) and Moore (1978), it is possible that the hierarchy of speech tasks may have introduced a treatment agent that was as responsible as reduced muscle tension for the therapy benefits. Any step-wise schedule containing graduated speaking tasks that are passed on the basis of reduced stuttering may have potential for modifying stuttering. The treatment principle is the same as has been used with some success in the GILCU programs (Chapter 9). But another potential treatment agent in many of these studies is a change in the subject's speech pattern. In some reports, there is evidence that the subject's reduced stuttering during biofeedback conditions was either accompanied by unusually slow speech rates (Hanna, Wilfling, & McNeil, 1975) or required only single-syllable production (Lanyon, 1977). But more obvious changes in speech quality were apparently evident in the subjects used in Moore's (1978) study: it was noted that vocal onsets, intensity, and pitch were all changed during the EMG-feedback conditions, and that these may have been the critical treatment factors. There was also another factor involved in Moore's study that might have helped alter a customary manner of speaking. In most EMG studies, the feedback signal is on continuously and, ostensibly, varies in frequency according to the tension level in the target-muscle region. But in Moore's study, the target EMG frequency range caused the feedback tone to be shut off. Hence, the subject experienced noncontinuous feedback under a negative-reinforcement schedule. It is quite possible that this type of feedback system produces relatively unusual effects when compared with the customary continuous feedback systems.

Among all of the procedures described thus far, perhaps none is more suited to a behavior therapy context than biofeedback. It carries the potential of permitting the clinician to almost completely operationalize the therapy process (with the exception of stuttering measurement) and systematically tailor the treatment to fit the individual—provided the modalities shown to be functionally associated with the individual's stuttering can also be fed back. The fact that the procedure has not yielded very many clinically useful findings carries a number of implications. It may be that the procedure is not as simple and efficient as others and, therefore, has only limited appeal. Another implication is that clinical applications of mainly EMG feedback have run into the problem that muscle-tension reduction, like relaxation, does *not* reliably reduce stuttering. Indeed, when EMG feedback is mainly used to produce relaxation effects with other disorders, then its benefits have not been shown to be better than those achieved by relaxation training (Andrasik, Coleman, & Epstein,1982; Burish,1981). As mentioned above, there appear to be many other forms of biofeedback methodology that might be more suited to stuttering treatment than those reported thus far. When these methods are investigated, then, in all likelihood, biofeedback methodology will become an essential feature of much stuttering therapy.

Hypnosis and Stuttering Therapy

Introduction

In his extensive review of the stuttering therapy literature, Van Riper (1973) chose to discuss hypnosis in the context of effects produced by suggestion. And there can be little doubt that this procedure fully exploits the amazing capacity of suggestion to influence behavior. It is also a procedure that is used to induce relaxation and remove the inhibiting impact on behavior of feared situations. For this reason, hypnosis has obvious relevance in a consideration of procedures designed to control the effects of tension on stuttering.

The alternative orientation to a biofeedback method of managing state anxiety, or stress-related behavior, is through procedures that rely upon other-person control. And, perhaps, hypnosis is the shining example of other-person control in the management of such behavior. For the essence of hypnosis is that the patient accepts and acts on another's suggestions regarding the self and the disorder. The effectiveness of this phenomenon in the treatment of various disorders has been a point of contention for more than two centuries. Nevertheless, it is now generally accepted that it may have a legitimate role in therapy for many disorders, even though its value in the treatment of stuttering continues to be uncertain.

The association between hypnosis and stuttering treatment is strange. There undoubtedly exists a strong belief in many quarters that hypnosis is an effective method for removing and curing stuttering. The belief is probably fostered by many professional hypnotherapists who enthusiastically advertise such claims. Yet, this belief is sustained by a surprisingly small and equivocal clinical literature, and an even smaller amount of treatment research. The use of hypnosis in stuttering therapy has been advocated for many years with varying degrees of enthusiasm. Mostly, it has been advocated as a method for inducing relaxation and overcoming excessive fear of certain speaking situations.

The hypnotic state has been regarded as a sleep-like condition (the term "hypnosis" derives from the Greek term *hypnos* meaning "sleep"), in which the subject is able to perform a range of behavioral responses only in response to suggestions from the hypnotist. During this state, the individual appears to be totally under the control of the hypnotist's suggestions and seems to have no will of his own. He may see, feel, smell, and taste in accordance with these suggestions, and in apparent contradiction to external stimuli. His memory and awareness of his own actions may also be altered by the hypnotist's suggestions. More significantly, the effects of these suggestions may extend into later waking activity and be displayed as posthypnotic suggestions. It is generally accepted that the subject's responses do not go beyond those available in his repertoire and that he cannot be hypnotized against his will. However, in this state, the person is usually able to alter a customary pattern of behavior (Kline, 1965).

There now exists a voluminous literature on hypnosis research and hypnotherapy (Burrows & Dennerstein, 1980; Wolberg, 1965) which is best summarized, for present purposes, by describing the features of hypnosis that appear relevant to stuttering therapy. The most generally accepted "explanation" of the hypnotic phenomenon is that it involves a state of hypersuggestibility (Hull, 1933). During this state, the subject is able to achieve substantial changes in variety of physiological functions including, for example, alterations to respiration and heart rate, plus a sensation of complete relaxation. Delusional states may also be produced; they may involve changes in mannerisms, attitudes, and speech that are consistent with the suggested imagery. Such states may also include age regression. The duration and extensiveness of posthypnotic suggestions are not entirely predictable, but the phenomenon is well established and has been used for therapeutic purposes.

In the course of these chapters, many phenomena have been found to modify stuttering without attracting very much research on the process involved. Chorus reading and shadowing are possibly the most obvious examples, but even more surprising is the anemic state of research into the effects of hypnosis on stuttering. A large measure of the problem can be attributed to the primitive state of therapy research during the period when hypnosis was introduced to stuttering therapy. However, while therapy research has now achieved a reasonable level of credibility, the problem still remains. It is only possible to guess at reasons why this is so. Some obvious possibilities are (1) the nonresponsiveness of a substantial part of the patient popultion to hypnosis, (2) the fact that it is not customary for speech-language pathologists to be trained to use hypnosis, and (3) the equivocal nature of early findings on hypnosis.

Therapy Applications of Hypnosis

There are a number of ways in which hypnosis has been recommended as a means of treating stuttering. Basically, they amount to its use in conjunction with other treatment techniques, or as the sole treatment technique (Falck, 1964). In either case, three general "suggestion techniques" are typically involved; relaxation, delusions relating to feared speaking situations, and posthypnotic activities designed to control speech situation difficulties.

The earliest discussion on the use of hypnosis for stuttering therapy appears to have been Gutzmann's (1898) account of its virtual impotence in treating stutterers. But in the years that followed, numerous reports appeared in the hypnosis literature claiming therapy success, particularly with cases in which the disorder was attributed to some traumatic incident. For example, Vogel was reported to have succeeded in curing stutterers by a method which "included revelation and aeration of the cause and suggestion to be patient under induced hypnosis" ("Stuttering Cured by Hypnotism," 1934, p. 311). A "successful" example of this treatment was described, but it was also indicated that some stuttering remained after therapy had ceased. Similar case descriptions occurred in the therapy literature throughout the 1940s and 1950s. Salter (1941) claimed that training in autohypnosis—the subject learned to self-administer posthypnotic suggestions—had helped to prevent relapse from hypnotherapy benefits for a female stutterer. Apparently, she "would speak impeccably for about two days, and then relapse to her old level. With auto hypnosis she had no occasion to revisit me" (p. 435). Watkins (1949) reported the successful use of posthypnotic suggestions to help a stutterer talk freely within therapy. A 21-year-old male soldier received this method, in conjunction with hypnotic treatment, for an underlying cause, the therapist's colleagues reported that the patient was much improved during several weeks following therapy. Madison (1954) claimed success in treating an 8-year-old boy who had an articulation and stuttering problem. During hypnosis, the child's stuttering apparently ceased, although the articulation difficulty remained unchanged. With continued treatment, the boy's stuttering decreased between hypnosis sessions, but no clear information is provided on the overall efficacy of the treatment. Rosen (1935) provided a very detailed account of the use of hypnosis as a support for psychoanalysis in treating a 21-year-old female who "had suddenly developed a stammer so severe as to make withdrawal from school necessary" (p. 83). The main focus of the treatment was on her obsessive sexual thoughts, which were claimed to be integrated with her stuttering. These thoughts were apparently resolved, and she was reported "symptom free" 6 years after this treatment ceased.

Many clinical reviews have been much less enthusiastic about the benefits of hypnosis with stutterers. Kroger (1963) considered that stuttering cannot be removed by simple posthypnotic suggestions. Estabrooks (1943) reported that his experiences had shown stuttering was remarkably resistent to hypnotherapy of all forms. Meares (1960) reviewed the use of hypnosis in treating stutterers and concluded that his experience with the "treatment of stuttering by suggestive therapy has not been consistent. Some patients have done remarkably well and others have not improved at all" (p. 317). The same conclusion appears to have been reached by Kline (1965); he claimed that hypnosis is only beneficial with disorders such as stuttering if it is used as an adjunct to treatment.

It is difficult to find any consistency in the clinical literature on the manner in which hypnosis should be used to benefit stutterers. Van Pelt (1956) claimed it could be used to cure stuttering by the expedient of "teaching people to relax perfectly and remove their fear" (p. 111). Others, such as Falck (1964), have reasoned that hypnotherapy should be used to provide information, break down conditioned stimuli, reinforce patterns of normal speech, minimize the effects of the original "primary" cause and reintegrate the personality. Rousey (1961) reviewed the (then) current literature on hypnosis and stuttering and argued that its benefits require the use of a deep trance in conjunction with speech therapy and hypnotherapy. Some behavior therapists have recommended that hypnosis be used to assist in applying reciprocal inhibition via relaxation. For example, Wolpe (1958) occasionally employed hypnosis to produce relaxation, but there is no indication that he used it to treat stuttering. Hussain (1966) also reported using hypnosis to reciprocally inhibit problematic responses and condition new responses. He claimed it helped to achieve more than 90% success with various types of disorders. Three of the treated subjects were described as displaying "speech disorders," but the nature of the disorders was not revealed. Small (1975) used behavioral rehearsal under hypnosis in the course of treating a 19-year-old stutterer by Azrin and Nunn's regulated breathing procedure, the value of hypnosis in this context was not obvious.

A frequently cited report, which is used to encourage the use of hypnosis with stutterers, is Moore's (1946) abridged description of the treatment of 31 stutterers (ages unspecified) who had responded to trance suggestions in varying degrees. Nine other stutterers were rejected from treatment because of their failure to respond to hypnosis or failure to respond in a sleep state. The therapy description merely indicates that the treated subjects were taught, individually, to relax via hallucination or posthypnotic suggestion. From the case reports of three male stutterers (two aged 14 years, and another aged 18 years), it is also evident that much of their treatment included the use of Iowa procedures such as the "bounce." In each case description, there is an account of a spectacular improvement in fluency due to the treatment, but this is essentially an informal account of therapy and is unfettered by data.

Remarkably, there are only two available reports on a stuttering treatment using hypnosis that include some form of speech-performance data. The first is a report by Dempsey and Granich (1978) on the "hypno-behavioral treatment" of a 41-year-old Korean War veteran who was reported to have begun stuttering after a traumatic accident. The treatment involved suggestions to either reduce or practice stuttering. The stuttering practice was based on Dunlap's (1942) negative-practice technique; it was designed to demonstrate to the subject that he was able to bring his stuttering under control. The limited data collected from this subject were obtained before and after treatment, but they were not supported by information about their source or reliability. They show that the subject's mean duration of stuttering and "repetitions per word" were reduced by about 80%. The subject's WPM rate increased from 5.1 to 24.8, which strongly suggests that he was still markedly debilitated by his stuttering.

Somewhat more information and data were provided in a report by Lockhart and Robertson (1977). They treated 30 stutterers (15-62 years) by either hypnosis alone, or the combination of hypnotherapy and speech therapy. Seven subjects were treated only by hypnosis because the severity of their disorder was relatively mild (it was assumed to be "a manifestation of normal nonfluency"). The treatment occurred at weekly intervals for 4 to 6 weeks, and consisted of repeated "ego-strengthening suggestions" and autohypnosis; subjects were "taught to recognize their own specific feared situations and to imagine the associated tension and anxiety symbolically concentrated in the clenched fist of their left hand" (p.98). Posthypnotic suggestions were given to carry out this instruction in the waking state, and by this means it was claimed that all subjects achieved complete fluency. The other 23 subjects were additionally trained to control their stuttering intervals by a system termed "block control." These subjects displayed more severe and frequent stuttering, which was considered to be "organic in nature." The description of the block control procedure reveals a system that is strikingly similar to that outlined by Webster (1974; 1980); it involved light articulatory contacts and gentle voicing over different classes of speech sounds. The hypnosis sessions were designed to assist the stutterer to use this altered speech pattern and to learn autohypnosis, in order to cope with feared speaking situations. The treatment was evaluated by counts of "words stammered" and reading rate on the Rainbow Passage (Fairbanks, 1960), which was given before treatment and after the majority of subjects had completed treatment. In the milder group, three of the seven subjects actually failed to stutter on this task before treatment. Nevertheless, at the final assessment all were stutter-free, and six had increased their reading rate. In addition, six subjects were reported to have been "fluent" for 2 to 3 months. The more severe group is more difficult to evaluate. Before treatment, their mean scores on the reading task were 22.23% WS (3.9-61.1%WS) and 88.7 WPM (6.2-180.0 WPM). But only ten subjects had completed treatment at the final assessment: all but one of the ten were fluent, and eight of these had increased their WPM rate. The rest were either continuing with the treatment or had discontinued therapy. Ratings were also made on the severity of blocks, and these were markedly reduced at the final assessment (for many subjects, this assessment was made part way through their treatment). It is one indication of the poverty-stricken state of hypnotherapy research on stuttering that this is the most data-supported study yet reported. But these data were not accompanied by reliability measures or assessments in conversational speech. There is also dubious value in brief oral readings made under unspecified conditions and at an unstated time relative to therapy.

Conclusions

The therapy evidence available to judge the merit, or otherwise, of using hypnosis for stuttering is woefully inadequate. The kindest interpretation of that evidence is that hypnosis may have some value in assisting stutterers to overcome certain feared speaking situations, speak under reduced state anxiety, and gain improved fluency under the influence of suggestion. It is incredible that there has been so little research and so few treatment studies investigating the contribution of hypnosis to stuttering. If the procedure is effective in reducing tension during speech production, or in the face of problematic speaking situations, then surely it should have some value in stuttering therapy. It certainly deserves much more serious attention than it has received thus far. In the absence of that attention, it will no doubt continue to be regarded as a fringe treatment that is normally used by less-qualified practitioners. There may be little evidence to support its use in a therapy context (even allowing for Lockhart and Robertson's vaguely promising data), but there is also nothing to contraindicate its use in treatment, particularly for the extraordinary difficulties that many stutterers experience in certain speaking situations. In this respect, hypnosis may yet have a very useful role in stuttering therapy.

Drug Treatment of Stuttering

Introduction

There has not been much enthusiasm for the application of drug treatment in the practice of behavior therapy, the obvious reason being that behavior therapy has been largely developed and used by clinicians who are not permitted to administer drug treatments. But, in principle, it is rather surprising that so little use has been made of some drugs. A huge pharmaceutical industry exists, which is substantially supported by the sale of drugs designed to change behavior, especially anxiety or stress. Many of these compounds are undoubtedly reliable agents for reducing state anxiety—reason enough to expect that behavior therapists might have shown more interest in pharmacology. Perhaps this also testifies to the overriding influence of environmental management or conditioning methodology on behavior therapy. Nevertheless, some clinicians have recognized that drug-based procedures may have utility in behavior therapy—especially with respect to anxiety reduction.

During behavior therapy's infancy, Wolpe and Lazarus (Wolpe 1958; Wolpe & Lazarus, 1966) reported using inhalations of carbon dioxide and oxygen to assist with reciprocal inhibition treatments for neurotic behavior. Some other clinicians employed drugs to assist relaxation, but their use was relatively restricted. At that time, however, drug treatments for many neurotic and psychotic conditions began to flourish with the advent of a number of powerful anti-anxiety, antipsychotic, and antidepressant compounds. These compounds made a modest contribution to behavior therapy practice—mainly via the anti-anxiety drugs—as is shown in reviews by Brady (1968) and Silverstone (1979), but they continued to have a limited role in behavior therapy. Some clinicians, such as Lazarus (1976), have recognized their place in a "multimodel" approach to problem behavior treatment. More significantly, others believed that the anxiety-reducing effects of some compounds could benefit stuttering treatment. Almost inevitably, therefore, most of the drugs advocated for anxiety-related conditions, or even psychotic conditions, were eventually tried with stutterers.

As a preface to this review of drug treatments of stuttering, the methods that have been devised to determine drug-treatment effects will be considered briefly. In some respects, drug-treatment evaluation shares much in common with hypnosis. For, just as hypnosis recognizes the strength of suggestion on behavior, so pharmacologists have long appreciated its potential role in any drug treatment effect. Indeed, the anticipated benefit of medication is a well-known treatment agent. These benefits are usually identified through the action of placebos; that is, a procedure or substance known to be without specific activity for the condition being treated. Actually, placebo effects are useful treatment agents in their own right (Shapiro & Morris, 1978), and may avoid some undesirable side effects of drug therapy, such as addiction. Placebo effects may also be generated by using demonstrably active compounds, but with ineffectual dosage levels.

The placebo effect has contributed much to the clinical evaluation of drug therapies, particularly through the use of the following methodologies. The simplest method is the single-blind procedure, in which the investigator administers a known placebo, and the subject is unaware that the substance is inert. But even investigator bias may contribute to treatment effects, and so the double-blind procedure was evolved. This method is normally used with groups of subjects, and neither the investigator nor the subject is aware of which subject group has received the placebo. The method is strengthened by the addition of a cross-over procedure, wherein both groups receive the allegedly active drug, or the placebo, at different times. More sophisticated experimental control is achieved by using different types of placebos. An inert placebo may be evident to a subject because of the absence of side effects, so active placebos (substances that mimic the experimental drug's side effects) are frequently preferred in evaluative studies. There are many limitations in such designs, not the least being that placebo effects may not be as reliable as true treatment effects. As a result, the treatment-evaluation method may hide a true difference. Another limitation is the difficulty in procuring an appropriate and active placebo. Hence, the final evaluation of a drug may involve comparisons between results from many experiments.

Behavior-therapy research can learn much from these drug-therapy-research methods. It is rather more difficult to translate the placebo-effect techniques into the methods that constitute much behavior therapy, but there are many procedures that can be varied in ways that should sufficiently deactivate the therapy process to permit tests for placebo factors. This is particularly relevant to stuttering treatments where DAF schedules, masking devices, and rhythmic stimulation techniques are prescribed without much consideration for their placebo components. Of course, the very introduction of a treatment procedure may incorporate numerous placebo factors.

One concern in this book's account of stuttering treatment has been the brevity of non-English reports on stuttering treatment. This is not always due to a bias towards accessible literature—it has mainly resulted from the limited number of relevant treatment reports in the non-English literature. But this is certainly not so for drug therapy: such therapies have been used extensively in Europe for many years. Some idea of its widespread use can be gained from Van Riper's (1973) therapy review, and from treatment practices such as those described by Sedlackova (1970) and Novak (1975). Derazne (1966) also described successfully treating "four thousand children" (younger than 7-8 years) in Russia by a combination of medication ("bromium and calcium chloride") and not less than 12 hours' sleep per day. Nevertheless, much of the available European literature has supplied little more than a general comment on therapy effects. Fortunately, this literature usually describes the use of drugs that have also been reported in English-language treatment reports. In other words, it is still possible to gain some general idea of their efficacy. Needless to say, therefore, the following review is necessarily abbreviated.

The Early Studies

Many of the English-language reports on drug treatments of stuttering do little more than record general clinical impressions. For example, Hogewind (1940) reported one of the first accounts of the use of sedation, and claimed that the preparation was occasionally "successful," especially in reducing "the duration and the gravity of the relapses" in older stutterers. Schaubel and Street (1949) argued that the muscle-spasm control achieved by prostigin would suggest its usefulness in therapy for some spastic conditions that might relate to stuttering. But their data-less report on the treatment of 10 stutterers with prostigin indicated little benefit. Hale (1951) also noted that spasticity may accompany Vitamin B_1 deficiency, and speculated that stuttering may be a related condition treatable by thiamin supplements. Hale reported that a child's stuttering was reduced by this means, and that this effect was replicated in a double-blind cross-over study—but no speech data accompanied the report.

During the 1950s, the increasing number of reports on drug therapies for ancillary behaviors in neurotic conditions included some that described their use with stutterers. Tuttle (1952) reported that a female stutterer, who also hyper-ventilated, was assisted by intravenous doses of methedrine: presumably her breathing pattern improved, and, "where stammering had previously interfered with communication, there was now little speech impediment" (p.780). Drake and Ebaugh (1955) treated a variety of patients with the tranquilizer reserpine and reported that a 22-year-old male stutterer showed "considerable obvious improvement in his speech," but they provided no other information. Burr and Mullendore (1960) also reported a single blind study on the use of reserpine to treat a "male adult stutterer." Their subject showed "a significant and steady drop in the percentage of stuttered words on both reading and conversation" when reserpine was taken regularly over two periods (5 and 13 weeks). The subsequent introduction of speech therapy produced no further improvements in his speech. But, again, no data or other information accompanied this report. Equally vague information accompanied two reports on the use of the antipsychotic drug chlorpromazine. Winkelman (1954) included five stutterers among a group of psychotics and neurotic patients who were treated over periods of 8 to 32 weeks. Ratings of their performance were based on self-appraisal, plus the comments from the patient's friends and family; they showed that one subject made "marked improvement" and another made "moderate improvement" (the rest showed "slight" or "no improvement"). Nichamin (1956) treated a 9-year-old male stutterer with chlorpromazine and found his speech improved, but apparently this gain was not maintained.

One of the few early studies to provide some speech data was conducted by Love (1955). This was a relatively brief experimental study in which 20 stutterers (18-30 years) were assessed in each of four conditions over 4 consecutive days; control, placebo (lactose), pentobarbital sodium (a depressant barbiturate), and amphetamine sulphate (a stimulant barbiturate). The assessment was a 200-word oral reading repeated eight times at the end of each day. No significant differences were reported between stuttering in each condition, but quite substantial side effects accompanied the active drug conditions.[3]

The evaluation of drug treatments for stuttering seemed to improve around the time Maxwell and Paterson (1958) reported beneficial effects from the anti-anxiety drug meprobamate. They provided a sketchy account of the treatment of 18 stutterers (18-50 years) for varying periods over 8 months: their "response to treatment" was described as merely "very good" for 33%, "good" for 44%, and slight or no improvement for the rest. Maxwell and Paterson's report prompted at least three evaluation studies. DiCarlo, Katz, and Batkin (1959) conducted a double-blind cross-over study on meprobamate with 30 stutterers (15-45 years). They were divided into three equal groups (meprobamate, placebo, and control) and were assessed via weekly oral readings (500-word passage). Their data revealed no significant difference between the treatment conditions. Almost identical findings were reported by Holliday (1959), who compared 30 stutterers (21-39 years) after they had been treated by either placebo or meprobamate. In this double-blind study, an oral-reading task was given before and after 3 weeks of daily ingestion of either substance; neither produced a change on number of words stuttered or durations of stuttering. There was, however, a reduction in ratings of physical tension in the meprobamate group. And, finally, Kent and Williams (1959) assessed the effects of meprobamate or a placebo on the performance of, respectively, eight and seven stutterers (18-29 years) who were also receiving speech therapy. Oral readings, spontaneous speech, and clinician judgments made before and after the 99-day treatment period showed nonsignificant changes in either group's speech. In retrospect, it now appears that the overall result of these studies was consistent with findings obtained from many studies on the use of meprobamate with other disorders. Shapiro (1976), for example, reported that the drug has been shown to be better than a placebo in only five out of 26 studies, and better than barbiturates in only one out of ten studies.

In many ways the meprobamate studies are a salutary reminder on the need for carefully controlled investigations of drug treatments. The pattern of these studies is almost identical to that which occurred with another almost-forgotten treatment for stuttering, and many other disorders—Carbon Dioxide Therapy. This inhalation procedure came to prominence with some reports by Meduna and colleagues in the late 1940s and early 1950s. The procedure was used with a wide variety of patients (usually neurotics), and involved 20 to 40 inhalations of a mixture of 30% carbon dioxide and 70% oxygen. These inhalation treatments were given three to six times a week, and could total from 20 to 150 depending on the clinician's judgment and the patient's reported response. The treatment's immediate effect was to cause loss of consciousness and "psychomotor excitement." There is no evidence that these side effects were particularly harmful,

[3]Of incidental interest here is a report by Palasek and Curtis (1960) on the effects of lactose on stuttering. They conducted a double-blind investigation of the use of lactose and calcium carbonate with nine stutterers. No significant differences were reported between their subjects' stutterings under either placebo during oral reading. They did, however, observe an improvement trend in favor of lactose.

and many clinical accounts of its use suggest that patients quite enjoyed the experience. In the first report of its use with stutterers, Meduna (1948) treated 32 subjects. He claimed that 16 "improved" and 16 were "not improved" as a result of this treatment. But no other details were provided. A little more information on this treatment regime was provided in the first edition of Meduna's book, *Carbon Dioxide Therapy,* (1950) which mentioned that 33 stutterers had been treated by this therapy, with 11 reported to have achieved 100% improvement. According to Meduna, the subjects were said to "no longer feel that they are stutterers. If one of them occasionally hesitates when speaking, he considers such a hesitancy a part of a normal speech pattern" (p.78). Three others showed 75% improvement, two showed 50% improvement, and the rest either less or no improvement. These assessments were global judgments made by a clinician who subsequently published the same findings (Smith, 1953). Meduna (1958) later reported that other clinicians had also found success in treating stutterers with carbon dioxide. Kent (1961), in her encouraging review of Carbon Dioxide Therapy, also reported that an Argentinian clinician (Goldenberg, 1953a; 1953b) had achieved "considerable success" in treating stutterers with this method. In this review, Kent also summarized a survey she had conducted on members of the "Carbon Dioxide Association, Inc." in the United States, who had reported using carbon dioxide to treat stutterers. She found that about half claimed no benefits. However the "15 members who reported favorable results did not report overwhelming success, but any report of success was considered a favorable report" (p.270).

The vague nature of the "successful" results of Carbon Dioxide Therapy and the absence of speech data implies that the treatment benefits were at best questionable—particularly since there was no indication that any benefits extended beyond the treatment interval. These doubts were enhanced by negative reports plus evidence from a controlled experiment on its use. Gaitonde (1954) followed Meduna's procedure with 11 stutterers and found that there was "no improvement" in nine subjects (two discontinued treatment). Weaver, Peterson, and Anderson (1951) also used Meduna's method in a case-report account of the treatment of two adult stutterers: one showed changes that were identical to routine variations in his stuttering, while the other showed no change whatsoever. But the most telling assessment of the therapy's effects emerged in the only controlled investigation on Carbon Dioxide Therapy. This was reported by Arthurs, Cappon, Douglass, and Quarrington (1954), who compared the performance of 16 stutterers who received Meduna's procedure (minus encouraging statements to subjects about its potential benefits) and six who received nitrous oxide (presumably an active placebo). Oral readings were given after six administrations of carbon dioxide, and at 2-week intervals over a variable treatment period. The experimenters also administered a test battery which included attitude scales and questionnaires for the subjects' friends and relatives. The resulting data revealed that no evident changes were associated with the treatment regime. Thus, in the absence of comparable (or any) speech-performance data from "successful" carbon dioxide treatments for stuttering, it is difficult to accept that this therapy had any clinical merit. This conclusion is also made credible by later reviews on this therapy in psychiatric practice, where it is now generally regarded as ineffectual (Shapiro,1976).

Later Developments

There is no clear demarcation between earlier and recent developments in drug treatments, except that the 1960s and 1970s saw the extensive development of many psychotropic compounds and, inevitably, their application to stuttering. More specifically, this era witnessed the extraordinary interest in one anxiolytic drug—haloperidol—for virtually the same questionable reasons that meprobamate and carbon dioxide were popularized in the previous decade. But the brief "haloperidol era" was preceded by a number of reports of treatments using other compounds. In retrospect, these compounds appear to have achieved effects that markedly resemble those associated with haloperidol.

The phenothiazine group of drugs has produced some of the most effective tranquilizers for treating psychotic and neurotic behavior, particularly chlorpromazine and trifluoperazine. The former drug has been used with some stutterers (Nichamin, 1956; Winkelman, 1954), but with little evident success. However, trifluoperazine has yielded some benefits. Aron (1965) reported evaluating trifluoperazine in conjunction with amylobarbitone (the latter being a barbiturate designed to reduce hyperexcitability). She conducted a double-blind cross-over study with 46 adult stutterers, who received daily doses of either the combination drug or a placebo. The 3-week-treatment periods were interspersed with equivalent no-treatment intervals. A variety of assessments were made, including tests for anxiety plus regular conversational and oral-reading tasks. The findings revealed that the active agent mainly produced reductions in severity, rather than frequency of stuttering, and some reduction in trait-anxiety scores. Also, about two-thirds of the subjects thought that they had improved during the drug condition. Fish and Bowling (1965) conducted a somewhat less-controlled study on the effects of amphetamine and trifluoperazine with stutterers who were also mentally retarded. No data were provided to support speech therapists' judgments that 22 of their 28 subjects (10-59 years; 21-77 IQ) were improved by either the amphetamine of trifluoperazine treatment.[4] More recently, Quinn and Peachey (1973a) treated a group of 10 stutterers for 3 weeks with daily doses (mean=4.0 mg) of trifluoperazine and reported little difference between their pre- and posttreatment stuttering frequency or speech rate during casual and prepared conversational speech tasks. This report, though, was not accompanied by reliability data.

Goldman (1966) and Goldman and Guth (1965) investigated the comparative effectiveness on stuttering of three major tranquilizers: thioridazine,

[4]It is noteworthy that Fish and Bowling's (1965) study is one of very few that has been concerned with treating suttering in the mentally retarded popultion—a population which, according to Bloodstein (1981), contains proportionately more stutterers "than in any other single identifiable group of people" (p.162).

meprobamate, and chlordiazepoxide. In preliminary investigations, thioridazine was found to produce beneficial changes in observer ratings of severity when compared with either a placebo or chlordiazepoxide. But, as Goldman states: "The findings were not spectacular in terms of reduction of frequency or severity of stuttering but more notable in the reported change in attitude and anxiety associated with stuttering behavior" (1966, p.1997). As a result, 20 stutterers (10-52 years) were divided into two equal groups and treated for 4 months either by placebo or thioridazine (40-100 mgs/day) in conjunction with speech therapy. The drug-treated group reduced its serverity ratings from severe-moderate down to moderate-mild, but the placebo group showed no change in these ratings over the treatment period. The former group also increased their oral-reading rate, while the placebo group showed no change in their rates. Unfortunately, no relevant data accompanied this report. Leanderson and Levi (1967) also compared two tranquilizers, opipramol and diazepam, with a placebo in a double-blind cross-over design with 44 stutterers (19-48 years). No speech data (other than "tendency to stutter" graphs) were presented, but the experimenters reported that "neither of the psychopharmaca appeared to have a particularly marked effect upon the percentage of wrongly spoken words or speech rate under stress" (p.315). The study incorporated a series of, allegedly, stressful speaking tasks that apparently presented as much difficulty in spite of the tranquilizers.

By the early 1970s, the results of a variety of mixed-quality studies on the use of tranquilizers had led to the belief (Perkins, 1971; Van Riper, 1973) that these compounds did not aid stuttering treatment, although there was some suggestion that they might reduce its severity. That appeared to change with some reports of success with the tranquilizer haloperidol. The rise and fall of this drug's promise actually demonstrates a number of interesting issues in stuttering-treatment research, especially the value of multidimensional assessment methods. It also demonstrates the remarkable amount of research that may be needed to counter poorly based claims for "successful" treatment.

Haloperidol was synthesized in 1957 (Shapiro, 1976), and quickly gained popularity because of its beneficial effects with acute psychotics—especially those showing psychomotor agitation—and with paranoid schizophrenics (Crane, 1967; Gerle, 1966). It was also reported to reduce various anxiety states (Gilbert, 1969). The drug achieved some special distinction because it is almost uniquely successful in treating Gilles de la Tourette's syndrome (Crane, 1967). Haloperidol's side effects are rather unpredictable, but they appear similar to those produced by many of the phenothiazines (mainly producing parkinsonism). These side effects have been reported in roughly 30% of patients at between one and four mg/day, and increase to 55% of patients when dosages range between four and eight mg/day (Crane, 1967).

The first reported use of haloperidol with stutterers was an Italian paper by Gattuso and Leocata (1962), who described its use in treating 50 children (5-12 years). They received varying doses (0.5-1.5 mg/day), and it was claimed that after 4 weeks "the symptomatology disappeared completely in 80% of children aged 5-8 years." The others improved, but the older children did not respond as well as the younger children.

In another Italian report, Cozzo and Gabrielli (1965) treated 48 stutterers with haloperidol and triperidol. They found that 16 showed marked improvement and 17 showed some slight improvement, but, apparently, there was no posttreatment carry-over effect. Tapia (1969) provided an equally vague, though less promising, account of the use of haloperidol with 12 child stutterers. Few details or data are provided, except that the dosages were 1.0 to 2.5 mg/day (calibrated by determining the "point of drowsiness"), and only two subjects (8- and 12-year-old girls) reduced their counts of " 'sticks' and hesitations" when compared with their responses to a placebo.

These initial reports on haloperidol excited some interest, but this increased dramatically following publication of Wells and Malcolm's (1971) study. This sparked considerable excitement because it appeared to provide a data-based and clinically significant demonstration of haloperidol's effect on stuttering. Thirty-six stutterers (15-60 years) were assigned to one of six groups that received various combinations of haloperidol, orphenadrine (used to prevent side effects) and speech therapy (Kingdon-Ward's relaxation procedures) over an 8-week period. In the haloperidol-treated groups, the dosage levels were gradually increased to an average of 4.5 mg per day. One hundred words of spontaneous speech were assessed before treatment, at 4 weeks, and after 8 weeks, for percentages of repetitions, percentages of interjections, and speaking time. The haloperidol groups' (n=12) mean scores showed that by the fourth week repetitions and interjections were reduced by, respectively, more than 50% and 80%, with a 200-300% increase in speech rate. Similar changes failed to appear in the other groups' scores. Furthermore, 10 of the 12 haloperidol-treated subjects showed their group's pattern of change. Eight of these subjects remained for the last 8 weeks and, as a group, sustained their improved performance. Some side effects (dry mouth, blurred vision, and drowsiness) were reported, and some subjects required reduced dosage levels. Wells and Malcolm's data certainly appeared impressive, but their study contained some questionable features that became extremely significant in the light of subsequent efforts to replicate its findings. The most prominent of these was the absence of reliability data, but equally important was the failure to specify details on the disfluencies. For example, it is not clear that the repetitions and interjections ("e.g., 'er'—'um' ") were necessarily stutterings (this concern is strengthened by a later report on this study), or whether each repetition, or words containing repetitions, was counted as a disfluency.

The first challenge to Wells and Malcolm's findings occurred with Quinn and Peachy's (1973a) account of the treatment of 28 stutterers (15-39 years) by either haloperidol (n=18) or trifluoperazine (n=10). They chose the latter drug in place of orphenodrine, which they had earlier found produced disabling side effects. They were also forced (because of side effects) to use only a maximum of 2.5 mg/day of haloperidol (compared with the 2.5-4.5 mg/day level used by Wells and Malcolm) over their 3-week treatment phase. Both treatment groups were assessed, before and after treatment, via 1000 syllables of spontaneous speech and 3 minutes of unobtrusively collected "causal conversational speech." The resulting data were not assessed for reliability. Nevertheless, Quinn and Peachy found no significant differences between the percentage of syllables stuttered before and after treatment from both drug-treated groups. Their speaking-rate data were not subjected to statistical analysis, but it is evident that the haloperidol group substantially increased their speech rate (33% to 24%), while marginal rate increases occurred in the trifluoperazine group. Quinn and Peachy also reported that only four of the haloperidol-treated subjects reduced their frequency of stuttering by 50% or more, while eight subjects actually increased their stuttering frequency, a finding which led Quinn and Peachy (1973b) to publish a caution against using haloperidol to treat stuttering.

In response to Quinn and Peachy, Cookson and Wells (1973) stated that they had followed up nine of Wells and Malcolm's haloperidol-treated subjects and that their "fluency alone remained significantly improved." They then added further confusion to the original study's measure of "fluency" by noting that "the other two measures, repetitions and interjections, though much improved failed to show significance or improvement" (Cookson & Wells, 1973, p.491). Cookson and Wells also recommended flupenthixol to reduce the acknowledged "serious problem" of side effects. Later, Wells (1975) pointed out that the efficacy of haloperidol may depend on gradually achieving a dosage level of 4.5 mg/day—or a level above that used by Quinn and Peachy (1973a).

The short-term effects of low doses of haloperidol were determined in a double-blind cross-over study by Burns, Brady, and Kuruvilla (1978). They arranged for 12 stutterers (16-43 years) to experience either no drug, saline, apomorphine (0.5-0.75 ma/day), or haloperidol (0.5 mg/day), on each of 4 consecutive days. The chosen drugs were also used to test the hypothesis that stuttering is mediated by the dopaminergic system.[5] It was postulated that haloperidol's benefits may derive from its dopamine-blocking effects, which should not be evident if the dopamine-recepters are stimulated via apomorphine. In theory, therefore, the latter drug should increase stuttering. Oral-reading and spontaneous-speech samples obtained about an hour after each drug was taken show that with haloperidol there was a significant decrease in percentage of "dysfluencies," relative to saline, during both types of speaking—this was true for nine of the 12 subjects. The apomorphine condition showed inconsistent trends: "reduced dysfluency" during oral reading and increased "dysfluency" during spontaneous speaking (relative to saline). But it is unclear as to whether these changes occured with stutterings, since the description of some "dysfluencies" included "fillers" such as " 'aw,' 'er,' 'like,' 'you know,' etc." (Burns, Brady & Kuruvilla, 1978, p. 258) These appear to be accessory features of stuttering (Wingate, 1964) that may have varied independently of other disfluencies—a possibility that becomes rather probable in the light of later findings.

Positive benefits of haloperidol were also reported in a double-blind study by Swift, Swift, and Arellano (1975). Their study compared groups treated with placebo (n=10) and haloperidol (n=7) over 3 weeks, using weekly assessments of spontaneous speech and oral reading (300 words). The study used benztropine

[5] Rosenberger (1980) has recently discussed the foundations of this hypothesis.

with both groups to induce dry mouths and blurred vision, thereby masking the placebo condition. The haloperidol group had 35-43% block reduction and 23-10% speech-rate increase, while the placebo group changed only slightly on these measures. Two weeks after treatment, there was a virtual return to base rate in the haloperidol group's performance. Three of four patients who chose to continue the haloperidol treatment (1.5-3.5 mg/day) apparently maintained improved performance for 3 months, though no data were reported.

In many ways the Swift et al. (1975) study produced odd findings, for, in the following 5 years, six haloperidol studies have failed to yield similar benefits for stutterers. A single-subject study by Martin and Hershey (1975) set the result pattern for many of these studies. They treated an extremely severe 22-year-old stutterer (stutterings were reported on almost "every syllable in multisyllable words and almost all monosyllabic words") by three mg/day doses over 4 months. His percentage of stuttered words (in spontaneous speaking, conversations, and oral readings) was only reduced by about 10% over this period; however, his speech rate did increase two- to five-fold. This rate improvement was reported to be "due to the decrease in multisyllabic stutterings and a decrease in the duration of blocks" (p.14). Unfortunately, these data failed to have the benefit of reliability measures. This was also true of a double-blind cross-over study by Rantala and Petri-Larma (1976) on 58 stutterers (6-66 years). Their subjects received haloperidol (1.5-3.0 mg/day for adults; 0.5-1.5 mg/day for children) for 4 weeks, plus equivalent time on a placebo. Essentially, they found no significant differences in frequency of "spasms" and "iterations" during oral readings under either condition, although the haloperidol condition produced an increased oral-reading rate. Rosenberger, Wheelden, and Kalotkin (1976) obtained virtually complementary findings in their assessment of haloperidol and placebo effects with eight stutterers (20-32 years). Each subject received either three mg/day of the drug or the placebo for six regular weekly or two-weekly periods. From various speaking tasks given each week, the experimenters derived measures of speech rate, plus the frequency and duration of "dysfluencies." The findings are difficult to interpret, but it appears that haloperidol probably reduced the "percent-time-dysfluent" score, though for only five subjects. Murray, Kelly, Campbell, and Stefanik (1977) provided some indication of the exigencies in using haloperidol as a treatment.[6] Twenty-six stutterers (16-49 years) were included in their double-blind cross-over study using haloperidol (3 mg/day) or a placebo over 6 weeks. Eight subjects retired from the study and only 12 completed 6 weeks on haloperidol without dosage reductions. A wide range of side effects were reported, including leg pains, blurred vision, nausea, agitation, dizziness, and frequent urination. The most serious side effect was extrapyramidal dyskinesia. The results, based on oral-reading and spontaneous-speech samples, reveal a significant increase in speech rate plus a slight reduction in the percentage of "dysfluencies" under haloperidol—but only during oral reading. Eleven subjects chose to continue using haloperidol after the study ceased, although only one

[6] The same study is summarized by Murray, Kelly, and Rosenberg (1977).

subject was still using it a year later. Yet another replication of many of the previous findings occurred in a two part study by Andrews and Dozsa (1977). The first part was an uncontrolled "clinical trial" with 25 stutterers who received 0.75-3.00 mg/day haloperidol over varying periods; 10 dropped out of the study (six because of side effects), and 15 (19-29 years) remained for at least 20 days. A 5-minute pretreatment monologue on these 15 subjects was compared with their mean score from similar samples obtained every 2 weeks (it is unclear how many scores were obtained in the treatment phase). This showed that there was a significant reduction in stuttering (20%SS at 76 SPM to 13%SS at 117 SPM) and six subjects apparently halved (or more) their pretreatment stuttering frequency. The second part of this investigation was a double-blind cross-over study on 27 stutterers, which was ultimately reduced to 15 (16-46 years), mainly because of haloperidol's side effects. The subjects experienced at least 20 days of three mg/day haloperidol or an unspecified period on a placebo (the conditions were separated by 2 weeks). No significant differences were reported between the %SS and SPM scores obtained during both conditions, although three subjects had at least 50% reductions in stuttering under haloperidol. This effect was apparently repeated when the subjects were reassessed during a period on diazepam followed by further haloperidol treatment. But no data were reported for these subjects. There is also a noteworthy absence of reliability data.

Across all the previous five studies, it is evident that haloperidol has shown, at best, remarkably similar effects to those found in so many other drug treatments —reduced severity of stuttering moments (for some stutterers), but little change in stuttering frequency. This effect is more clearly described in perhaps the most detailed investigation of haloperidol's effect on stuttering—a study by Prins, Mandelkorn, and Cerf (1980).

The distinguishing feature of Prins, Mandlekorn, and Cerf's (1980) study is that it evaluated haloperidol's effects on a wide range of disfluency categories. Their data were derived from a double-blind cross-over study with 14 stutterers—the "survivors" of an original pool of 21 stutterers (7-41 years). Six received 4 weeks of haloperidol (gradually increased over 7 days to three mg/day) followed by 4 weeks of a placebo. The conditions were reversed for the other eight subjects. The compounds were supplemented by cogentin (one mg/day) to suppress haloperidol's side effects (despite this, five of the original subjects dropped out of the study because of various side effects). Spontaneous-speech and oral-reading samples obtained throughout the experiment were used to derive Wingate's (1976) "core features of stuttering" (elemental repetitions, sound prolongations, and silent prolongations) and "accessory features of stuttering" (whole-word repetitions, phrase repetitions, interjections, and revisions). In general, Prins et al. found haloperidol failed to produce clinically significant effects—although it did produce statistically significant reductions in disfluency frequency and increased speech rate, but only during spontaneous speech. Quite the most interesting findings related to the disfluency categories: "From this point of view using criteria for stuttering proposed by Wingate (1977), Haloperidol actually had no effect on stuttering at all, but rather had its impact for most subjects upon their use of accessory features" (Prins, Mandelkorn, & Cerf, 1980, p.627). In other words, if this result relates to those from other haloperidol studies, then their reported reductions in severity of stuttering may largely stem from changes in disfluencies that are not always regarded as stutterings. Incidentally, Prins et al. reasoned that because these accessory features are generally thought to be conditioned avoidance responses to stuttering, then their response to haloperidol may be similar to the drug's affect on many other conditioned responses. Bobon, Janssen, and Bobon (1969), for example, reported that haloperidol and many other neuroleptics are useful inhibitors of many conditioned-avoidance behaviors.

It now seems possible, at last, to place haloperidol's effect on stuttering in reasonable perspective. There is now almost irrefutable evidence that the drug may have beneficial effects on either the severity of moments of stuttering, or some of stuttering's accessory features. It is not clear whether it is this effect that, in turn, produces increased speech rates, but it seems likely. It *is* clear, however, that very few stutterers show clinically significant changes under the drug, and its side effects are often sufficient to contraindicate its use. Perhaps the only aspect of the drug that has yet to be resolved is its efficacy with very young children. In view of the range of alternative treatments for this age group (see Chapter 10), this does not seem to be an urgent consideration.

Before closing this section, and for completeness, it should be mentioned that there have been some recent reports which also contain some pertinent information regarding drug therapy for stutterers. Rustin, Kuhr, Cook, and James (1981) claimed to have assessed the effects of the drug oxprenolol on stutterers. The drug, which is a beta-adrenergic blocking agent, is said to improve performance on skilled tasks under stressful conditions. Their stutterers were assessed under presumably stressful conditions after having taken the drug or a placebo. However, no data accompanied their report of a nonsignificant drug effect on stuttering performance. But drug effects reported in some recent case reports do appear to have clinical significance. Baratz and Mesulam (1981) reported the appearance of stuttering in the conversational speech of a 42-year-old female following a head injury. She achieved "adequate control" over her stuttering after receiving treatment with the anticonvulsant compounds phenytoin and carbamazepine. Other case reports have described drug treatments that may exacerbate stuttering. Nurnberg and Greenwald (1981) reported that phenothiazine treatments of two schizophrenic patients had activated stuttering. And McCarthy (1981) reported that whenever an asthmatic 4-year-old boy was given oral doses of theophylline, there was an evident increase in stuttering-like behaviors (the child repeated some words eight to ten times before saying the next word). These reports serve to highlight an aspect of pharmacotherapy that is in need of much more investigation.

Conclusions on Drug Treatments

For the present, it is safe to conclude there is little evidence that stuttering can be usefully treated by drug therapy. That is not to imply that individual stutterers may not be assisted by certain compounds, particularly where handicapping anxiety is a complicating factor. It is also not meant to imply that effective drug treatments may not be possible. Conceivably, certain compounds will eventually emerge with highly specific sites of action that might be relevant to, for example, the alleged timing difficulties of stutterers (see Chapter 10), although that seems less likely as long as stuttering continues to be subjected to drug investigations using compounds designed for other conditions. In all probability, though, stutterers will continue to be "tried out" on all manner of compounds. It is to be hoped, therefore, that the "haloperidol story" will be a salutary reminder of the need for carefully conducted investigations of their efficacy.

General Conclusions

This chapter has brought together three different general approaches to stuttering treatment that have been based mainly on the notion that stuttering is fostered or aggravated by anxiety or stress. In many respects the results of these approaches have been remarkably similar to those obtained by the anxiety-reduction treatments reported in Chapter 6.

Until now, it has appeared that most of the biofeedback treatments have assumed that reductions in certain muscle areas will achieve concomitant effects on stuttering. Thus far, the results of this approach have been very disappointing. Much of this disappointment may be due to an untoward reliance on a simple muscle-tension-reduction principle. There are numerous ways in which the biofeedback principle could be used to enhance many other treatment procedures. The anxiety-reduction principle has also dictated therapeutic applications of hypnosis. But in this case, any estimation of its value appears to have been thwarted by the wholesale absence of data-based therapy reports. The same is true of drug therapy for stutterers. The difference here, however, is that poor evaluation has meant that many stutterers may have been subjected to quite unnecessary and even distressing medication. It is becoming evident that one useful legacy of behavior therapy is that it has brought to stuttering therapy increased demand for data-based evaluations of treatments, whatever their type or mode of action. It is hoped, therefore, that the strengths and weaknesses of many of the peripheral treatments, such as the drug therapies, can be more rapidly identified, so that stutterers are not subject to so many unrewarding experiences.

In an earlier review of anxiety-reduction procedures, it was observed that to assume that a heightened anxiety state is necessarily debilitating is questionable. This assumption has often dictated the course and development of many stuttering treatments, and has been prominent among procedures reviewed in this chapter. The biofeedback procedures, in particular, almost presume that high arousal states and/or excessive muscle tension are clinically undesirable. This presumption continues despite the now unflattering record of stuttering treatments based on this premise. Actually, there is increasing evidence that heightened arousal (a condition that is often difficult to distinguish physiologically from state anxiety) may be quite desirable. Arguing the same point,

Svebak and Stoyva (1980) suggest that we need only think of the avidity with which individuals pursue sporting and recreational activities that involve high levels of arousal. In fact, clinicians may well be training irrelevant or counterproductive skills by limiting fluency to behavior states characterized by low arousal. More to the point, it could be that certain anxiety- or tension-modifying procedures have not had their clinical possibilities fully exploited. Thus far, only Pachman et al. (1978) have shown that increased muscle tension during biofeedback may also reduce some stuttering behaviors. That finding also has some connection with Ingham and Andrews's (1971) report that stuttering may be reduced during sustained periods of high-state anxiety. It may ultimately emerge that such alternative considerations of tension and arousal provide useful options for some stuttering treatments.

References

Ancoli, S., & Kamiya, J. Methodological issues in alpha biofeedback. *Biofeedback and Self-Regulation*, 1978, *3*, 159-183.

Andrasik, F., Coleman, D., & Epstein, L.H. Biofeedback: Clinical and research considerations. In D.M. Doleys, R.L. Meredith, & A.R. Cimero (Eds.), *Behavioral medicine: Assessment and treatment strategies.* New York: Plenum, 1982.

Andrews, G., & Dozsa, M. Haloperidol and the treatment of stuttering. *Journal of Fluency Disorders*, 1977, *2*, 217-224.

Aron, M.L. The effects of the combination of trifluoperazine and amylobarbitone on adult stutterers. *Medical Proceedings South African Journal for the Advancement of Medical Science* 1965, *11*, 227-233.

Arthurs, R.G.S., Cappon, D., Douglass, E., & Quarrington, B. Carbon dioxide therapy with stutterers. *Disorders of the Nervous System*, 1954, *15*, 123-126.

Azrin, N.H., & Nunn, R.G. A rapid method of eliminating stuttering by a regulated breathing approach. *Behaviour Research and Therapy*, 1974, *12*, 279-286.

Baratz, R., & Mesulam, M.M. Adult onset stuttering treated with anticonvulsants. *Archives of Neurology*, 1981, *38*, 132.

Basmajian, J.V. Control and training of individual motor-units. *Science*, 1963, *144*, 440-441.

Basmajian., J.V., & Newton, W.J. Feedback training of parts of buccinator muscle in man. *Psychophysiology*, 1974, *11*, 92.

Basmajian, J.V., & White, E.R. Neuromuscular control of trumpeters' lips. *Nature*, 1973, *241*, 70.

Beaty, D.T. A multimodal approach to elimination of stuttering. *Perceptual and Motor Skills*, 1980, *50*, 51-55.

Bloodstein, O. *A handbook on stuttering.* (3rd ed.) Chicago: National Easter Seal Society, 1981.

Bobon, D., Janssen, P., & Bobon, J. *The neuroleptics.* New York: Liege S. Karger, 1969.

Brady, J.P. Drugs in behavior therapy. In D.H. Efrom (Ed.), *Psychopharmacology: A review of progress, 1957-1967.* Washington Public Health Services. Publication No.1836, 1968.

Budzynski, T.H., & Stoyva, J.M. An instrument for producing deep muscle relaxation by means of analog information feedback. *Journal of Applied Behavior Analysis*, 1969, *2*, 231-237.

Budzynski, T.H., Stoyva, J.M., & Adler, C.S. Feedback-induced muscle relaxation: Application to tension headache. *Journal of Behavior Therapy and Experimental Psychiatry,* 1970, *1,* 205-211.

Budzynski, T.H., Stoyva, J.M., Adler, C.S., & Mullaney, D.M. EMG biofeedback and tension headache: A controlled outcome study. *Psychosomatic Medicine,* 1973, *35,* 484-496.

Burish, T.G. EMG, biofeedback in the treatment of stress-related disorders. In C.K. Prokop & L.A. Bradley (Eds.), *Medical psychology: Contributions to behavioral medicine.* New York: Academic Press, 1981.

Burns, D., Brady, J.P., & Kuruvilla, K. The acute effect of haloperidol and apomorphine on the severity of stuttering. *Biological Psychiatry,* 1978, *13,* 255-264.

Burr, H.G., & Mullendorf,J.M. Recent investigations on tranquilizers and stuttering. *Journal of Speech and Hearing Disorders,* 1960, *25,* 33-37.

Burrows, G.D., & Dennerstein, L. (Eds.), *Handbook of hypnosis and psychosomatic medicine.* Amsterdam: Elsevier North-Holland, 1980.

Carlsoo, S., & Edfeldt, A.W. Attempts at muscle control with visual and auditory impulses as auxiliary stimuli. *Scandinavian Journal of Psychology,* 1963, *4,* 231-235.

Conture, E.G., McCall, G.N., & Brewer, D.W. Laryngeal behavior during stuttering. *Journal of Speech and Hearing Research,* 1977, *20,* 661-668.

Cookson, L.B., & Wells, P.G. Haloperidol in the treatment of stutterers. *British Journal of Psychiatry,* 1973, *123,* 491.

Cozzo, G., & Gabrielli, L. La thérapie du begayement avec les butyrophenones. *De Therapia Vocis et Loquelae (Eighth Congress, International Society of Logopedics and Phoniatrics),* 1965, *1,* 415-419.

Crane, G.E., A review of clinical literature on haloperidol. *International Journal of Neuropsychiatry,* 1967, *3,* suppl. I, 110-127.

Cross, D.E. Effects of false increasing, decreasing, and true electromyographic biofeedback on the frequency of stuttering. *Journal of Fluency Disorders,* 1977, *2,* 109-116.

Dempsey, G.L., & Granich, M. Hypno-behavioral therapy in the case of a traumatic stutterer: A case study. *The International Journal of Clinical and Experimental Hypnosis,* 1978, *26,* 125-133.

Derazne, J. Speech pathology in the U.S.S.R. In R.W. Rieber & R.S. Brubaker (Eds.), *Speech pathology.* Amsterdam: North Holland, 1966.

DiCarlo, L.M., Katz, J., & Batkin, S. An exploratory investigation of the effect of meprobamate on stuttering behavior. *Journal of Nervous and Mental Diseases,* 1959, *128,* 558-561.

Drake, F.R., & Ebaugh, F.G. The use of reserpine in office psychiatry: Preliminary report. *Annals of the New York Academy of Science,* 1955, *61,* 198-205.

Dunlap, K. The technique of negative practice. *American Journal of Psychology,* 1942, *55,* 270-273.

Estabrooks, G.H. *Hypnotism.* New York: Dutton, 1943.

Fairbanks, G. *Voice and articulation drillbook.* (2nd ed.) New York: Harper & Row, 1960.

Falck, F.J. Stuttering and hypnosis. *International Journal of Clinical and Experimental Hypnosis,* 1964, *12,* 67-74.

Fish, B.H., & Bowling, E. Stuttering: The effect of treatment with d-amphetamine and a tranquilizer agent trifluoperazine. *California Medicine,* 1965, *103,* 337-339.

Freeman, F.J., & Ushijima, T. Laryngeal muscle activity during stuttering. *Journal of Speech and Hearing Research,* 1978, *21,* 532-562.

Gaitonde, M.R. Stammering: Treatment of 27 cases. *Indian Journal of Medical Science,* 1954, *8,* 831-835.

Gattuso, R., & Leocata, A. Haloperidol in the treatment of stuttering. *La Clinica*

Otorinolaringoiatrica, 1962, *14,* 227-234.

Gerle, B. Haloperidol — clinical experience. *Clinical Trials Journal,* 1966, *3,* 380-384.

Gilbert, M. Haloperidol in the treatment of anxiety-tension states. *Current Therapy Research,* 1969, *11,* 520-523.

Goldenburg, L.R. Resultados obtenidos en el tratamiento de la tartamundez con la terapeutica del anhidrido carbonico (metado de van Meduna). *Otolaringologica, Buenos Aires,* 1953, *3,* 312-317. (a)

Goldenberg, L.R. Tartamundez: apartaciones a su tratamiento mediante el anhidrido carbonico. *Dia Medico, Buenos Aires,* 1953, *25,* 1242-1244. (b)

Goldman, R. The use of Mellaril as an adjunct to the treatment of stuttering. *Excerpta Medica, International Congress Series,* 1966, *150,* 1996-1998.

Goldman, R., & Guth, P. The effects of psychotherapeutic drugs on stuttering. *De Therapia Vocis et Loquelae (Eighth Congress, International Society of Logopedics and Phoniatrics),* 1965, *1,* 411-414.

Gray, B.B., & England G. Some effects of anxiety deconditioning upon stuttering frequency. *Journal of Speech and Hearing Research,* 1972, *15,* 114-122.

Guitar, B. Reduction of stuttering frequency using analog electromyographic feedback. *Journal of Speech and Hearing Research,* 1975, *18,* 672-685.

Gutzmann, H. *Das Stottern: Eine Monographie fur Aerzte, Pedagogen und Rehorden.* Frankfort: Rosenheim, 1898.

Hale,L.L. A consideration of thiamin supplement in prevention of stuttering in preschool children. *Journal of Speech and Hearing Disorders,* 1951, *16,* 327-333.

Hanna, R., Wilfling, F., & McNeil, B. A biofeedback treatment for stuttering. *Journal of Speech and Hearing Disorders,* 1975, *40,* 270-273.

Hatch, J.P., & Gatchel,R.J. The role of biofeedback in the operant modification of human heart rate. *Biofeedback and Self-Regulation,* 1981, *6,* 139-167.

Hefferline, R.F. The role of proprioception in the control of behavior. *Transactions of the New York Academy of Science,* 1958, *20,* 739-764.

Hogewind, F. Medical treatment of stuttering. *Journal of Speech Disorders,* 1940, *5,* 203-208.

Holliday, A.R. Effect of meprobamate on stuttering. *Northwest Medicine,* 1959, *58,* 837-841.

Hull, C.L. *Hypnosis and suggestibility.* New York: Appleton-Century, 1933.

Hussain, A. Behavior therapy using hypnosis. In J. Wolpe, A. Salter, & L.J. Reyna (Eds.), *The conditioning therapies.* New York: Holt, Rinehart & Winston, 1966.

Ingham, R.J., & Andrews, G. The relation between anxiety reduction and treatment. *Journal of Communication Disorders,* 1971, *4,* 289-301.

Jacobson, E. *Progressive relaxation.* Springfield, IL: Charles C. Thomas, 1938.

Jones, B.A. Modified regulated-breathing in treatment of a single case of stuttering. *Perceptual and Motor Skills,* 1981, *52,* 130.

Kalotkin, M., Manschreck, T., & O'Brien, D. Electromyographic tension levels in stutterers and normal speakers. *Perceptual and Motor Skills,* 1979, *49,* 109-110.

Kent, L.R. Carbon dioxide therapy as a medical treatment for stuttering. *Journal of Speech and Hearing Disorders,* 1961, *26,* 268-271.

Kent, L.R., & Williams, D.E. Use of meprobamate as an adjunct to stuttering therapy. *Journal of Speech and Hearing Disorders,* 1959, *24,* 64-69.

Kline, M.V. Hypnotherapy. In B.B. Wolman (Ed.), *Handbook of clinical psychology.* New York: McGraw-Hill, 1965.

Kroger, W.S. *Clinical and experimental hypnosis in medicine, dentistry and psychology.* Philadelphia: Lippincott, 1963.

Lanyon, R.I. Effect of biofeedback-based relaxation on stuttering during reading and spontaneous speech. *Journal of Consulting and Clinical Psychology*, 1977, *45*, 860-866.

Lanyon, R.I. Behavioral approaches to stuttering. In M. Hersen, R.M. Eisler, & P.M. Miller (Eds.), *Progress in behavior modification.* (Vol.6). New York: Academic Press, 1978.

Lanyon, R.I., Barrington, C.C., & Newman, A.C. Modification of stuttering through EMG biofeedback: A preliminary study. *Behavior Therapy*, 1976, *7*, 96-103.

Lanyon, R.I., Lanyon, B.P., & Goldsworthy, R.J. Outcome predictors in the behavioral treatment of stuttering. *Journal of Fluency Disorders*, 1979, *4*, 131-139.

Lazarus, A.A. *Multimodal behavior therapy*. New York: Springer, 1976.

Leanderson, R., & Levi, L. A new approach to the experimental study of stuttering and stress. *Acta Otolaryngology*, 1967, *224*, (Suppl.), 311-316.

Legewie, H., Cleary, P., & Rackensperger, W. EMG recording and biofeedback in the diagnosis and therapy of stuttering: A case study. *European Journal of Behavioral Analysis and Modification*, 1975, *1*, 137-143.

Lockhart, M., & Robertson, A.W. Hypnosis and speech therapy as a combined therapeutic approach to the problem of stuttering. *British Journal of Disorders of Communication*, 1977, *12*, 97-108.

Love, W.R. The effect of pentobarbital sodium (nembutal) and amphetamine sulphate (benzedrine) on the severity of stuttering. In W. Johnson & R.R. Leutenegger (Eds.), *Stuttering in children and adults*. Minneapolis: University of Minnesota Press, 1955.

Madison, L. The use of hypnosis in the differential diagnosis of a speech disorder. *Journal of Clinical and Experimental Hypnosis*, 1954, *2*, 305-317.

Manschreck, T.C., Kalotkin, M., & Jacobson, A.M. Utility of electromyographic biological feedback in chronic stuttering: A clinical study with follow-up. *Perceptual and Motor Skills*, 1980, *51*, 535-540.

Martin, S., & Hershey, L.G. The use of haloperidol in the management of stuttering: A case study. *Journal of Fluency Disorders*, 1975, *1*, 13-17.

Maxwell, R.D.H., & Paterson, J.W. Meprobamate in the treatment of stuttering. *British Medical Journal*, 1958, *5075*, 873-874.

McCarthy, M.M. Speech effect of theophylline. *Pediatrics*, 1981, *68*, 749-750.

McLean, A.E., & Cooper, E.B. Electromyographic indications of laryngeal-area activity during stuttering expectancy. *Journal of Fluency Disorders*, 1978, *3*, 205-219.

Meares, A. *A system of medical hypnosis*. London: W.B. Saunders, 1960.

Meduna, L.J. Alteration of the neurotic pattern by use of carbon-dioxide inhalations. *Journal of Nervous and Mental Disorders*, 1948, *108*, 373-379.

Meduna, L.J. *Carbon dioxide therapy* (1st ed.). Springfield, IL: Charles C. Thomas, 1950.

Moduna, L.J. (Ed.), *Carbon dioxide therapy* (2nd ed.). Springfield, IL: Charles C. Thomas, 1958.

Moore, W.E. Hypnosis in a system of therapy for stutterers. *Journal of Speech and Hearing Disorders*, 1946, *11*, 117-122.

Moore, W.H., Jr. Some effects of progressively lowering electromyographic levels with feedback procedures on the frequency of stuttered verbal behaviors. *Journal of Fluency Disorders*, 1978, *3*, 127-138.

Moore, W.H., Jr., Cunko, C., & Flowers, P. Cumulative integrated electromyographic activity of selected speech-related muscle groups of nonstutterers during massed oral readings. *Journal of Fluency Disorders*, 1979, *4*, 149-161.

Moore, W.H., Jr., Dunster,J.R., & Lang, M.K. The effects of alpha biofeedback conditioning on stuttered verbal behavior: A case report and some clinical implications. *Journal of*

Biofeedback, 1975, *2*, 19-28.

Murray, T.J., Kelly, P., Campbell, L., & Stefanik, K. Haloperidol in the treatment of stuttering. *British Journal of Psychiatry*, 1977, *130*, 370-373.

Murray, T.J., Kelly, P., & Rosenberg, E. The treatment of stuttering with haloperidol. *Canadian Journal of Neurological Science*, 1977, *4*, 219.

Myers, F.L. Relationship between eight physiological variables and severity of stuttering. *Journal of Fluency Disorders*, 1978, *3*, 181-191.

Nichamin, S.J. Chlorpromazine in the treatment of mild behavior disturbances. *Journal of the Michigan Medical Society*, 1956, *55*, 1469-1471.

Novak, A. Results of the treatment of severe forms of stuttering in adults. *Folia Phoniatrica*, 1975, *27*, 278-282.

Nurnberg, H.G., & Greenwald, B. Stuttering: An unusual side effect of phenothiazines. *American Journal of Psychiatry*, 1981, *138*, 386-387.

Pachman, J.S., Oelschlaeger, M.L., Hughes, A., & Hughes, H. Toward identifying effective agents in use of biofeedback to decelerate stuttering behavior. *Perceptual and Motor Skills*, 1978, *46*, 1006.

Palasek, J.R., & Curtis, W.S. Sugar placebos and stuttering. *Journal of Speech and Hearing Research*, 1960, *3*, 223-226.

Perkins, W.H. *Speech pathology. An applied behavioral science*. St.Louis: C.V. Mosby, 1971.

Platt, L.J., & Basili, A. Jaw tremor during stuttering block: An electromyographic study. *Journal of Communication Disorders*, 1973, *6*, 102-109.

Prins, D., Mandelkorn, T., & Cerf, F.A. Principal and differential effects of haloperidol and placebo treatments upon speech disfluencies in stutterers. *Journal of Speech and Hearing Research*, 1980, *23*, 614-629.

Quinn, P.T., & Peachy, C. Stuttering: An investigation of haloperidol. *The Medical Journal of Australia*, 1973, *2*, 809-811. (a)

Quinn, P.T., & Peachy, C. Haloperidol in the treatment of stutterers. *British Journal of Psychiatry*, 1973, *123*, 247-255. (b)

Rantala, S.L., & Petri-Larma, M. Haloperidol (serenase) in the treatment of stuttering. *Folia Phoniatrica*, 1976, *28*, 354-361.

Reed, C.G., & Lingwall, J.B. Some relationships between punishment, stuttering and galvanic skin responses. *Journal of Speech and Hearing Research*, 1976, *19*, 197-205.

Reed, C.G., & Lingwall, J.B. Conditioned stimulus effects on stuttering and GSR's. *Journal of Speech and Hearing Research*, 1980, *23*, 336-343.

Resick, P.A., Wendiggensen, P., Ames, S., & Meyer, V. Systematic slowed speech: A new treatment for stuttering. *Behaviour Research and Therapy*, 1978, *16*, 161-167.

Rosen, H. *Hypnotherapy in clinical psychiatry*. New York: Julian, 1953.

Rosenberger, P.B. Dopaminergic systems and speech fluency. *Journal of Fluency Disorders*, 1980, *5*, 255-267.

Rosenberger, P., Wheelden, J., & Kalotkin, M. The effects of haloperidol on stuttering. *American Journal of Psychiatry*, 1976, *133*, 331-334.

Rousey, C.L., Hypnosis in speech pathology and audiology. *Journal of Speech and Hearing Disorders*, 1961, *26*, 258-262.

Rustin, L., Kuhr, A., Cook, P.J., & James, I.M. Controlled trial of speech therapy versus oxprenolol for stammering. *British Medical Journal*, 1981, *283*, 517-519.

Salter, A. Three techniques of autohypnosis. *Journal of General Psychology*, 1941, *24*, 423-438.

Schaubel, H.J., & Street, R.F. Prostigmin and the chronic stutterer. *Journal of Speech and Hearing Disorders*, 1949, *14*, 143-146.

Sedlackova, E. A contribution to pharmacotherapy of stuttering and cluttering. *Folia Phoniatrica*, 1970, *22*, 354-375.

Shapiro, A.I. An electromyographic analysis of the fluent and dysfluent utterances of several types of stutterers. *Journal of Fluency Disorders*, 1980, *5*, 203-231.

Shapiro, A.K. Psychochemotherapy. In R.G. Grenell & S.Gabay (Eds.), *Biological foundations of psychiatry*. New York: Raven Press, 1976.

Shapiro, A.K., & Morris, L.A. The placebo effect in medical and psychological therapies. In S.L. Garfield & A.E. Bergin (Eds.), *Handbook of psychotherapy and behavior change: An empirical analysis*. New York: Wiley, 1978.

Shapiro, D., & Surwit, R.S. Learned control of physiological function and disease.In H.Leitenberg (Ed.), *Handbook of behavior modification and behavior therapy*. Englewood Cliffs, NJ: Prentice-Hall, 1976.

Sheehan, J.G., & Voas, R.B. Tension patterns during stuttering in relation to conflict, anxiety-binding, and reinforcement. *Speech Monographs*, 1954, *21*, 272-279.

Silverstone, T. The use of drugs in behavior therapy. *Behavior Therapy*, 1970, *1*, 487-497.

Small, M.M. Treatment of stuttering: A case history. *Perceptual and Motor Skills*, 1975, *41*, 812.

Smith, A.M. Treatment of stutterers (on basis of psychoneurotic personality) with carbon dioxide. *Diseases of the Nervous System*, 1953, *14*, 243-244.

Snidecor, J.C. Tension and facial appearance in stuttering. In W. Johnson & R.R. Leutenegger (Eds.), *Stuttering in children and adults*. Minneapolis: Universitiy of Minnesota Press,1955.

St. Louis, K.O., Clausell, P.L., Thompson, J.N., & Rife, C.C. Preliminary investigation of EMG biofeedback induced relaxation with a preschool aged stutterer. *Perceptual and Motor Skills*, 1982, *55*, 195-199.

Stuttering cured by hypnotism. *Scientific American*, 1934, *151*, 311.

Svebak, S., & Stoyva, J. High arousal can be pleasant and exciting. *Biofeedback and Self-Regulation*, 1980, *5*, 439-444.

Swift, W.J., Swift, E.W., & Arellano, M. Haloperidol as a treatment for adult stuttering. *Comprehensive Psychiatry*, 1975, *16*, 61-67.

Tapia,F. Haldol in the treatment of children with tics and stutterers—and an incidental finding. *Psychiatric Quarterly*, 1969, *43*, 647-649.

Tarler-Benlolo, L. The role of relaxation in biofeedback training: A critical review of the literature. *Psychological Bulletin*, 1978, *85*, 727-755.

Travis, L.E. Dissociation of the homologous muscle function: Stuttering. *Archives of Neurology and Psychiatry*, 1934, *31*, 127-133.

Treon, M., & Tamayo, F.M.V. The separate and combined effects of GSR biofeedback and delayed auditory feedback on stuttering: A preliminary study. *Journal of Fluency Disorders*, 1974, *1*, 3-9.

Tuttle, E. Hyperventilation in a patient who stammered: Methedrine as an adjunct to psychotherapy. *American Journal of Medicine*, 1952, *13*, 777-779.

Van Pelt, S.J. *Hypnotism and the power within*. New York: Fawcett, 1956.

Van Riper, C. *The treatment of stuttering*. Englewood Cliffs, NJ: Prentice-Hall, 1973.

Watkins, J.G. *Hypnotherapy of war neuroses*. New York: Ronald Press, 1949.

Weaver, O.M., Peterson, D.B., & Anderson, W.H. Carbon dioxide therapy of psychoneuroses. *Disorders of the Nervous System*, 1951, *12*, 355-361.

Webster, R.L. A behavioral analysis of stuttering: Treatment and theory. In K.S. Calhoun, H.E. Adams, & K.M. Mitchell (Eds.), *Innovative treatment methods in psychopathology*. New York: Wiley, 1974.

Webster, R.L. Evolution of a target-based behavioral therapy for stuttering. *Journal of*

Fluency Disorders, 1980, *5*, 303-320.
Weiner, A.E. Vocal control therapy for stutterers. *Journal of Fluency Disorders*, 1978, *3*, 115-126.
Wells, P.G. Haloperidol in the treatment of stutter. *British Journal of Psychiatry*, 1975, *126*, 491-492.
Wells, P.G., & Malcolm, M.T. Controlled trial of the treatment of 36 stutterers. *British Journal of Psychiatry*, 1971, *119*, 603-604.
Williams, D.E. Masseter action potentials in stuttered and nonstuttered speech. *Journal of Speech and Hearing Disorders*, 1955, *20*, 242-261.
Williamson, D.A., Epstein, L.H., & Coburn, C.C. Multiple baseline analysis of the regulated breathing procedure for the treatment of stuttering. *Journal of Fluency Disorders*, 1981, *6*, 327-339.
Wingate, M.E. A standard definition of stuttering. *Journal of Speech and Hearing Disorders*, 1964, *29*, 484-489.
Wingate, M.E. *Stuttering: Theory and treatment*. New York: Irvington, 1976.
Wingate, M.E. Criteria for stuttering. *Journal of Speech and Hearing Research*, 1977, *20*, 596-607.
Winkelman, N.W., Jr. Chlorpromazine in the treatment of neuropsychiatric disorders. *Journal of the American Medical Association*, 1954, *155*, 18-21.
Wolberg, L.R. *Short-term psychotherapy*. New York: Grune & Stratton, 1965.
Wolff, H.G. *Headache and other head pain*. New York: Oxford University Press, 1963.
Wolpe, J. *Psychotherapy by reciprocal inhibition*. Palo Alto, CA: Stanford University Press, 1958.
Wolpe, J., & Lazarus, A.A. *Behavior therapy techniques*. Palo Alto, CA: Stanford University Press, 1966.
Yates, A.J. *Biofeedback and the modification of behavior*. New York: Plenum, 1980.
Yonovitz, A., Shepherd, W.T., & Garrett, S. Hierarchical simulation: Two case studies of stuttering modification using systematic desensitization. *Journal of Fluency Disorders*, 1977, *2*, 21-28.

12

Some Reflections and Suggestions

Introduction

Whatever conclusions may be drawn from the preceding chapters, at least one is compelling: behavior therapy has indeed made a plentiful contribution to stuttering treatment. This review of treatments reported over the last decade and a half has revealed nearly 250 studies that can be described as "mainstream" behavior therapy approaches to stuttering. Not all are unblemished examples of the application of experimental method to treatment, but most have integrated reasonably replicable procedures and, to a lesser extent, systems for evaluating those procedures. They have also served to introduce an alternative treatment orientation to stuttering—a "behavioral preparadigm." The treatment studies in this preparadigm are beginning to provide clinicians with a rich array of techniques that should help most stutterers achieve improved speech. At the same time, the increasing sophistication of therapy method is revealing the strengths and weaknesses of the techniques used in those therapies. In drawing together this burgeoning therapy literature, it is to be hoped that such considerations have been adequately highlighted for clinicians and researchers alike, and; moreover, that this has also been aided by overviewing the research that underpins these techniques. In general, the aim has been to assist in some way the development of clinically viable and effective treatments for this disorder.

This book's review of stuttering treatments, loosely related under the banner of behavioral approaches, has been attempted with a constant and ill-disguised bias: to determine clinical value by critically evaluating methodology. This is particularly true of those therapies that claim clinical benefits. It should be evident by now that such claims are difficult to sustain in the light of the complexities of outcome evaluation. So, to end on a more positive note, much of this final chapter will be concerned with formulating a viable and valid approach to therapy evaluation.

It may seem like putting the cart before the horse to reserve a review of treatment evaluation until the last chapter. However the simple truth is that, as yet, there is little agreement on just what *is* necessary for evaluation. In fact, most notions of stuttering therapy evaluation are in a state of evolution, largely prompted by the developments in different treatment procedures. It often transpires, for instance that a treatment's peculiarities generate special variables that are seemingly less important to the evaluation of other types of treatment. This has been most apparent in efforts to evaluate the numerous varieties of "prolonged speech" treatments. For instance, the important evaluation issues for this type of therapy involve such matters as the speaker's "naturalness" and "automaticity": such dimensions are rarely mentioned in the evaluations of treatments that use only response-contingent techniques.

The State of the Art

Before the evaluation issues are explored further, the main general findings from the preceding chapters will be summarized. There are many ways of ascertaining the contribution that the behavioral preparadigm has brought to stuttering. One simple way is to look across the reported treatments and identify the number of adequately documented "successes" and "failures." The difficulty with this approach is that however many successful treatments are reported, it is unlikely that they will represent the total number of stutterers who failed in such treatments. It is an unfortunate fact that the treatment literature tends to favor reports of success rather than failure. In any event there are, as yet, no suitably controlled comparisons among stuttering treatments that would justify concluding that one treatment is always superior to another, or all others.

The most ambitious recent attempt to compare stuttering treatments was conducted by Andrews, Guitar, and Howie (1980). They applied Smith and Glass's (1977) meta-analysis technique on a selection of stuttering-treatment studies. The Andrews et al. study, which was discussed in Chapter 10, concluded that therapies employing "prolonged speech" and "gentle onsets" were superior to others in terms of the size and duration of treatment effects. They reached this conclusion from comparisons between the results of therapy studies that used varying numbers of stutterers. But the problems with the Andrews et al. study are manifold, perhaps the most important being that it simply excluded all single-subject treatment reports. In other words, it virtually ignored the response-contingent treatment literature, and, in the process, bypassed masking and biofeedback treatments. In many respects, therefore, Andrews and his colleagues' conclusions were, in the wider sense of the term, foolish. For such conclusions are likely to fool clinicians into believing that other procedures cannot succeed as well as those that use "prolonged speech" or "gentle onsets." These findings are also likely to fool the unwary into believing that the data base for their conclusions are entirely credible—and that is palpably untrue. In view of the questionable status of therapy evaluation, the current literature can only reveal that certain procedures have been used with some stutterers to produce some therapeutic benefits. At best, that literature should be used to derive some very tentative conclusions about current trends, with full awareness of the limitations of the techniques that constitute these trends.

The current treatment literature is beginning to make it possible to extract some idea of the advantages and difficulties associated with some techniques. The chapter reviews show, for example, that there has been a virtual demise in the use of rhythmic stimulation techniques. It is difficult to fully understand why this has occurred, especially since rhythmic stimulation remains one of *the* most reliable methods for briefly removing stuttering. The most obvious explanation is that some comparative studies (Andrews & Ingham, 1972; Helps & Dalton, 1979) have encouraged the belief that another speech pattern technique, prolonged speech, achieves more favorable results. Presumably, also, many clinicians who had reported using rhythmic stimultion (Andrews, Azrin, Brady, Ingham, and others) have since turned to one or another of the variants of prolonged speech. Nevertheless, there have been remarkably few attempts to investigate ways of changing the less desirable aspects of rhythmic speech into more desirable or normal speech.

The procedures that are predicated on an association between anxiety and stuttering also seem to have lost favor. There is very little persuasive evidence that the modification of state anxiety or related characteristics—such as tension or speech situation fears—has assisted stuttering treatment. There are scattered reports, albeit poorly documented, of stutterers obtaining some improvements via the combination of reciprocal inhibition and relaxation. Alternative approaches to anxiety reduction, such as biofeedback, hypnosis, and drug therapy, have also yielded only limited benefits. But the overall impression, from all such treatments, is that they produce improved, rather than completely stutter-free, speech. This is a dubious advantage considering the reliability with which other procedures may actually remove stuttering (albeit temporarily). One of the surprising features among the anxiety-reduction treatment reports is that they rarely report investigations on stutterers who are quite incapacitated by anxiety, in whatever form. And there are clearly many stutterers who fit this category. It is almost incontestable that the combination of relaxation and systematic desensitization has improved treatment for numerous disabling conditions (Kazdin & Wilcoxon, 1976). The most obvious disability for stutterers, which lends itself to this type of treatment, is their use of the telephone. Yet, surprisingly little reported use has been made of anxiety-reduction techniques in treating telephone fears. On the other hand, the systematic desensitization (or successive approximation) principle is probably integral to treatments that oblige stutterers to master increasingly more "difficult" speaking situations. These controlled and graduated exposures to demanding speaking situations may have functional characteristics integral to those used in anxiety-reduction treatments.

The possibility that the conceptual basis for most anxiety-reduction procedures in stuttering treatment is misplaced has already been discussed at length (Chapter 11). Suffice to say that there is a continuing need for research into the clinical utility of stress or anxiety manipulation. It may be the case that some stutterers should learn to sustain fluency under the situational stresses that normal speakers are supposed to withstand, but with minimal threat to their fluency. Another conceptual issue, relevant to this form of treatment, concerns its role in a treatment regime. Many studies report using anxiety-reduction procedures to supplement other treatment techniques (Azrin & Nunn, 1974; Resick, Wendiggensen, Ames, & Meyer, 1978; Treon & Tamayo, 1974), which suggests that many clinicians believe that anxiety reduction contributes something to the therapeutic process. However, the nature of that contribution is still unclear—a somewhat amazing situation considering the length of time that anxiety-reduction has been used in stuttering treatment.

Chorus reading and shadowing procedures have also made unspectacular contributions to stuttering therapy. This is quite disappointing, for, although the reason for their effects on stuttering is puzzling, they are nevertheless reliable modifiers of stuttering. Indeed, there is virtually no evidence that while in use they have ever failed to reduce, or eliminate, stuttering. Shadowing has been mainly employed in therapy settings, but, like chorus reading, it has been disadvantaged by fairly unimaginative applications in a therapy context. Some inventive uses of both techniques have been described by Shelton (1975) and Lee, McGough, and Peins (1973), but in the context of relatively uncontrolled studies. The fact that the chorus-reading effect does not always depend on identical material might suggest that fading procedures could be used to sustain their effects. Perhaps the most clinically significant feature of this technique is that it appears not to depend upon reduced speech rate or abnormal-sounding speech.

Chorus reading and shadowing have emerged as the least researched, though, possibly, the most interesting of all stuttering modification procedures. This paradox may actually embody its own explanation; for the continuing paucity of reported treatments using these techniques may mean that they have been tried and found wanting in unreported research. There is one interesting role for these techniques that has not been explored—their diagnostic value. There may be much clinical value in procedures that reliably reduce stuttering, but fail to produce similar effects on other speech disorders. Could it be that the chorus-reading/shadowing effect is unique to stuttering? If this were so, then it may serve to distinguish the disorder's characteristics from those of, say, dysarthric or dysphasic speech. If this were true, then these techniques might have immense clinical value.

Almost the same considerations apply to masking. Like chorus reading and shadowing, this procedure has also been infrequently reported as an effective treatment agent. In recent years, the publicity surrounding a voice-activated portable masking unit, known as the "Edinburgh Masker," has suggested that masking may yet have some therapeutic potential. The claims made for masking procedures have usually been modest, primarily because masking is simply unpleasant. Nevertheless, the Edinburgh Masker has gained widespread acceptance, presumably because it helps *some* stutterers achieve *some* benefits. It therefore merits consideration as a technique that could be used in conjunction with other treatment techniques. It would certainly warrant much more consideration if only a small portion of the time and money devoted to its publicity were dedicated to collecting data on its claimed therapy benefits.

The contribution of operant-conditioning methodology to stuttering treatment is now so extensive that, arguably, few treatments do *not* incorporate contingency arrangements in one form or another. Response-contingent procedures have been shown to reduce stuttering frequency, shape fluency-enhancing responses, or help sustain treatment gains. But their impact on much stuttering treatment has been much more profound. For example, their use led to the disorder being conceptualized as a composite of responses, or response classes, whose frequency is modifiable by environmental contingencies. In turn, this has led to an awareness that the disorder may be treated, or at least brought under control, by managing critical environmental stimuli. Of equal importance has been the move to integrate measurement and treatment—an overlooked contribution of operant methodology that will be discussed later. This has prompted some clinical researchers and clinicians to regard the disorder's dimensions, or stuttering therapy objectives, as measurable concepts that may be directly integrated with punishment and/or reinforcement schedules. Another important consequence has emerged from the success of operant-conditioning methodology in treating children. There is now ample evidence that childhood stuttering may be treated effectively by procedures that were previously accepted (almost without question) as likely to aggravate the disorder. This may ultimately prove to be contingency management's greatest contribution to stuttering therapy. There is even a reasonable possibility that "spontaneous recovery" from stuttering, particularly in childhood, might be due to the informal use of contingencies.

There remains a great need for carefully controlled studies on treatments that employ operant-conditioning principles. Nevertheless, it may not be too early to suggest that many of them, particularly those using time-out or the GILCU technique (see Chapter 9), are emerging as preferred initial stuttering treatments for children. At this stage, those treatments that use only response contingencies have not shown the same promise with older stutterers. On the other hand, the recent developments in self-management technology suggest that this technique has much therapeutic potential for this age group. Actually, the most successful applications of response-contingent techniques for adult stutterers have occurred when they are combined with other techniques, especially prolonged speech and its variants. In addition, response-contingent techniques are finally making a positive contribution to one of the perenial therapy problems—maintenance of treatment effects.

In some ways, it is difficult to disentangle the reasons for the current enthusiasm over various "prolonged speech treatments" from the evolution of contingency-management procedures. Virtually all of the main developments in the therapies that employ this speech-pattern technique have used different types of contingency schedules. In fact, it may well be one reason why this type of speech pattern has been accepted in therapy practice while rhythmic speech has become less acceptable. This situation might not have transpired if more attempts had been made to marry operant-conditioning methodologies and rhytnmic stimulation.

The various manifestations of prolonged speech seem to infest most currently reported treatments for stuttering, particularly for adults. The phenomenal number of treatment reports that claim success (in varying forms) with this procedure is, at least, some testimony to the reliability with which stuttering is reduced by certain modifications to the speech pattern. In general, treatment studies have shown that these modifications can be used to produce reasonably durable reductions in stuttering that are sustained for at least 1 to 2 years. The technique's impact has not been confined to treatment. It has also been largely responsible for a revived interest in respiration, articulation, and prosodic factors in stuttering. But in the midst of the excitement about prolonged speech and its offspring, few efforts have been made to determine their necessary features. Presumably, these techniques depend on inducing the stutterer to increase the duration of phonation intervals, reduce articulatory contrasts, and, possibly, slightly reduce speech rate. And, at long last, some attempts are being made to develop replicable methods for achieving these these features. Possibly, this development will help to isolate the necessary and sufficient conditions for the effective use of these techniques. Another important need is for information on whether some or all of the technique's features must be continued in order to "support" the subject's posttreatment speech. It has been argued (Chapter 10) that the failure to resolve these issues has been responsible for an increasing number of "fringe therapies": therapies that pay lip service to behavioral principles in order to give patients the dubious advantage of short-term relief from stuttering. Arguably, the most interesting byproduct of the growing legitimate use of these techniques have been the efforts to ensure that these short-term gains become long-term benefits. The task of shaping this speech pattern towards normally fluent speech that *completely* replaces the stuttering speech pattern is finally beginnning to receive appropriate research attention.

Therapy-Evaluation Issues

A Consideration of Bloodstein's Criteria

The clinical value of the measurement methodology and treatment-evaluation strategies in the reviewed treatments have emerged as major concerns throughout this book. Much of the concern over the merit of many stuttering treatments can be traced to the absence of agreed criteria for evaluating treatment effects. Some efforts to resolve this problem have been mentioned at various points (for example, Andrews & Ingham, 1972; Ingham, 1981; Ryan, 1974; Silverman, 1981), but none has been entirely satisfactory. One attempt to bring together all the relevant variables is Bloodstein's (1981, pp.386-390) recent listing of 11 criteria for evaluating stuttering therapy. So, in what follows, these criteria will be partially or completely listed and reviewed for their contribution. (The interested reader is urged to read Bloodstein's justification for each criterion).

1. The method must be shown to be effective with an ample and representative group of stutterers. The single-subject design has a place in scientific research. It has been widely misused, however in the area of research on stuttering therapy, where most single cases written up for publication are apparently chosen for the precise reason that they were successes. This practice produces a distorted picture. In the end we learn little from it beyond what we already know—that somewhere, at sometime almost any therapy can achieve a remarkable result for some stutterers (p.386).

This is not so much a criterion as a recommendation that therapy evaluation should not depend on single-subject research. This is an extremely important issue, since it challenges the value of single-subject research designs. Actually, the point at issue is the external validity of these designs. Single-subject-research designs entered therapy research for a variety of reasons; foremost was the failure of parametrics to reflect critical aspects of the clinical process (Hersen & Barlow, 1976). For, not only do group trends fail to reflect the pattern of an individual's response to treatment, they may also overlook treatments that succeed for certain individuals. It is certainly true that single-subject studies can only show that a treatment has produced some profitable results for some stutterers; but that is far from a trivial finding, particularly if the study is internally valid and reveals the total dimension of results. At this point in the struggle to find reliable treatments, a great deal has been gained from carefully managed time-series investigations that probe the relationship between a procedure and its clinical effects. Bloodstein's claim that a method must be effective across "representative" stutterers may, unwittingly, subscribe to the "uniformity assumption myth" (Kiesler, 1966)—the notion that there should be a uniform treatment suitable for a uniform patient. There is some indication that some treatment techniques, most notably, the prolonged speech procedures, are useful for many stutterers, but they too have benefited from controlled single-subject investigations (see Chapters 9, 10, and 11).

2. Results must be demonstrated by objective measures of speech behavior such as frequency of stuttering or rate of speech, and by judges' ratings of severity. Such measurements should be made before, during, and after treatment by observers other than the experimenters themselves or without knowledge that might influence their judgment, and due account must be taken of the observers' reliability (Bloodstein,1981, p.386).

There are two aspects to this criterion—the types of measures and their reliability. The first refers mainly to the construct validity of measures currently used to assess stutterers during treatment. Frequency counts of stuttering and, to a lesser extent, ratings of stuttering severity have become almost descriptive datum for this disorder. It is also quite significant that Bloodstein should recommend counts of stutterings, rather than measures of disfluencies or dysfluencies. Another interesting aspect of this criterion is that no reference is made to different disfluency categories; a method of measuring stuttering that is beginning to fade in its treatment utility. Severity ratings present a number of problems, mainly because there is no agreed method for rating severity (Chapter 2). The principal purpose of severity ratings during the course of treatment is to ensure that frequency reduction is not offset by worsening severity. One common method for determining severity is to measure the duration of individual moments of stuttering. The difficulty with such a measure is that it too may lack construct validity; for duration may not be integral to the type of behavior that clinicians or patients regard as stuttering's severity. Speech-rate measures are under challenge for similar reasons. At best, syllables-per-minute, or articulation-rate scores, only broadly indicate whether the subject is speaking unnaturally fast or slow. And for this reason there may also be merit in accompanying this measure with perceptual judgments of the naturalness of the subject's speech (see below).

The importance of independently assessing or, at the very least, cross-checking these measures against an independent assessor's measurements, is seemingly self-evident. Yet that does not seem self-evident to many researchers, nor to many journal editors. The preceding chapters revealed a staggering number of treatment and experimental studies that fail to report such data, a fact that destroys the credibility of much of the current treatment literature. Even when reliability data are reported, they are rarely justified as sufficient to retain confidence in the reported results. Hawkins and Dotson (1975), for example, have shown that high agreement between the experimenter's and independent assessor's scores may be deceptive: the difference between their scores may well be the difference between a data trend consistent with a treatment effect and one that fails to demonstrate that effect. Quite obviously, it is almost essential for treatment studies to report independently gathered data trends that alone (or in concert with the experimenter's data trends) justify a study's conclusions.

One other issue concerns the methods used to obtain stuttering counts and speech rate. There is now a growing body of evidence that clinicians are able to use electronic counters to count both of these variables "on-line" and reliably. Stuttering treatment would undoubtedly advance in leaps and bounds if these variables could be counted automatically.

3. Reports of therapeutic success must be based on repeated evaluations and adequate samples of speech. The great variability of stuttering from time to time and under different conditions is liable to result in assessments that are unrepresentative (Bloodstein, 1981, p.386).

This criterion is simple to justify, but less simple to prescribe. It is far from clear how frequently such evaluations should be made, or what represents an "adequate" sample of speech. The main purpose of repeated evaluation is to help decide whether within- and between-condition variability has been unambiguously and significantly modified by treatment. This means that the duration of evaluation cannot always be standardized across individuals. In turn, of course, this presents difficulties for the use of group designs in therapy research. The same issue applies to sample size, although there is increasing acceptance of a method used by Ryan (1971; 1974); that is, 5-minute samples of conversation, monologue, and oral reading.

One attempt to derive a methodology that prescribes minimal frequency and sample-size parameters will be outlined below. But this attempt is also hindered by the relatively impoverished state of research into stuttering variability. That should not be so in view of developments in recording technology. The problems involved in recording stuttering in "natural" circumstances have certainly received insufficient attention (Ingham, 1981). However, the advent of portable micro-cassette recorders has helped make it possible to obtain repeated speech samples in representative speaking situations.

The method of choosing "representative" speaking situations has also received very little attention in the treatment literature. One obvious method is to derive these situations from speaking log books that the subject could prepare in advance of the treatment study. This information would surely help specify sample sizes that represent average speaking time in certain situations.

A presumption in most treatment research is that stuttering variability is only affected by situational factors. That may not be so. One feature of variability occasionally noticed by this writer is a tendency for time factors to influence variability (Ingham, 1981). The duration of time that the subject spends speaking in certain situations, or even the time of day that assessments are made, might be sources of variability worthy of investigation.

4. Improvement must be shown to carry over to speaking situations outside the clinical setting. (Bloodstein, 1981, p.386).

This is much related to Criterion 3. Most clinicians are aware that vast differences may occur between clinic and nonclinic speech performance, but evidence showing this difference is surprisingly small. Studies by Resick et al. (1978), Ingham and Packman (1977), and Ingham (1982a) go some way towards illustrating this criterion's importance.

A much more interesting factor is the boundary of the "clinical setting." The mere presence of a recorder or an assessor in the subject's nonclinic setting may evoke clinic-related speech performance (Ingham, 1981). For example, subjects may be assessed via telephone conversations from home or elsewhere, but unless the assessment components are absent they may not typify customary telephone conversations (Ingham, 1981; 1982a). Unfortunately, the only available solution to this problem is occasional covert assessment.

5. The stability of the results must be demonstrated by long-term follow-up investigations. Any number of methods for making stuttering disappear have been known for many years: the great and persistent problem of stuttering therapy is how to keep the stutterer from relapsing. Relatively little is known about the subject of relapse. (Bloodstein, 1981, p. 387).

Long-term investigations of stuttering-treatment effects are becoming increasingly frequent in spite of their enormous technical and conceptual problems. Not the least of these is the length of time needed to prove the treatment has produced a durable improvement. Some of the issues associated with maintenance of treatment effects have been discussed elsewhere by this author (Ingham, 1981), but will be taken up again later in this chapter.

Bloodstein (1981) suggests that "Perhaps 18 months to 2 years is the shortest interval after which most experienced clinicians would not feel unduly optimistic in hoping that the improvement was lasting" (p.387). But their optimism should be tempered by information on what has transpired in that period. Most current treatment programs employ a wide variety of strategies that are designed to prevent relapse. These include speech practice, routine clinic visits, and continuing involvement with previously treated patients. These may well be useful techniques for sustaining improvement, but they may also confound the most clinically desirable effect—sustained improvement with the same level of attention to speech that is used by normal speakers. That is not to deny the advantages of "aided" maintenance; it simply suggests that clinicians should recognize that there are different types of sustained improvement.[1] Needless to say that this topic is in dire need of investigation.

There is now much attention to both the measurement and management of the maintenance process (Boberg, 1981). There may be some value in "booster" treatments, and in treatment schedules designed to sustain treatment gains for increasingly longer intervals. Another interesting area of treatment research concerns the use of self-management techniques. There are also numerous suggested approaches to maintenance that need to be researched (Boberg, Howie, & Woods, 1979; Hanna & Owen, 1977; Ingham, 1981; Shames, 1981). These mainly include self-help groups, regular speech practice schedules, and the assistance of "significant others." A large number of other ostensibly useful approaches have been reviewed by Stokes and Baer (1977).

One aspect of relapse that has claimed some attention concerns the stutterer's attitude towards communication at the end of treatment. The shaky foundations of studies which claim that poor communication attitudes (as measured by the S24 Scale) may influence long-term outcome have been discussed in Chapter 10. Nevertheless, it is highly likely that patients who show little interest in sustaining speech practice or continuing with treatment schedules will be strong candidates for posttreatment relapse. The complex factors that enjoin patients to seek treatment and complete its often-demanding requirements deserve much more attention. It may well emerge that these variables can be manipulated by controlling such factors as the duration of waiting times for treatment. This is a much overlooked variable in the overall treatment process. Some treatments, such as those reported by this writer, have required (usually out of necessity) that patients wait up to 3 years for enrollment in treatment programs. The comparative clinical value of different pretreatment intervals certainly merits investigation.

6. Suitable control groups or control conditions must be used to show that reductions in stuttering are the result of treatment. (Bloodstein, 1981, p.389).

This criterion highlights the need for treatment designs that overcome threats to their internal validity. The advantage of time-series designs is that the effect of most nontreatment-related variables can be identified by the judicious choice of a base-rate(s) duration and data sources. The difficulty is to be certain that all

[1]This author's experience in treating childhood stuttering has yielded one powerful, but informal, indicator of sustained improvement. At the end of lengthy follow-up assessments, some stutter-free children appear to have completely forgotten the reason why they were brought for therapy.

validity threats have been controlled before, during, or even after treatment. For instance, base-rate variablity may not include placebo effects, unless these are specifically introduced. Far more important is the amount of "control" the subject is able to exert over stuttering frequency or severity. Arguably, it should be incumbent on the researcher to demonstrate that the treatment's effects are independent of the extent and/or duration of such factors. This is a much-overlooked consideration and merits the use of appropriate conditions, be they placebo or otherwise, in order to test for this factor.

Group designs can only partially avoid some of the problems of assessing treatment effects, since most fail to identify individual treatment responses. One compromise is a multiple-baseline design, using subjects rather than, say, situations with each introduction of the treatment. Another difficulty with group designs is the choice of an appropriate control group or treatment control. Most group designs presume that roughly equivalent stuttering frequency, speech rate, and, perhaps, age and sex will ensure that the groups have potentially equivalent reactions to the treatment condition. There are literally no data that justify this assumption of uniformity.

Another interesting issue concerns the use of treatment designs that determine when treatments become impotent, or when their effects generalize. These effects have been identified through the use of multiple baselines or within-session designs, such as those used by Costello (1975). This also means there is a need to determine the time required to decide when a treatment has *not* been effective or, conversely, the size of change which indicates that clinically significant treatment effects are present.

7. The subjects' speech must sound natural and spontaneous to listeners, and the subjects must be free from the need to monitor their speech (Bloodstein, 1981, p.389).

This criterion has become increasingly important in recent years because of therapies that rely on changing the subject's customary (stutter-free) speech pattern. A number of investigators have measured naturalness by using listeners to rate speech samples for either normalcy or naturalness (Jones & Azrin, 1969; Perkins, Rudas, Johnson, Michael, & Curlee, 1974). Another way has been to test whether listeners are able to distinguish between recordings of the stutterer's post-treated speech among speech samples from normally fluent speakers (Ingham, & Packman, 1978; Runyan & Adams, 1978; 1979). Others have approached this task by measuring aspects of speech, such as vowel duration or rate, in order to relate the subject's speech to normal speech (Metz, Onufrak, & Ogburn, 1979). One of the most interesting approaches to this task has emerged from some recent research by Martin (1981), who reported that listeners could rate speech samples for naturalness on five-point scales with remarkably high levels of reliability. In consequence, both Martin and this author have begun researching the effects on stuttering and speech quality of feeding back speech naturalness ratings every 30 seconds during spontaneous speech. The preliminary results suggest that the rater is also able to perform this task reliably, and that for some stutterers, it does influence their observed speech quality. Similar endeavors have not been made to measure for spontaneity but, in principle, there is no reason why listener judgments could not be used in the same fashion.

Shames and Florance (1980) have described an attempt to measure "monitored" and "unmonitored speech" in the course of their treatment program. Their procedure requires speakers to indicate whether intervals of speech will be monitored or unmonitored. Unfortunately, the absence of an independent measure of this variable(s) makes it difficult to determine whether speakers do manipulate speech monitoring. In fact it is not clear how much, or what form of monitoring, is either desirable or, more importantly, customary for normal speakers. Webster (1974) has attempted to evaluate outcome from the Hollins program by asking listeners to respond to, "How much attention must you pay to the task of speaking fluently?" This may help determine whether posttreatment effects oblige speakers to concentrate excessively on their "fluency." But, at present, it is unclear how to measure the "spontaneity" that most clinicians believe is necessary for normally fluent speech.

8. Treatment must remove not only stuttering, but also the sense of handicap and the person's self-concept as a stutterer. (Bloodstein, 1981, p.389).

This type of criterion is often presumed to present a special challenge to treatments mainly concerned with modifying or removing the impediment to normal speech. It is assumed that a "sense of handicap," or a stutterer's "self concept," are constructs that either retain the problem or are the essence of the problem—and, more significantly, that their removal or alteration is necessary to the treatment's success. The simple fact is that no data have ever been gathered which demonstrate that changes in stuttering do not influence the "sense of handicap," or change the speaker's concept of himself as a speaker. That is not to suggest that patterns of behavior associated with stuttering will readily and immediately change when the disorder is modified. It would be rather surprising, for example, if circumstances long regarded as sources of embarrassment, or constantly avoided, were suddenly of no concern when stuttering was no longer prominent. However, no data exist to show that these reactions are essentially abnormal and need to be removed before the speaker is regarded as normally fluent.

Ironically, Bloodstein (1981) partly justifies this criterion by referring to Andrews and Cutler's (1974) claim that the removal of stuttering in one circumstance was not sufficient to change stutterers' attitudes towards speaking. Subsequent investigations on the attitude scale used in the Andrews and Cutler study by Ulliana and Ingham (1984) have shown that the scale scores are probably strongly influenced by the frequency of stuttering that occurs in situations described in the scale. In other words, it is highly likely that the attitudinal factors measured by this scale are affected by stuttering frequency. There is no reason to expect that a "sense of handicap," or "self-concept," might not also change in the same manner. In short, there is no evidence that such variables need particular attention within treatment in order to ensure therapy success.

9. The success of a program of therapy should not be inflated by ignoring dropouts. (Bloodstein, 1981, p.390).

Numerous examples of this problem have been mentioned in the previous chapters. This is a problem in almost all areas of psychotherapy research and, when excessive, presents an insurmountable barrier to meaningful conclusions from a study. The problem may well be much greater than is evident in the many studies in which large-scale dropouts have been reported. For example, in single-subject studies it is very rarely indicated that the subject(s) treated in the study were the *only* subjects on whom the procedure was tried. This information can be exceedingly important, as is demonstrated by numerous subjects who dropped out of haloperidol treatment programs. Their loss often reflected the less savory effects of this treatment and even served to contraindicate haloperidol as a treatment for stuttering. It hardly needs mentioning that the true clinical value of many treatments can only emerge when clinical researchers carefully ascertain the reasons for dropouts, and also report on subjects who failed to respond in the course of single-subject research.

10. The method must be shown to be effective in the hands of essentially any qualified clinician, including those without unusual status, prestige, or force of personality.

and

11. The method must continue to be successful when it is no longer new and the initial wave of enthusiasm over it has died away (Bloodstein, 1981, p.390).

These are much-related criteria that refer to the treatment's replicability and viability in normal clinical circumstances. Actually, these criteria have been met by some of the procedures reviewed in earlier chapters. But most of the "replication" studies invariably highlight the contribution of additional treatment factors or therapy variations, and are, of course, presented by equally enthusiastic clinicians. At the same time, an increasing number of treatment reports reveal the limitations of certain procedures, especially those using prolonged speech and its variants. This is a vital change in the pattern of much stuttering-therapy research and meets the spirit of Bloodstein's criteria. However, many of the response-contingent treatments and the prolonged speech programs continue to produce benefits despite a decline in the "initial wave of enthusiasm" over their use.

Bloodstein's (1981) criteria highlight most of the critical issues that need consideration in evaluating stuttering therapy. Some of the criteria are questionable, most notably Criteria 1 and 8, but they are useful pointers towards gauging the merit of a stuttering therapy. However, they only provide topic areas that need recognition in designing and evaluating stuttering therapy research. They fail to specify minimum requirements for satisfactory research or, more importantly, for assisting clinicians to evaluate the merit of their therapy endeavors. The purpose of clinical research is not only to design and evaluate treatments, but also to improve therapy practice. So, in what follows, an attempt will be made to develop a set of guidelines that clinicians may use to determine their treatment's efficacy. These guidelines will embrace most of the factors that Bloodstein highlighted, plus a distillation of information derived from clinical research. Of course, these are necessarily temporary guidelines, since they will inevitably change as stuttering research continues to influence treatment technology and evaluation.

Towards a Therapy-Evaluation System

Introduction

The purpose here is to develop a therapy-evaluation system suitable for the stuttering-therapy procedures reviewed in this book. This may seem a less-than-satisfactory ending to a book concerned with evaluating treatments. The reader might be justified in expecting to read an account of recommended techniques or methods of applying techniques after traversing the previous chapters. Unfortunately, to date, there is little to reward that effort, for there is no clear-cut evidence that any treatment technique has been sufficiently refined so that a definite form(s) of treatment can be recommended. But there is sufficient information to begin outlining some necessary operations that should accompany therapy.

Searching for an all-purpose, completely acceptable treatment-evaluation design seems to have about as much chance of success as the search for the Holy Grail. The problem is that it is not at all clear that we would know success when we found it. For, if the object of stuttering therapy is to produce normally fluent speech, then there are no operationalized concepts that will detect this phenomenon. Indeed, there are virtually no measures (or sets of measures) that can be used to describe normal fluency (Starkweather, 1980). But if we are prepared to settle for an assessment strategy that shows when stuttering is changing relative to treatment, and when some of the important parameters of normal fluency are evident, then perhaps the search will not be fruitless.

Another impediment to the search appears to be the different formats that are used in stuttering therapy. These obviously differ among treatments, particularly those treatments concerned with controlling, but not removing stuttering, or those that treat stuttering by modifying other behaviors. That is not a major impediment, since, in each case, the main objective is to modify stuttering, and so their success, or otherwise, can be related to frequency counts of stuttering. More of a problem is whether the treatment is delivered intensively or in the typical once- or twice-weekly-clinic-visit format. Since it is expected that intensive treatments will change stuttering more rapidly, the format will need flexibility in order to accommodate different expected rates of change. Nevertheless, even this problem is surmountable provided the principal components of the format are common to both approaches, and the guidelines of a less-intensive format derive from the slowest expected improvements that result from treatment. A final source of difficulty might be the age of patients; there are various indicators in the preceding chapters that children may be more responsive to certain treatments than either adolescents or adults. It is possible that this difference might extend to rates of change, plus any criteria used for determining clinically significant changes in speech. The same arguments could apply to differences in the intellectual level of patients, for there is some indication that retardates have a relatively slower response to treatment. This resolution is reasonably straightforward if the format is derived empirically. In other words, where data exist that demand exceptional formats, then those formats should be found. There is probably some justification for developing separate formats for child therapy and adolescent/adult therapy. This will be attempted in the proposals to follow.

The Initial Assessment

The most important initial-assessment factor concerns those procedures that permit the clinician to decide whether a child, adolescent, or adult is suitable for therapy. A considerable amount of recent literature has been devoted to determining whether a child requires stuttering therapy. And, oddly enough, many of the factors are pertinent to older-aged subjects, along with some necessary additional factors.

There is remarkably little research on what factors are relevant in deciding to offer therapy to any persons displaying stuttering. In the case of stutterers, other than children, the person's decision to seek treatment should be almost sufficient reason to offer therapy. There is certainly insufficient indication that certain types of subjects are unlikely to benefit from treatment, but the requirements of therapy evaluation mean that the clinician and subject (or subject's parent) will need to reach a number of agreements—even contractural arrangements. The minimum features of those agreements will be acceptance of the multiple requirements of the evaluation and treatment process.

Some reasonable consensus has been reached that certain forms of speech are relevant in determining the likelihood that a child will develop into a chronic stutterer. Certain types and frequencies of disfluencies are expected events during speech development, but their form, frequency, and variability probably distinguish young children who are identified as stutterers. Adams (1977) and Curlee (1980) have recently provided worthwhile reviews of the pertinent literature in this area, and have outlined some useful guidelines to help distinguish the nonfluent child who is at risk. To paraphrase Adams, the child diagnosed as an "incipient stutterer" exhibits at least 10% of disfluent words that are characterized by part-word repetitions, audible silent prolongations, and broken words. The *schwa* vowel is perceived, and there is difficulty in starting and/or sustaining voicing, or air-flow, which is evident at transitions from voiceless to voice sounds. These speech problems may also be accompanied by bodily movements, and the whole diagnosis should be supplemented by pertinent information from the parents and child. Essentially the same recommendations are made by Curlee (1980), with the additional interesting suggestion that the child should be assessed under different speaking conditions. For, unlike normally disfluent children (Martin, Haroldson, & Kuhl, 1972a; 1972b), the incipient stutterer's disfluencies tend to vary under different speaking conditions.

In the case of young children, there may also be some advantages in arranging for spectrographic analyses of disfluencies that parents label "stutterings." Some years ago, Stromsta (1965) provided some provocative data which suggested that comparisons between disfluent and fluent tokens from young children served to distinguish between those who were stuttering 10 years later and those who were not. The data were based on observations as to whether or not the disfluencies showed "lack of formant transitions and/or abnormal terminations of phonation" (p.317). Ten years later, most of the children who displayed these features remained stuttering and those who did not were stutter-free. Unfortunately, the level of confidence we can have in these data is somewhat questionable since, as Curlee (1980) noted, the analysis criteria for the spectrograms were not adequately operationalized, and it is not known which of these children received therapy during the following decade. Furthermore, the study still awaits the benefit of replication.

Curlee's (1980) recommendation that the child's speech be assessed under different conditions brings us back to the task of choosing speaking conditions that will identify variability, this time within the clinic. Some useful guidelines have been suggested by Ryan and Costello. Ryan (1974) has developed a "Stuttering Interview" which contains tasks suitable mainly for school-age stutterers. Costello (1981) has also provided a set of within-clinic procedures that can be employed to test for variability as well as gauge responsiveness to potential therapy procedures. Many of these within-clinic measures of variability have multiple advantages, especially if it can be shown that they correlate with counterpart beyond-clinic conditions. For example, repeated within-clinic assessments of the child speaking with "significant others" may match counterpart ratings of the child's speech with the same persons outside the clinic. The most obvious gain from this happy coincidence would be the possibility of confining the treatment to the clinic, rather than extending to beyond-clinic conditions with their attendant organizational difficulties. With young children, Ryan (1974) recommends a variety of tasks including monologues, oral reading (if possible), telephone conversations, and conversations that incorporate questions. These seem to be particularly worthwhile tasks in view of Ryan's finding of very different stuttering frequencies across these tasks.

From all the foregoing, what should be regarded as necessary? The most obvious contenders are conversational speech, monologues, and oral reading, since they are useful for assessment and treatment. Perhaps the main reason that oral reading is included is because of its utility in certain therapies; otherwise it is strange that stuttering assessments have placed so much store on a task that is rarely performed in the natural environment (except occasionally in the school setting). Nevertheless, it does have the presumed advantage of controlling for word avoidance. Clinician-client conversations, heavily laced with questions, and telephone conversations are obviously good choices. The latter is especially useful because of its viability for beyond-clinic treatment and assessment, particularly with older-age stutterers. The ideal duration of each of these tasks is yet another "unknown," but in the context of demands on clinician time, perhaps each should be around 3 minutes.

Most of the current stuttering-assessment systems place great emphasis on questionnaires. Their purpose is to highlight factors such as an abnormal health history, unusual reactions to speaking situations, the patterns of parent behavior, and aspects considered relevant to treatment. And all may serve a useful function. But most of this information can be gained during the course of an interview that simply overviews these areas of the subject's life. There is even less certainty that any of the questionnaires currently recommended for clinicians contribute anything to treatment or evaluation that cannot be derived from suitably obtained speech-performance data. For instance, there is no evidence that responses on the available questionnaires have benefited a treatment program. Thus far, it seems that they have about as much functional value as a description of the color of the patient's hair. Perhaps the only exception to this dismissive note, as will be mentioned later, are posttreatment questionnaires that rate the subject's reaction to treatment (Webster, 1974).

Formulating the Evaluation Design

The most significant lesson from the checkered history of stuttering therapy is that a useful treatment-evaluation design must be able to account for the known and expected variability of stuttering. It must be a design capable of demonstrating that therapy progress or outcome evaluation is not confounded by the known untreated variability of the subject's stuttering. Treatment-evaluation formats, suitable for this purpose, have begun to emerge from the time-series quasi-exerimental designs (Hersen & Barlow, 1976) typically used in single-subject research. They are especially suitable, because they not only permit the analysis of variability, but they also help deal with concerns such as accountability, decision making, and outcome evaluation. Furthermore, they are not only the most powerful designs available for determining sources of within-subject variability, but also the only ones that will enable the clinician to discern whether therapy produces generalized changes in the object of treatment.

The strength, or internal and external validity, of these designs in therapy depends on repeated data collection within and beyond the therapy setting. They are also enhanced by suitable data, collected at clinically relevant intervals before, during, and after treatment. In short, the foundation of the recommended format is an integration of the now-familiar multibaseline and ABA design. But the clinical viability of this format depends on finding some basis for determining the clinically significant frequency, duration, and content of the measures that should be incorporated in the format's design. The rationale for the basis of a proposed format will now be outlined.

The Data Base

There is probably little argument that an appropriate evaluation design requires access to audio-recorded speech within relevant speaking situations. It would be useful if these recordings could be supplemented by video recordings, if only to ensure that the visual aspects of stuttering (especially with respect to severity measurement) were taken into account. In the absence of this facility, there is value in utilizing observed performance data.

Perhaps the minimal acceptable clinical data are stuttering-frequency counts and words-or-syllables-spoken during talking time. They provide the basic necessities for gauging changes in stuttering, and the contribution that the amount and rate of speaking make to stuttering variability.

A frequency count of "moments of stuttering" may not fully depict the extent of disability caused by stuttering, but it has certainly passed the test of time as a treatment measure—probably for the same reasons that measures of stuttering intervals or disfluency categories are less frequently used in treatment. The virtue of frequency counts of stuttering is that they can be integrated in treatment via "on-line" measurement, as well as indicating the treatment's success (or otherwise) in removing the crux of the disorder. Most current therapy programs are designed to remove all instances of stuttering, so it is becoming less important that those instances to be described as "severe" or "part-word repetitions." It also makes little sense now to confound stuttering counts with counts of normal disfluencies. There is increasing acceptance that clinicians and (certainly lay observers) are able to distinguish between disfluencies and stutterings (MacDonald & Martin, 1973). This is an important point since there is no obvious advantage in a treatment that removes normal disfluencies, but is less successful in removing stutterings. Conversely, a treatment that removes all disfluencies, normal or abnormal, may actually succeed in producing an unusual form of fluency.

There are at least two dangers in relying on frequency counts of stuttering alone in order to evaluate treatment. The first relates to severity. Occasionally, a relatively low frequency of stuttering, certainly less than the much-touted 3% of words (Shine, 1980; Webster, 1979), may contain exceptionally long blocks (Ingham, 1981). Because of this, there is good reason to record the nature of low-frequency stuttering. The second reason concerns the role of word-avoidance. This must be the least-researched stuttering phenomenon, yet one of the best-known features of the disorder — especially in adults. Perhaps the only way of measuring its presence is the subject's report and instructional tests for its influence. The latter may be ascertained by asking the subject to try to minimize stuttering for an interval, possibly by "avoiding stutterings" during spontaneous speech, and then comparing this interval with another in which the reverse instruction is given.

It is generally accepted that reduced speech rate may be sufficient to cause reductions in stuttering. Of course, reduced speaking as such may also have the same effect. Less publicized is the possibility that abnormally fast speech rate may also reduce stuttering (Ingham, Martin, & Kuhl, 1971). But there is no accepted method for measuring speech rate. The principal point of contention is the relationship between the measure and normally fluent speech rate. The issue of speech rate, as Starkweather (1980) has recently pointed out, is much more complex than simple counts of words- or syllables-per-minute. What is perceived as "fast" or "slow" turns out to be partially relative, and also dependent upon variables such as sound durations, pause durations, co-articulation, and rate of syllable production. Consequently, the currently used clinical measures of rate only approximate what is perceived as rate, or what might be normal rate. In light of this, what options are available?

For some years, this writer and colleagues have used 170 to 210 syllables per minute as a target normal speech rate (Ingham, 1981). But this measure (allowing for its imperfections) is based on relatively unusual speech—a monologue that is not interrupted by the conversational exchanges that typify speech in the natural environment. It is also the speech rate of young adults. Furthermore, it is neither as useful nor, probably, as valid as Perkins's (1975) measure of articulation rate which excludes pauses and stutterings. However, in the absence of pertinent speech-rate research, both measures probably provide clinically useful methods for measuring rate during therapy. Another reflection of the need for research in this area is that there is little to indicate what the relevant target-speech rates should be for treatment, particularly with respect to the subject's age. There are some data from school children which indicate that the average syllables-per-minute rates in normal speech progressively increase throughout childhood. Kowal, O'Connell, and Sabin (1975) have shown that in kindergarten years this rate is about 50% of adult rates and rises to near adult rates by around 12 years. At present, that might provide the best guide for estimating the expected syllable-per-minute rates for different age groups at the end of treatment. Perhaps a better alternative, certainly one worthy of investigation, is the subject's speech rate during stutter-free intervals. Admittedly, these intervals (depending on their length) may be influenced by stuttering frequency, but they may also be a more appropriate basis for determining the speaker's "normally" fluent rate. Actually, the clinician's perceptual judgment on what is an acceptable and normal rate may ultimately translate into the most clinically suitable syllable-per-minute scores for the individual case—especially if normalcy or naturalness is, in the final analysis, a reliable basis for determining this measure.

There are numerous reasons why speech-rate and stuttering-frequency measures are only partially satisfactory in assessing speech performance in treatment, even though they are necessary measures. The most important is the imperfect connection between zero stuttering at "normal" speech rate and normally fluent speech (Ingham, 1981; Perkins, 1981). The need to improve this connection stems mainly from the proliferation of treatments that procure "fluency" via unusual speech patterns, such as the variants of prolonged speech. Adams (1982), for example, has been particularly concerned about the need to gain much more information on the indices needed to identify normally fluent speech. Starkweather (1980) also explored the issues in the above-mentioned review and concluded that fluent speech "is the quality of speech that includes rapid and easy, as well as smooth production" (p.195). But, as yet, the combination of measurement operations that would quantify that form of speaking is unknown.

A number of approaches to the task of measuring speech quality have already been mentioned. These include ratings of naturalness (Jones & Azrin, 1969) prosody, rate, and fluency (Perkins et al., 1974), plus perceptual analysis of differences between speech samples from normally fluent speakers and post-treated stutterers. The difficulty with these measures is that they may evaluate the results of treatment, but cannot be readily integrated with the treatment process in the same fashion as rate and stuttering counts. However, one promising approach to this task, as was previously described, is to use on-line ratings of naturalness, provided it is possible to establish the reliability and validity of such ratings.

In general terms, therefore, the measurement process that has maximum utility in a therapy context is one that yields data with dual functions: (1) provide a basis for establishing within- and beyond-clinic treatment effects, and (2) contribute to treatment operations. Such dual function measures may not be useful to all types of therapy, but in many of the reviewed therapies they would serve the first function. In passing, it is interesting to observe that there has been a gradual recognition of the importance of measures that do more than passively chart the subject's progress through therapy. The most useful measures permit decisions about the efficacy of therapy, and may have an integral role as treatment agents. It is this latter function of such measures which is being used lately to assist the transfer and maintenance of therapy effects.

Where and When to Collect Data

The choice of the situations in which the subject's speech should be measured will be conditioned by the recordability of the situation as much as its validity. The recording process has been greatly assisted by the availability of exceedingly small, good-quality micro-cassette recorders that should not be beyond the resources of a clinic, or indeed, many clients. They can be worn comfortably and equipped with remote hand controls that simplify recording in most situations. The choice of recordable assessment situations, especially for children, presents some complicated, but not unsolvable, difficulties. There are some logical choices; with parents, peers, and significant others in the subject's speaking environment. However, the validity of these situations may be aided by two other factors: the subject's choice of "difficult" but recordable situations, and the relative frequency with which these situations occur. These additional considerations should certainly be included within the decision base for choosing samples from the subject's environment. One logical starting point for deciding on sample sizes is that they should reflect the typical speaking time that occurs in any of the settings. If the subject's speech with his parents occupies more than 50% of estimated speaking time (speaking time could be derived with reasonable precision from logs kept by the subject or, in the case of children, their parents), then this should be represented proportionately in the sampling arrangements.

Reaching an agreeable decision about the frequency and duration of samples in a repeated-measures-assessment design involves at least three considerations: identifying variability, establishing that a treatment is "working," and data management. However, taking account of these considerations in a generally acceptable therapy format is like putting together a jigsaw puzzle with pieces shaped by special interest groups whose members can never agree. And we certainly have plenty of those groups. Nevertheless there may be some parts of the puzzle that can be solved by compromise pieces.

Perhaps the first puzzle piece should come from the ranks of clinical researchers who show little agreement over the minimum number of data points that are needed to reflect variability. For compromise purposes, therefore, perhaps the much-referenced text by Hersen and Barlow (1976) should be a guide. They recommend at least three "data points" in any phase of an evaluation design employing data-trend comparisons, although many of Hersen and Barlow's examples use four or more data points for this purpose. But if the seemingly small number of four is acceptable, then does this translate into four consecutive days, once every 4 weeks, or perhaps, once every 4 months? This piece of the puzzle should probably come from two interest groups; practicing clinicians and the editors of journals reporting treatment studies. For it relates to the frequency with which treatment is offered, and the interval of time needed to convince peers that treatment efficacy has been established. Presumably, the object of treatment is to show that reductions or increases (in whatever the behavior) unambiguously differ from those found during a base-rate period. It is therefore necessary to decide on what will be regarded as a significant treatment benefit. But perhaps the search for that puzzle piece should be deferred for a moment. The third, and most overlooked factor, is the sheer task of assessing data obtained from audio-recordings, and the subject's ability to obtain such recordings. Actually, the indeterminate number and size of the puzzle's pieces start to take shape at this point, since much of their shape depends on a decision about frequency-of-therapy contact. If conventional individual therapy is used as a guide, then such therapy is usually offered twice weekly for a maximum of 1 hour per session. Within or between these times, there needs to be sufficient time to process beyond-clinic data.

Determining a Treatment Effect

The next task is to find a suitable time-frame that can be used to decide whether therapy is beneficial or not beneficial. This could lead to a veritable Pandora's Box—comparing different therapies and their effects. Fortunately, the interior of the box is not as daunting as might be expected. We can now take advantage of a body of therapy literature that should help us estimate the rate of change in target behaviors from successfully treated clients. Indeed, if that literature cannot be used for this purpose, then it has virtually no external validity (Birnbrauer, 1981). At the very least, it should teach us the expected rate of change in stuttering if a client responds to a particular treatment. For example, if the chosen treatment was one of the response-contingent procedures, then perhaps a very much less dramatic decline in stuttering frequency should be expected when compared with rhythm or any of the numerous variants of prolonged speech. On the other hand, the relevant target behavior for these speech-pattern techniques is usually restoration of normal speech rate, thus extending the time needed to determine responsiveness to that treatment.

There is no reason to skirt the "treatment-effect time" issue with generalities, since much of the reviewed treatment literature, at least that which provides single-subject data, can be summarized for this purpose. Tables 12.1 and 12.2 provide summaries of the treatment studies that permit an estimation to be made of the treatment time required for stuttering or disfluencies (sometimes "dysfluencies") to decrease by at least 50% relative to the base rate and "successful outcome." The term "successful outcome" is used in a very broad sense. It refers to those subjects who were reported, at the end of their treatment, to have reduced stuttering by at least 50% and, when speech-rate data are provided, not decreased their speed of speaking. The successfully treated subjects have been divided into children, those 12 years of age or younger (Table 12.1), and adults (Table 12.2). This is for no special reason, other than the recurring suggestion in the literature that children appear to respond more rapidly to some treatments. In general terms, the tables show that children respond a little more rapidly to most treatment procedures, particularly the response-contingent techniques. The rate of response to the GILCU and speech-pattern techniques are more difficult to translate, since there is no clear indication of the time taken to reach 50% improvement. For this reason it was decided to use half the treatment or talking time required to reach the final target behavior as equivalent to 50% improvement. This is probably the main reason why these treatments appear to take longer to reach the treatment-effect criterion.

Resolving the Treatment-Design Puzzle

The next task is to translate the preceding information into solution pieces for the treatment-format puzzle. The pieces are easier to construct if it is accepted that treatment-effect time and base-rate periods need to incorporate similar data-collection intervals if the most credible comparison is to be made between the variabililty in both phases of the therapy format. In other words, if treatment is offered twice weekly then base-rate, treatment, and posttreatment data should be collected twice weekly. This task is also aided if some of the extreme scores are regarded as less probable representations of expected durations. Consequently, if the 95th percentile is used as the upper duration point, then, for children this turns out to be 12.65 hours, and for adults 23 hours. In other words, these durations might be used to indicate the maximum treatment time that should be offered before the clinician should decide that the treatment is, or is not, producing clinical benefits. The base-rate period might be constructed on the basis of some data collected by Andrews and Harvey (1981). They reported that pretreatment speech measures in groups of stutterers do not show substantial changes over a 6-week period. Thus, the most conservative treatment design might incorporate up

Table 12.1
This table summarizes the results of a survey of stuttering treatments involving *children 12 years of age or younger.*

Method	*Procedure*	*Study*	*Hours Required for 50% Reduction in Target Behavior*	*Number of Subject/ Age Range*
Response Contingent	GILCU	Costello (1980)	15.50	1/11
		Johnson et al. (1978)	10.50	1/6
		Ryan (1974)	3.30-30.50	6/7-9
		Mowrer (1975)	5.00	1/10
	Positive Reinforce-ment	Peters (1977)	0.60	2/8,8
		Shaw & Shrum (1972)	0.67	3/9-10
	Combined Punishment and Reinforce-ment	Ryan (1974)	1.00-6.00	2/9
	Punishment	Martin & Berndt (1970)	0.67	1/12
		Martin et al. (1972)	1.33-2.00	2/3 & 4
		McDermott (1971)	1.20	1/9
		Reed & Godden (1977)	1.33-1.67	2/3 & 5
Masking	Continuous	MacCulloch et al. (1970)	6.00	4/11.9
Speech Pattern	Rhythmic Stimulation	Herscovitch & Le Bow (1973)	2.00	2/12 & 12
	MCSR	Brady (1971)	4.00	1/12
Speech Pattern	DAF/ Prolonged Speech	Ryan (1971)	2.00	1/8
		Ryan (1974)	5.65-20.25	2/8 & 12
		Turnbaugh & Guitar (1981)	4.50	1/12
Speech Pattern	Regulated Breathing	Hee & Holmes (1976)	1.50	1/10
Speech Pattern	Shadowing	Ottoni (1974)	1.00	1/9
Traditional	Programmed	Ryan (1974)	2.30	1/10

The survey was designed to identify studies in which it was possible to discern the treatment time needed for individual subjects to reduce stuttering or disfluencies by more than 50% relative to pretreatment performance. That point was established when the target behavior reached the 50% reduction level on two assessment occasions. In the case of the Gradual Increase in Length and Complexity of Utterance (GILCU), the 50% reduction level was regarded as equivalent to half the time required to achieve the designated treatment target. For the speech-pattern procedures, the 50% reduction level was regarded as equivalent to half the time required to complete the treatment's instatement phase.

Table 12.2
This table incorporates the same information as Table 12.1, but for subjects older than 12 years.

Method	*Procedure*	*Study*	*Hours Required for 50% reduction in target behavior*	*Number of subjects/ age range*
Response Contingent	GILCU	Mowrer (1975)	5.00-9.75	2/23 & 31
		Ryan (1974)	5.25-19.30	3/16-35
	Punishment	Costello (1975)	1.83	1/18
		Ryan (1974)	3.05-5.15	2/15 & 20
	Self-management	James (1981)	23.00	1/18
		LaCroix (1973)	1.00	2/★
Anxiety Reduction	Reciprocal Inhibition	Boudreau & Jeffrey (1973)	12.00	4/16-22
Speech Pattern	Rhythmic Stimulation	Brady (1971)	5.00-31.00	17/14-53
Speech Pattern	Prolonged Speech	Andrews (1973)	5.00	1/2★
		Boberg & Fong (1980)	15.00	1/19
	DAF/ Prolonged Speech	Goldiamond (1965)	3.08	2/40, ★
		Ingham & Andrews (1973)	1.63-4.60	11/18-56
		Ryan (1974)	1.00-88.60	23/14-45
		Webster (1970)	5.00-20.00	8/15-45
Biofeedback	EMG	Guitar (1975)	2.67	1/32
Traditional	Programmed	Ryan (1974)	1.45-12.05	9/14-43

★Age unknown.

to 6 weeks of twice-weekly recordings of the subject's speech within and beyond the clinic. The least conservative approach might utilize the four-data-point principle, and use a minimum of 2 weeks of twice-weekly recordings in both settings. If the spirit of compromise prevails, then the most practical alternative would be 4 weeks of twice-weekly recordings.

Thus, the preceding formulations would suggest that for all practical purposes the base-rate phase should be around 4 weeks. The treatment phase for almost all current data-based treatments should not exceed about 12 hours for children, or 23 hours for adults, before a decision is made as to whether the treatment should continue or be changed. Presumably, quite discernible trends in relevant data should be expected by the fifth hour, if some treatments are likely to be beneficial. It should be recognized, of course, that this does not mean the treatment will be successful, since it is likely that many treatment failures showed evidence of responsiveness within this time-frame. But relatively few successful treatments demonstrated their benefits outside of these intervals.

The next important issue is whether 4 weeks of twice-weekly recordings of "natural-situation" behavior provides a reliable estimate of variability. The simple fact is that there are almost no data that can be used to address the issue. Perhaps the sole exception is a study by Ingham and Packman (1977) on an adult stutterer. But this is certainly one circumstance in which group data would be preferable. All that can be stated is that 4 weeks merely has the "ring" of face validity. It also has the advantage of suitability for time-series analyses of behavior change.

Another issue concerns the point at which treatment should cease. In the context of the broad format developed thus far, perhaps stability over four weeks of nontreatment might be one rational basis for that decision. This would ensure that the subject's improved performance has been sustained long enough to determine that it differs unambiguously from pretreatment performance. However, there are more complex issues associated with assessing treatment outcome that will be discussed later.

Treatment-Choice-Assessment Procedures

One of the paradoxes of the current treatment literature concerns the method by which a therapy is chosen. As yet, there is virtually no research-based information that will help clinicians choose an appropriate treatment for either a child or adult. On the other hand, there is a growing literature that indicates some procedures may benefit children, while for adults some treatments have shown more success than others. Consequently, it may be of interest to review some reported decision-making processes for those treatments. Virtually all of these processes refer to the treatment of children, but they also have some relevance for adults.

Costello (1980; 1981) has suggested that the initial evaluation should include three brief tests to determine the modifiability of a child's stuttering; instructions to "talk as perfectly as possible" (Costello, 1980, p.19), speaking in rhythm, and using prolonged speech. The first of these obviously indicates the extent to which the child may modify stuttering under "demand" conditions. Presumably, this also provides an opportunity to discern the forms of speaking the child may adopt that could confound any therapy gains. The other two probes are also recommended to gain some notion of the child's responsiveness to potential therapy strategies. In most respects, this procedure resembles the suggestions made by Guitar and Peters (1980).

Riley and Riley (1979; 1983) have introduced an interesting assessment strategy. They have devised a procedure for assessing children (3-11 years) in terms of four "neurologic" and five "traditional" components of stuttering, the neurologic being "attending disorders," "auditory-processing disorders," "sentence-formulation disorders," and "oral-motor disorders." The traditional components are "high self-expectations," "manipulative stuttering," "disruptive communication environment," "unrealistic parental expectations," and "abnormal parental need for the child to stutter." The child (and parents) are rated on each of these components; a treatment is then formulated to deal with each of the more problematic components. The general results of the treatments, based on these components, have been favorable according to data presented by the Rileys, but these data give no evidence that progress in treatment or outcome actually depends upon the inclusion of treatment procedures derived from these components. In other words, at present, these pretreatment tasks are little more than sensible suggestions, for there are no data that show that they accurately (or even inaccurately) predict a child's responsiveness to these procedures in therapy.

Another interesting approach to the therapy-choice issue is offered by Adams (1980). For example, with children who exhibit "problems in commencing and sustaining voicing or air flow" (p.291), Adams recommends a variation of Perkins's (1973) breathstream-management technique. This may be supplemented by Ryan's (1974) GILCU procedure. If the child's stuttering is not characterized by difficulties in commencing and maintaining vocalization, then another option is that he may have "slowness and uncertainty in the operation of various aspects of the language-encoding process (for example, word retrieval)" (Adams, 1980, p.293). The GILCU procedure is also recommended for such cases since it gives "the child more time to manage the control integrative aspects of communication" (p.293). Recently, Adams and Runyan (1981) have provided more detailed recommendations that flow from evaluation of the acoustic signal. But as this writer has argued (Ingham, 1982b), the clinical merit of these recommendations is in dire need of a data-based investigation.

In the absence of relevant data on the therapy decision-making process there appears to be virtue in the suggestions offered by Costello, Guitar and Peters, Adams, and the Rileys. The current treatment literature also provides some plausible guidelines (Costello, 1983). In the case of young children, there is every indication that the contingency-management procedures may be of benefit, and may not demand significant alterations in the child's manner of speech production. In effect, the response-contingent punishment schedules suggested in the studies by Martin, Kuhl, and Haroldson (1972) and Reed and Godden (1977), or the GILCU procedures used in studies by Ryan (1974), Mowrer (1975), and Costello (1980) are useful starting points. So, too, might be the modeling strategies described by Johnson (1980) and Gregory and Hill (1980) for very young children, although these require much more supportive research. These seem preferable initial interventions over those that require marked alterations to the speech pattern. In other words, the procedures described in Chapter 10 might form a useful second-stage intervention.

The methods available for choosing treatment techniques for adult or adolescent stutterers are even less satisfactory. There are some suggested diagnostic approaches that have ample face validity. For instance, Brutten (1975) and Webster and Brutten (1974) have described a Behavior Assessment Battery that distinguishes certain features of the stuttering problem, but there are no data to demonstrate in any convincing way that this has improved the choice of therapy. Various approaches to pretreatment assessment are well summarized by Williams (1978), but, as well, there is nothing to indicate that the subject's responses to these assessments improves treatment choice.

Some clinicians have virtually cut the Gordian Knot by recommending one treatment as suitable for virtually all stutterers. For example, Webster (1979) claims that his Precision Fluency Shaping Program contains the essential ingredients for treating most stutterers: "We have found that 19 carefully structured, consecutive days of [Precision Fluency Shaping] treatment provide a standard interval that is effective with a large majority of cases" (p.219). In fact, it is not clear what makes a subject unsuitable for this treatment. In many ways, Webster's recommendation probably typifies the approach adopted by many prominent clinical researchers, for few report the tailoring of treatments to the individual's pretreatment pattern of behavior. The clinician can be rightly excused for believing that the treatments these authorities report are the treatments advocated for all clients who enter their clinics.

There are, however, some endeavors to use diagnostic strategies to determine the client's suitability for some of the reported treatments. Perkins (1979), for example, has built much of his therapy around the stutterer's ability to manage coordination: "The effects of simplifying these coordinations has been so stable that the procedure has been a diagnostic tool for us." (p.105). In other words, the subject's failure to reduce stuttering via simplified adjustments to respiration, phonation, and articulation has contraindicated the use of breathstream management approaches to therapy.

The decision to use, or not use, variants of prolonged speech is probably the basis for most current therapy endeavors with adults. Guitar and Peters (1980), for instance, believe the decision is between offering stuttering modification therapy—procedures advocated by Luper and Mulder (1964), Sheehan (1970), Van Riper (1973), and Williams (1971)—and Fluency Shaping Therapy (variants of prolonged speech). The choice, for Guitar and Peters (1980), is mainly based on responses to the S24 Scale (Andrews & Cutler, 1974), and trial therapy. Fluency Shaping is recommended as "very effective when the client has relatively low communication attitude and avoidance scores and responds well to prolonged speech during trial fluency shaping therapy. This would be true regardless of the severity of the stuttering, and especially true when there is minimal avoidance behavior" (Guitar & Peters, 1980, p.35). It should be evident by now, however, that there are no available data that support these recommendations.

Ryan's (1974) investigations on different treatment techniques might have yielded some pointers to factors relevant in choosing among, say, GILCU, prolonged speech, punishment, or the programmed offering of Van Riper's (1963) procedures. But, again, there is little to suggest that any particular pretreatment behavior relates to the successful use of any of these treatments.

Against that background, it is probably foolhardy to make any recommendations. Nevertheless, there are some factors that might be useful in establishing the choice of treatment. Perhaps the most important decision, with respect to the current therapies for adult stutterers, is whether they should be offered intensively or on a distributed schedule (the distinction between these offerings is often unclear and usually relative). There are numerous exigencies that could influence such a decision, not the least being the subject's preference. However, when the treatment of choice involves reorganizing the subject's speech pattern, then there could be advantages in managing this process in an intensive or continuous treatment setting. Otherwise, the method of choosing a treatment technique for adults and adolescents would still seem to have much in common with that recommended for children. In other words, there appears to be less immediate demand on the subject and clinician if the initial treatment does not alter the subject's speech pattern. Thus, all things being equal, the preferred initial treatments would probably be the response-contingent stimulation techniques, or, in those cases where state anxiety needs attention, possibly the anxiety-reduction techniques. The failure to respond to these first-stage approaches would then suggest the need to use speech-pattern-change procedures, such as prolonged speech or any of its variants. This second stage might also involve masking or even shadowing. Each of the second stage approaches might also be tried in a nonintensive context before proceeding to the use of intensive strategies.

Dismantling Therapy

It may well be that a number of treatments are tried before a therapy strategy is found which will achieve within- and beyond-clinic treatment gains. These will be strategies that establish and transfer treatment gains. It is therefore necessary for the assessment process to incorporate strategies which will indicate when the initial phase of treatment should be replaced by maintenance strategies.

There is general agreement that maintenance strategies are necessary components of the therapy process, although it is often difficult to believe that—considering the slight amount of research they have attracted. There are some very limited data available that demonstrate the efficacy of current maintenance techniques (Boberg, 1981; Boberg, Howie, & Woods, 1977), though they give no guidance on how to choose assessment procedures for this phase. To some extent, the task has been eased by some useful data which suggest that when beyond-clinic generalization occurs in the treatment of preschool children, then unassisted maintenance will follow (Prins & Ingham, 1983). But the evidence is certainly not so persuasive in the case of older-age children.

Actually the evaluation format might be useful in helping to establish the necessity, or otherwise, of maintenance treatment. The logical reference source is the assessment format used in base rate and the initial treatment phase. In other words, the immediate posttreatment phase should be seen as a counterpart to the base-rate phase. By this principle, repeated assessments should continue for at least 4 weeks. This should provide a reasonable basis for estimating the initial stability of these gains.

The dismantling of the therapy process may also blend with treatment and assessment procedures. One internally valid method of establishing when treatment should be withdrawn is to use a period when assessment and therapy-controlled measures of speech performance begin to merge. Martin, Kuhl, and

Haroldson (1972) used this strategy to compare the treatment- and nontreatment-setting performance of two preschool stutterers treated by contingency arrangements. Costello (1975) also used this strategy to good effect during therapy sessions by comparing nontreatment and treatment intervals over contingency-managed therapy sessions.

Another strategy has been used by this writer in recent years (Ingham, 1980; 1981; 1982a). It involves the systematic withdrawal of regular assessment sessions contingent upon sustained performance, plus comparisons with intermittent covert assessments. This is also an example of how beyond-clinic (or within-clinic) assessments can serve dual functions; that is, they decrease the contact frequency with the client, but remain a useful source of speech control.

The above-mentioned method for continuing maintenance and evaluation actually serves to illustrate how maintenance and outcome-evaluation strategies can be gradually integrated. The core procedure has been referred to in Chapter 10. The subject is required to return to the clinic initially for two once-weekly assessments, and if the target behavior (0% syllables stuttered at between 170 and 210 SPM) is maintained in all within- and beyond-clinic assessments, then the subject "earns" a 2-week rest from assessments. If these 2-week-apart assessments achieve the target behavior, then the subject earns a 4-week "rest" from assessments. This systematic and performance-contingent withdrawal of assessment continues until two 32-week-apart assessments are passed successfully. If the subject fails on any assessment (that is, has one stuttering or departs from the target-speech rate on any task), then the subject returns to the weekly assessments. In the most recent applications of this procedure (Ingham, 1982a), it has been used in conjunction with a self-managment technique (specifically, self-evaluation training) in order to shift the responsibility for conducting this performance-contingent assessment strategy to the subject. In the main, these procedures have been used with some success on adults. They have also been useful with older-age children (Ingham, 1980). The data from these studies have been supplemented by nonperformance-contingent assessments made in beyond-clinic conditions, which thereby serve to establish the point when the nontreatment-related assessments blend with the treatment-related assessments. They have also been supplemented by a wide variety of covert assessments which have shown, in some cases, that overt and covert assessments differ markedly. To a large extent, though, these concurrent assessments have suggested that the maintenance strategy may be phased out well before the 32-week-apart assessment point.

Undoubtedly, covert-assessment procedures are among the most contentious assessment techniques used in stuttering therapy. But in their defense, it should be noted that they have the potential of providing the most clinically valid treatment-assessment data, particularly when used in conjunction with relevant overt assessment data. Their claim to validity, however, is only as strong as their claims to be unobtrusive—and these claims are often difficult to demonstrate. There are various degrees of "covertness," or varieties of techniques that might be free of the reactive features found in overt assessments, features that many clinicians suspect produce unrealistic or "artificial" posttreatment data. Perhaps the most useful is the "unplanned telephone call," made (ideally) by a person not associated with the treatment. Other relevant information may be obtained from the subject's associates, which can then be validated by carefully arranged recordings. Admittedly, this all sounds uncomfortably unethical, but it need not be. In the case of older-age children, adolescents, and adults, it is unlikely that the assessment's validity will be threatened if, before treatment, the client agrees that such assessments will be made from time to time to test the treatment's worth. This writer has used this procedure on numerous occasions over the past decade, and has yet to meet one client who found it to be distasteful or disconcerting. More importantly, it has often provided an immensely useful clinical service. For instance, in the current applications of this maintenance schedule, clinicians intermittently telephone subjects. If the clinician detects stuttering, then, regardless of whether the subject "passed" the previous assessment, the subject automatically fails that assessment and returns to the initial step in the maintenance schedule.

How should covert assessments be organized within an assessment schedule? Like all other assessment decisions, the decision to use covert assessment should be guided, where possible, by treatment and evaluation considerations. However, the difficulty with this form of assessment is that it may lose its "cover" if it is used too frequently. This type of assessment probably carries adequate treatment and assessment value if it occurs four times during the transfer phase and four times during the immediate posttreatment assessment phase. This allows the clinician to decide whether the subject's assessed speech performance is indeed reflected in less stimulus-bound conditions. Probably the most practical procedure for this purpose is an unannounced telephone conversation with a person unconnected with the treatment. It is up to the clinician to decide how this should be recorded, but there is no reason why it cannot be rated on-line by a trained clinician. The frequency with which covert assessments should be made during the maintenance phase largely depends on the duration of that phase. Of course, in turn, this raises the issue of time spans for posttreatment assessments, the final phase of this suggested format.

Follow-up Assessment

To date, our literature has little to offer as justification for prescribed follow-up intervals or assessments. The typical recommendations are that post-treatment assessments should occur at intervals ranging from a few weeks to 5 years (Silverman, 1981). What this reflects is yet another area of confusion; this time, about the function of posttreatment evaluation. The primary purpose of follow-up evaluation is surely to establish whether the subject is unimproved, improved, or free of his problem after a period in which variables likely to influence the problem have had every opportunity to occur. The difficulty is that there is very little information available on the nature of these variables. But the fact that a subject has improved or not improved speech performance at follow-up may have very little to do with treatment. Quite clearly, the longer the interval between cessation of treatment and follow-up evaluation, the more likely it is that this interval will be filled with variables of far more relevance to current performance than the original treatment. Of course, there is also little information available on the nature of these variables. But there are some logical contenders; practice regimes, "significant other" control of speech performance, and even additional treatment are good prospects for consideration.

At best, it would appear that follow-up evaluation may give the clinician and client knowledge about the current state of the disorder and some useful hypotheses about the durability of the treatment's effects. For this reason, perhaps the most practical guideline for follow-up evaluation is to schedule assessments over the following year. At least, this probably accommodates to a clinic's annual time-tabling arrangements, and is consistent with the intervals used in many clinical studies.

The frequency of follow-up assessments presents another imponderable. Perhaps the logical solution is to use the "four-data-point" principle from the previously mentioned therapy assessment format. This means that follow-up assessments should occur at 3-month intervals. And in order to determine the validity of this trend, perhaps these assessments should be interspersed with another four covert assessments.

The content of these posttreatment assessments warrants a few additional comments. The logical contenders are the within- and beyond-clinic assessments used over the initial therapy phases. Perhaps the most practical option for covert assessment is a 3-to-5-minute surprise telephone call involving a question-answer conversation with a stranger. But at least two other assessments may be important—some form of assessment of the subject's speech quality and a questionnaire similar to that devised by Webster (1974). The main value of Webster's questionnaire is that it solicits the subject's judgments on the extent to which he must attend to his speech in order to continue to speak fluently. At present, no other means is available for determining the extent to which therapy gains are sustained at the cost of unusual levels of attention to speaking. Once again, there are no available norms for this part of Webster's questionnaire, but it might be expected that over the follow-up period there should be some evidence that the subject's level of attention to his speech declines in concert with sustained improvements. That would seem to be one final clinically valid indication of treatment success.

Conclusions

Let us now try to put together all the pieces of our therapy assessment puzzle. It begins with a series of diagnostic sessions designed to establish the subject's suitability for therapy. This is followed by a base-rate period, containing repeated within- and beyond-clinic recorded assessments conducted once-weekly over at least 4 weeks. These assessments continue at this frequency throughout the establishment and transfer phases of therapy, and for at least 4 more weeks into the maintenance phase. The maintenance phase may include decreasingly frequent assessments that might also be tied to the treatment process. The pattern of maintenance assessment should continue until they occur at 3-month intervals. At this point, they should fade into follow-up assessments made at 3-month intervals over a year. The overt assessment procedure should be supplemented by at least four unobtrusive or covert assessments made during both the treatment and transfer phases, plus another four during the immediate posttreatment phase. In addition, perhaps covert assessments (of one form or another) should be made at regular intervals over the maintenance and follow-up periods. The content of the overt assessments should include representative speech samples from the speaker's natural environment, oral readings, monologues, and telephone conversations within the clinic. The minimum data should be syllable or articulation rate and percentage of words or syllables stuttered. These data should be supplemented by ratings of speech quality. Finally, the posttreatment phase of therapy should be supplemented by a questionnaire reporting the subject's estimate of his or her speech performance.

Quite obviously, this is an unrealistic format for very young children—indeed it is probably suitable only for school-age and older subjects. However, it should be equally obvious that the components not suitable for young children can be removed or modified without too much threat to the format. For example, parent recordings may replace subject-collected recordings, and the duration of post-treatment assessments may be reduced. Nevertheless, there is no reason why the format's substance cannot be used with young children.

It is hoped that the suggested therapy format will be given serious consideration as one means of shifting stuttering therapy towards a reasonably common pattern of assessment, which might make it possible to gain a clearer understanding of the therapy process—an understanding that will be of immense benefit to all concerned with this disorder. There is an almost desperate need for a data base from field clinicians on current stuttering-therapy procedures. If clinicians could be encouraged to gather and report data within the suggested format, then the profession should be considerably advanced in solving that need. For, only clinicians can show the strengths and weaknesses of these treatments in the field, rather than in the research "laboratory."

References

Adams, M.R. A clinical strategy for differentiating the normally nonfluent child and the incipient stutterer. *Journal of Fluency Disorders*, 1977, *2*, 141-148.

Adams, M.R. The young stutterer: Diagnosis, treatment and assessment of progress. *Seminars in Speech, Language and Hearing*, 1980, *1*, 289-299.

Adams, M.R. Fluency, nonfluency, and stuttering in children. *Journal of Fluency Disorders*, 1982, *7*, 171-185.

Adams, M.R., & Runyan, C.M. Stuttering and fluency: Exclusive events or points on a continuum? *Journal of Fluency Disorders*, 1981, *6*, 197-218.

Andrews, G. Stuttering therapy: How simple can an effective treatment programme become? *Australian Journal of Human Communication Disorders*, 1973, *1*, 44-46.

Andrews, G., & Cutler, J. Stuttering therapy: The relation between changes in symptom level and attitudes. *Journal of Speech and Hearing Disorders*, 1974, *39*, 312-319.

Andrews, G., Guitar, B., & Howie, P. Meta-analysis of the effects of stuttering treatment. *Journal of Speech and Hearing Disorders*, 1980, *45*, 287-307.

Andrews, G., & Harvey, R. Regression to the mean in pretreatment measures of stuttering. *Journal of Speech and Hearing Disorders*, 1981, *46*, 204-207.

Andrews, G., & Ingham, R.J. An approach to the evaluation of stuttering therapy. *Journal of Speech and Hearing Research*, 1972, *15*, 296-302.

Azrin, N.H., & Nunn, R.G. A rapid method of eliminating stuttering by a regulated breathing approach. *Behaviour Research and Therapy*, 1974, *12*, 279-286.

Birnbrauer, J.S. External validity and experimental investigation of individual behavior. *Analysis and Intervention in Developmental Disabilities*, 1982, *1*, 117-132.

Bloodstein, O. *A handbook on stuttering*. (3rd ed.) Chicago: National Easter Seal Society, 1981.

Boberg, E. *Maintenance of fluency*. New York: Elsevier, 1981.

Boberg, E., & Fong, L. Therapy program for young retarded stutterers. *Human Communication*, 1980, *2*, 95-102.

Boberg, E., Howie, P., & Woods, L. Maintenance of fluency: A review. *Journal of Fluency Disorders*, 1979, *4*, 93-116.

Boudreau, L.A., & Jeffrey, C.J. Stuttering treated by desensitization. *Journal of Behavior Therapy and Experimental Psychiatry*, 1973, *4*, 209-212.

Brady, J.P. Metronome-conditioned speech retraining for stuttering. *Behavior Therapy*, 1971, *2*, 129-150.

Brutten, G.J. Stuttering: Topography, assessment, and behavior-change strategies. In J. Eisenson (Ed.), *Stuttering: A second symposium*. New York: Harper & Row, 1975.

Costello, J.M. The establishment of fluency with time-out procedures: Three case studies. *Journal of Speech and Hearing Disorders*, 1975, *40*, 216-231.

Costello, J.M. Operant conditioning and the treatment of stuttering. *Seminars in Speech, Language and Hearing*, 1980, *1*, 311-325.

Costello, J.M. Pretreatment assessment of stuttering in young children. *Communicative disorders. An audio journal for continuing education*. New York: Grune & Stratton, 1981.

Costello, J.M. Current behavioral treatments for children. In D. Prins & R.J. Ingham (Eds.), *Treatment of stuttering in early childhood: Methods and issues*. San Diego: College-Hill Press, 1983.

Curlee, R.F. A case selection strategy for young disfluent children. *Seminars in Speech, Language and Hearing*, 1980, *1*, 277-287.

Goldiamond, I. Stuttering and fluency as manipulatable operant response classes. In L. Krasner & L.P. Ullmann (Eds.), *Research in behavior modification*. New York: Holt, Rinehart & Winston, 1965.

Gregory, H.H., & Hill, D. Stuttering therapy for children. *Seminars in Speech, Language and Hearing*, 1980, *1*, 351-363.

Guitar, B. Reduction of stuttering frequency using analog electromyographic feedback. *Journal of Speech and Hearing Research*, 1975, *18*, 672-685.

Guitar, B., & Peters, T.J. *Stuttering: An integration of contemporary therapies*. Memphis: Speech Foundation of America, 1980.

Hanna, R., & Owen, N. Facilitating transfer and maintenance of fluency in stuttering therapy. *Journal of Speech and Hearing Disorders*, 1977, *42*, 65-76.

Hawkins, R.P., & Dotson, V.A. Reliability scores that delude: An Alice in Wonderland trip through the misleading characteristics of interobserver agreement scores in interval recording. In E. Ramp & G. Semb (Eds.), *Behavior analysis: Areas of research and application*. Englewood Cliffs, NJ: Prentice-Hall, 1975.

Hee, J.C., & Holmes, P.A. Elimination of stuttering by a regulated breathing approach. *Journal of Communication Pathology*, 1976, *8*, 40-44.

Helps, R., & Dalton, P. The effectiveness of an intensive group speech therapy programme for adult stammerers. *British Journal of Disorders of Communication*, 1979, *14*, 17-30.

Herscovitch, A., & Lebow, M.D. Imaginal pacing in the treatment of stuttering. *Journal of Behavior Therapy and Experimental Psychiatry*, 1973, *4*, 357-360.

Hersen, M., & Barlow, D.H. *Single-case experimental designs*. New York: Pergamon, 1976.

Ingham, R.J. Modification of maintenance and generalization in stuttering treatment. *Journal of Speech and Hearing Research*, 1980, *23*, 732-745.

Ingham, R.J. Evaluation and maintenance in stuttering treatment: A search for ecstasy with nothing but agony. In E. Boberg (Ed.), *Maintenance of fluency*. New York: Elsevier, 1981.

Ingham, R.J. The effects of self-evaluation training on maintenance and generalization during stuttering treatment. *Journal of Speech and Hearing Disorders*, 1982, *47*, 271-280. (a)

Ingham, R.J. Some comments on "Stuttering and fluency": Exclusive events or points on a continuum? *Journal of Fluency Disorders*, 1982, *7*, 303-307. (b)

Ingham, R.J., & Andrews, G. An analysis of a token economy in stuttering therapy. *Journal of Applied Behavior Analysis*, 1973, *6*, 219-229.

Ingham, R.J., Martin, R.R., & Kuhl, P. Modification and control of rate of speaking by stutterers. *Journal of Speech and Hearing Research*, 1974, *17*, 489-496.

Ingham, R.J., & Packman, A. Treatment and generalization effects in an experimental treatment for a stutterer using contingency management and speech rate control. *Journal of Speech and Hearing Disorders*, 1977, *42*, 394-407.

Ingham, R.J., & Packman, A. Perceptual assessment of normalcy of speech following stuttering therapy. *Journal of Speech and Hearing Research*, 1978, *21*, 63-73.

Ingham, R.J., & Packman, A. A further evaluation of the speech of stutterers during chorus- and nonchorus-reading conditions. *Journal of Speech and Hearing Research*, 1979, *22*, 784-793.

James J.E. Behavioral self-control of stuttering using time-out from speaking. *Journal of Applied Behavior Analysis*, 1981, *14*, 25-37.

Johnson, G.F., Coleman, K., & Rasmussen,K. Multidays: Multidimensional approach for the young stutterer. *Language, Speech and Hearing Services in Schools*, 1978, *9*, 129-132.

Johnson, L.J. Facilitating parental involvement in therapy of the disfluent child. *Seminars in Speech, Language and Hearing*, 1980, *1*, 301-309.

Jones, R.J., & Azrin, N.H. Behavioral engineering: Stuttering as a function of stimulus duration during speech synchronization. *Journal of Applied Behavior Analysis*, 1969, *2*, 223-229.

Kazdin, A.E., & Wilcoxon, L.A. Systematic desensitization and nonspecific treatment effects: A methodological evaluation. *Psychological Bulletin*, 1976, *83*, 729-758.

Kiesler, D.J. Some myths of psychotherapy research and the search for a paradigm. *Psychological Bulletin*, 1966, *65*, 110-136.

Kowal, S., O'Connell, D.C., & Sabin, E.F. Development of temporal patterning and vocal hesitations in spontaneous narratives. *Journal of Psycholinguistic Research*, 1975, *4*, 195-207.

LaCroix, Z.E. Management of disfluent speech through self-recording procedures. *Journal of Speech and Hearing Disorders*, 1973, *38*, 272-274.

Lee, B.S., McGough, W.E., & Peins, M. A new method for stutter therapy. *Folia Phoniatrica*, 1973, *25*, 186-195.

Luper, H.L., & Mulder, R.L. *Stuttering: Therapy for children.* Englewood Cliffs, NJ: Prentice-Hall, 1964.

MacCulloch, M.J., Eaton, R., & Long, E. The longterm effect of auditory masking on young stutterers. *British Journal of Disorders of Communication,* 1970, *5,* 165-173.

MacDonald, J.D., & Martin, R.R. Stuttering and disfluency as two reliable and unambiguous response classes. *Journal of Speech and Hearing Research,* 1973, *16,* 691-699.

Martin, R.R. Appercus. In E. Boberg (Ed.), *Maintenance of fluency.* New York: Elsevier, 1981.

Martin, R.R., & Berndt, L.A. The effects of time-out on stuttering in a 12-year-old boy. *Exceptional Children,* 1970, *36,* 303-304.

Martin, R.R., Haroldson, S.K., & Kuhl, P. Disfluencies in child-child and child-mother speaking situations. *Journal of Speech and Hearing Research,* 1972, *15,* 753-756. (a)

Martin, R.R., Haroldson, S.K., & Kuhl, P. Disfluencies of young children in two speaking situations. *Journal of Speech and Hearing Research,* 1972, *15,* 831-836. (b)

Martin, R.R., Kuhl, P., & Haroldson, S.K. An experimental treatment with two preschool stuttering children. *Journal of Speech and Hearing Research,* 1972, *15,* 743-752.

McDermott, L.D. Clinical management of stuttering behavior: A case study. *Feedback,* 1971, *1,* 6-7.

Metz, D.E., Onufrak, J.A., & Ogburn, R.S. An acoustical analysis of stutterer's speech prior to and at the termination of therapy. *Journal of Fluency Disorders,* 1979, *4,* 249-254.

Mowrer, D. An instructional program to increase fluent speech of stutterers. *Journal of Fluency Disorders,* 1975, *1,* 25-35.

Ottoni, T.M. Uso de la tecnica delineamento del habla para cambiar la conducta verbal. *Revisita Interamericana de Psicologia,* 1974, *8,* 3-4.

Perkins, W.H. Replacement of stuttering with normal speech: II. Clinical procedures. *Journal of Speech and Hearing Disorders,* 1973, *38,* 295-303.

Perkins, W.H. Articulatory rate in the evaluation of stuttering treatments. *Journal of Speech and Hearing Disorders,* 1975, *40,* 277-278.

Perkins, W.H. From psychoanalysis to discoordination. In H.H. Gregory (Ed.), *Controversies about stuttering therapy.* Baltimore: University Park Press, 1979.

Perkins, W.H. Measurement and maintenance of fluency. In E. Boberg, (Ed.), *Maintenance of fluency.* New York: Elsevier, 1981.

Perkins, W.H., Rudas, J., Johnson, L., Michael, W.B., & Curlee, R.F. Replacement of stuttering with normal speech: III. Clinical effectiveness. *Journal of Speech and Hearing Disorders,* 1974, *39,* 416-428.

Peters, A.D. The effect of positive reinforcement on fluency: Two case studies. *Language, Speech and Hearing Services in Schools,* 1977, *8,* 15-22.

Prins, D., & Ingham, R.J. *Treatment of stuttering in early childhood: Methods and issues.* San Diego: College-Hill Press, 1983.

Reed, C.G., & Godden, A.L. An experimental treatment using verbal punishment with two preschool stutterers. *Journal of Fluency Disorders,* 1977, *2,* 225-233.

Resick, P.A., Wendiggensen, P., Ames, S., & Meyer, V. Systematic slowed speech: A new treatment for stuttering. *Behaviour Research and Therapy,* 1978, *16,* 161-167.

Riley, G.D., & Riley, J. A component model for diagnosing and treating children who stutter. *Journal of Fluency Disorders,* 1979, *4,* 279-293.

Riley, G.D., & Riley, J. Evaluation as a basis for intervention. In D.Prins & R.J. Ingham (Eds.), *Treatment of stuttering in early childhood: Methods and issues.* San Diego: College-Hill Press, 1983.

Runyan, C.M., & Adams, M.R. Perceptual study of the speech of "successfully therapeutized" stutterers. *Journal of Fluency Disorders,* 1978, *3,* 25-39.

Runyan, C.M., & Adams, M.R. Unsophisticated judges' perceptual evaluations of the speech of "successfully treated" stutterers. *Journal of Fluency Disorders*, 1979, *4*, 29-38.

Ryan, B.P. Operant procedures applied to stuttering therapy for children. *Journal of Speech and Hearing Disorders*, 1971, *36*, 264-280.

Ryan, B.P. *Programmed therapy for stuttering in children and adults*. Springfield, IL: Charles C. Thomas, 1974.

Shames, G.H. Relapse in stuttering. In E. Boberg (Ed.), *Maintenance of fluency*. New York: Elsevier, 1981.

Shames, G.H., & Florance, C.L. *Stutter-free speech: A goal for therapy*.Columbus, OH: Charles E. Merrill, 1980.

Shaw, C.K., & Shrum, W.F. The effects of response-contingent reward on the connected speech of children who stutter. *Journal of Speech and Hearing Disorders*, 1972, *37*, 75-88.

Sheehan, J.G. *Stuttering: Research and therapy*. New York: Harper & Row, 1970.

Shelton, J.L. The elimination of persistent stuttering by the use of homework assignments involving speech shadowing: A case report. *Behavior Therapy*, 1975, *6*, 392-393.

Shine, R.E. Direct management of the beginning stutterer. *Seminars in Speech, Language and Hearing*, 1980, *1*, 339-350.

Silverman, F.H. Relapse following stuttering therapy. In N.J. Lass (Ed.), *Speech and language: Advances in basic research and practice*, (Vol. 5). New York: Academic Press, 1981.

Smith, L.M., & Glass, G. Meta-analysis of psychotherapy outcome studies. *American Psychologist*, 1977, *32*, 752-760.

Starkweather, C.W. Speech fluency and its development in normal children. In N.J. Lass (Ed.), *Speech and language: Advances in basic research and practice*, (Vol. 4). New York: Academic Press, 1980.

Stokes, T.F., & Baer, D.M. An implicit technology of generalization. *Journal of Applied Behavior Analysis*, 1977, *10*, 349-367.

Stromsta, C. A spectrographic study of dysfluencies labeled as stuttering by parents. *De Therapia Vocis et Loquelae (Proceedings XIII International Congress of Logopedics and Phoniatrics, Vienna), Vol. 1*, 1965, 317-319.

Treon, M., & Tamayo, F.M.V. The separate and combined effects of GSR biofeedback and delayed auditory feedback on stuttering: A preliminary study. *Journal of Fluency Disorders*, 1974, *1*, 3-9.

Turnbaugh, K.R., & Guitar, B.E. Short-term intensive stuttering treatment in a public school setting. *Language, Speech and Hearing Services in the Schools*, 1981, *12*, 107-114.

Ulliana, L., & Ingham, R.J. Behavioral and non-behavioral variables in the measurement of stutterers' communication attitudes. *Journal of Speech and Hearing Disorders*, in press.

Van Riper, C. *Speech correction: Principles and methods*. Englewood Cliffs, NJ: Prentice-Hall, 1963.

Van Riper, C. *The treatment of stuttering*. Englewood Cliffs, NJ: Prentice-Hall, 1973.

Webster, L.M., & Brutten, G.J. The modification of stuttering and associated behaviors. In S. Dickson (Ed.), *Communication disorders*, Glenview, IL: Scott Foresman, 1974.

Webster, R.L. Stuttering: A way to eliminate it and a way to explain it. In R. Ulrich, T. Stachnik, & J. Mabry (Eds.), *Control of human behavior*, (Vol. 2), Glenview, IL: Scott Foresman, 1970.

Webster, R.L. *The precision fluency shaping program: Speech reconstruction for stutterers*. Roanoke, VA: Hollins Communication Research Institute, 1974.

Webster, R.L. Empirical considerations regarding stuttering therapy. In H.H. Gregory (Ed.), *Controversies about stuttering therapy*. Baltimore: University Park Press, 1979.

Williams, D.E. Stuttering therapy for children. In L.E. Travis (Ed.), *Handbook of speech pathology and audiology*. New York: Appleton-Century-Crofts, 1971.

Williams, D.E. The problem of stuttering. In F.L. Darley & D.C. Spriestersbach (Eds.), *Diagnostic methods in speech pathology*. New York: Harper & Row, 1978.

Author Index

Subject Index

C

D

E

F

G

H

I

J

L

M

N

O

P

V

W